D0838584

Nursing

RAPID-FIRE
DRUG FACTS

Nursing

RAPID-FIRE
DRUG FACTS

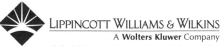

LIPPINCOTT WILLIAMS & WILKINS
A **Wolters Kluwer** Company

Philadelphia • Baltimore • New York • London
Buenos Aires • Hong Kong • Sydney • Tokyo

PART IV
DRUG THERAPY IN COMMON DISEASES AND DISORDERS

PART V
SPECIAL SKILLS

PART VI
HERBAL THERAPY

CONTRIBUTORS AND CONSULTANTS

Lauren D. Blough, RN, BSN, CRNI
Clinical Specialist and Educator, Infusion Therapy
Florida Hospital
Orlando, Fla.

Lawrence Carey, PharmD
Assistant Professor, Physician Assistant Program
Philadelphia University
Philadelphia

Noreen Coyne, RN, MSN, CRNI, OCN
National Director of Clinical Standards & Development
Tender Loving Care, Staff Builders Home Health Care
Lake Success, N.Y.

Jennifer D. Faulkner, PharmD, BCPP
Clinical Pharmacy Specialist
Central Texas Veterans Health Care System
Temple, Tex.

Christopher A. Fausel, PharmD, BCPS, BCOP
Clinical Pharmacist
Indiana University Hospital
Indianapolis, Ind.

Tatyana Gurvich, PharmD
Clinical Pharmacologist
Glendale Adventist FPRP
Glendale, Calif.

Nicole M. Maisch, RPh, PharmD
Assistant Clinical Professor of Pharmacy Practice
St. John's University College of Pharmacy and Allied Health Professions
Jamaica, N.Y.

Jeffrey B. Purcell, PharmD
Clinical Lead Pharmacist
Harborview Medical Center
Seattle

Barbara Reville, CRNP, MS, BC, AOCN
Clinical Instructor
University of Pennsylvania School of Nursing
Philadelphia

Susan Sard, PharmD
Clinical Pharmacist
Anne Arundel Medical Center
Annapolis, Md.

Elizabeth J. Scharman, PharmD, DABAT, BCPS, FAACT
Director, West Virginia Poison Center
Associate Professor, West Virginia University School of Pharmacy
Charleston, W.Va.

Wendy J. Smith, RN, MSN, ACNP,
   AOCN
Nurse Practitioner
The West Clinic
Memphis, Tenn.

Joanne Whitney, RPH, PHARMD, PHD
Director, Drug Products Laboratory
Associate Clinical Professor
University of California
San Francisco

Barbara S. Wiggins, PHARMD, BCPS
Pharmacy Clinical Specialist,
   Cardiology
University of Virginia Health System
Charlottesville, Va.

FOREWORD

If you search for a drug therapy book, you discover that there are two main types of books—drug references and administration manuals. The problem, however, is that drug references leave out administration information every clinician needs, and administration manuals leave out the important details of individual drugs. What's more, both references may be difficult and cumbersome to read.

That's why I think *Nursing Rapid-Fire Drug Facts* will make such a valuable addition to every nurse's library. This book is specifically targeted on essential information—the most important, clinically relevant facts about all aspects of drug therapy. This quick-scan book lightens the labor of reading by providing most of its information in easy-to-read bulleted lists and handy tables. It covers all the major aspects of drug therapy in six intuitive sections.

The first section reviews fundamental facts about drug therapy in four key chapters. It's a unique section not found in most drug books. Chapter 1 offers an overview of more than 40 major drug classes, focusing on indications, actions, adverse reactions, contraindications and cautions, nursing considerations, and patient teaching. Chapter 2 reviews vital considerations for drug therapy in pregnant women, breastfeeding women, children, and geriatric patients. The chapter also includes strategies for preventing adverse drug reactions in older patients and recognizing adverse reactions misinterpreted as age-related changes. Chapter 3 provides Spanish translations for key drug-related assessment and patient-teaching topics. And Chapter 4 reviews the most important dosage calculation methods.

The book's second section reviews the details of drug administration and monitoring. Chapter 5 highlights important aspects of administering drugs by all major routes. Chapter 6 compiles key tools for providing and troubleshooting I.V. therapy. And Chapter 7 includes handy guides to therapeutic drug ranges and normal laboratory values.

The third section, which includes chapters 8 through 11, contains the essential facts you'll need to recognize and manage the complications of drug therapy. It includes chapters on medication errors, adverse and allergic reactions, overdose, and interactions.

The fourth section presents the critical information you need to understand drug therapy for all major diseases and disorders. Encompassing 11 chapters, the section reviews contraindications, cautions, and key points for each drug used to treat disorders in all major body systems, including the cardiovascular, endocrine, gastrointestinal, genitourinary, immune, musculoskeletal, respiratory, and neurologic systems. The section also reviews drug therapy for infectious disorders, mood disorders, and neoplastic disorders.

The fifth section guides you through the special management skills needed to care for patients receiving chemotherapy and patients dealing with pain.

The final section includes everything you need to know about popular herbal medicines, plus handy references to toxic herbs, herb-drug interactions, and key steps in monitoring patients who take herbs.

A very helpful feature of the book is its use of an "Alert" icon and a "Clinical tip" icon to draw your attention to especially crucial information—information that could save your patient from a dangerous adverse effect or save you from making a clinical error.

This fact-filled book manages to be both practical and factual, detailed and comprehensive. It does so by focusing on the most important, clinically relevant information about drug therapy and weeding out unnecessary information. This book makes a useful companion to any drug dosage book. Clearly, it is written with the thinking clinician in mind. *Nursing Rapid-Fire Drug Facts* will prove to be a key reference for every nurse who delivers drug therapy, and I recommend it highly.

Michael Ackerman, DNS, RN, APRN-CS, FCCM, FNAP
Professor
University of Rochester
School of Nursing
Rochester, N.Y.

GUIDE TO ABBREVIATIONS

ACE	angiotensin-converting enzyme	EEG	electroencephalogram
ADH	antidiuretic hormone	EENT	eyes, ears, nose, throat
AIDS	acquired immunodeficiency syndrome	FDA	Food and Drug Administration
ALT	alanine transaminase	g	gram
AST	aspartate transaminase	G	gauge
AV	atrioventricular	GFR	glomerular filtration rate
b.i.d.	twice daily	GGT	gamma-glutamyltransferase
BPH	benign prostatic hyperplasia	GI	gastrointestinal
BSA	body surface area	G6PD	glucose-6-phosphate dehydrogenase
BUN	blood urea nitrogen	gtt	drops
cAMP	cyclic 38, 58 adenosine monophosphate	GU	genitourinary
CBC	complete blood count	H_1	histamine$_1$
CK	creatine kinase	H_2	histamine$_2$
CMV	cytomegalovirus	HDL	high-density lipoprotein
CNS	central nervous system	HIV	human immunodeficiency virus
COPD	chronic obstructive pulmonary disease	HMG-CoA	3-hydroxy-3-methylglutaryl coenzyme A
CSF	cerebrospinal fluid	h.s.	at bedtime
CV	cardiovascular	I.D.	intradermal
CVA	cerebrovascular accident	I.M.	intramuscular
D_5W	dextrose 5% in water	INR	international normalized ratio
DIC	disseminated intravascular coagulation	IPPB	intermittent positive-pressure breathing
dl	deciliter	I.V.	intravenous
DNA	deoxyribonucleic acid	kg	kilogram
ECG	electrocardiogram		

L	liter	RSV	respiratory syncytial virus
lb	pound	SA	sinoatrial
LDH	lactate dehydrogenase	S.C.	subcutaneous
LDL	low-density lipoprotein	sec	second
M	molar	SIADH	syndrome of inappropriate antidiuretic hormone
m^2	square meter		
MAO	monoamine oxidase		
mcg	microgram	S.L.	sublingual
mEq	milliequivalent	SSRI	selective serotonin reuptake inhibitor
mg	milligram		
MI	myocardial infarction	T_3	triiodothyronine
min	minute	T_4	thyroxine
ml	milliliter	t.i.d.	three times daily
mm^3	cubic millimeter	tsp	teaspoon
msec	millisecond	USP	United States Pharmacopeia
NSAID	nonsteroidal anti-inflammatory drug		
		UTI	urinary tract infection
OTC	over-the-counter	WBC	white blood cell
PABA	para-aminobenzoic acid	wk	week
PCA	patient-controlled analgesia		
P.O.	by mouth		
P.R.	by rectum		
p.r.n.	as needed		
PT	prothrombin time		
PTT	partial thromboplastin time		
PVC	premature ventricular contraction		
q	every		
q.i.d.	four times daily		
RBC	red blood cell		
RDA	recommended daily allowance		
REM	rapid eye movement		
RNA	ribonucleic acid		

PART I

GENERAL INFORMATION

1 / DRUG CLASSES

ALKYLATING DRUGS

altretamine
busulfan
carboplatin
carmustine
chlorambucil
cisplatin
cyclophosphamide
dacarbazine
ifosfamide
lomustine
mechlorethamine
   hydrochloride
melphalan
thiotepa

Indications
■ Various tumors, especially those with a large volume and slow cell-turnover rate

Actions
Alkylating drugs seem to act independently of cell-cycle phase. They're polyfunctional compounds that can be divided chemically into five groups:
■ alkyl sulfonates
■ ethylenimines
■ nitrogen mustards
■ nitrosoureas
■ triazines.
  Highly reactive, these drugs mainly target nucleic acids and form links with the nuclei of different molecules. This allows them to cross-link double-stranded DNA and prevent strands from separating for replication, which may contribute to their ability to destroy cells.

Adverse reactions
Adverse reactions may include anxiety, bone marrow depression, chills, diarrhea, fever, flank or joint pain, hair loss, leukopenia, nausea, redness or pain at the injection site, sore throat, swelling of feet or lower legs, thrombocytopenia, and vomiting.

Contraindications and cautions
■ Contraindicated in patients hypersensitive to these drugs.

■ Use cautiously in patients receiving other cell-destroying drugs or radiation therapy.

LIFESPAN

■ *Pregnant women.* Advise these patients to consult the prescriber because alkylating drugs may harm a fetus.

■ *Breast-feeding women.* Discourage breast-feeding because alkylating drugs appear in breast milk.

■ *Children.* Safety and efficacy of many alkylating drugs aren't known.

■ *Geriatric patients.* These patients have an increased risk of adverse reactions; monitor them closely.

Nursing considerations

■ Perform a complete assessment before therapy begins.

■ Monitor patient for adverse reactions throughout therapy.

■ Check hematocrit, platelet count, total and differential leukocyte counts, and blood urea nitrogen, alanine transaminase, aspartate transaminase, lactate dehydrogenase, bilirubin, creatinine, uric acid, and other levels as needed.

■ Assess vital signs and patency of catheter or I.V. line throughout therapy.

■ Follow established procedures for safe and proper handling, administration, and disposal of chemotherapeutic drugs.

■ Treat extravasation right away.

■ While giving carboplatin or cisplatin, keep epinephrine, corticosteroids, and antihistamines available in case of anaphylactoid reaction.

■ Maintain adequate hydration before and for 24 hours after giving cisplatin.

■ Give ifosfamide with mesna to prevent hemorrhagic cystitis.

■ Give lomustine 2 to 4 hours after meals. Nausea and vomiting usually last less than 24 hours, although loss of appetite may last several days.

■ Allopurinol may be used to prevent drug-induced hyperuricemia.

Patient teaching

■ Tell patient to avoid people with bacterial or viral infections because chemotherapy can increase susceptibility. Urge him to report possible infection promptly.

■ Advise women of childbearing age to avoid becoming pregnant during therapy.

■ Review proper oral hygiene, including cautious use of toothbrush, dental floss, and tooth-picks.

■ Advise patient to complete dental work before therapy begins or to delay it until blood counts are normal.

■ Warn patient that he may bruise easily.

ALPHA BLOCKERS (PERIPHERALLY ACTING)

**doxazosin mesylate
(non-selective)**
**prazosin hydrochloride
(non-selective)**
**tamsulosin hydrochloride
(selective)**
**terazosin hydrochloride
(non-selective)**

Indications

■ Hypertension
■ Mild to moderate urinary obstruction in men with benign prostatic hyperplasia (BPH)

Actions

Selective alpha blockers decrease vascular resistance and increase venous capacity, thereby lowering blood pressure and causing nasal and scleroconjunctival congestion, ptosis, orthostatic and exercise hypotension, mild to moderate miosis, interference with ejaculation,

and pink, warm skin. They also relax nonvascular smooth muscle, especially in the prostate capsule, which reduces urinary problems in men with BPH. Because alpha$_1$ blockers don't block alpha$_2$ receptors, they don't cause transmitter overflow.

Non-selective alpha blockers antagonize both alpha$_1$ and alpha$_2$ receptors. Generally, alpha-adrenergic blockade results in tachycardia, palpitations, and increased renin secretion because of abnormally large amounts of norepinephrine (from transmitter overflow) released from adrenergic nerve endings as a result of the blockade of alpha$_1$ and alpha$_2$ receptors. Norepinephrine's effects are counterproductive to the major uses of non-selective alpha blockers.

Adverse reactions

Alpha blockers may cause severe orthostatic hypotension and syncope, especially the first few doses—commonly called the "first-dose effect." The most common adverse effects of alpha$_1$ blockade are dizziness, drowsiness, headache, malaise, and somnolence. These drugs also may cause fluid retention (from excess renin secretion), orthostatic hypotension, nasal and ocular congestion, palpitations, tachycardia, and worsening of respiratory tract infection.

Contraindications and cautions

■ Contraindicated in patients hypersensitive to these drugs or their components and in patients with myocardial infarction (MI), coronary insufficiency, or angina.

LIFESPAN

■ *Pregnant women.* Use cautiously.
■ *Breast-feeding women.* Use cautiously.
■ *Children.* Safety and efficacy of many alpha blockers aren't known; use cautiously.
■ *Geriatric patients.* Hypotensive effects may be more pronounced.

Nursing considerations

■ Monitor vital signs, especially blood pressure.
■ Watch closely for adverse reactions.
■ Give drug at bedtime to minimize dizziness or lightheadedness.
■ Start with a small dose to avoid first-dose syncope.

Patient teaching

■ Warn patient not to rise suddenly from a lying or sitting position.
■ Urge patient to avoid hazardous tasks until the drug's full effects are known.
■ Advise patient that alcohol, excessive exercise, prolonged standing, and heat exposure will intensify adverse effects.
■ Tell patient to promptly report dizziness or irregular heartbeat.

AMINOGLYCOSIDES

amikacin sulfate
gentamicin sulfate
neomycin sulfate
streptomycin sulfate
tobramycin sulfate

Indications

■ Aerobic gram-negative bacillary meningitis that isn't susceptible to other antibiotics
■ Anaerobic infections involving *Bacteroides fragilis*
■ Enterococcal infections
■ Initial empiric therapy in febrile, leukopenic patients
■ Intra-abdominal infection
■ Nosocomial pneumonia
■ Postoperative infection
■ Pulmonary infection
■ Septicemia

- Serious staphylococcal, *Pseudomonas aeruginosa*, and *Klebsiella* infections
- Skin, soft tissue, bone, and joint infections
- Tuberculosis
- Urinary tract infection

Actions

Aminoglycosides are bactericidal. They bind directly and irreversibly to 30S ribosomal subunits, inhibiting bacterial protein synthesis. They're active against many aerobic gramnegative and some aerobic gram-positive organisms.

Susceptible gram-negative organisms include *Acinetobacter, Citrobacter, Enterobacter, Escherichia coli, Klebsiella,* indole-positive and indole-negative *Proteus, Providencia, Pseudomonas aeruginosa, Salmonella, Serratia,* and *Shigella.* Streptomycin is also active against *Brucella, Calymmatobacterium granulomatis, Pasteurella multocida,* and *Yersinia pestis.*

Susceptible gram-positive organisms include *Staphylococcus aureus* and *epidermidis.* Streptomycin is also active against *Nocardia, Erysipelothrix,* and some mycobacteria, including *Mycobacterium tuberculosis, M. marinum,* and certain strains of *M. kansasii* and *M. leprae.*

Adverse reactions

Ototoxicity and nephrotoxicity are the most serious complications. Neuromuscular blockade also may occur. Oral forms most commonly cause diarrhea, nausea, and vomiting. Parenteral drugs may cause phlebitis, sterile abscess, and vein irritation.

Contraindications and cautions

- Contraindicated in patients hypersensitive to aminoglycosides.
- Use cautiously if patient has hearing loss or a neuromuscular disorder, such as myasthenia gravis or parkinsonism.
- Use cautiously in patients receiving neuromuscular blockers because prolonged respiratory depression may occur.
- Reduce dosage if patient has renal impairment. (See *Aminoglycosides: Renal function and half-life,* page 8.)

LIFESPAN

- *Pregnant women.* Advise pregnant patients that aminoglycosides cross the placenta and may harm a fetus.
- *Breast-feeding women.* Safety isn't known.
- *Neonates and premature infants.* Half-life of aminoglyco-

Indications

- Diabetic nephropathy (captopril)
- Heart failure
- Hypertension
- Left ventricular dysfunction
- Myocardial infarction (ramipril and lisinopril)

Actions

Angiotensin-converting enzyme (ACE) inhibitors prevent conversion of angiotensin I to angiotensin II, a potent vasoconstrictor. Besides reducing peripheral arterial resistance by decreasing vasoconstriction, inhibiting angiotensin II decreases adrenocortical secretion of aldosterone, which reduces sodium and water retention and extracellular fluid volume. ACE inhibition also increases bradykinin levels, resulting in vasodilation and decreased heart rate and systemic vascular resistance. (See *Comparing doses of ACE inhibitors.*)

Adverse reactions

Adverse effects of ACE inhibitors include angioedema of face and limbs; a dry, persistent cough; dysgeusia; fatigue; headache; hyperkalemia; hypotension; photosensitivity; proteinuria; rash; and tachycardia. Severe hypotension may occur at toxic levels.

Contraindications and cautions

- Contraindicated in patients hypersensitive to ACE inhibitors.
- Use cautiously in patients with impaired renal function or serious autoimmune disease and in those taking other drugs known to decrease white blood cell (WBC) count or immune response.

LIFESPAN

- *Women of childbearing age.* Tell patient to report suspected pregnancy immediately. ACE inhibitor therapy should stop during pregnancy because it can cause fetal birth defects or death, especially in the second and third trimesters.
- *Breast-feeding women.* Some ACE inhibitors appear in breast milk; patient should stop breast-feeding during therapy.
- *Children.* Safety and efficacy aren't known; give drug only if potential benefit outweighs risk.
- *Geriatric patients.* These patients may need lower doses because of impaired drug clearance.

Nursing considerations

- Observe patient for adverse reactions.

COMPARING DOSES OF ACE INHIBITORS

DRUG	TARGET ADULT DAILY DOSE	DOSAGE ADJUSTMENTS
benazepril	10–40 mg in single or divided doses	Creatinine clearance <30 ml/min or patient on concurrent diuretic: initially, 5 mg daily
captopril	6.25–150 mg b.i.d. or t.i.d.	Renal impairment, hyponatremia, or hypovolemia: 6.25–12.5 mg b.i.d. or t.i.d.
enalapril	P.O.: 10–40 mg in single or divided doses I.V.: 1.25 mg q 6 hours	Creatinine clearance 30 ml/min or patient on concurrent diuretic: initially, 2.5 mg daily
fosinopril	20–40 mg in single or divided doses	Use cautiously if patient on concurrent diuretic: initially, 10 mg daily
lisinopril	10–40 mg in a single dose	Creatinine clearance 10–30 ml/min or patient on concurrent diuretic: initially, 5 mg daily Creatinine clearance <10 ml/min: initially, 2.5 mg daily
moexipril	7.5–30 mg in single or divided doses	Creatinine clearance <40 ml/min: initially, 3.75 mg daily
perindopril	4–8 mg in single or divided doses	Creatinine clearance 30–60 ml/min: initially, 2 mg daily
quinapril	20–80 mg in single or divided doses	Creatinine clearance 30–60 ml/min or patient on concurrent diuretic: initially, 5 mg daily Creatinine clearance 10–30 ml/min: initially, 2.5 mg daily
ramipril	2.5–20 mg in single or divided doses	Creatinine clearance <40 ml/min or serum creatinine >2.5 mg/dl: initially, 1.25 mg daily
trandolapril	1–4 mg in a single dose	Creatinine clearance <30 ml/min, concurrent diuretic therapy, or hepatic cirrhosis: initially, 0.5 mg daily

■ Monitor vital signs regularly and WBC count and electrolyte level periodically.

■ Stop diuretic 2 to 3 days before beginning ACE inhibitor to reduce risk of hypotension. If drug doesn't adequately control blood pressure, diuretics may be restarted.

■ Give a reduced dosage if the patient has impaired renal function.

■ Give potassium supplements and potassium-sparing diuretics cautiously because ACE inhibitors may cause potassium retention.

■ Give captopril and moexipril 1 hour before meals.

Patient teaching

■ Tell patient that therapy may cause a dry, persistent, tickling cough that stops when therapy stops.

■ Urge patient to report lightheadedness, especially in the first few days of therapy, so the dosage can be adjusted; evidence of infection (such as sore throat and fever) because these drugs may decrease WBC count; facial swelling or trouble breathing because these drugs may cause angioedema; and loss of taste, for which therapy may stop.

■ Advise patient to avoid sudden position changes to minimize orthostatic hypotension.

■ Warn patient to seek medical approval before taking self-prescribed cold preparations.

■ Warn patient to consume potassium-containing salt substitutes cautiously because ACE inhibitors may cause potassium retention.

■ Advise women of childbearing age to avoid becoming pregnant during therapy.

ANTACIDS

aluminum hydroxide
calcium carbonate
magaldrate
magnesium hydroxide
magnesium oxide
sodium bicarbonate

Indications

■ Hyperacidity

Actions

Antacids reduce the total acid load in the gastrointestinal (GI) tract and elevate gastric pH to reduce pepsin activity. They also strengthen the gastric mucosal barrier and increase esophageal sphincter tone.

Adverse reactions

Aluminum-containing antacids may cause aluminum intoxication, constipation, hypophosphatemia, intestinal obstruction, and osteomalacia.

Magnesium-containing antacids may cause diarrhea or hypermagnesemia (in renal failure).

Calcium carbonate, magaldrate, magnesium oxide, and sodium bicarbonate may cause milk-alkali syndrome or rebound hyperacidity.

Contraindications and cautions

■ *Aluminum preparations.* Use cautiously in elderly patients; those receiving antidiarrheals, antispasmodics, or anticholinergics; and those with dehydration, fluid restriction, chronic renal disease, or suspected intestinal absorption.

■ *Calcium carbonate, magaldrate.* Contraindicated in patients with severe renal disease. Use cautiously in elderly patients; those receiving antidiarrheals, antispasmodics, or anticholinergics; and those with dehydration, fluid restriction, chronic renal disease, or suspected intestinal absorption.

■ *Magnesium oxide.* Contraindicated in severe renal disease.

Use cautiously in mild renal impairment.

■ *Sodium bicarbonate.* Contraindicated in patients with hypertension, renal disease, or edema; patients who are vomiting; patients receiving diuretics or continuous GI suction; and patients on sodium-restricted diets.

LIFESPAN

■ *Pregnant women.* Advise patient to consult her health care provider before taking an antacid.

■ *Infants.* Monitor patient closely; serious adverse effects possible from changes in fluid and electrolyte balance.

■ *Geriatric patients.* Give drug cautiously and monitor patient closely because of increased risk of adverse reactions.

Nursing considerations

■ Assess patient's condition before therapy and regularly thereafter.

■ Record number and consistency of stools.

■ Observe patient for adverse reactions.

■ Monitor patient receiving long-term, high-dose aluminum carbonate and hydroxide for fluid and electrolyte imbalance, especially if patient is following a sodium-restricted diet.

■ Monitor phosphate level if patient takes aluminum carbonate or hydroxide.

■ Watch for evidence of hypercalcemia if patient takes calcium carbonate.

■ Monitor magnesium level if patient has mild renal impairment and takes magaldrate.

■ Manage constipation with laxatives or stool softeners, or switch patient to a magnesium preparation.

■ If patient has diarrhea, give an antidiarrheal and switch patient to an antacid that contains aluminum.

■ Shake container well, and give with small amount of water or juice to facilitate passage.

■ When giving through a nasogastric tube, make sure the tube is patent and placed correctly. After instilling the drug, flush the tube with water to ensure passage to the stomach and to clear the tube.

Patient teaching

■ Because antacids may interact with certain drugs, warn patient not to select an antacid or switch antacids without consulting a health care provider.

■ Tell patient not to take calcium carbonate with milk or other foods high in vitamin D.

■ If patient takes sodium bicarbonate, warn against taking it with milk because doing so could cause hypercalcemia.

ANTIANGINALS

BETA BLOCKERS
atenolol
metoprolol
nadolol
propranolol hydrochloride

CALCIUM CHANNEL BLOCKERS
amlodipine besylate
diltiazem hydrochloride
nicardipine hydrochloride
nifedipine
verapamil hydrochloride

NITRATES
isosorbide dinitrate
isosorbide mononitrate
nitroglycerin

Indications

■ Acute angina (S.L. nitroglycerin and S.L. or chewable isosorbide dinitrate)

■ Classic, effort-induced angina and Prinzmetal's angina (calcium channel blockers)

■ Moderate to severe angina (beta blockers)

■ Recurrent angina (long-acting nitrates and topical, transdermal, transmucosal, and oral extended-release nitroglycerin)

■ Unstable angina (I.V. nitroglycerin)

Actions

Beta blockers decrease catecholamine-induced increases in heart rate, blood pressure, and myocardial contraction.

Calcium channel blockers inhibit the flow of calcium through muscle cells, which dilates coronary arteries and decreases systemic vascular resistance, known as afterload.

Nitrates decrease afterload and preload (left ventricular end-diastolic pressure) and increase blood flow through collateral coronary vessels.

Adverse reactions

Beta blockers may cause bradycardia, cough, diarrhea, disturbing dreams, dizziness, dyspnea, fatigue, fever, heart failure, hypotension, lethargy, nausea, peripheral edema, and wheezing.

Calcium channel blockers may cause bradycardia, confusion, constipation, depression, diarrhea, dizziness, edema, elevated liver enzyme levels (transient), fatigue, flushing, headache, hypotension, insomnia, nervousness, and rash.

Nitrates may cause alcohol intoxication (from I.V. preparations containing alcohol), flushing, headache, orthostatic hypotension, reflex tachycardia, rash, syncope, and vomiting.

Contraindications and cautions

■ *Beta blockers.* Contraindicated in patients hypersensitive to them and in patients with cardiogenic shock, sinus bradycardia, heart block greater than first degree, bronchial asthma, or heart failure unless failure results from tachyarrhythmia treatable with propranolol. Use cautiously in patients with nonallergic bronchospastic disorders, diabetes mellitus, or impaired hepatic or renal function.

■ *Calcium channel blockers.* Contraindicated in patients with severe hypotension or heart block greater than first degree (except with functioning pacemaker). Use cautiously in patients with hepatic or renal impairment, bradycardia, heart failure, or cardiogenic shock.

■ *Nitrates.* Contraindicated in patients with severe anemia, cerebral hemorrhage, head trauma, glaucoma, or hyperthyroidism. Use cautiously in patients with hypotension or recent myocardial infarction.

LIFESPAN

■ *Pregnant women.* Use beta blockers cautiously.

- *Breast-feeding women.* Recommendations vary by drug; use beta blockers and calcium channel blockers cautiously.
- *Children.* Safety and efficacy aren't known. Check with prescriber before giving these drugs to children.
- *Geriatric patients.* Increased risk of adverse reactions; use cautiously.

Nursing considerations

- Don't give a beta blocker or calcium channel blocker to relieve acute angina.
- Have patient sit or lie down when receiving the first nitrate dose.
- Take pulse and blood pressure before giving first nitrate dose and when drug action starts.
- Withhold dose and notify prescriber if patient's heart rate is lower than 60 beats/minute or systolic blood pressure is lower than 90 mm Hg.
- Monitor vital signs. With I.V. nitroglycerin, monitor blood pressure and pulse rate every 5 to 15 minutes while adjusting dosage and every hour thereafter.
- Monitor drug effectiveness.
- Observe patient for adverse reactions.

Patient teaching

- Warn patient not to stop drug abruptly without prescriber's approval.
- Teach patient to take his pulse before taking a beta blocker or calcium channel blocker. Tell him to withhold the dose and alert the prescriber if his pulse rate is below 60 beats/minute.
- Instruct patient taking nitroglycerin S.L. to go to the emergency department if three tablets taken 5 minutes apart don't relieve angina.
- Tell patient to report serious or persistent adverse reactions.
- Warn patient against taking drugs for erectile dysfunction while taking nitrates.

ANTIARRHYTHMICS

CLASS IA
disopyramide
moricizine hydrochloride
procainamide hydrochloride
quinidine bisulfate
quinidine gluconate
quinidine sulfate

CLASS IB
lidocaine hydrochloride
mexiletine hydrochloride
phenytoin sodium
tocainide hydrochloride

Class Ic
flecainide acetate
propafenone hydrochloride

Class II (beta blockers)
acebutolol
esmolol hydrochloride
propranolol hydrochloride

Class III
amiodarone hydrochloride
dofetilide
ibutilide fumarate
sotalol hydrochloride

Class IV (calcium channel blocker)
verapamil hydrochloride

Indications
■ Atrial and ventricular arrhythmias

Actions
Class I drugs reduce the inward current carried by sodium ions, which stabilizes neuronal cardiac membranes.

Class Ia drugs depress phase 0, prolong the action potential, and stabilize cardiac membranes.

Class Ib drugs depress phase 0, shorten the action potential, and stabilize cardiac membranes.

Class Ic drugs block the transport of sodium ions, which decreases conduction velocity but not repolarization rate.

Class II drugs decrease heart rate, myocardial contractility, blood pressure, and atrioventricular node conduction.

Class III drugs prolong the action potential and refractory period.

Class IV drugs decrease myocardial contractility and oxygen demand by inhibiting calcium ion influx; they also dilate coronary arteries and arterioles.

Adverse reactions
Most antiarrhythmics can aggravate existing arrhythmias or cause new ones. They also may produce hypersensitivity reactions; hypotension; gastrointestinal problems, such as nausea, vomiting, or altered bowel elimination; and central nervous system (CNS) disturbances, such as dizziness or fatigue. Some antiarrhythmics may worsen heart failure. Class II drugs may cause bronchoconstriction.

Contraindications and cautions
■ Contraindicated in patients hypersensitive to drug.
■ Many antiarrhythmics are contraindicated or require cautious use in patients with cardiogenic shock, digitalis toxici-

ty, and second- or third-degree heart block (unless patient has a pacemaker).

LIFESPAN

■ *Pregnant women.* Use only if potential benefits to mother outweigh risks to fetus.

■ *Breast-feeding women.* Use cautiously. Many antiarrhythmics appear in breast milk.

■ *Children.* Monitor patient closely because of increased risk of adverse reactions.

■ *Geriatric patients.* Use cautiously because these patients may have physiologic changes in the cardiovascular system.

Nursing considerations

■ Monitor electrocardiogram continuously when therapy starts and dosage is adjusted.

■ Check vital signs frequently, and assess patient for evidence of toxicity and adverse reactions.

■ Measure apical pulse rate before giving drug.

■ Monitor drug level as indicated.

■ Don't crush sustained-release tablets.

■ Take safety precautions if adverse CNS reactions occur.

■ Notify prescriber about adverse reactions.

Patient teaching

■ Stress the importance of taking drug exactly as prescribed.

■ Teach patient to take his pulse before each dose and to notify prescriber if it's irregular or less than 60 beats/minute.

■ Instruct patient to avoid hazardous activities if adverse CNS reactions occur.

■ Tell patient to limit fluid and salt intake if drug causes fluid retention.

ANTIBIOTIC ANTINEOPLASTICS

bleomycin sulfate
daunorubicin hydrochloride
doxorubicin hydrochloride
epirubicin hydrochloride
idarubicin hydrochloride
mitomycin
mitoxantrone hydrochloride
procarbazine hydrochloride

Indications

■ Various tumors

Actions

Although classified as antibiotics, these drugs destroy cells and disrupt proliferation of malignant cells, thus ruling out their use as antimicrobials alone. Some act like alkylating drugs or antimetabolites. Their action may be specific to cell-cycle phase, not specific to cell-cycle phase, or both. By binding to or complexing with DNA, these drugs directly or indirectly inhibit DNA, RNA, and protein synthesis.

Adverse reactions

Antibiotic antineoplastics may cause anxiety, bone marrow depression, chills, confusion, diarrhea, fever, flank or joint pain, hair loss, leukopenia, nausea, redness or pain at the injection site, sore throat, swelling of the feet or lower legs, and vomiting.

Contraindications and cautions

■ Contraindicated in patients hypersensitive to drug.

LIFESPAN

■ *Pregnant women.* These patients should avoid antineoplastics.
■ *Breast-feeding women.* Breast-feeding isn't recommended during therapy.
■ *Children.* Safety and efficacy of some drugs aren't known.
■ *Geriatric patients.* Use cautiously because of increased risk of adverse reactions.

Nursing considerations

■ Perform a complete assessment before therapy starts.

■ Try to ease patient and family anxiety before treatment.
■ Monitor hemoglobin, hematocrit, platelet count, total and differential leukocyte counts, and levels of alanine transaminase, aspartate transaminase, lactate dehydrogenase, bilirubin, creatinine, uric acid, and blood urea nitrogen.
■ Assess vital signs and patency of catheter or I.V. line.
■ Watch for adverse reactions.
■ Treat extravasation right away.
■ Follow established procedures for safe and proper handling, administration, and disposal of chemotherapeutic drugs.
■ *Bleomycin.* Keep epinephrine, corticosteroids, and antihistamines available in case of anaphylactoid reaction. Monitor pulmonary function tests, and assess lung function regularly.
■ *Daunorubicin, doxorubicin.* Assess patient's electrocardiogram before and during treatment.
■ *Idarubicin.* Ensure adequate hydration during therapy.
■ *Procarbazine.* Stop drug and notify prescriber if patient becomes confused or develops neuropathies.

Patient teaching

- Urge patient to complete dental work before therapy begins or to delay it until blood counts are normal.
- Tell patient to report redness, pain, or swelling at injection site immediately. Local tissue injury and scarring may result if I.V. infiltration occurs.
- Advise patient to avoid people who have bacterial or viral infections because chemotherapy increases susceptibility. Urge patient to report evidence of infection immediately.
- Warn patient that he may bruise easily.
- Review proper oral hygiene, including cautious use of toothbrush, dental floss, and toothpicks. Chemotherapy can increase the risk of microbial infection, delayed healing, and bleeding gums.
- *Procarbazine*. Warn patient to avoid hazardous activities until CNS effects of drug are known. Also, advise taking drug at bedtime and in divided doses to reduce nausea and vomiting.
- *Daunorubicin, doxorubicin, or idarubicin*. Explain that urine may turn orange or red for 1 to 2 days after therapy begins.

ANTICHOLINERGICS

atropine sulfate
benztropine mesylate
dicyclomine hydrochloride
scopolamine
scopolamine butylbromide
scopolamine hydrobromide

Indications

- Adjunct treatment of peptic ulcers and other gastrointestinal (GI) disorders
- Blockage of cholinomimetic effects of cholinesterase inhibitors or other drugs
- Preoperative reduction of secretions and blockage of cardiac reflexes
- Prevention of motion sickness
- Various spastic conditions, including acute dystonic reactions, muscle rigidity, parkinsonism, and extrapyramidal disorders (benztropine). (See *Comparing systemic anticholinergics*.)

Actions

Anticholinergics competitively antagonize the actions of acetylcholine and other cholinergic agonists at muscarinic receptors.

COMPARING SYSTEMIC ANTICHOLINERGICS

Drug	Plasma half-life (hr)	Onset of action	Duration of action
atropine, oral	2½	Inhibition of saliva occurs in 30–60 min	4–6 hr
atropine, parenteral	2½	Peak increase in heart rate occurs after 2–4 min	Brief
benztropine	Unknown	P.O. 1–2 hr I.V., I.M.: 15 min	24 hr
dicyclomine	9–10	Unknown	Unknown
glycopyrrolate	I.V.: ½ – 4½ I.M.: 15–30 min	I.V.: 1 min I.M.: 30–40 min	2–7 hr 2–7 hr
homatropine	Unknown	40–60 min	1–3 days
hyoscyamine, oral	3½ Sustained-release: 7	20–30 min	4–6 hr Sustained-release: 12 hr
hyoscyamine, parenteral	3½	2–3 min	4–6 hr
oxybutynin	Unknown	30–60 min	6–10 hr
propantheline	1½	1½ hr	6 hr
scopolamine, oral	1	1–2 hr	Unknown
scopolamine, parenteral	½	Varies	Varies
tolterodine	Unknown	1 hr	5 hr
trihexyphenidyl	Unknown	Within 1 hr	6 – 12 hr

Adverse reactions

Therapeutic doses may cause blurred vision, constipation, cycloplegia, decreased sweating or anhidrosis, dry mouth, headache, mydriasis, palpitations, tachycardia, and urinary hesitancy and retention. These reactions usually disappear when therapy stops.

Toxicity can cause blurred vision; changes resembling psychosis (agitation, anxiety, confusion, delusions, disorientation, hallucinations, restlessness); decreased or absent bowel sounds; dilated, nonreactive pupils; dry mucous membranes; dysphagia; hot, dry, flushed skin; hypertension; hyperthermia; increased respirations; tachycardia; and urine retention.

Contraindications and cautions

■ Contraindicated in patients hypersensitive to drug and in those with angle-closure glaucoma, renal or GI obstructive disease, reflux esophagitis, or myasthenia gravis.

■ Use cautiously in patients with autonomic neuropathy, GI infection, heart disease, hiatal hernia with reflux esophagitis, hypertension, hyperthyroidism, open-angle glaucoma, prostatic hypertrophy, or ulcerative colitis.

LIFESPAN

■ *Women of childbearing age.* Advise patient to report suspected pregnancy.

■ *Breast-feeding women.* Avoid anticholinergics because these drugs may decrease milk production, appear in breast milk, or cause infant toxicity.

■ *Children.* Safety and efficacy aren't known.

■ *Adults over age 40.* These patients may be more sensitive to these drugs.

■ *Geriatric patients.* Use cautiously and give a reduced dosage as indicated.

Nursing considerations

■ Monitor patient regularly for adverse reactions.

■ Check vital signs at least every 4 hours.

■ Measure urine output; check for urine retention.

■ Assess patient for changes in vision and for signs of impending toxicity.

■ Provide ice chips, cool drinks, or hard candy to relieve dry mouth.

■ Relieve constipation with stool softeners or bulk laxatives.

■ Give a mild analgesic for headache.

■ Notify prescriber of urine retention, and be prepared for catheterization.

Patient teaching

■ Teach patient how and when to take the drug; caution against taking other drugs unless prescribed.

■ Warn patient to avoid hazardous tasks if drug causes dizziness, drowsiness, or blurred vision. Inform patient that the drug may increase sensitivity to or intolerance of high temperatures, resulting in dizziness.

■ Advise patient to avoid alcohol because it may cause additive central nervous system effects.

■ Urge patient to drink plenty of fluids and to eat a high-fiber diet to prevent constipation.

■ Tell patient to notify prescriber promptly about development of confusion, a rapid or pounding heartbeat, dry mouth, blurred vision, rash, eye pain, significant change in urine volume, or pain or difficulty with urination.

ANTICOAGULANTS

COUMARIN DERIVATIVE
warfarin sodium

HEPARIN DERIVATIVE
heparin sodium

LOW−MOLECULAR-WEIGHT HEPARINS
dalteparin sodium
enoxaparin sodium
tinzaparin sodium

SELECTIVE FACTOR XA INHIBITOR
fondaparinux sodium

THROMBIN INHIBITORS
argatroban
bivalirudin

Indications

■ Atrial fibrillation
■ Blood clotting
■ Deep vein thrombosis
■ Disseminated intravascular coagulation
■ Myocardial infarction
■ Pulmonary emboli
■ Thrombus
■ Unstable angina

Actions

Heparin derivatives accelerate formation of an antithrombin III–thrombin complex that inactivates thrombin and prevents conversion of fibrinogen to fibrin.

The coumarin derivative, warfarin, inhibits vitamin-K–dependent activation of clotting factors II, VII, IX, and X, which are formed in the liver.

- Prevention of seizures after trauma or craniotomy
- Seizure disorders
- Status epilepticus

Actions

Anticonvulsants include six drug classes and two miscellaneous drugs:

- acetazolamide, which inhibits carbonic anhydrase
- barbiturates, which limit seizure activity by increasing the threshold for motor cortex stimuli.
- benzodiazepines, which may increase inhibition of gamma aminobutyric acid (GABA) in brain neurons.
- carboxylic acid derivatives, which may increase inhibition of GABA in brain neurons.
- iminostilbene derivatives (carbamazepine), which inhibit the spread of seizure activity in the motor cortex.
- magnesium sulfate, which interferes with release of acetylcholine at the myoneural junction
- selected hydantoin derivatives, which inhibit the spread of seizure activity in the motor cortex.
- succinimides, which limit seizure activity by increasing the threshold for motor cortex stimuli.

Adverse reactions

Anticonvulsants can cause adverse central nervous system (CNS) effects, such as confusion, somnolence, tremor, and ataxia. Many anticonvulsants also cause gastrointestinal (GI) effects, such as vomiting; cardiovascular disorders, such as arrhythmias and hypotension; and hematologic disorders, such as leukopenia, bone marrow depression, thrombocytopenia, and agranulocytosis. Stevens-Johnson syndrome and other severe rashes and abnormal liver function tests may occur with certain anticonvulsants.

Contraindications and cautions

- Contraindicated in patients hypersensitive to anticonvulsants.
- Carbamazepine is contraindicated within 14 days of monoamine oxidase inhibitor use.

LIFESPAN

- *Breast-feeding women.* Safety of many anticonvulsants hasn't been established.
- *Children.* Use cautiously; children, especially young ones, are sensitive to the CNS depression of some anticonvulsants.

■ *Geriatric patients.* May need lower doses because of increased sensitivity to CNS effects. Some anticonvulsants may take longer to be eliminated because of decreased renal function. Parenteral use is more likely to cause apnea, hypotension, bradycardia, and cardiac arrest.

Nursing considerations
■ Monitor drug level and patient's response as indicated.
■ Adjust dosage according to patient's response.
■ Assess patient for adverse reactions. Take safety precautions if patient has adverse CNS reactions.
■ Give oral forms with food to reduce GI irritation.
■ Assess patient's compliance with therapy at each follow-up visit.
■ Phenytoin binds with tube feedings, decreasing its absorption. Stop tube feedings for 2 hours before and after giving phenytoin, according to your facility's policy.

Patient teaching
■ Instruct patient to take drug exactly as prescribed and not to stop without medical supervision.

■ Urge patient to avoid hazardous activities if adverse CNS reactions occur.
■ Advise patient to wear or carry medical identification at all times.

ANTIDEPRESSANTS, TRICYCLIC

amitriptyline hydrochloride
amitriptyline pamoate
amoxapine
clomipramine hydrochloride
desipramine hydrochloride
doxepin hydrochloride
imipramine hydrochloride
imipramine pamoate
nortriptyline hydrochloride

Indications
■ Anxiety (doxepin hydrochloride)
■ Depression
■ Enuresis in children over age 6 (imipramine)
■ Obsessive-compulsive disorder (clomipramine)

Actions
Tricyclic antidepressants may inhibit reuptake of norepinephrine and serotonin in central nervous system nerve terminals (presynaptic neurons), thus increasing the level and activity of neurotransmitters in the synaptic cleft. These drugs also have

antihistamine, sedative, anticholinergic, vasodilatory, and quinidine-like effects.

Adverse reactions

Adverse reactions include sedation, anticholinergic effects, and orthostatic hypotension.

Tertiary amines (amitriptyline, doxepin, and imipramine) exert the strongest sedative effects; tolerance usually develops in a few weeks.

Amoxapine is most likely to cause seizures, especially with overdose.

Contraindications and cautions

■ Contraindicated in patients hypersensitive to tricyclic antidepressants and in patients with urine retention or angle-closure glaucoma.

■ Tricyclic antidepressants are contraindicated in patients taking monoamine oxidase inhibitors.

■ Use cautiously in patients with suicidal tendencies, schizophrenia, paranoia, seizure disorders, cardiovascular disease, or impaired hepatic function.

LIFESPAN

■ *Pregnant women.* Safety isn't known. Use only if potential benefit to mother outweighs possible harm to fetus.

■ *Breast-feeding women.* Safety isn't known; use cautiously.

■ *Children under age 12.* Not recommended.

■ *Geriatric patients.* Reduce dosage; these patient are more sensitive to drug effects.

Nursing considerations

■ Observe patient for mood changes to monitor drug effectiveness; benefits may not appear for 3 to 6 weeks.

■ Check vital signs regularly for tachycardia or decreased blood pressure; observe patient carefully for other adverse reactions and report changes. Check electrocardiogram in patients over age 40 before starting therapy.

■ Monitor patient for adverse anticholinergic effects, such as urine retention or constipation, which may require dosage reduction.

■ Make sure patient swallows each dose; a depressed patient may hoard pills for suicide attempt, especially when symptoms begin to improve.

■ Don't withdraw drug abruptly; instead, gradually reduce dosage over several weeks to avoid rebound effect or other adverse reactions.

Patient teaching

■ Explain the rationale for therapy and its anticipated risks and benefits. Inform patient that full therapeutic effect may not occur for several weeks.

■ Teach patient how and when to take the drug. Warn against increasing the dosage, stopping the drug, or taking any other drug, including over-the-counter medicines and herbal supplements, without medical approval.

■ Advise patient not to take drug with milk or food to minimize gastrointestinal distress. Suggest taking full dose at bedtime if daytime sedation is a problem.

■ Tell patient to avoid alcohol.

■ Advise patient to avoid hazardous tasks until full effects of drug are known.

■ Recommend sugarless gum or hard candy, artificial saliva, or ice chips to relieve dry mouth.

■ Warn patient that excessive exposure to sunlight, heat lamps, or tanning beds may cause burns and an abnormal increase in pigmentation.

■ Advise patient to report adverse reactions promptly.

■ Urge diabetic patient to monitor glucose levels carefully because drug may change them.

■ Because overdose with tricyclic antidepressants is commonly fatal, entrust a reliable family member with the drug, and warn him to store drug safely away from children.

ANTIDIARRHEALS

bismuth subgallate
bismuth subsalicylate
calcium polycarbophil
diphenoxylate hydrochloride
   and atropine sulfate
kaolin and pectin mixtures
loperamide
octreotide acetate
opium tincture
opium tincture, camphorated

Indications

■ Diarrhea caused by tumors (octreotide acetate)

■ Mild, acute, or chronic diarrhea

Actions

Bismuth preparations may have a mild water-binding capacity, may absorb toxins, and provide a protective coating for the intestinal mucosa.

Kaolin and pectin mixtures decrease fluid in the stool by absorbing bacteria and toxins that cause diarrhea.

Opium preparations increase smooth muscle tone in the gastrointestinal tract, inhibit motility and propulsion, and decrease digestive secretions.

Adverse reactions

Bismuth preparations may cause salicylism (with high doses) or temporary darkening of tongue and stools.

Kaolin and pectin mixtures may cause constipation and fecal impaction or ulceration.

Opium forms may cause dizziness, light-headedness, nausea, physical dependence (with long-term use), and vomiting.

Contraindications and cautions

■ Contraindicated in patients hypersensitive to these drugs.

LIFESPAN

■ *Breast-feeding patients.* Some antidiarrheals may appear in breast milk; check individual drugs for specific recommendations.
■ *Infants under age 2.* Don't give kaolin and pectin mixtures.
■ *Children or teenagers recovering from flu or chickenpox.* Consult prescriber before giving bismuth subsalicylate.
■ *Geriatric patients.* Use caution when giving antidiarrheals, especially opium preparations.

Nursing considerations

■ Assess patient's condition before therapy and regularly thereafter.
■ Monitor fluid and electrolyte balance.
■ Observe patient for adverse reactions.
■ Take safety precautions if patient experiences adverse central nervous system (CNS) reactions.
■ Don't substitute opium tincture for paregoric.
■ Notify prescriber about serious or persistent adverse reactions.

Patient teaching

■ Instruct patient to take drug exactly as prescribed; warn that excessive use of opium preparations can lead to dependence.
■ Instruct patient to notify prescriber if diarrhea lasts more than 2 days and to report adverse reactions.
■ Warn patient to avoid hazardous activities if CNS depression occurs.

ANTIHISTAMINES

azelastine hydrochloride
brompheniramine maleate
**cyproheptadine
  hydrochloride**

desloratadine
diphenhydramine
   hydrochloride
fexofenadine hydrochloride
hydroxyzine embonate
hydroxyzine hydrochloride
hydroxyzine pamoate
loratadine
meclizine hydrochloride
promethazine hydrochloride
promethazine theoclate
triprolidine hydrochloride

Indications

- Allergic rhinitis
- Dyskinesia
- Motion sickness
- Nausea and vomiting
- Parkinsonism
- Pruritus
- Sedation
- Urticaria
- Vertigo

Actions

Antihistamines are structurally related chemicals that compete with histamine for histamine H_1-receptor sites on smooth muscle of bronchi, gastrointestinal (GI) tract, and large blood vessels, binding to cellular receptors and preventing access to and subsequent activity of histamine. They don't directly alter histamine or prevent its release.

Adverse reactions

Many antihistamines cause drowsiness and impaired motor function early in therapy. They also can cause dry mouth and throat, blurred vision, and constipation. Some antihistamines, such as promethazine, may cause cholestatic jaundice, which may be a hypersensitivity reaction, and may predispose patients to photosensitivity.

Contraindications and cautions

- Contraindicated in patients hypersensitive to drug and in those with angle-closure glaucoma, stenosing peptic ulcer, pyloroduodenal obstruction, or bladder neck obstruction. Also contraindicated in those taking monoamine oxidase inhibitors.

LIFESPAN

- *Pregnant women.* Safety isn't known. Use only when clearly needed. Avoid use during the third trimester because of the risk of severe reactions in newborns and premature infants.
- *Breast-feeding women.* Antihistamines shouldn't be used; many drugs appear in breast milk and may cause unusual excitability in the infant.

■ *Neonates, especially premature infants.* Antihistamines may cause seizures.

■ *Children, especially those under age 6.* Antihistamines may cause paradoxical hyperexcitability with restlessness, insomnia, nervousness, euphoria, tremors, and seizures; administer cautiously.

■ *Geriatric patients.* Use cautiously and monitor patient closely because of increased sensitivity to adverse drug effects, especially dizziness, sedation, hypotension, and urine retention.

Nursing considerations

■ Assess patient for adverse reactions.

■ Monitor blood counts during long-term therapy; watch for evidence of blood dyscrasia.

■ Reduce GI distress by giving antihistamines with food.

■ Provide sugarless gum, hard candy, or ice chips to relieve dry mouth.

■ Increase fluid intake or humidify air to decrease adverse effect of thickened secretions.

Patient teaching

■ Advise patient to take drug with meals or snacks to prevent GI upset.

■ Suggest that patient use warm water rinses, artificial saliva, ice chips, or sugarless gum or candy to relieve dry mouth. Advise against overusing mouthwash, which may worsen dryness and destroy normal flora.

■ Warn patient to avoid hazardous activities until full central nervous system effects of drug are known.

■ Tell patient to seek medical approval before using alcohol, tranquilizers, sedatives, pain relievers, or sleeping medications.

■ For accurate diagnostic skin test results, advise patient to stop taking antihistamines 4 days before test.

ANTIHYPERTENSIVES

ANGIOTENSIN-CONVERTING ENZYME INHIBITORS
benazepril hydrochloride
captopril
enalaprilat
enalapril maleate
fosinopril sodium
lisinopril
moexipril hydrochloride
perindopril erbumine
quinapril hydrochloride
ramipril
trandolapril

ALPHA BLOCKERS, CENTRALLY ACTING (SYMPATHOLYTICS)
clonidine hydrochloride
guanfacine hydrochloride
methyldopa

ALPHA BLOCKERS, PERIPHERALLY ACTING
doxazosin mesylate
prazosin hydrochloride
tamsulosin hydrochloride
terazosin hydrochloride

ANGIOTENSIN II RECEPTOR BLOCKERS
candesartan cilexetil
eprosartan mesylate
irbesartan
losartan potassium
telmisartan
valsartan

BETA BLOCKERS
acebutolol
atenolol
bisoprolol fumarate
carvedilol
labetalol hydrochloride
metoprolol tartrate
nadolol
pindolol
propranolol hydrochloride
timolol maleate

CALCIUM CHANNEL BLOCKERS
amlodipine besylate
diltiazem hydrochloride
felodipine
nicardipine hydrochloride
nifedipine
nisoldipine
verapamil hydrochloride

RAUWOLFIA ALKALOID
reserpine

VASODILATORS
diazoxide
hydralazine hydrochloride
minoxidil
nitroprusside sodium

Indications
■ Essential and secondary hypertension

Actions
Antihypertensives reduce blood pressure through various mechanisms. For more on the action of angiotensin-converting enzyme inhibitors, alpha blockers, angiotensin II receptor blockers, beta blockers, calcium channel blockers, and diuretics, see their individual drug class entries in this chapter.

Centrally acting sympatholytics stimulate central alpha-adrenergic receptors, reducing cerebral sympathetic outflow, thereby decreasing peripheral vascular resistance and blood pressure.

Rauwolfia alkaloids bind to and gradually destroy storage vesicles containing norepinephrine in central and peripheral adrenergic neurons.

Vasodilators act directly on smooth muscle to reduce blood pressure.

Adverse reactions

Antihypertensives may cause orthostatic hypotension, changes in heart rate, headache, nausea, and vomiting. Other reactions vary greatly among different drug types.

Centrally acting sympatholytics may cause constipation, depression, dizziness, drowsiness, dry mouth, headache, palpitations, severe rebound hypertension, and sexual dysfunction; methyldopa also may cause aplastic anemia and thrombocytopenia.

Rauwolfia alkaloids may cause anxiety, depression, drowsiness, dry mouth, hyperacidity, impotence, nasal stuffiness, and weight gain.

Vasodilators may cause heart failure, electrocardiogram changes, diarrhea, dizziness, palpitations, pruritus, and rash.

Contraindications and cautions

■ Contraindicated in patients hypersensitive to antihypertensives and in those with hypotension.

■ Use cautiously in patients with hepatic or renal dysfunction.

LIFESPAN

■ *Breast-feeding women.* Use cautiously; some antihypertensives appear in breast milk.

■ *Children.* Safety and efficacy of many antihypertensives aren't known; give these drugs cautiously, and monitor patient closely.

■ *Geriatric patients.* Monitor patient closely because of increased risk of adverse reactions; give lower maintenance doses as needed.

Nursing considerations

■ Obtain baseline blood pressure and pulse rate and rhythm; recheck regularly.

■ Assess patient for adverse reactions.

■ Monitor patient's weight and fluid and electrolyte status.

■ Check patient's compliance with treatment.

■ Give drug with food or h.s., as indicated.

■ Follow manufacturer's guidelines when mixing and administering parenteral drugs.

■ Take steps to prevent or minimize orthostatic hypotension.

■ Monitor patient's nondrug therapy, such as sodium restriction, calorie reduction, stress management, and exercise program.

Patient teaching

■ Instruct patient to take drug exactly as prescribed. Warn against stopping drug abruptly.

■ Review adverse reactions caused by drug, and urge patient to notify prescriber about serious or persistent reactions.

■ Advise patient to avoid sudden changes in position to prevent dizziness, light-headedness, or fainting.

■ Warn patient to avoid hazardous activities until full effects of drug are known. Also, warn patient to avoid physical exertion, especially in hot weather.

■ Advise patient to consult prescriber before taking any over-the-counter medications or herbal supplements; serious drug interactions can occur.

■ Encourage patient to comply with therapy.

ANTILIPEMICS

BILE-SEQUESTERING DRUGS
cholestyramine
colesevelam hydrochloride

CHOLESTEROL ABSORPTION INHIBITOR
ezetimibe

FIBRIC ACID DERIVATIVES
fenofibrate
gemfibrozil

HMG-CoA REDUCTASE INHIBITORS
atorvastatin calcium
fluvastatin sodium
lovastatin
pravastatin sodium
rosuvastatin calcium
simvastatin

Indications
■ Hypercholesterolemia
■ Hyperlipidemia

Actions
Antilipemics lower elevated lipid levels.

Bile-sequestering drugs form insoluble complexes with bile salts, thus triggering cholesterol to leave the bloodstream and other storage areas to make new bile acids.

The cholesterol absorption inhibitor ezetimibe inhibits absorption of cholesterol in the intestine.

Fibric acid derivatives reduce cholesterol formation, increase sterol excretion, and decrease lipoprotein and triglyceride synthesis.

COMPARING HMG-CoA REDUCTASE INHIBITORS

DRUG	USUAL DOSE	ABSOLUTE BIOAVAILABILITY (%)	METABOLISM ENZYMES
atorvastatin	10–80 mg/day	14	CYP 3A4
fluvastatin	20–80 mg/day h.s.	24	CYP 2C9
lovastatin	20–80 mg/day with evening meal	< 5	CYP 3A4
pravastatin	10–40 mg/day h.s.	17	Not reported
rosuvastatin	5–40 mg/day	20	CYP 2C9
simvastatin	10–80 mg/day in evening	< 5	CYP 3A4

The 3-hydroxy-3-methyl-glutaryl coenzyme A (HMG-CoA) reductase inhibitors interfere with enzymes that generate cholesterol in the liver. (See *Comparing HMG-CoA reductase inhibitors.*)

Adverse reactions

Antilipemics commonly cause GI upset.

Bile-sequestering drugs may cause cholelithiasis, constipation, bloating, and steatorrhea.

Fibric acid derivatives may cause cholelithiasis and GI or CNS effects. Use of gemfibrozil with lovastatin may cause myopathy.

HMG-CoA reductase inhibitors may affect liver function or cause rash, pruritus, increased creatine kinase (CK) levels, rhabdomyolysis, and myopathy.

Contraindications and cautions

■ Contraindicated in patients hypersensitive to drug.

■ Bile-sequestering drugs are contraindicated in patients with complete biliary obstruction. Use cautiously in constipated patients.

■ Fibric acid derivatives are contraindicated in patients with primary biliary cirrhosis or significant hepatic or renal dys-

Active metabolite	Excretion (%)	Protein binding (%)	Half-life (hr)	LDL-C lowering (%)
Yes	<2 (urine)	≥98	~ 14	26.5–60
Yes	<6 (urine) ~ 90 (feces)	98	<1	18.9–35
No	10 (urine) 83 (feces)	>95	3–4	21–40
No	~ 20 (urine) 70 (feces)	~ 50	1½	22–34
Yes	90 (feces)	88	19	45–63
No	13 (urine) 60 (feces)	~ 95	3	14–47

function. Use cautiously in patients with peptic ulcer.

■ HMG-CoA reductase inhibitors are contraindicated in patients with active liver disease or persistently elevated transaminase levels. Use cautiously in patients who consume large amounts of alcohol or who have a history of liver or renal disease.

LIFESPAN

■ *Pregnant women.* Use bile-sequestering drugs and fibric acid derivatives cautiously. Avoid HMG-CoA reductase inhibitors.

■ *Breast-feeding women.* Give bile-sequestering drugs cautiously. Avoid fibric acid derivatives and HMG-CoA reductase inhibitors.

■ *Children ages 10 to 17.* Certain antilipemics are approved to treat heterozygous familial hypercholesterolemia in adolescent boys and girls at least one year post-menarche.

■ *Geriatric patients.* Use bile-sequestering drugs cautiously and monitor patient closely because of increased risk of severe constipation.

Nursing considerations

■ Monitor cholesterol and lipid levels before and periodically during therapy.

■ Check CK level when therapy begins and every 6 months thereafter.

■ Assess patient for adverse reactions.

■ *Bile-sequestering drugs.* Mix powder form with 120 to 180 ml of liquid. Never give dry powder alone because patient may inhale it accidentally.

■ *HMG-CoA reductase inhibitors.* Check CK level if patient complains of muscle pain.

■ *Lovastatin.* Give with evening meal.

■ *Simvastatin.* Give in the evening.

■ *Fluvastatin, pravastatin.* Give at bedtime.

Patient teaching

■ Instruct patient to take drug exactly as prescribed. If he takes a bile-sequestering drug, warn him never to take the dry form.

■ Stress the importance of diet in controlling lipid levels.

■ Advise patient to drink 2 to 3 L of fluid daily and to report persistent or severe constipation.

ANTIMETABOLITE ANTINEOPLASTICS

capecitabine
cytarabine
cytarabine liposomal
fludarabine phosphate
fluorouracil
hydroxyurea
mercaptopurine
methotrexate
pentostatin
thioguanine

Indications

■ Various tumors

Actions

Antimetabolites are structurally similar to naturally occurring metabolites and can be divided into three subcategories:

■ folic acid antagonists

■ purine analogues

■ pyrimidine analogues.

Most of these drugs interrupt cell reproduction at a specific phase of the cell cycle.

Purine analogues are incorporated into DNA and RNA, interfering with nucleic acid synthesis (by miscoding) and replication. They also may inhibit synthesis of purine bases through pseudofeedback mechanisms.

Pyrimidine analogues inhibit enzymes in metabolic pathways that interfere with biosynthesis of uridine and thymine.

Folic acid antagonists prevent conversion of folic acid to tetrahydrofolate by inhibiting the enzyme dihydrofolic acid reductase.

Adverse reactions

The most common adverse effects include nausea, vomiting, diarrhea, fever, chills, hair loss, flank or joint pain, redness or pain at injection site, anxiety, bone marrow depression, leukopenia, thrombocytopenia, anemia, and swelling of the feet or lower legs.

Contraindications and cautions

■ Contraindicated in patients hypersensitive to drug.

LIFESPAN

■ *Pregnant women.* Inform patient about risks to fetus.
■ *Breast-feeding women.* Breast-feeding isn't recommended when taking these drugs.
■ *Children.* Safety and efficacy of some drugs aren't known.
■ *Geriatric patients.* Monitor patient closely because of increased risk of adverse reactions.

Nursing considerations

■ Perform a complete assessment before therapy begins.
■ Assess patient for adverse reactions.
■ Monitor vital signs and patency of catheter or I.V. line throughout administration.
■ Check hematocrit, platelet and total and differential leukocyte counts, and levels of alanine transaminase, aspartate transaminase, lactate dehydrogenase, bilirubin, creatinine, uric acid, and blood urea nitrogen.

■ Follow established procedures for safe and proper handling, administration, and disposal of drugs.
■ Try to ease anxiety in patient and family before treatment.
■ Give an antiemetic before giving drug to lessen nausea.
■ Treat extravasation right away.
■ *Cytarabine.* Give with allopurinol to decrease the risk of hyperuricemia. Encourage patient to drink fluids.
■ *Cytarabine, fluorouracil, methotrexate.* Provide patient with diligent mouth care to prevent stomatitis.
■ *Fluorouracil.* Anticipate diarrhea, possibly severe, with prolonged therapy.
■ *High-dose methotrexate therapy.* Anticipate the need for leucovorin rescue.

Patient teaching

■ Teach patient proper oral hygiene, including cautious use of toothbrush, dental floss, and toothpicks. Chemotherapy can increase the risk of microbial infection, delayed healing, and bleeding gums.

■ Advise patient to complete dental work before therapy begins or to delay it until blood counts are normal.

■ Warn patient that he may bruise easily because of drug's effect on platelets.

■ Advise patient to avoid close contact with persons who have been exposed to bacterial or viral infection because chemotherapy may increase susceptibility. Urge patient to notify prescriber promptly if evidence of infection develops.

■ Instruct patient to report redness, pain, or swelling at injection site. Local tissue injury and scarring may result from tissue infiltration at infusion site.

■ Tell patient to defer immunizations if possible until hematologic stability is confirmed.

ANTIPARKINSONIANS

amantadine hydrochloride
benztropine mesylate
bromocriptine mesylate
diphenhydramine
    hydrochloride
entacapone
levodopa
levodopa and carbidopa
levodopa, carbidopa, and
    entacapone
pergolide mesylate

pramipexole dihydrochloride
ropinirole hydrochloride
selegiline hydrochloride
tolcapone
trihexyphenidyl
    hydrochloride

Indications
■ Drug-induced extrapyramidal reactions
■ Signs and symptoms of Parkinson's disease

Actions
Antiparkinsonians include synthetic anticholinergics and dopaminergics and the antiviral, amantadine.

Anticholinergics probably prolong the action of dopamine by blocking its reuptake into presynaptic neurons and by suppressing central cholinergic activity.

Dopaminergics act in the brain by increasing dopamine availability, thus improving motor function. Entacapone is a reversible inhibitor of peripheral catechol-O-methyltransferase, which is responsible for elimination of various catecholamines, including dopamine. Blocking this pathway when giving carbidopa and levodopa should result in higher levels of levodopa, thereby allowing greater dopaminergic stimulation in the central nervous system (CNS) and leading to a greater effect in treating parkinsonian symptoms.

Amantadine is thought to increase dopamine release in the substantia nigra.

Adverse reactions

Anticholinergics may cause decreased sweating or anhidrosis, dry mouth, headache, mydriasis, blurred vision, cycloplegia, urinary hesitancy and urine retention, constipation, palpitations, and tachycardia.

Dopaminergics may cause nausea, vomiting, muscle cramps, dystonias, headache, orthostatic hypotension, confusion, arrhythmias, hallucinations, and disturbing dreams.

Amantadine also causes irritability, insomnia, and livedo reticularis (with prolonged use).

Contraindications and cautions

■ Contraindicated in patients hypersensitive to drug.
■ Use cautiously in patients with prostatic hyperplasia or tardive dyskinesia and in debilitated patients.
■ Abrupt withdrawal may cause a neuroleptic malignant–like syndrome involving muscle rigidity, increased body temperature, and mental status changes.

Lifespan

■ *Pregnant patients.* Safety isn't known.
■ *Breast-feeding patients.* Because antiparkinsonians may appear in breast milk, a decision should be made to stop the drug or stop breast-feeding based on the importance of the drug to the mother.
■ *Children.* Safety and efficacy aren't known.
■ *Geriatric patients.* Monitor patient closely because of increased risk of adverse reactions.

Nursing considerations

■ Obtain baseline assessment of patient's impairment, and reassess regularly to monitor drug effectiveness.
■ Assess patient for adverse reactions.
■ Monitor vital signs, especially during dosage adjustments.
■ Give drug with food to prevent gastrointestinal (GI) irritation.
■ Adjust dosage according to patient's response and tolerance.
■ Never withdraw drug abruptly.
■ Institute safety precautions.
■ Provide ice chips, drinks, or sugarless hard candy or gum to relieve dry mouth. Increase fluid and fiber intake to prevent constipation, as appropriate.

■ Notify prescriber about urine retention; the patient may need to be catheterized.

Patient teaching

■ Instruct patient to take drug exactly as prescribed and not to stop drug suddenly.

■ Advise patient to take drug with food to prevent GI upset.

■ Teach patient how to manage anticholinergic effects, if needed.

■ Caution patient to avoid hazardous tasks if adverse CNS effects occur.

■ Urge patient to avoid alcohol during therapy.

■ Encourage patient to report severe or persistent adverse reactions.

ANTIVIRALS

abacavir sulfate
acyclovir sodium
amantadine hydrochloride
amprenavir
atazanavir sulfate
cidofovir
delavirdine mesylate
didanosine
efavirenz
emtricitabine
enfuvirtide
famciclovir
fosamprenavir calcium
foscarnet sodium
ganciclovir
indinavir sulfate
lamivudine
lamivudine and zidovudine
lopinavir and ritonavir
nelfinavir mesylate
nevirapine
oseltamivir phosphate
ribavirin
rimantadine hydrochloride
ritonavir
saquinavir mesylate
stavudine
valacyclovir hydrochloride
valganciclovir
zalcitabine
zanamivir
zidovudine

Indications

■ Viral infections

Actions

Abacavir, amprenavir, atazanavir, fosamprenavir, indinavir, lopinavir and ritonavir, nelfinavir, ritonavir, saquinavir, and stavudine inhibit the activity of human immunodeficiency virus (HIV) protease.

Acyclovir, cidofovir, didanosine, famciclovir, ganciclovir, valacyclovir, valganciclovir, and zalcitabine interfere with DNA synthesis and replication. Ribavirin may also act in this way.

Amantadine and rimantadine prevent the release of infectious viral nucleic acid into the host cell and possibly prevent viruses from penetrating cells.

Delavirdine, efavirenz, emtricitabine, lamivudine, nevirapine, and zidovudine inhibit reverse transcriptase.

Foscarnet blocks the pyrophosphate-binding site.

Oseltamivir and zanamivir inhibit neuraminidase, thus preventing the virus's release from the host cell.

Enfuvirtide blocks the entry of HIV-1 into cells by inhibiting the fusion of viral and cellular membranes.

Adverse reactions

Antivirals may cause anorexia, chills, confusion, depression, diarrhea, dry mouth, edema, fatigue, hallucinations, headache, nausea, and vomiting.

Contraindications and cautions

■ Contraindicated in patients hypersensitive to drug.

LIFESPAN

■ *Pregnant women.* Use only if potential benefits to mother justify risk to fetus.
■ *Breast-feeding women.* Some antivirals are contraindicated; others require cautious use.
■ *Infants and children.* Recommendations vary with the antiviral prescribed.

■ *Geriatric patients.* Monitor patient closely because of increased risk of adverse reactions.

Nursing considerations

■ Obtain baseline assessment of patient's viral infection, and reassess regularly to monitor drug's effectiveness.
■ Monitor renal and hepatic function, complete blood count, and platelet count regularly.
■ Inspect patient's I.V. site regularly for signs of irritation, phlebitis, inflammation, or extravasation.
■ Adjust dosage of selected antiviral if patient has decreased renal function, especially during parenteral therapy.
■ Follow manufacturer's guidelines for reconstituting and giving an antiviral.
■ Obtain an order for an antiemetic or antidiarrheal, if needed.
■ Take safety precautions if patient has adverse central nervous system reactions. For example, place bed in low position, raise bed rails, and supervise ambulation and other activities.
■ Notify prescriber about serious or persistent adverse reactions.
■ *Amantadine.* If patient has a history of heart failure, watch

closely for worsening or recurrence.

■ *Foscarnet.* Monitor levels of electrolytes, such as calcium, phosphate, magnesium, and potassium.

■ *Ribavirin.* Monitor patient's cardiac status.

Patient teaching

■ Instruct patient to take drug exactly as prescribed, even if he feels better.

■ Urge patient to notify prescriber promptly about severe or persistent adverse reactions.

■ Encourage patient to keep appointments for follow-up care.

BARBITURATES

amobarbital
amobarbital sodium
pentobarbital sodium
phenobarbital
phenobarbital sodium
primidone
secobarbital sodium

Indications

■ Preanesthesia
■ Sedation
■ Seizure disorders
■ Short-term treatment of insomnia

Actions

Barbiturates act throughout the central nervous system (CNS), especially in the mesencephalic reticular activating system, which controls the CNS arousal mechanism. The main anticonvulsant actions are reduced nerve transmission and decreased excitability of the nerve cell. Barbiturates decrease presynaptic and postsynaptic membrane excitability by promoting the actions of gamma-aminobutyric acid. They also depress respiration and gastrointestinal motility and raise the seizure threshold.

Adverse reactions

Drowsiness, lethargy, vertigo, headache, and CNS depression are common with barbiturates. High fever, severe headache, stomatitis, conjunctivitis, or rhinitis may precede potentially fatal skin eruptions. Withdrawal symptoms may occur after as little as 2 weeks of uninterrupted therapy.

At hypnotic doses, a hangover effect, subtle distortion of mood, and impaired judgment and motor skills may continue for many hours. After dosage reduction or discontinuation, rebound insomnia or increased dreaming or nightmares may occur.

At subhypnotic doses, barbiturates cause hyperalgesia. They also can cause paradoxical excitement, confusion in elderly patients, and hyperactivity in children.

Contraindications and cautions

■ Contraindicated in patients hypersensitive to drug and in those with bronchopneumonia, other severe pulmonary insufficiency, or liver dysfunction.

■ Use cautiously in patients with blood pressure alterations, pulmonary disease, and cardiovascular dysfunction.

LIFESPAN

■ *Pregnant women.* Barbiturates can cause fetal abnormalities; avoid use.

■ *Breast-feeding patients.* Barbiturates appear in breast milk and cause CNS depression in the infant; use cautiously.

■ *Premature infants.* These patients are more susceptible to depressant effects of barbiturates because of their immature hepatic metabolism.

■ *Children.* Use cautiously and monitor patient closely because of possible hyperactivity, excitement, or hyperalgesia.

■ *Geriatric patients.* Use cautiously because of possible hyperactivity, excitement, or hyperalgesia.

Nursing considerations

■ Assess patient's level of consciousness and sleeping patterns before and during therapy to evaluate drug effectiveness. Monitor neurologic status for alteration or deterioration.

■ Check vital signs frequently, especially during I.V. administration.

■ Monitor seizure character, frequency, and duration for changes.

■ Observe patient to prevent hoarding or self-dosing, especially if patient is depressed, suicidal, or drug-dependent.

■ When giving parenteral drug, avoid extravasation, which may cause local tissue damage and tissue necrosis; inject I.V. or deep I.M. only. Don't exceed 5 ml for any I.M. injection site to avoid tissue damage.

■ Keep resuscitation supplies available. Too-rapid I.V. administration may cause respiratory depression, apnea, laryngospasm, or hypotension.

■ Take seizure precautions, as needed.

■ Institute safety measures to prevent falls and injury. Raise side rails, assist patient out of bed, and keep call light within easy reach.

■ Stop drug slowly. Abrupt discontinuation may cause withdrawal symptoms.

Patient teaching
■ Explain that barbiturates can cause physical or psychological dependence.

■ Instruct patient to take drug exactly as prescribed. Warn against changing the dosage or taking other drugs, including over-the-counter medications or herbal supplements, without prescriber's approval.

■ Reassure patient that a morning hangover is common after barbiturate use.

■ Advise patient to avoid hazardous tasks, including driving a car, while taking drug and to review other safety measures to prevent injury.

■ Instruct patient to report skin eruption or other significant adverse effects.

BETA BLOCKERS

BETA₁ BLOCKERS
acebutolol
atenolol
betataxol
bisoprolol fumarate
esmolol hydrochloride
metoprolol tartrate

NON-SELECTIVE BETA BLOCKERS
carteolol
carvedilol
labetalol hydrochloride
nadolol
pindolol
propranolol hydrochloride
sotalol hydrochloride
timolol maleate

Indications
■ Angina pectoris (atenolol, metoprolol, nadolol, propranolol)

■ Arrhythmias (acebutolol, esmolol, propranolol, sotalol)

■ Glaucoma (betaxolol, timolol)

■ Heart failure (atenolol, bisoprolol, carvedilol, metoprolol)

■ Hypertension (most drugs)

■ Pheochromocytomas or essential tremors (selected drugs)

■ Prevention of myocardial infarction (atenolol, metoprolol, propranolol, timolol)

■ Prevention of recurrent migraine and other vascular headaches (propranolol, timolol)

Actions
Beta blockers compete with beta agonists for available beta receptors; individual drugs differ in their ability to affect beta receptors. Some drugs are considered non-selective: they

block beta$_1$ receptors in cardiac muscle and beta$_2$ receptors in bronchial and vascular smooth muscle. Several drugs are cardioselective and, in lower doses, inhibit mainly beta$_1$ receptors. Some beta blockers have intrinsic sympathomimetic activity and stimulate and block beta receptors, thereby decreasing cardiac output. Others stabilize cardiac membranes, which affects cardiac-action potential. (See *Comparing beta blockers*, pages 48 and 49.)

Adverse reactions

Therapeutic doses may cause bradycardia, fatigue, and dizziness; some may cause other central nervous system disturbances, such as nightmares, depression, memory loss, and hallucinations. Toxic doses can produce severe hypotension, bradycardia, heart failure, or bronchospasm.

Contraindications and cautions

■ Contraindicated in patients hypersensitive to drug and in patients with cardiogenic shock, sinus bradycardia, heart block greater than first degree, bronchial asthma, and heart failure unless failure is caused by tachyarrhythmia treatable with propranolol.

■ Use cautiously in patients with nonallergic bronchospastic disorders, diabetes mellitus, or impaired hepatic or renal function.

LIFESPAN

■ *Pregnant women.* Use cautiously.

■ *Breast-feeding women.* These drugs appear in breast milk.

■ *Children.* Safety and efficacy aren't known; use only if potential benefits outweigh potential risks.

■ *Geriatric patients.* Use cautiously and at reduced maintenance doses, if needed, because of increased bioavailability, delayed metabolism, and increased adverse effects.

Nursing considerations

■ Check apical pulse rate daily; alert prescriber about extremes, such as a rate lower than 60 beats/minute.

■ Monitor blood pressure, electrocardiogram, and heart rate and rhythm frequently; be alert for progression of atrioventricular block or bradycardia.

■ If patient has heart failure, obtain body weight regularly; watch for weight gain of more than 2.25 kg (5 lb) per week.

■ Observe diabetic patients for sweating, fatigue, and hunger.

COMPARING BETA BLOCKERS

DRUG	HALF–LIFE (HR)	LIPID SOLUBILITY	MEMBRANE-STABILIZING ACTIVITY
Non-selective			
carteolol	6	Low	0
carvedilol	7–10	High	Unknown
labetalol	6–8	Moderate	0
nadolol	20	Low	0
penbutolol	5	High	0
pindolol	3–4	Low	0
propranolol	4	High	++
timolol	4	Low to moderate	0
Beta$_1$-selective			
acebutolol	3–4	Low	+
atenolol	6–7	Low	0
betaxolol	14–22	Low	+
bisoprolol	9–12	Low	0
esmolol	¼	Low	0
metoprolol	3–7	Moderate	*

* Only in higher-than-usual doses.
+ Activity that drug possesses in comparison to other beta blockers.

INTRINSIC SYMPATHOMIMETIC ACTIVITY
++
0
0
0
+
+++
0
0
+
0
0
0
0
0

Signs of hypoglycemic shock may be masked.
■ Keep glucagon nearby to reverse beta blocker overdose.
■ Discontinue a beta blocker before surgery for pheochromocytoma. Before any surgical procedure, notify anesthesiologist that patient is taking a beta blocker.

Patient teaching
■ Teach patient to take drug exactly as prescribed, even when he feels better.
■ Warn against stopping drug suddenly, which can worsen angina or trigger MI.
■ Tell patient not to take over-the-counter medications or herbal supplements without prescriber's approval.
■ Explain potential adverse reactions, and stress importance of reporting unusual effects.

CALCIUM CHANNEL BLOCKERS

amlodipine besylate
diltiazem hydrochloride
felodipine
nicardipine hydrochloride
nifedipine
nisoldipine
verapamil hydrochloride

Indications
- Arrhythmias
- Chronic stable angina
- Mild-to-moderate hypertension
- Prinzmetal's variant angina
- Unstable angina

Actions
The main physiologic action of calcium channel blockers is to inhibit calcium influx across the slow channels of myocardial and vascular smooth muscle cells. By inhibiting calcium flow into these cells, calcium channel blockers reduce intracellular calcium levels. This, in turn, dilates coronary arteries, peripheral arteries, and arterioles and slows cardiac conduction.

When used to treat Prinzmetal's variant angina, calcium channel blockers inhibit coronary spasm, which then increases oxygen delivery to the heart. Peripheral artery dilation decreases total peripheral resistance, which reduces afterload. This, in turn, decreases the amount of oxygen used by the myocardium. Inhibiting calcium flow into the specialized cardiac conduction cells (specifically, those in the sinoatrial and atrioventricular [AV] nodes) slows conduction through the heart. Of the calcium channel blockers, verapamil and diltiazem have the greatest effect on the AV node, which slows the ventricular rate in atrial fibrillation or flutter and converts supraventricular tachycardia to a normal sinus rhythm. (See *Comparing oral calcium channel blockers.*)

Adverse reactions
Adverse reactions vary among the drugs.

Diltiazem's most common adverse reactions are anorexia and nausea, and the drug may also induce various degrees of heart block, bradycardia, heart failure, and peripheral edema.

Nifedipine may cause hypotension, peripheral edema, flushing, light-headedness, and headache.

Verapamil may cause bradycardia, various degrees of heart block, worsening of heart failure, and hypotension after rapid I.V. administration. Prolonged oral verapamil therapy may cause constipation.

Contraindications and cautions
- Contraindicated in patients hypersensitive to drug and in those with second- or third-degree heart block (except those with a pacemaker) and cardiogenic shock.

COMPARING ORAL CALCIUM CHANNEL BLOCKERS

DRUG	ONSET OF ACTION	PEAK SERUM LEVEL (HR)	HALF-LIFE (HR)
amlodipine	Unknown	6–12	30–50
diltiazem	15 min	½	3–4
felodipine	2–5 hr	2½–5	11–16
isradipine	20 min	1½	8
nicardipine	20 min	½–2	8⅔
nifedipine	10 min	½	2
nimodipine	Unknown	< 1	1–2
nisoldipine	Unknown	6–12	7–12
verapamil	30 min	1–2	6–12

LIFESPAN

■ *Pregnant women.* Use cautiously.

■ *Breast-feeding women.* Calcium channel blockers may appear in breast milk; instruct patient to stop breast-feeding during therapy.

■ *Neonates and infants.* Adverse hemodynamic effects of parenteral verapamil are possible, but safety and efficacy of other calcium channel blockers haven't been established; avoid use, if possible.

■ *Geriatric patients.* Half-life of calcium channel blockers may be increased from decreased clearance; use cautiously.

Nursing considerations

■ Assess cardiac rate and rhythm and blood pressure carefully when therapy starts or dosage increases.

■ Monitor fluid and electrolytes.

■ Observe patient for adverse reactions.

■ Don't give calcium supplements while patient takes a calcium channel blocker; they may decrease the drug's effectiveness.

■ Expect to decrease dosage gradually; don't stop calcium channel blockers abruptly.

Patient teaching

■ Teach patient to take drug exactly as prescribed, even if he feels better.

■ Instruct patient to take a missed dose as soon as possible, unless it's almost time for his next dose. Warn him never to double the dose.

■ Warn patient not to stop drug suddenly because serious adverse effects are possible.

■ Urge patient to report irregular heartbeat, shortness of breath, swelling of hands and feet, dizziness, constipation, nausea, or hypotension.

CEPHALOSPORINS

FIRST GENERATION
cefadroxil monohydrate
cefazolin sodium
cephalexin monohydrate

SECOND GENERATION
cefaclor
cefotetan disodium
cefoxitin sodium
cefprozil
cefuroxime axetil
cefuroxime sodium
loracarbef

THIRD GENERATION
cefdinir
cefditoren pivoxil
cefoperazone sodium

cefotaxime sodium
cefpodoxime proxetil
ceftazidime
ceftibuten
ceftizoxime sodium
ceftriaxone sodium

Indications

■ Ampicillin-resistant middle ear infection caused by *Haemophilus influenzae*

■ Central nervous system infections caused by susceptible strains of *Neisseria meningitidis*, *H. influenzae*, and *Streptococcus pneumoniae*

■ Infections of the lungs, skin, soft tissue, bones, joints, urinary and respiratory tracts, blood, abdomen, and heart

■ Infections that develop after surgical procedures classified as contaminated or potentially contaminated

■ Otitis media

■ Penicillinase-producing *Neisseria gonorrhoeae*

■ Meningitis caused by *Escherichia coli* or *Klebsiella* (See *Comparing cephalosporins*.)

Actions

Cephalosporins are chemically and pharmacologically similar to penicillin; they act by inhibiting bacterial cell wall synthesis, causing rapid cell destruction. They act on enzymes known as penicillin-binding proteins. The

Comparing cephalosporins

Drug and route	Elimination half-life (hr): Normal renal function	End-stage renal disease	Sodium (mEq/g)	Cerebrospinal fluid penetration
cefaclor P.O.	½–1	2–3	Unknown	No
cefadroxil P.O.	1–2	20–25	Unknown	No
cefazolin I.M., I.V.	1¼–2¼	3–7	2	No
cefdinir P.O.	1½	16	Unknown	Unknown
cefepime I.M., I.V.	2	17–21	Unknown	Yes
cefoperazone I.M., I.V.	1½–2½	1⅓–3	1.5	Sometimes
cefotaxime I.M., I.V.	1–1½	3–11	2.2	Yes
cefotetan I.M., I.V.	2¾–4⅔	13–35	3.5	No
cefoxitin I.M., I.V.	½–1	20	2.3	No
cefpodoxime P.O.	2–3	9¾	Unknown	Unknown
cefprozil P.O.	1–1½	5¼–6	Unknown	Unknown
ceftazidime I.M., I.V.	1½–2	14–30	2.3	Yes

(continued)

COMPARING CEPHALOSPORINS (continued)

DRUG AND ROUTE	ELIMINATION HALF-LIFE (HR)		SODIUM (mEq/g)	CEREBRO-SPINAL FLUID PENETRATION
	NORMAL RENAL FUNCTION	END-STAGE RENAL DISEASE		
ceftibuten P.O.	2⅓	13½–22⅓	Unknown	Unknown
cefti-zoxime I.M., I.V.	1½–2	25–30	2.6	Yes
ceftriax-one I.M., I.V.	5½–11	15.7	3.6	Yes
cefurox-ime I.M., I.V.	1–2	15–22	2.4	Yes
cephalexin P.O.	½–1	19–22	Unknown	No
cephra-dine P.O., I.M., I.V.	½–2	8–15	6	No

affinity of certain cephalosporins for these proteins in various microorganisms helps explain the differing actions of these drugs. They are bactericidal; they act against many aerobic gram-positive and gram-negative bacteria and some anaerobic bacteria but don't kill fungi or viruses.

First-generation cephalosporins act against many gram-positive cocci, including penicillinase-producing *Staphylococcus aureus* and *Staphylococcus epidermidis*; *Streptococcus pneumoniae*, group B streptococci, and group A beta-hemolytic streptococci; susceptible gram-negative organisms include *Klebsiella pneu-*

moniae, E. coli, Proteus mirabilis, and *Shigella.*

Second-generation cephalosporins are effective against all organisms attacked by first-generation drugs and have additional activity against *Moraxella catarrhalis, H. influenzae, Enterobacter, Citrobacter, Providencia, Acinetobacter, Serratia,* and *Neisseria.* Bacteroides fragilis is susceptible to cefotetan and cefoxitin.

Third-generation cephalosporins are less active than first- and second-generation drugs against gram-positive bacteria, but are more active against gram-negative organisms, including those resistant to first- and second-generation drugs. They have the greatest stability against beta-lactamases produced by gram-negative bacteria. Susceptible gram-negative organisms include *E. coli, Klebsiella, Enterobacter, Providencia, Acinetobacter, Serratia, Proteus, Morganella,* and *Neisseria.* Some third-generation drugs are active against *B. fragilis* and *Pseudomonas.*

Adverse reactions

Many cephalosporins have similar adverse effects. Hypersensitivity reactions range from mild rashes, fever, and eosinophilia to fatal anaphylaxis and are more common in patients with penicillin allergy.

Adverse gastrointestinal (GI) reactions include nausea, vomiting, diarrhea, abdominal pain, glossitis, dyspepsia, and tenesmus.

Hematologic reactions include positive direct and indirect antiglobulin in Coombs' test, thrombocytopenia or thrombocythemia, transient neutropenia, and reversible leukopenia.

Minimal elevation of liver function test results occurs occasionally.

Adverse renal effects may occur with any cephalosporin; they are most common in older patients, those with decreased renal function, and those taking other nephrotoxic drugs.

Local venous pain and irritation are common after I.M. injection; these reactions occur more often with higher doses and long-term therapy.

Disulfiram-type reactions occur when cefoperazone or cefotetan are given within 3 days of alcohol use.

Bacterial and fungal superinfections may result from suppression of normal flora.

Contraindications and cautions

■ Contraindicated in patients hypersensitive to drug.

■ Use cautiously in patients with renal or hepatic impairment, history of GI disease, or allergy to penicillins.

LIFESPAN

■ *Pregnant women.* Safety isn't known.

■ *Breast-feeding women.* Use cautiously because drugs appear in breast milk.

■ *Neonates and infants.* Half-life is prolonged; use cautiously.

■ *Geriatric patients.* Use cautiously; these patients are susceptible to superinfection and coagulopathies, commonly have renal impairment, and may need a lower dosage.

Nursing considerations

■ Review patient's history of allergies. Try to determine whether previous reactions were true hypersensitivity reactions or adverse effects (such as GI distress) that patient interpreted as allergy.

■ Monitor patient continuously for possible hypersensitivity reactions or other adverse effects.

■ Obtain culture and sensitivity specimen before giving first dose; check test results periodically to assess drug's effectiveness.

■ Evaluate renal function; dosage of certain cephalosporins must be lowered in a patient with severe renal impairment. In patient with decreased renal function, monitor blood urea nitrogen and creatinine levels and urine output for significant changes.

■ Assess patient receiving long-term therapy for possible bacterial and fungal superinfection, especially elderly and debilitated patients and those receiving immunosuppressants or radiation therapy.

■ Monitor at-risk patients for fluid retention while they are taking sodium salts of cephalosporins.

■ Give these drugs at least 1 hour before bacteriostatic antibiotics, such as tetracyclines, erythromycins, and chloramphenicol; the antibiotics keep bacteria from growing by decreasing cephalosporin uptake by bacterial cell walls.

■ Refrigerate oral suspensions, which are stable for 14 days; shake well before giving to ensure correct dosage.

■ Follow manufacturer's directions for reconstitution, dilution, and storage of drugs; check expiration dates.

■ Give I.M. dose deep into gluteal muscle mass or midlateral thigh; rotate injection sites to minimize tissue injury.

■ Don't add or mix other drugs with I.V. infusions, particularly aminoglycosides, which will be inactivated if mixed with cephalosporins. If other drugs must be given I.V., temporarily stop infusion of primary drug.

■ Ensure adequate dilution of I.V. infusion, and rotate site every 48 hours to help minimize local vein irritation; using a small-gauge needle in a larger available vein may be helpful.

■ *Cefoperazone, cefotetan, ceftriaxone.* Monitor prothrombin time and platelet count, and assess patient for signs of hypoprothrombinemia, which may occur with or without bleeding. It usually occurs in elderly, debilitated, malnourished, and immunocompromised patients and in patients with renal impairment or impaired vitamin K synthesis.

Patient teaching

■ Make sure patient understands how and when to take drug. Urge compliance with instructions for around-the-clock dosing and completing the prescribed regimen.

■ Advise patient to take oral drug with food if GI irritation occurs.

■ Review proper storage and disposal of drug, and remind patient to check expiration date.

■ Teach signs and symptoms of hypersensitivity and other adverse reactions, and emphasize importance of reporting unusual effects.

■ Teach signs and symptoms of bacterial and fungal superinfection, especially if patient is elderly or debilitated or has low resistance from immunosuppressants or irradiation. Emphasize importance of reporting signs and symptoms promptly.

■ Warn patient not to ingest alcohol in any form within 3 days of treatment with cefoperazone or cefotetan.

■ Advise patient to add yogurt or buttermilk to diet to prevent intestinal superinfection from suppression of normal intestinal flora.

■ Advise diabetic patient to monitor glucose level with Diastix, not Clinitest.

■ Urge patient to keep follow-up appointments.

CORTICOSTEROIDS

betamethasone
betamethasone sodium
phosphate
cortisone acetate
dexamethasone
dexamethasone acetate
dexamethasone sodium
phosphate
fludrocortisone acetate
hydrocortisone
hydrocortisone acetate
hydrocortisone cypionate
hydrocortisone sodium
phosphate
hydrocortisone sodium
succinate
methylprednisolone
methylprednisolone acetate
methylprednisolone sodium
succinate
prednisolone
prednisolone acetate
prednisolone sodium
phosphate
prednisolone steaglate
prednisolone tebutate
prednisone
triamcinolone
triamcinolone diacetate
triamcinolone hexacetonide

Indications

- Dermatologic diseases
- Hypersensitivity
- Inflammation, particularly of eye, nose, and respiratory tract
- Initiation of immunosuppression
- Replacement therapy in adrenocortical insufficiency
- Respiratory disorders
- Rheumatic disorders

Actions

Corticosteroids suppress cell-mediated and humoral immunity in three ways:

- by reducing levels of leukocytes, monocytes, and eosinophils
- by decreasing immunoglobulin binding to cell-surface receptors
- by inhibiting interleukin synthesis.

They reduce inflammation by preventing hydrolytic enzyme release into the cells, preventing plasma exudation, suppressing polymorphonuclear leukocyte migration, and disrupting other inflammatory processes.

Adverse reactions

Systemic corticosteroid therapy may suppress the hypothalamic-pituitary-adrenal axis. Excessive use may cause cushingoid symptoms and various systemic disorders, such as diabetes and osteoporosis. Other effects may include euphoria, psychosis, insomnia, edema, hypertension, peptic ulcer, increased appetite, weight gain, fluid and electrolyte imbalances, dermatologic disorders, and immunosuppression.

Contraindications and cautions

■ Contraindicated in patients hypersensitive to drug or its components and in those with systemic fungal infection.

■ Use cautiously in patients with GI ulceration, renal disease, hypertension, osteoporosis, varicella, vaccinia, exanthema, diabetes mellitus, hypothyroidism, thromboembolic disorder, seizures, myasthenia gravis, heart failure, tuberculosis, ocular herpes simplex, hypoalbuminemia, emotional instability, or psychosis.

LIFESPAN

■ *Pregnant women.* Avoid use, if possible, because of risk to fetus.

■ *Breast-feeding women.* Advise woman to stop breast-feeding because these drugs appear in breast milk and could cause serious adverse effects in infant.

■ *Children.* Avoid long-term use, if possible, because growth may be stunted.

■ *Geriatric patients.* Monitor patient closely; risk of adverse reactions may be increased.

Nursing considerations

■ Establish baseline blood pressure, fluid and electrolyte status, and weight; reassess regularly.

■ Monitor patient closely for adverse reactions.

■ Evaluate drug effectiveness at regular intervals.

■ Give drug early in the day to mimic circadian rhythm.

■ Give drug with food to prevent gastrointestinal irritation.

■ Take precautions to avoid exposing patient to infection.

■ Don't stop drug abruptly.

■ Notify prescriber of severe or persistent adverse reactions.

■ Avoid prolonged use of corticosteroids, especially in children.

Patient teaching

■ Teach patient to take drug exactly as prescribed, and warn him never to stop the drug suddenly.

■ Tell patient to notify prescriber if stress level increases; dosage may need to be temporarily increased.

■ Instruct patient to take oral drug with food.

■ Urge patient to report black tarry stools, bleeding, bruising, blurred vision, emotional changes, or other unusual effects.

COMPARING LOOP DIURETICS

DRUG AND ROUTE	ONSET (MIN)	PEAK (HR)	DURATION (HR)
bumetanide			
I.V.	≤ 5	¼–½	½–1
P.O.	30–60	1–2	4–6
ethacrynic acid			
I.V.	5–15	¼–½	2
P.O.	≤ 30	2	6–8
furosemide			
I.V.	≤ 5	½	2
P.O.	30–60	1–2	6–8
torsemide			
I.V.	≤ 10	≤ 1	6–8
P.O.	≤ 60	1–2	6–8

■ Encourage patient to wear or carry medical identification at all times.

DIURETICS, LOOP

bumetanide
ethacrynate sodium
ethacrynic acid
furosemide
torsemide

Indications

■ Acute pulmonary edema or hypertensive crisis (adjunct treatment)

■ Edema from heart failure, hepatic cirrhosis, or nephrotic syndrome

■ Mild to moderate hypertension

Actions

Loop diuretics inhibit sodium and chloride reabsorption in the ascending loop of Henle, thus increasing excretion of sodium, chloride, and water. Like thiazide diuretics, loop diuretics increase potassium excretion. They produce more diuresis and electrolyte loss than thiazide diuretics. (See *Comparing loop diuretics*.)

USUAL DOSAGE	I.V. INJECTION TIME (MIN)
0.5–1 mg 0.5–2 mg/day	1–2
0.5–1 mg/kg 50–200 mg/day	Several
20–40 mg 20–80 mg/day	1–2
10–20 mg/day 10–20 mg/day	2

Adverse reactions

Therapeutic doses commonly cause metabolic and electrolyte disturbances, particularly potassium depletion. They also may cause hypochloremic alkalosis, hyperglycemia, hyperuricemia, and hypomagnesemia. Rapid parenteral administration may cause hearing loss (including deafness) and tinnitus. High doses can produce profound diuresis, leading to hypovolemia and cardiovascular collapse. Photosensitivity also may occur.

Contraindications and cautions

■ Contraindicated in patients hypersensitive to drug and in patients with anuria, hepatic coma, or severe electrolyte depletion.

■ Use cautiously in patients with severe renal disease.

■ Use cautiously in patients with severe hypersensitivity to sulfonamides because allergic reaction may occur.

LIFESPAN

■ *Pregnant women.* Use cautiously.

■ *Breast-feeding women.* Don't use.

■ *Neonates.* Use cautiously. Usual pediatric dose can be given, but dosage intervals should be extended.

■ *Geriatric patients.* Monitor patient closely because of possible increased susceptibility to drug-induced diuresis. Reduced dosages may be indicated.

Nursing considerations

■ Monitor blood pressure and pulse rate, especially during rapid diuresis. Establish baseline values before therapy begins, and watch for significant changes.

■ Establish baseline complete blood count (including white blood cell count), liver function test results, and electrolytes, carbon dioxide, magnesium, blood urea nitrogen, and creatinine levels. Review periodically.

■ Assess patient for evidence of excessive diuresis: hypotension, tachycardia, poor skin turgor, excessive thirst, or dry and cracked mucous membranes.

■ Monitor patient for edema and ascites. Observe the legs of ambulatory patients and the sacral area of patients on bed rest.

■ Weigh patient each morning immediately after voiding and before breakfast, in the same type of clothing, and on the same scale. Weight provides a reliable indicator of patient's response to diuretic therapy.

■ Monitor and record patient's intake and output daily.

■ Give diuretics in morning to ensure that major diuresis occurs before bedtime. To prevent nocturia, give diuretics before 6 p.m.

■ Take safety measures for all ambulatory patients until response to diuretic is known.

■ Consult dietitian about need for potassium supplements.

■ Keep urinal or commode readily available.

■ Decrease dosage if patient has hepatic dysfunction. Increase dosage if patient has renal impairment, oliguria, or decreased diuresis. Inadequate urine output may result in circulatory overload, which causes water intoxication, pulmonary edema, and heart failure. Increase dosage of insulin or oral hypoglycemic in diabetic patient, and reduce dosage of other antihypertensives.

Patient teaching

■ Explain rationale for therapy and importance of following prescribed regimen.

■ Review adverse effects, and urge patient to report symptoms promptly, especially chest, back, or leg pain; shortness of breath; dyspnea; increased edema or weight; and excess diuresis evidenced by weight loss of more than 2 lb daily.

■ Encouragee patient to eat potassium-rich foods and to avoid high-sodium foods, such as lunch meat, smoked meats, and processed cheeses. Caution him not to add table salt to foods.

■ Encourage patient to keep follow-up appointments to monitor the effectiveness of therapy.

DIURETICS, THIAZIDE AND THIAZIDE-LIKE

THIAZIDE
chlorothiazide
hydrochlorothiazide

THIAZIDE-LIKE
indapamide
metolazone

Indications
■ Diabetes insipidus, particularly nephrogenic
■ Edema and ascites from hepatic cirrhosis
■ Edema from right-sided heart failure, mild-to-moderate left-sided heart failure, or nephrotic syndrome
■ Hypertension

Actions
Thiazide and thiazide-like diuretics interfere with sodium transport across the tubules of the cortical diluting segment in the nephron, thereby increasing renal excretion of sodium, chloride, water, potassium, and calcium.

Thiazide diuretics also have an antihypertensive effect, possibly in part from direct arteriolar dilation. In diabetes insipidus, thiazides cause a paradoxical decrease in urine volume and an increase in renal concentration of urine, possibly because of sodium depletion and decreased plasma volume. This increases water and sodium reabsorption in the kidneys.

Adverse reactions
Therapeutic doses cause electrolyte and metabolic disturbances, most commonly potassium depletion. Other abnormalities include hypochloremic alkalosis, hypomagnesemia, hyponatremia, hypercalcemia, hyperuricemia, hyperglycemia, and elevated cholesterol levels. Photosensitivity also may occur.

Contraindications and cautions
■ Contraindicated in patients hypersensitive to drug and in those with anuria.
■ Use cautiously in patients with severe renal disease, impaired hepatic function, or progressive liver disease.

LIFESPAN
■ *Pregnant women.* Use cautiously.
■ *Breast-feeding women.* Thiazides are contraindicated because they appear in breast milk.
■ *Children.* Safety and efficacy haven't been established.
■ *Geriatric patients.* Monitor patient closely because of possi-

ble increased susceptibility to drug-induced diuresis. Reduced dosage may be needed.

Nursing considerations

■ Monitor patient's intake, output, and electrolyte level regularly.

■ Weigh patient each morning immediately after voiding and before breakfast, in the same type of clothing, and on the same scale. Weight provides a reliable indicator of patient's response to diuretic therapy.

■ Monitor diabetic patient's glucose level. Diuretics may cause hyperglycemia.

■ Check creatinine and blood urea nitrogen levels regularly. Drug isn't as effective if these levels are more than twice normal. Also, monitor uric acid level.

■ Give drug in the morning to prevent nocturia.

■ Provide a high-potassium diet.

■ Give potassium supplements to maintain acceptable potassium level.

■ Keep urinal or commode readily available to patient.

Patient teaching

■ Explain the rationale for therapy and the importance of following the prescribed regimen.

■ Tell patient to take drug at the same time each day to prevent nocturia. Suggest taking drug with food to minimize gastrointestinal irritation.

■ Urge patient to seek prescriber's approval before taking any other drug, including over-the-counter medications and herbal remedies.

■ Advise patient to record his weight each morning after voiding and before breakfast, in the same type of clothing, and on the same scale.

■ Review adverse effects, and urge the patient to report symptoms promptly, especially chest, back, or leg pain; shortness of breath; dyspnea; increased edema or weight; or excess diuresis evidenced by weight loss of more than 2 lb daily. Warn patient about photosensitivity reactions that usually occur 10 to 14 days after initial sun exposure.

■ Encourage patient to eat potassium-rich foods and to avoid high-sodium foods, such as lunch meat, smoked meats, processed cheeses. Caution against adding table salt to foods.

■ Encourage patient to keep follow-up appointments to monitor the effectiveness of therapy.

ESTROGENS

esterified estrogens
estradiol
estradiol cypionate
estradiol valerate
estrogenic substances,
   conjugated
estrone
estropipate

Indications

- Contraception
- Female castration
- Female hypogonadism
- Inhibition of hormone-sensitive cancer growth
- Menopausal vasomotor symptoms
- Ovulation control
- Primary ovulation failure
- Stimulation of vaginal tissue development, cornification, and secretory activity

Actions

Estrogens promote the development and maintenance of the female reproductive system and secondary sexual characteristics. They inhibit the release of pituitary gonadotropins and have various metabolic effects, including retention of fluid and electrolytes, retention and deposition in bone of calcium and phosphorus, and mild anabolic activity. Of the six naturally oc-curring estrogens in humans, estradiol, estrone, and estriol are present in significant quantities.

Estrogens and estrogenic substances given as drugs have effects related to endogenous estrogen's mechanism of action. They can mimic the action of endogenous estrogen when used as replacement therapy and can inhibit ovulation or the growth of certain hormone-sensitive cancers. Conjugated estrogens and estrogenic substances are normally obtained from the urine of pregnant mares. Other estrogens are manufactured synthetically.

Adverse reactions

Acute adverse reactions include abdominal cramps, swollen feet or ankles, bloating caused by fluid and electrolyte retention, breast swelling and tenderness, weight gain, nausea, loss of appetite, headache, photosensitivity, loss of libido, and changes in menstrual bleeding patterns, such as spotting and prolongation or absence of bleeding.

Long-term effects include elevated blood pressure (sometimes into the hypertensive range), cholestatic jaundice, benign hepatomas, endometrial carcinoma (rare), and thromboembolic disease (risk increases markedly with cigarette smoking, especially in women over age 35).

Contraindications and cautions

■ Contraindicated in women with thrombophlebitis or thromboembolic disorders, unexplained abnormal genital bleeding, or estrogen-dependent neoplasia.

■ Use cautiously in patients with hypertension; metabolic bone disease; migraines; seizures; asthma; cardiac, renal, or hepatic impairment; blood dyscrasia; diabetes; family history of breast cancer; or fibrocystic disease.

LIFESPAN

■ *Pregnant women.* Patient should stop taking drug immediately if she becomes pregnant because estrogens can harm fetus.

■ *Breast-feeding women.* Contraindicated.

■ *Adolescents with incomplete bone growth.* Use cautiously because of effects on epiphyseal closure.

■ *Postmenopausal women.* Increased risk of endometrial cancer with long-term estrogen use and increased risk of breast cancer, heart attack, cerebrovascular accident, and blood clots with long-term use of estrogen and progestin.

Nursing considerations

■ Assess patient regularly to detect improvement or worsening of symptoms; observe patient for adverse reactions.

■ If patient has diabetes mellitus, watch closely for loss of diabetes control.

■ Monitor prothrombin time of patient receiving warfarin-type anticoagulant. Adjust anticoagulant dosage.

■ Notify pathologist of patient's estrogen therapy when sending specimens for evaluation.

■ Give drug once daily for 3 weeks, followed by 1 week without drugs; repeat as needed.

Patient teaching

■ Urge patient to read the package insert describing adverse reactions, and also provide a verbal explanation. Tell patient to keep the package insert for later reference.

■ Advise patient to take drug with meals or at bedtime to relieve nausea. Reassure her that nausea usually disappears with continued therapy.

■ Teach patient how to apply estrogen ointments or transdermal estrogen. Review symptoms that accompany a systemic reaction to ointments.

■ Teach patient how to insert intravaginal estrogen suppository. Advise her to use sanitary pads instead of tampons when using suppository.

■ Teach patient how to perform routine monthly breast self-examination.

■ If patient is receiving cyclic therapy for postmenopausal symptoms, explain that withdrawal bleeding may occur during the week off, but that fertility hasn't been restored and ovulation won't occur.

■ Explain that medical supervision is essential during prolonged therapy.

■ Instruct patient to notify prescriber immediately if she experiences abdominal pain; pain, numbness, or stiffness in legs or buttocks; pressure or pain in chest; shortness of breath; severe headaches; visual disturbances, such as blind spots, flashing lights, or blurriness; vaginal bleeding or discharge; breast lumps; swelling of hands or feet; yellow skin and sclera; dark urine; or light-colored stools.

■ Urge diabetic patient to report symptoms of hyperglycemia or glycosuria.

■ Tell man on long-term therapy about possible temporary gynecomastia and impotence, which will disappear when therapy ends.

FLUOROQUINOLONES

ciprofloxacin
gatifloxacin
levofloxacin
lomefloxacin
moxifloxacin
norfloxacin
ofloxacin
sparfloxacin

Indications

■ Acute sinusitis
■ Bacterial bronchitis
■ Bone and joint infections
■ Chancroid
■ Endocervical and urethral chlamydia and gonorrhea
■ Febrile neutropenia (empiric therapy)
■ Gastroenteritis
■ Intra-abdominal infections
■ Meningococcal carrier state
■ Pelvic inflammatory disease
■ Pneumonia
■ Prostatitis
■ Septicemia
■ Skin and soft tissue infections
■ Typhoid fever

■ Urinary tract infections (prevention and treatment)

Actions

Fluoroquinolones are broad-spectrum, systemic antibacterial drugs active against a wide range of aerobic gram-positive and gram-negative organisms. (See *Comparing fluoroquinolones*, pages 70 and 71.)

Gram-positive aerobic bacteria include *Staphylococcus aureus, Staphylococcus epidermis, Staphylococcus hemolyticus, Staphylococcus saprophyticus;* penicillinase- and non–penicillinase-producing staphylococci and some methicillin-resistant strains; *Streptococcus pneumoniae;* group A (beta) hemolytic streptococci *(Streptococcus pyogenes);* group B streptococci *(Streptococcus agalactiae);* viridans streptococci; groups C, F, and G streptococci and nonenterococcal group D streptococci; and *Enterococcus faecalis.*

These drugs also are active against gram-positive aerobic bacilli, including *Corynebacterium* species, *Listeria monocytogenes,* and *Nocardia asteroides.*

Fluoroquinolones are effective against such gram-negative aerobic bacteria as *Neisseria meningitidis* and most strains of penicillinase- and non–penicillinase-producing *Haemophilus ducreyi, Haemophilus influenzae, Haemophilus parainfluenzae, Moraxella catarrhalis, Neisseria gonorrhoeae,* and most clinically important *Enterobacteriaceae, Pseudomonas aeruginosa, Vibrio cholerae,* and *Vibrio parahaemolyticus.*

Certain fluoroquinolones are active against *Chlamydia trachomatis, Legionella pneumophila, Mycobacterium avium-intracellulare, Mycoplasma hominis,* and *Mycoplasma pneumoniae.*

Fluoroquinolones produce a bactericidal effect by inhibiting intracellular DNA topoisomerase II (DNA gyrase) or topoisomerase IV—enzymes essential in catalyzing the duplication, transcription, and repair of bacterial DNA.

Adverse reactions

Fluoroquinolones may cause central nervous system (CNS) reactions (dizziness, drowsiness, headache, insomnia, nervousness), gastrointestinal reactions, and photosensitivity. These reactions require no medical attention unless they persist or become intolerable.

Rarely, fluoroquinolones may cause CNS stimulation (acute psychosis, agitation, hallucinations, tremors), hepatotoxicity, hypersensitivity reactions, interstitial nephritis, phlebitis, pseudomembranous colitis, and tendinitis or tendon rupture. These reactions do warrant medical attention.

Contraindications and cautions

■ Contraindicated in patients hypersensitive to fluoroquinolones or other quinolones, those who have experienced tendinitis or tendon rupture with quinolone use, those taking QTc-prolonging antiarrhythmics (such as class Ia or class III drugs), and those whose lifestyle or profession prevents them from following the required phototoxicity safety precautions.

■ Avoid use in patients with a prolonged QT interval.

■ Use cautiously in patients with renal impairment, a seizure disorder, or cerebral ischemia.

LIFESPAN

■ *Pregnant women*. Adequate studies haven't been completed, but these drugs cross the placental barrier and may cause arthropathies.

■ *Breast-feeding women*. Because it isn't known whether fluoroquinolones appear in breast milk, avoid giving them to breast-feeding mothers because of the risk of arthropathies in their infants.

■ *Children*. Not recommended because of the risk of joint problems.

■ *Geriatric patients*. Daily dose may need reduction because of these patients' slower renal function.

Nursing considerations

■ Monitor renal function in patients with renal impairment.

■ Achilles and other tendon ruptures have been reported. Notify prescriber immediately if patient reports pain, inflammation, or rupture of a tendon.

■ Assess patient for adverse reactions and drug interactions.

Patient teaching

■ Instruct patient to take drug as prescribed and to finish the full course of therapy.

■ Tell patient to take drug with an 8-oz (240-ml) glass of water.

■ Caution patient that norfloxacin should be taken on an empty stomach.

■ If patient misses a dose, advise taking the next dose as soon as possible. Advise against doubling the dose.

■ Urge patient to avoid taking an antacid or sucralfate with an oral fluoroquinolone. If coadministration can't be avoided, tell patient to take the fluoroquinolone at least 2 hours be-

COMPARING FLUOROQUINOLONES

DRUG	ORAL BIOAVAILABILITY (%)	PLASMA PROTEIN– BINDING (%)	HALF–LIFE (HR)
ciprofloxacin	70–80 (with food)	20–40	Normal renal function: 4–6 Severe renal failure: 6–8
gatifloxacin	96 (without regard to food)	20	Normal renal function: 714 Severe renal failure: 36
levofloxacin	100 (without regard to food)	24–38	Normal renal function: 6 Severe renal failure: 76
lomefloxacin	95–98 (without regard to food)	10	Normal renal function: 8 Severe renal failure: 21–45
moxifloxacin	90 (without regard to food)	50	Normal renal function: 10–14
norfloxacin	30–40 (without regard to food)	10–15	Normal renal function: 3–4 Severe renal failure: 9–10
ofloxacin	98 (without regard to food)	32	Normal renal function: 4½–7 Severe renal failure: 28–37
sparfloxacin	92 (without regard to food)	45	Normal renal function: 16–30 Severe renal failure: 38⅕

Peak Concentration (hr)	Elimination	Dosage Adjustment	Dialyzability
1–2	40–70% of drug is cleared unchanged by the kidneys in 24 hr	Renal impairment	< 10% removed by hemodialysis
1–2	70% unchanged by the kidneys	Renal impairment	Not defined
1	Almost entirely eliminated unchanged in the urine	Renal impairment	Not defined
1½	60–80% of drug is cleared unchanged by the kidneys in 48 hr	Renal impairment	< 3% removed by hemodialysis
1–3	45% unchanged (20% in urine, 25% in feces)	None	Not defined
1–2	26% of drug is cleared unchanged by the kidneys in 24 hr	Renal impairment	< 10% removed by hemodialysis
1–2	70–90% of drug is cleared unchanged by the kidneys in 36 hr	Renal impairment	< 10–30% removed by hemodialysis
3–6	10% is excreted unchanged in the urine	Renal impairment	Not defined

fore or 6 hours after the antacid.

■ Caution patient not to take additional drugs without medical approval.

HEMATINICS, ORAL

ferrous fumarate
ferrous gluconate
ferrous sulfate

Indications
■ Prevention and treatment of iron-deficiency anemia

Actions
Iron is an essential component of hemoglobin. It's needed in adequate amounts for erythropoiesis and for efficient oxygen transport in the blood. After absorption into the blood, iron is immediately bound to transferrin, a plasma protein that transports iron to bone marrow, where it's used during hemoglobin synthesis. Some iron is also used during synthesis of myoglobin and other nonhemoglobin heme units.

Adverse reactions
Because iron is corrosive, gastrointestinal intolerance occurs in 5% to 20% of patients; symptoms include nausea, vomiting, anorexia, constipation, and dark stools. Liquid forms may stain teeth.

Contraindications and cautions
■ Contraindicated in patients with hemochromatosis, hemolytic anemia, or hemosiderosis.

■ Use cautiously in patients with peptic ulcer disease, regional enteritis, ulcerative colitis, or sensitivity to sulfites or tartrazine.

LIFESPAN
■ *Breast-feeding women.* Iron supplements are commonly recommended; no adverse effects are known.

■ *Children.* Caution parents about possible lethal effects of iron overdose.

■ *Geriatric patients.* Iron-induced constipation is common; stress a proper diet high in fiber to minimize this effect. Elderly patients also may need higher doses because reduced gastric secretions and achlorhydria may lower their capacity for iron absorption.

Nursing considerations
■ Assess patient for adverse reactions, especially those related to bowel function.

■ Monitor patient's hemoglobin and reticulocyte count during therapy.

■ Dilute liquid forms in juice (preferably orange juice, which promotes iron absorption) or water, but not in milk or antacids. To avoid staining teeth, give liquid preparations through a straw. Don't give antacids within 1 hour before or 2 hours after an iron product, if possible, to prevent interference with absorption.

■ Don't crush tablets or capsules; if patient has trouble swallowing, use a liquid form.

Patient teaching

■ Explain rationale for therapy, and urge patient to follow the prescribed regimen.

■ Tell patient to resume the regular dosage schedule after missing a dose; warn against doubling the dose.

■ Advise patient to dilute liquid form in juice (preferably orange juice) or water. Suggest using a straw to avoid staining teeth.

■ Review possible adverse effects. Tell patient that oral iron may turn stools black; explain that this is harmless. Teach dietary measures to help prevent constipation.

■ Explain the toxicity of iron, and stress the need to keep iron away from children to prevent poisoning. As few as three or four tablets can cause serious iron poisoning.

■ Urge patient to report diarrhea or constipation because prescriber may want to adjust dosage, modify diet, or order further tests.

■ Explain that iron therapy may be required for 4 to 6 months after anemia resolves. Encourage compliance.

HISTAMINE₂– RECEPTOR ANTAGONISTS

cimetidine
famotidine
nizatidine
ranitidine hydrochloride

Indications

■ Acute duodenal or gastric ulcer
■ Gastroesophageal reflux
■ Zollinger-Ellison syndrome

Actions

All H_2-receptor antagonists inhibit the action of H_2-receptors in gastric parietal cells, reducing gastric acid output and concentration, regardless of stimulants—such as histamine, food, insulin, and caffeine—or basal conditions. (See *Adult*

ADULT DOSAGES OF HISTAMINE$_2$-RECEPTOR ANTAGONISTS

INDICATION	CIMETIDINE	FAMOTIDINE
Duodenal ulcer	P.O.: 800 mg h.s. or 300 mg q.i.d. with meals and h.s. or 400 mg b.i.d. I.M., I.V.: 300 mg q 6–8 hr (maximum, 2,400 mg/day)	P.O.: 40 mg h.s. or 20 mg b.i.d.
Duodenal ulcer maintenance	P.O.: 400 mg h.s. I.M., I.V.: 300 mg q 6–8 hr (maximum, 2,400 mg/day)	P.O.: 20 mg h.s.
Gastric ulcer	P.O.: 800 mg h.s. or 300 mg q.i.d. with meals and h.s.	P.O.: 40 mg h.s.
Gastric ulcer maintenance	NA	NA
Gastroesophageal reflux disease	P.O.: 400 mg q.i.d. or 800 mg b.i.d.	P.O.: 20 mg b.i.d.
Erosive esophagitis	P.O.: 400 mg q.i.d. or 800 mg b.i.d.	P.O.: 20–40 mg b.i.d.
Erosive esophagitis healing maintenance	NA	NA
Pathological hypersecretory conditions	P.O.: 300 mg q.i.d. with meals and h.s. I.V.: 300 mg q 6–8 hr (maximum, 2,400 mg/day)	P.O.: 20 mg q 6 hr up to 160 mg q 6 hr I.V.: 20 mg q 12 hr
Prevention of upper GI bleeding	I.V.: 50 mg/hr continuous infusion	NA
Heartburn, acid indigestion, sour stomach (over-the-counter use)	P.O.: 200 mg, p.r.n., up to 200 mg b.i.d.	P.O.: 10 mg, p.r.n., up to 10 mg b.i.d.

NA: No approved dosage.

NIZATIDINE	RANITIDINE
P.O.: 300 mg h.s. or 150 mg b.i.d.	P.O.: 150 mg b.i.d. or 300 mg once daily after evening meal or h.s. I.M., I.V.: 50 mg q 6–8 hr
P.O.: 150 mg h.s.	P.O.: 150 mg h.s.
P.O.: 300 mg h.s. or 150 mg b.i.d.	P.O.: 150 mg b.i.d. I.M., I.V.: 50 mg q 6–8 hr
NA	P.O.: 150 mg h.s.
P.O.: 150 mg b.i.d.	P.O.: 150 mg b.i.d.
P.O.: 150 mg b.i.d.	P.O.: 150 mg q.i.d.
NA	P.O.: 150 mg b.i.d.
NA	P.O.: 150 mg b.i.d. I.M., I.V.: 50 mg q 6–8 hr (maximum, 6 g/day)
NA	NA
P.O.: 75 mg, p.r.n., up to 75 mg b.i.d.	P.O.: 75 mg p.r.n., up to 75 mg b.i.d.

dosages of histamine$_2$-receptor antagonists.)

Adverse reactions

H$_2$-receptor antagonists rarely cause adverse reactions. Mild and transient diarrhea, thrombocytopenia, dizziness, fatigue, headache, cardiac arrhythmias, and gynecomastia are possible.

Contraindications and cautions

■ Contraindicated in patients hypersensitive to drug.
■ Use cautiously in patients with impaired renal or hepatic function.

LIFESPAN

■ *Pregnant women.* Use cautiously.
■ *Breast-feeding women.* Contraindicated because drug may appear in breast milk.
■ *Children.* Safety and efficacy haven't been established.
■ *Geriatric patients.* Increased risk of adverse reactions, particularly those affecting the central nervous system; use cautiously.

Nursing considerations

■ Monitor patient for adverse reactions, especially hypotension and arrhythmias.

improving insulin sensitivity. These drugs are potent and highly selective agonists for receptors in insulin-sensitive tissues, such as adipose, skeletal muscle, and liver.

Adverse reactions

Sulfonylureas cause dose-related reactions that usually respond to decreased dosage: headache, nausea, vomiting, anorexia, heartburn, weakness, and paresthesia. Hypoglycemia may follow excessive dosage, increased exercise, decreased food intake, or alcohol use.

The most serious adverse reaction linked to metformin is lactic acidosis. It's rare and most likely to occur in patients with renal dysfunction. Other reactions to metformin include gastrointestinal upset, megaloblastic anemia, rash, dermatitis, and unpleasant or metallic taste.

Contraindications and cautions

■ Contraindicated in patients hypersensitive to drug and in patients with diabetic ketoacidosis with or without coma.

■ *Alpha-glucosidase inhibitors.* Use cautiously in patients with mild to moderate renal insufficiency.

■ *Metformin.* Contraindicated in patients with renal disease or metabolic acidosis. Avoid using it in patients with hepatic disease. Use it cautiously in patients with adrenal or pituitary insufficiency and in debilitated and malnourished patients.

■ *Sulfonylureas.* Use cautiously in patients with renal or hepatic disease.

■ *Thiazolidinediones.* Use cautiously in patients with edema or heart failure.

LIFESPAN

■ *Pregnant women.* Contraindicated.

■ *Breast-feeding women.* Contraindicated; oral hypoglycemics appear in small amounts in breast milk and may cause hypoglycemia in the infant.

■ *Children.* Oral hypoglycemics aren't effective in type 1 diabetes mellitus.

■ *Geriatric patients.* These patients may be more sensitive to these drugs, usually need lower dosages, and are more likely to develop neurologic symptoms of hypoglycemia; monitor patient closely. Avoid chlorpropamide because of its long duration of action.

Nursing considerations

■ Assess patient's glucose level regularly. Assess more often during periods of increased stress, such as infection, fever, surgery, or trauma.

■ Monitor patient for adverse reactions.

■ Assess patient's compliance with drug therapy and other aspects of diabetic treatment.

■ Keep in mind that a patient transferring from one oral hypoglycemic to another (except chlorpropamide) usually needs no transition period.

■ Anticipate patient's need for insulin during periods of increased stress.

■ *Alpha-glucosidase inhibitors.* Give with the first bite of each main meal three times daily.

■ *Metformin.* Give with morning and evening meals.

■ *Sulfonylureas.* Give 30 minutes before morning meal for once-daily dosing or 30 minutes before morning and evening meals for twice-daily dosing.

■ *Thiazolidinediones.* Have liver enzyme levels measured at the start of therapy, every 2 months for the first year of therapy, and periodically thereafter.

Patient teaching

■ Emphasize importance of following the prescribed regi-men. Urge patient to adhere to diet, weight reduction, exercise, and personal hygiene recommendations.

■ Explain that therapy relieves symptoms but doesn't cure the disease.

■ Teach patient how to recognize and treat hypoglycemia.

LAXATIVES

BULK-FORMING
calcium polycarbophil
methylcellulose
psyllium

EMOLLIENT
docusate calcium
docusate potassium
docusate sodium

HYPEROSMOLAR
glycerin
lactulose
magnesium citrate
magnesium hydroxide
magnesium sulfate
sodium phosphates

STIMULANT
bisacodyl
senna

Indications

■ Constipation
■ Diverticulosis

- Irritable bowel syndrome

Actions

Laxatives promote movement of intestinal contents through the colon and rectum in several ways: bulk-forming, emollient, hyperosmolar, and stimulant.

Adverse reactions

All laxatives may cause flatulence, diarrhea, abdominal discomfort, weakness, and dependence.

Bulk-forming laxatives may cause intestinal obstruction, impaction, or (rarely) esophageal obstruction.

Emollient laxatives may cause a bitter taste or throat irritation.

Hyperosmolar laxatives may cause fluid and electrolyte imbalances.

Stimulant laxatives may cause urine discoloration, malabsorption, and weight loss.

Contraindications and cautions

- Contraindicated in patients with gastrointestinal (GI) obstruction or perforation, toxic colitis, megacolon, nausea and vomiting, or acute surgical abdomen.
- Use cautiously in patients with rectal or anal conditions,

such as rectal bleeding or large hemorrhoids.

LIFESPAN

- *Breast-feeding women.* Recommendations vary for individual drugs.
- *Infants and children.* Use cautiously because of the increased risk of fluid and electrolyte disturbances.
- *Geriatric patients.* Dependence is more likely because of age-related changes in GI function; monitor these patients closely.

Nursing considerations

- Obtain baseline assessment of patient's bowel patterns and GI history before giving drug.
- Assess patient for adverse reactions.
- Monitor bowel pattern throughout therapy. Assess bowel sounds and color and consistency of stools.
- Check patient's fluid and electrolyte status during administration.
- Don't crush enteric-coated tablets.
- Time administration so that bowel evacuation doesn't interfere with sleep.
- Make sure patient has easy access to bedpan or bathroom.
- Institute measures to prevent constipation.

Patient teaching

■ Advise patient that therapy should be short-term. Point out that overuse or prolonged use can cause nutritional imbalances.

■ Teach patient about including foods high in fiber into diet.

■ *Bulk-forming laxatives.* Explain that results may take several days. Encourage patient to remain active and to drink plenty of fluids.

■ *Stimulant laxatives.* Mention that urine may be discolored, a harmless change.

■ *Stool softeners.* Explain that results may take several days.

NONSTEROIDAL ANTI-INFLAMMATORY DRUGS

celecoxib
diclofenac potassium
diclofenac sodium
diflunisal
etodolac
ibuprofen
indomethacin
indomethacin sodium
  trihydrate
ketoprofen
ketorolac tromethamine
mefenamic acid
meloxicam
nabumetone
naproxen
naproxen sodium
oxaprozin
piroxicam
rofecoxib
sulindac
valdecoxib

Indications

■ Mild to moderate pain, inflammation, stiffness, swelling, or tenderness caused by headache, arthralgia, myalgia, neuralgia, dysmenorrhea, rheumatoid arthritis, juvenile arthritis, osteoarthritis, or dental or surgical procedures

Actions

The analgesic effect of nonsteroidal anti-inflammatory drugs (NSAIDs) may result from interference with the prostaglandins involved in pain. Prostaglandins appear to sensitize pain receptors to mechanical stimulation or to other chemical mediators. NSAIDs inhibit synthesis of prostaglandins peripherally and possibly centrally.

Like salicylates, NSAIDs exert an anti-inflammatory effect that may result in part from inhibition of prostaglandin synthesis and release during inflammation. The exact mechanism isn't clear.

Adverse reactions

Adverse reactions chiefly involve the gastrointestinal (GI) tract, particularly erosion of the gastric mucosa. The most common symptoms are dyspepsia, heartburn, epigastric distress, nausea, and abdominal pain. Central nervous system reactions also may occur. Flank pain with other evidence of nephrotoxicity occurs occasionally. Fluid retention may aggravate hypertension or heart failure.

Contraindications and cautions

■ Contraindicated in patients with GI lesions or GI bleeding and in patients hypersensitive to drug.
■ Use cautiously in patients with cardiac decompensation, hypertension, fluid retention, or coagulation defects.

LIFESPAN

■ *Pregnant women.* Use cautiously in the first and second trimesters; don't use in the third trimester.
■ *Breast-feeding women.* NSAIDs aren't recommended.
■ *Children under age 14.* Safety of long-term therapy isn't known.
■ *Adults over age 60.* These patients may be more susceptible to toxic effects because of decreased renal function.

Nursing considerations

■ Assess patient's level of pain and inflammation before therapy begins, and evaluate drug effectiveness after administration.
■ Monitor patient for signs and symptoms of bleeding. Assess bleeding time if patient needs surgery.
■ Assess ophthalmic and auditory function before and periodically during therapy to detect toxicity.
■ Check complete blood count (CBC), platelet count, prothrombin time, and hepatic and renal function studies periodically to detect abnormalities.
■ Watch for bronchospasm in patients with aspirin hypersensitivity, rhinitis or nasal polyps, and asthma.
■ Administer oral NSAIDs with 8 oz (240 ml) of water to ensure adequate passage into the stomach. Have patient sit up for 15 to 30 minutes after taking drug to prevent lodging in esophagus.
■ Crush tablets or mix with food or fluid to aid swallowing. Give with antacids to minimize GI upset.

Patient teaching

■ Encourage patient to take drug as directed to achieve desired effect. Explain that benefits of drug therapy may take 2 to 4 weeks.

■ Review methods to prevent or minimize GI upset.

■ Work with patient on long-term therapy to arrange for monitoring of laboratory values, especially blood urea nitrogen and creatinine levels, liver function test results, and CBC.

■ Instruct patient to notify prescriber about severe or persistent adverse reactions.

OPIOIDS

alfentanil hydrochloride
codeine phosphate
codeine sulfate
difenoxin
diphenoxylate
fentanyl citrate
hydromorphone
    hydrochloride
meperidine hydrochloride
methadone hydrochloride
morphine sulfate
oxycodone hydrochloride
oxymorphone hydrochloride
propoxyphene hydrochloride
propoxyphene napsylate
sufentanil citrate

Indications

■ Anesthesia support
■ Diarrhea
■ Dry, nonproductive cough
■ Management of opiate dependence
■ Moderate to severe pain
■ Sedation

Actions

Opioids act as agonists at specific opiate-receptor binding sites in the central nervous system (CNS) and other tissues, altering the patient's perception of and emotional response to pain. (See *Comparing opioids*, pages 84 and 85.)

Adverse reactions

Respiratory and circulatory depression (including orthostatic hypotension) are the major hazards of opioids. Other adverse CNS effects include dizziness, visual disturbances, mental clouding, depression, sedation, coma, euphoria, dysphoria, weakness, faintness, agitation, restlessness, nervousness, and seizures.

Adverse gastrointestinal (GI) effects include nausea, vomiting, constipation, and biliary colic.

Urine retention or hypersensitivity also may occur.

COMPARING OPIOIDS

DRUG	ROUTE	ONSET (MIN)
alfentanil	I.V.	Immediate
codeine	I.M., P.O., S.C.	15–30
fentanyl	I.M., I.V. Transdermal P.O. (Actiq)	7–8 Gradual Rapid
hydrocodone	P.O.	30
hydromorphone	I.M., I.V., S.C. P.O., rectal	15 30
meperidine	I.M. P.O. S.C.	10–15 15–30 10–15
methadone	I.M., P.O., S.C.	30–60
morphine	I.M. P.O., P.R. S.C.	≤ 20 ≤ 20 ≤ 20
oxycodone	P.O.	15–30
oxymorphone	I.M., S.C. I.V. P.R.	10–15 5–10 15–30
propoxyphene	P.O.	20–60
remifentanil	I.V.	Immediate
sufentanil	I.V.	1–3

*Because of cumulative effects, duration of action increases with repeated doses.

Tolerance to the drug and psychological or physical dependence may follow prolonged therapy.

Contraindications and cautions

■ Contraindicated in patients hypersensitive to drug and in those who have recently taken a

Peak	Duration (hr)
Not available	Not available
30–60 min	4–6
Not available	1–2
12–24 hr	Unknown
20–40 min	Unknown
60 min	4–6
30 min	4–5
60 min	4–5
30–50 min	2–4
60 min	2–4
40–60 min	2–4
30–60 min	4–6*
30–60 min	3–7
≤ 60 min	3–7
50–90 min	3–7
30–60 min	4–6
30–60 min	3–6
30–60 min	3–6
30–60 min	3–6
2–2½ hr	4–6
Immediate	Not available
Not available	Not available

monoamine oxidase inhibitor. Also contraindicated in those with acute or severe bronchial asthma or respiratory depression.

■ Use cautiously in patients with head injury, increased intracranial or intraocular pressure, hepatic or renal dysfunction, mental illness, emotional disturbance, or drug-seeking behaviors.

LIFESPAN

■ *Pregnant women.* Use cautiously.

■ *Breast-feeding women.* Use cautiously; codeine, meperidine, methadone, morphine, and propoxyphene appear in breast milk. Methadone could cause physical dependence in infant.

■ *Children.* Safety and efficacy aren't known.

■ *Geriatric patients.* These patients may be more sensitive to opioids; lower doses are usually indicated.

Nursing considerations

■ Obtain baseline assessment of patient's pain, and reassess frequently to determine drug effectiveness.

■ Evaluate patient's respiratory status before each dose; watch for respiratory rate below patient's baseline level and for restlessness, which may be compensatory signs of hypoxia. Respiratory depression may last longer than the analgesic effect.

■ Monitor patient for other adverse reactions.

COMPARING PENICILLINS

Drug	Route	Adult dosage	Penicillinase-resistant
amoxicillin	P.O.	250–500 mg q 8 hr 3 g with 1 g probenecid for gonorrhea as single dose	No
amoxicillin and potassium clavulanate	P.O.	250 mg q 8 hr 500 mg q 12 hr	Yes
ampicillin	I.M., I.V.	150–200 mg/kg daily in divided doses given q 3–4 hr (for septicemia, bacterial meningitis)	No
	I.M., I.V., P.O.	250–500 mg q 6 hr	
	P.O.	3.5 g with 1 g probenecid (for gonorrhea) as single dose	
ampicillin sodium and sulbactam sodium	I.M., I.V.	1.5–3 g q 6–8 hr	Yes
dicloxacillin	P.O.	125–500 mg q 6 hr	Yes
nafcillin	I.M., I.V.	250 mg–2 g q 4–6 hr	Yes
	P.O.	500 mg–1 g q 6 hr	
oxacillin	I.M., I.V.	250 mg–2 g q 4–6 hr	Yes
	P.O.	500 mg–1 g q 6 hr	
penicillin G benzathine	I.M.	1.2–2.4 million units as single dose	No
penicillin G potassium	I.M., I.V.	200,000–4 million units q 4 hr	No
penicillin G procaine	I.M.	600,000–1.2 million units q 1–3 days 600,000 units/day for 8 days for primary, secondary, and early latent syphilis and 10–15 days for late latent syphilis	No

COMPARING PENICILLINS (continued)

DRUG	ROUTE	ADULT DOSAGE	PENICILLINASE-RESISTANT
penicillin G sodium	I.M., I.V.	200,000–4 million units q 4 hr	No
penicillin V potassium	P.O.	250–500 mg q 6–8 hr	No
piperacillin sodium and tazobactam sodium	I.V.	3.375 g q 6 hr	Yes
ticarcillin	I.M., I.V.	150–300 mg/kg daily as divided doses given q 3–6 hr	No
ticarcillin and clavulanate potassium	I.V.	3.1 g q 4–6 hr	Yes

tidis and non–penicillinase-producing *Neisseria gonorrhoeae.*

Susceptible aerobic gram-positive bacilli include *Corynebacterium*, *Listeria*, and *Bacillus anthracis.* Susceptible anaerobes include *Peptococcus, Peptostreptococcus, Actinomyces, Clostridium, Fusobacterium, Veillonella,* and non–beta-lactamase–producing strains of *Streptococcus pneumoniae.* Susceptible spirochetes include *Treponema pallidum, Treponema pertenue, Leptospira, Borrelia recurrentis,* and, possibly, *Borrelia burgdorferi.*

AMINOPENICILLINS

Aminopenicillins have uses against more organisms, including many gram-negative organisms. Like natural penicillins, aminopenicillins are vulnerable to inactivation by penicillinase. Susceptible organisms include *Escherichia coli, Proteus mirabilis, Shigella, Salmonella, S. pneumoniae, N. gonorrhoeae, Haemophilus influenzae, S. aureus, Staphylococcus epidermidis* (non–penicillinase-producing *Staphylococcus*), and *Listeria monocytogenes.*

PENICILLINASE-RESISTANT PENICILLINS

Penicillinase-resistant penicillins are semisynthetic penicillins designed to remain stable against hydrolysis by most staphylococcal penicillinases and thus are the drugs of choice for susceptible penicillinase-producing staphylococci. They also act against most organisms susceptible to natural penicillins.

EXTENDED-SPECTRUM PENICILLINS

Extended-spectrum penicillins offer a wider range of bactericidal action than the other classes and usually are given with aminoglycosides. Susceptible strains include *Enterobacter, Klebsiella, Citrobacter, Serratia, Bacteroides fragilis, Pseudomonas aeruginosa, Proteus vulgaris, Providencia rettgeri,* and *Morganella morganii.* These drugs are also vulnerable to beta-lactamase and penicillinases.

Adverse reactions

With all penicillins, hypersensitivity reactions range from mild rash, fever, and eosinophilia to fatal anaphylaxis. Hematologic reactions include hemolytic anemia, transient neutropenia, leukopenia, and thrombocytopenia.

Certain adverse reactions are more common with specific classes. For example, bleeding episodes are usually seen with high doses of extended-spectrum penicillins, whereas GI adverse effects are most common with ampicillin.

In patients with renal disease, high doses, especially of penicillin G, irritate the central nervous system (CNS) and cause confusion, twitching, lethargy, dysphagia, seizures, and coma.

Hepatotoxicity may occur with penicillinase-resistant penicillins; hyperkalemia and hypernatremia have been reported with extended-spectrum penicillins.

Local irritation from parenteral therapy may be severe enough to warrant administration by subclavian or centrally placed catheter or discontinuation of therapy.

Contraindications and cautions

■ Contraindicated in patients hypersensitive to drug.

■ Use cautiously in patients with history of asthma or drug allergy, mononucleosis, renal impairment, cardiovascular diseases, hemorrhagic condition, or electrolyte imbalance.

LIFESPAN

■ *Pregnant women.* Use cautiously.

■ *Breast-feeding patients.* Recommendations vary depending on the drug.

■ *Children.* Dosage recommendations have been established for most penicillins.

■ *Geriatric patients.* Use cautiously and at lower dosage because these patients are susceptible to superinfection and renal impairment, which decreases excretion of penicillins.

Nursing considerations

■ Assess patient's history of allergies. Try to find out whether previous reactions were true hypersensitivity reactions or adverse reactions (such as GI distress) that patient interpreted as allergy.

■ Keep in mind that a patient who has never had a penicillin hypersensitivity reaction may still have future allergic reactions; monitor patient continuously for possible allergic reactions or other adverse effects.

■ Obtain culture and sensitivity tests before giving first dose; repeat tests periodically to assess drug's effectiveness.

■ Monitor vital signs, electrolytes, and renal function studies.

■ Assess patient's consciousness and neurologic status when giving high doses; CNS toxicity can occur.

■ Coagulation changes, even frank bleeding, can follow high doses, especially of extended-spectrum penicillins. Monitor prothrombin time, international normalized ratio, and platelet counts. Assess patient for signs of occult or frank bleeding.

■ Monitor patients receiving long-term therapy for possible superinfection, especially elderly patients, debilitated patients, and patients receiving immunosuppressants or radiation.

■ Give penicillin at least 1 hour before bacteriostatic antibiotics, such as tetracyclines, erythromycins, and chloramphenicol; these drugs inhibit bacterial cell growth and decrease rate of penicillin uptake by bacterial cell walls.

■ Follow manufacturer's directions for reconstituting, diluting, and storing drugs; check expiration dates.

■ Give oral penicillin at least 1 hour before or 2 hours after meals to enhance GI absorption.

■ Refrigerate oral suspensions, which will be stable for 14 days; shake well before giving to ensure correct dosage.

■ Give I.M. dose deep into gluteal muscle mass or midlateral thigh, rotate injection sites to minimize tissue injury, and apply ice to injection site to relieve pain. Don't inject more than 2 g of drug per injection site.

■ With I.V. infusions, don't add or mix another drug, especially an aminoglycoside, which will become inactive if mixed with a penicillin. If other drugs must be given I.V., temporarily stop infusion of primary drug.

■ Infuse I.V. drug continuously or intermittently over 30 minutes. Rotate infusion site every 48 hours. Intermittent I.V. infusion may be diluted in 50 to 100 ml sterile water, normal saline solution, D_5W, D_5W and half-normal saline solution, or lactated Ringer's solution.

Patient teaching

■ Make sure patient understands how and when to take drug. Urge him to complete the prescribed regimen, comply with instructions for around-the-clock scheduling, and keep follow-up appointments.

■ Teach patient signs and symptoms of hypersensitivity and other adverse reactions. Urge him to report unusual reactions.

■ Tell patient to check drug's expiration date and to discard unused drug. Warn him not to share drug with family or friends.

PHENOTHIAZINES

chlorpromazine hydrochloride
fluphenazine
mesoridazine besylate
perphenazine
prochlorperazine
promazine hydrochloride
promethazine
thioridazine hydrochloride
thiothixene
trifluoperazine hydrochloride

Indications

■ Acute intermittent porphyria
■ Agitated psychotic states
■ Behavioral problems caused by chronic organic mental syndrome
■ Bipolar disorder
■ Excessive motor and autonomic activity
■ Hallucinations
■ Intractable hiccups
■ Itching
■ Moderate anxiety
■ Nausea and vomiting
■ Symptomatic rhinitis
■ Tetanus

Actions

Phenothiazines are believed to function as dopamine antagonists by blocking postsynaptic dopamine receptors in various parts of the central nervous system (CNS). Their antiemetic effects result from blockage of the chemoreceptor trigger zone. They also produce varying degrees of anticholinergic effects and alpha-adrenergic–receptor blocking.

Adverse reactions

Phenothiazines may produce extrapyramidal symptoms, such as dystonic movements, torticollis, oculogyric crises, parkinsonian symptoms, ranging from akathisia during early treatment to tardive dyskinesia after long-term use. A neuroleptic malignant syndrome resembling severe parkinsonism may occur, most often in young men taking fluphenazine.

The progression of elevated liver enzyme levels to obstructive jaundice usually indicates an allergic reaction.

Other adverse reactions include orthostatic hypotension with reflex tachycardia, fainting, dizziness, confusion, agitation, hallucinations, arrhythmias, anorexia, dry mouth, urine retention, nausea, vomiting, abdominal pain, constipation, local gastric irritation, seizures, endocrine effects, hematologic disorders, visual disturbances, skin eruptions, and photosensitivity.

Contraindications and cautions

■ Contraindicated in patients with CNS depression, bone marrow suppression, heart failure, circulatory collapse, coronary artery or cerebrovascular disorders, subcortical damage, or coma. Also contraindicated in patients receiving spinal and epidural anesthetics and adrenergic blockers.

■ Use cautiously in debilitated patients and in those with hepatic, renal, or cardiovascular disease; respiratory disorders; hypocalcemia; seizure disorders; suspected brain tumor or intestinal obstruction; glaucoma; and prostatic hyperplasia.

LIFESPAN

■ *Pregnant women.* Use only if clearly needed; safety hasn't been established.

■ *Breast-feeding women.* Discourage breast-feeding during therapy because most phenothiazines appear in breast milk and directly affect prolactin levels.

■ *Children under age 12.* Usually not recommended. Use cautiously for nausea and vomiting. Acutely ill children, such as those with chickenpox, measles, CNS infections, or dehydration have a greatly increased risk of dystonic reactions.

■ *Geriatric patients.* Use cautiously and at reduced dosage, adjusted to patient response, because these patients are more sensitive to therapeutic and adverse effects, especially cardiac toxicity, tardive dyskinesia, and other extrapyramidal effects.

Nursing considerations

■ Check vital signs regularly for decreased blood pressure, especially before and after parenteral therapy, or tachycardia; observe patient carefully for other adverse reactions.

■ Check intake and output for urine retention or constipation, which may require dosage reduction.

■ Monitor bilirubin level weekly for the first 4 weeks. Establish baseline complete blood count, electrocardiogram (for quinidine-like effects), liver and renal function test results, electrolyte level (especially potassium), and eye examination findings. Monitor these findings periodically thereafter, especially in patients receiving long-term therapy.

■ Observe patient for mood changes, and monitor progress.

■ Monitor patient for involuntary movements. Check patient receiving prolonged treatment at least once every 6 months.

■ Don't stop drug abruptly. Although physical dependence doesn't occur with antipsychotic drugs, rebound worsening of psychotic symptoms may occur, and many drug effects may persist.

■ Follow manufacturer's guidelines for reconstitution, dilution, administration, and storage of drugs; slightly discolored liquids may or may not be acceptable for use. Check with pharmacist.

Patient teaching

■ Teach patient how and when to take drug. Advise against increasing the dosage or stopping the drug without prescriber's approval. Suggest taking the full dose at bedtime if daytime sedation occurs.

■ Explain that full therapeutic effect may not occur for several weeks.

■ Teach signs and symptoms of adverse reactions, and urge patient to report unusual effects, especially involuntary movements.

■ Instruct patient to avoid beverages and drugs containing alcohol, and warn against taking other drugs, including over-the-counter or herbal products, without prescriber's approval.

■ Advise patient to avoid hazardous tasks until full effects of drug are established. Explain that sedative effects will lessen after several weeks.

■ Inform patient that excessive exposure to sunlight, heat lamps, or tanning beds may cause photosensitivity reactions. Advise him to avoid exposure to extreme heat or cold.

■ Explain that phenothiazines may cause pink or brown discoloration of urine.

SELECTIVE SEROTONIN REUPTAKE INHIBITORS

citalopram hydrobromide
escitalopram
fluoxetine
fluvoxamine maleate
paroxetine
sertraline

Indications
■ Bulimia nervosa
■ Major depression
■ Obsessive-compulsive disorder
■ Panic disorders

■ Premenstrual dysphoric disorder

(See *Comparing selective serotonin reuptake inhibitors*, pages 96 and 97.)

Actions
The action of selective serotonin reuptake inhibitors (SSRIs) probably relates to the potent and selective inhibition of serotonin, but not norepinephrine or dopamine, uptake in the central nervous system. These drugs lack affinity for alpha-adrenergic receptors and muscarinic receptors.

Adverse reactions
Common adverse effects include headache, tremor, dizziness, sleep disturbances, gastrointestinal disturbances, and sexual dysfunction.

Less common adverse effects include bleeding (red spots on skin, nose bleeds), restlessness, breast tenderness or enlargement, extrapyramidal effects, dystonia, fever, hyponatremia, mania or hypomania, palpitations, serotonin syndrome, weight gain or loss, rash, hives, or itching.

Contraindications and cautions
■ Contraindicated in patients hypersensitive to SSRIs or their

COMPARING SELECTIVE SEROTONIN REUPTAKE INHIBITORS

DRUG	ADULT DOSAGE	DOSAGE ADJUSTMENT	BIOAVAIL-ABILITY
citalopram	20–40 mg/day	Reduced dose recommended in geriatric patients.	No food effect
escitalopram	10–20 mg/day	Reduced dose recommended for hepatic impairment and geriatric patients.	80%; no food effect
fluoxetine	20–80 mg/day in single or divided doses; 90 mg/week with delayed-release form	Reduced dose recommended for hepatic impairment and geriatric patients.	Well absorbed; no food effect
fluvoxamine	50–300 mg/day h.s. Total daily dose > 100 mg should be divided and given in two doses	Reduce initial dosage and modify subsequent doses in renal and hepatic impairment.	No food effect
paroxetine	10–60 mg/day in single or divided doses	Reduce dose in severe renal or hepatic impairment. Reduced dose recommended for geriatric patients.	50–100%; no food effect
sertraline	25–50 mg once daily	Reduce dose or increase interval in severe hepatic impairment.	Food increases rate and extent of absorption

Plasma protein–binding (%)	Half-life (HR)	Onset of action (WK)	Peak concentration (HR)	Elimination
80	35	1–4	4 (after a single dose)	35% in urine 65% in feces
56	27–32	1–4	5 (after a single dose)	7% in urine
94½	1–3 days for fluoxetine 4–16 days for norfluoxetine	1–3; may be 5 for obsessive-compulsive disorder	6–8 (after a single dose)	80% in urine 15% in feces
80	13½–15½	4–5	3–8	94% in urine
95	Average of 21–24	1–3	2–8	64% in urine 36% in feces
98	sertraline: 24–26 N-desmethyl-sertraline: 62–104	2–4	4½–8½	45% in urine 45% in feces

months of therapy, but reassure them that this is temporary.

■ Urge patient to keep follow-up appointments and have regular laboratory testing of thyroid levels.

XANTHINE DERIVATIVES

aminophylline
theophylline

Indications

■ Asthma and bronchospasm from emphysema and chronic bronchitis

Actions

Xanthine derivatives are structurally related; they directly relax smooth muscle, stimulate the central nervous system (CNS), induce diuresis, increase gastric acid secretion, inhibit uterine contractions, and exert weak inotropic and chronotropic effects on the heart. Of these drugs, theophylline exerts the greatest effect on smooth muscle.

The action of xanthine derivatives isn't completely caused by inhibition of phosphodiesterase. Current data suggest that inhibition of adenosine receptors or unidentified mechanisms may be responsible for therapeutic effects. By relaxing smooth muscle of the respiratory tract, they increase airflow and vital capacity. They also slow onset of diaphragmatic fatigue and stimulate the respiratory center in the CNS.

Adverse reactions

Adverse effects are dose-related, except for hypersensitivity, and can be controlled by dosage adjustment. Common reactions include hypotension, palpitations, arrhythmias, restlessness, irritability, nausea, vomiting, urine retention, and headache.

Contraindications and cautions

■ Contraindicated in patients hypersensitive to xanthines.

■ Use cautiously in patients with arrhythmias, cardiac or circulatory impairment, cor pulmonale, hepatic or renal disease, active peptic ulcers, hyperthyroidism, or diabetes mellitus.

LIFESPAN

■ *Pregnant women.* Use cautiously.

■ *Breast-feeding women.* These drugs appear in breast milk and may cause serious adverse reactions in infants.

■ *Small children.* Monitor patient closely for excessive CNS stimulation.

■ *Geriatric patients.* Use cautiously.

Nursing considerations

■ Monitor theophylline level closely; therapeutic level ranges from 10 to 20 mcg/ml.

■ Assess patient for adverse reactions, especially toxicity.

■ Check vital signs.

■ Don't crush or allow patient to chew timed-release preparations.

■ Calculate dosage from lean body weight because theophylline doesn't distribute into fatty tissue.

■ Adjust daily dosage in elderly patients and in those with heart failure or hepatic disease.

Patient teaching

■ Tell patient to take drug exactly as prescribed.

■ Advise patient to check with prescriber before using any other drug, including over-the-counter medications or herbal remedies, or before switching brands.

■ If patient smokes, explain that doing so may decrease the theophylline level. Urge patient to notify prescriber if he quits smoking because the dosage will need adjustment to avoid possible toxicity.

Four types of patients need special consideration before and during drug therapy: pregnant, breast-feeding, pediatric, and geriatric patients. In these patients, developmental changes or immature or declining body systems can cause pharmacokinetic and pharmacodynamic differences that make drug effects less predictable than in typical adult patients. Keep these differences in mind when giving a drug to a patient with these lifespan considerations.

PREGNANT WOMEN

Based on clinical and preclinical information, the Food and Drug Administration assigns a pregnancy risk category to systemically absorbed drugs. The five categories (A, B, C, D, and X) reflect a drug's potential to cause birth defects. Although a pregnant woman should avoid drugs as a general rule, this rating system permits rapid assessment of the risk-benefit ratio if she needs drug therapy. Drugs in category A generally are safe to use during pregnancy; drugs in category X are contraindicated. (See *Pregnancy risk categories*, page 110.)

Several pregnancy-related changes and structures can alter a drug's absorption, distribution, metabolism, and excretion. The fetus also can significantly influence drug distribution and disposition.

Because a pregnant woman may become a breast-feeding mother, the safety of a drug taken by the mother should be considered for her breast-fed infant as well.

Absorption
During pregnancy, gastrointestinal (GI) tone and motility decrease, probably because of increased progesterone production and a decreased level of motilin (a hormone that increases intestinal motility and stimulates pepsin secretion). These

Pregnancy risk categories

This list summarizes the Food and Drug Administration risk-factor categories for drugs used during pregnancy.

Category A: Controlled studies in women haven't shown a risk to the fetus in any trimester. Harm to the fetus seems unlikely.

Category B: Either animal studies haven't shown a risk to the fetus and no controlled studies have been done in pregnant women or animal studies have shown an adverse effect (other than decreased fertility) that wasn't confirmed in controlled studies with women in their first trimester and no evidence of a risk in later trimesters exists.

Category C: Either animal studies show adverse effects to the fetus and no controlled studies in women exist or no studies in women or animals exist. The drug should be given only if the potential benefit to the woman justifies the potential risk to the fetus.

Category D: The drug may cause risk to the fetus but use in pregnant women may be acceptable despite the risk (for example, if the drug is needed in a life-threatening situation or if safer drugs can't be used or are ineffective for a serious disease).

Category X: Studies in animals or women show fetal abnormalities, evidence of fetal risk exists based on studies in pregnant women, or both, and the risk clearly outweighs any possible benefit. The drug is contraindicated in women who are or may become pregnant.

Category NR: No rating available.

effects prolong gastric emptying and intestinal transit. Hydrochloric acid formation in the stomach also decreases. All these factors delay the absorption of oral drugs that need an acidic environment or that are absorbed in the small intestine.

Parenteral drug absorption also may change during pregnancy. Because of peripheral vasodilation, drugs given by the S.C., I.M., or intradermal route may be absorbed more rapidly.

Distribution

The physiologic changes of pregnancy also alter drug distribution. Influencing factors include increased interstitial and cellular water and increased blood volume, elevated nearly 45% by the end of gestation. These increases change the ratios of blood constituents that affect drug distribution. For example, the ratio of albumin to water decreases during pregnancy, altering protein-binding capacity.

During pregnancy, estrogen and progesterone levels rise, as do those of free fatty acids (triglycerides, cholesterol, and phospholipids) from increased fatty tissue metabolism. These effects are accompanied by greater competition for protein-binding sites. With fewer binding sites, a larger percentage of a drug remains free to move to receptor sites or across the placenta.

The term "placental barrier" can be misleading because it implies that the placenta protects the fetus from drug effects. In fact, although some drugs, such as insulin, don't cross the placenta, many do cross it when given at therapeutic levels. Placental transport of substances to and from the fetus begins around the fifth week of gestation. Later in the pregnancy, when the placenta thins, drugs with high lipid solubility or low protein-binding ability pass more easily through the placental barrier.

Long-term adverse effects may occur in the child of a mother who was given certain drugs during pregnancy. For example, maternal use of diethylstilbestrol has been noted as the cause of vaginal adenocarcinoma in young girls, a disease that had previously been considered rare in this population.

Metabolism

Because the placenta is metabolically active, it can affect drug disposition. The placenta may perform several enzymatic reactions that can reduce the potency of a drug's metabolites. Conversely, these reactions may produce a more potent and toxic metabolite, thereby increasing danger to the fetus.

Excretion

Many pregnancy-induced changes in the urinary system can affect drug excretion. Glomerular filtration rate (GFR) and renal plasma flow increase early in pregnancy; the increased GFR persists until delivery. Because of the increased renal plasma flow, drugs that normally are excreted easily may be eliminated even more rapidly.

A fetus has slower drug clearance than an adult, and drugs persist longer in fetal tissues and blood than in the mother's tissues and blood.

BREAST-FEEDING WOMEN

Breast-feeding confers many health benefits on the infant, such as a decreased risk of diarrhea, bacterial infections, tooth decay, and allergies. However, a woman who breast-feeds during drug therapy may subject her infant to the drug's effects. Unlike a fetus, an infant can't depend on the placenta to metabolize and excrete drugs ingested by the mother. Therefore, although few drugs require a woman to stop breast-feeding, the prescriber must consider which ones offer the greatest safety for the infant.

Infant sucking behavior, the amount consumed per feeding, and the frequency of breast-feeding affect the amount of drug ingested. In an infant, low gastric acidity and a slow absorption rate affect the amount of drug absorbed. Changes in protein binding in an infant may alter the drug level at receptor sites. Also, drugs that are metabolized insufficiently and excreted with difficulty by immature body systems may accumulate, increasing the risk of toxicity.

To help minimize the infant's exposure to a drug that reaches a detectable level in breast milk, teach the mother how to help protect her infant. Because these steps may vary with the drug used, consult a pharmacist as needed before the teaching session. To ensure success, cover these simple steps, and suggest ways to accommodate daily routines and minimize disruptions.

■ Avoid breast-feeding during times that milk will contain peak drug levels by feeding the infant at the end of a dosing interval or by taking the drug just after breast-feeding.

■ Take the drug before the infant's longest sleep period to allow sufficient time for the drug to clear from the milk before the next feeding. This is especially useful for a drug that readily diffuses into breast milk.

■ Pump and discard breast milk if the drug has a short half-life. (This step isn't appropriate for drugs with a long half-life.)

CHILDREN

A child's age, physiologic state, body composition, immature organ function, and other factors can affect drug absorption, distribution, metabolism, and excretion.

Absorption

A young child's gastric pH is higher, or less acidic, than an adult's. As the child develops, gastric pH decreases, acidity increases, and drug absorption is altered. For example, an infant absorbs nafcillin and penicillin G better than an adult because of lower gastric acidity. Milk and formula also can affect gastric pH and may alter absorption. Therefore, unless otherwise indicated, plan to give a drug when the child's stomach is empty.

Other factors can influence drug absorption from the GI tract and make absorption less predictable or less efficient in a child under age 2. The shortness of the intestine and the presence of diarrhea can reduce the amount of time a drug is available for absorption. Decreased transit time through the GI tract also can decrease drug absorption.

Absorption of an I.M. drug may be unpredictable in an infant because of vasomotor instability and decreased muscle tone. Percutaneous absorption of an S.C. drug is increased in an infant because of an underdeveloped epidermal barrier and increased skin hydration.

Distribution

A drug's distribution is affected by its dilution in the body. The higher percentage of water in neonates and infants dilutes water-soluble drugs, reducing their levels in the blood. That's why a neonate or infant may need a higher mg/kg dosage to achieve a therapeutic drug level.

Body composition affects the distribution and effects of water-soluble drugs. Most drugs travel through extracellular fluid to reach their receptors. Because children have a higher percentage of fluid in their bodies, their distribution area is proportionately greater than an adult's.

To a lesser degree, body composition also affects the distribution of lipid-soluble drugs. As the percentage of body fat increases with age, so does the distribution of lipid-soluble drugs. Therefore, distribution of these drugs is more limited in children than in adults.

An infant's immature liver may affect drug distribution by decreasing plasma protein formation, which results in a lower plasma protein level and a higher fluid volume than in an adult. This reduces the number of plasma proteins for drugs to bind with. Because only unbound, or free, drugs produce

RECOGNIZING GRAY BABY SYNDROME

New, safer antibiotics have dramatically reduced the use of chloramphenicol in infants. However, if an infant must receive chloramphenicol, be alert for evidence of gray baby syndrome, which usually appears 2 to 9 days after treatment begins and may develop in this order:

- ■ Vomiting
- ■ Refusal to suck
- ■ Loose, green stools
- ■ Hypotension
- ■ Cyanosis
- ■ Hypothermia
- ■ Cardiovascular collapse
- ■ Death

pharmacologic effects, an infant's decreased protein binding can intensify drug effects and possibly cause toxicity.

Several disorders, such as nephrotic syndrome and malnutrition, may decrease the plasma protein level and increase the unbound drug level, intensifying the drug's effects or producing toxicity.

Metabolism

An infant's immature liver may inefficiently metabolize drugs. As the liver matures during the first year of life, drug metabolism improves. This consideration guides the choice of drugs and dosages for a child. For example, the antibiotic chloramphenicol is used in adults to treat gram-positive and gram-negative bacterial infections. However, it shouldn't be prescribed for neonates, especially premature ones, because it can be fatal. In neonates, the liver doesn't have the enzymes needed for appropriate metabolism. So the drug accumulates, causing toxicity known as gray baby syndrome. (See *Recognizing gray baby syndrome*.) I.V. drugs and flush solutions that contain the preservative benzyl alcohol also shouldn't be given to neonates because their inability to metabolize it properly can also lead to toxicity.

Excretion

Because most drugs are excreted in the urine, the degree of renal development can affect drug excretion and, ultimately, dosage requirements for a child.

At birth, the kidneys are immature, renal excretion is slow, and drug dosages must be adjusted carefully. As the kidneys mature during the first few months after birth, renal excretion of drugs increases, although the rate of increase is slow for a premature neonate.

Some drugs, such as nafcillin, are excreted by the biliary tract into the intestines. In the first few days after birth, however, biliary blood flow is low, which can prolong the drug's effects.

GERIATRIC PATIENTS

Aging is usually accompanied by a decline in organ function, which can profoundly affect drug distribution and clearance, among other things. This physiologic decline is likely to be worsened by a disease or chronic disorder. Such a combination can significantly increase the geriatric patient's risk of drug toxicity and adverse reactions.

Absorption

Several age-related changes in the GI system can alter drug absorption. Decreased gastric acidity may affect drug solubility and alter drug absorption. Reduced blood flow to the GI tract and the decreased number of cells available for absorption also can delay drug absorption. However, because the GI transit time is slowed, drugs remain in the system longer, which in-

creases absorption. Overall, the effects of aging slow the absorption rate, but allow absorption to be as complete as in a younger patient.

Distribution

Proportions of fat, lean tissue, and water in the body change with age. Total body mass and lean body mass, for example, decrease with age. These changes lead to a relative increase in body fat and decrease in body water, altering the distribution of most drugs. Highly lipid-soluble drugs, such as diazepam, have an increased volume of distribution and prolonged distribution, leading to a longer half-life and duration of action. Highly water-soluble drugs, such as gentamicin, aren't distributed to fat cells. Because an elderly patient has relatively less lean tissue than a younger patient, more drug remains in the older patient's bloodstream and increases the risk of a toxic reaction.

Aging also reduces the level of albumin, a blood protein that binds with and transports many drugs. As a result, more unbound drugs may circulate, which typically increases the effects of drugs that are highly protein-bound.

COMMON CHARACTERISTICS AFFECTING DRUG DISTRIBUTION IN GERIATRIC PATIENTS

- Declining cardiac output
- Dehydration
- Electrolyte and mineral imbalances
- Extremes of body weight
- Inactivity
- Poor nutrition
- Prolonged bed rest

Other factors can alter drug distribution. (See *Common characteristics affecting drug distribution in geriatric patients*.) Perhaps the most significant factor is size: Geriatric patients are typically smaller than younger patients. So if a geriatric patient receives the same dose as a younger patient, the older patient's smaller volume may result in a higher drug level.

Metabolism

Aging reduces the liver's ability to metabolize drugs. Liver disease may further compromise its functioning. So may other diseases that reduce hepatic blood flow, such as heart failure.

Drug metabolism depends primarily on two processes: hepatic blood flow and metabolic enzyme action. Because aging decreases hepatic blood flow, a smaller amount of the drug is delivered to the liver for metabolism to inactive compounds. Hepatic enzymes metabolize

drugs in two major phases. Aging reduces the efficiency of both phases, but phase I reactions (oxidation, reduction, or hydrolysis of drug molecules) are affected more than phase II reactions (coupling of the drug or its metabolite with an acid to produce an inactive compound). Aging leads to different effects depending on whether a drug is metabolized in phase I, phase II, or both.

Excretion

With aging, glomerular filtration and tubular secretion decline progressively. Also, dehydration and cardiovascular and renal diseases may cause renal impairment. Keep in mind that a geriatric patient has a smaller renal reserve than a younger patient, even if his blood urea nitrogen and creatinine levels appear normal.

When a geriatric patient receives a drug that isn't metabolized, watch for evidence of toxicity because drug excretion may be delayed. Be particularly cautious with potentially nephrotoxic drugs, such as the aminoglycoside gentamicin, because they may cause severe nephrotoxicity quickly in a geriatric patient.

Drug receptors

Aging reduces the efficiency of many drug receptors and the density of beta receptors. As a result, geriatric patients show diminished response to drugs, such as isoproterenol, and increased toxicity from beta blockers, such as propranolol. With age comes a decline in parasympathetic control, which enhances the effects of anticholinergic drugs. Aging also reduces the number of neurotransmitters, particularly dopamine and acetylcholine, which may affect drugs such as phenothiazines and chlorpromazine.

Adverse drug reactions

Geriatric patients experience adverse drug reactions two to seven times more frequently than younger patients. Age-related physiologic changes account for many of these adverse reactions. (See *Preventing adverse drug reactions in older patients*, pages 118 to 127.)

Age-related central nervous system (CNS) changes may cause drug-related problems. These changes include increased sensitivity to depressants and decreased cerebral blood flow, which increase the risk of sedation and diminished cognitive function during drug therapy. Other CNS changes may include deterioration of the blood-brain barrier, which may allow a greater concentration in the CNS for some drugs and may account for many drug-induced behavioral changes in geriatric patients. One such change, paradoxical excitement, can happen with the use of sedatives and anxiety-relieving drugs.

Age-related cardiovascular changes that may affect drug response include decreased cardiac output, increased total peripheral resistance, increased circulating norepinephrine, and decreased sensitivity and function of baroreceptors. These changes may contribute to adverse reactions, such as orthostatic hypotension and heart failure.

Several endocrine changes may influence drug therapy in geriatric patients. For example, a decline in glucose tolerance may cause greater hyperglycemia in response to a thiazide

(Text continues on page 130.)

PREVENTING ADVERSE DRUG REACTIONS IN OLDER PATIENTS

A drug's action in the body and its interaction with body tissues (pharmacodynamics) change significantly in older people. In the table below, you'll find the information you need to help prevent adverse drug reactions in your elderly patients.

PHARMACOLOGY	INDICATIONS	SPECIAL CONSIDERATIONS
Adrenergics, direct- and indirect-acting ■ Exert excitatory actions on the heart, glands, and vascular smooth muscle and peripheral inhibitory actions on smooth muscles of the bronchial tree	■ Hypotension ■ Cardiac stimulation ■ Bronchodilation ■ Shock	■ An elderly patient may be more sensitive to therapeutic and adverse effects of some adrenergics and may require lower doses.
Adrenocorticoids, systemic ■ Stimulate enzyme synthesis needed to decrease the inflammatory response	■ Inflammation ■ Immunosuppression ■ Adrenal insufficiency ■ Rheumatic and collagen diseases ■ Acute spinal cord injury	■ These drugs may aggravate hyperglycemia, delay wound healing, or contribute to edema, insomnia, or osteoporosis in an elderly patient. ■ Decreased metabolic rate and elimination may cause increased plasma levels and increase the risk of adverse effects. Monitor the elderly patient carefully.
Alpha blockers ■ Block the effects of peripheral neurohormonal transmitters (norepinephrine, epinephrine) on adrenergic receptors in various effector systems	■ Peripheral vascular disorders ■ Hypertension ■ Benign prostatic hyperplasia	■ Hypotensive effects may be more pronounced in an elderly patient. ■ These drugs should be administered at bedtime to reduce potential for dizziness or lightheadedness.

PREVENTING ADVERSE DRUG REACTIONS IN OLDER PATIENTS (continued)

PHARMACOLOGY	INDICATIONS	SPECIAL CONSIDERATIONS
Aminoglycosides ■ Inhibit bacterial protein synthesis	■ Infection caused by susceptible organisms	■ Decreased renal function may increase the risk of nephrotoxicity, ototoxicity, and superinfection (common).
Angiotensin-converting enzyme (ACE) inhibitors ■ Prevent the conversion of angiotensin I to angiotensin II ■ Decrease vasoconstriction and adrenocortical secretion of aldosterone	■ Hypertension ■ Heart failure	■ Diuretic therapy should be discontinued before ACE inhibitors are started to reduce the risk of hypotension. ■ An elderly patient may need lower doses because of impaired drug clearance.
Anticholinergics ■ Exert antagonistic action on acetylcholine and other cholinergic agonists within the parasympathetic nervous system	■ Hypersecretory conditions ■ Gastrointestinal tract disorders ■ Sinus bradycardia ■ Dystonia and parkinsonism ■ Perioperative use ■ Motion sickness	■ These drugs should be used cautiously in an elderly adult, who may be more sensitive to the effects of these drugs; a lower dosage may be indicated.
Antihistamines ■ Prevent access and subsequent activity of histamine	■ Allergy ■ Pruritus ■ Vertigo ■ Nausea and vomiting ■ Sedation ■ Cough suppression ■ Dyskinesia	■ An elderly patient is usually more sensitive to the adverse effects of antihistamines; he's especially likely to experience a greater degree of dizziness, sedation, hypotension, and urine retention.

(continued)

PREVENTING ADVERSE DRUG REACTIONS
IN OLDER PATIENTS (continued)

PHARMACOLOGY	INDICATIONS	SPECIAL CONSIDERATIONS
Barbiturates ■ Decrease presynaptic and postsynaptic excitability, producing central nervous system (CNS) depression	■ Seizure disorders ■ Sedation (including preanesthesia) ■ Hypnosis	■ An elderly patient and a patient receiving subhypnotic doses may experience hyperactivity, excitement, or hyperanalgesia. Use with caution.
Benzodiazepines ■ Act selectively on polysynaptic neuronal pathways throughout the CNS; synthetically produced sedative-hypnotic	■ Seizure disorders ■ Anxiety, tension, insomnia ■ Surgical adjuncts for conscious sedation or amnesia ■ Skeletal muscle spasm, tremor	■ These drugs should be used cautiously in an elderly patient sensitive to the drugs' CNS effects; parenteral administration is more likely to cause apnea, hypotension, bradycardia, and cardiac arrest.
Beta blockers ■ Compete with beta agonists for available beta-receptor sites; individual drugs differ in their ability to affect beta receptors	■ Hypertension ■ Angina ■ Arrhythmias ■ Glaucoma ■ Myocardial infarction (MI) ■ Migraine prophylaxis	■ Increased bioavailability or delayed metabolism in the elderly patient may warrant a lower dosage; an elderly patient may also experience enhanced adverse effects.
Calcium channel blockers ■ Inhibit calcium influx across the slow channels of myocardial and vascular smooth muscle cells, causing dilation of coronary arteries, peripheral arteries, and arterioles and slowing cardiac conduction	■ Angina ■ Arrhythmias ■ Hypertension	■ These drugs should be used cautiously in an elderly patient because the half-life of calcium channel blockers may be increased as a result of decreased clearance.

Preventing adverse drug reactions in older patients (continued)

Pharmacology	Indications	Special Considerations
Cardiac glycosides ■ Directly increase myocardial contractile force and velocity, atrioventricular node refractory period, and total peripheral resistance ■ Indirectly depress sinoatrial node and prolong conduction to the atrioventricular node	■ Heart failure ■ Arrhythmias ■ Paroxysmal atrial tachycardia or atrioventricular junctional rhythm ■ MI ■ Cardiogenic shock ■ Angina	■ These drugs should be used cautiously in an elderly patient with renal or hepatic dysfunction or with electrolyte imbalance that may predispose him to toxicity.
Cephalosporins ■ Inhibit bacterial cell wall synthesis, causing rapid cell lysis	■ Infection caused by susceptible organisms	■ Because the elderly patient commonly has impaired renal function, he may need a lower dosage. ■ An older adult is more susceptible to superinfection and coagulopathies.
Coumarin derivatives ■ Interfere with the hepatic synthesis of vitamin K–dependent clotting factors II, VII, IX, and X, decreasing the blood's coagulation potential	■ Treatment for or prevention of thrombosis or embolism	■ An older adult has an increased risk of hemorrhage because of altered hemostatic mechanisms or age-related hepatic and renal deterioration.
Diuretics, loop ■ Inhibit sodium and chloride reabsorption in the ascending loop of Henle and increase excretion of potassium, sodium, chloride, and water	■ Edema ■ Hypertension	■ An elderly or debilitated patient is more susceptible to drug-induced diuresis and can quickly develop dehydration, hypovolemia, hypokalemia, and hyponatremia, which may cause circulatory collapse.

(continued)

PREVENTING ADVERSE DRUG REACTIONS IN OLDER PATIENTS (continued)

PHARMACOLOGY	INDICATIONS	SPECIAL CONSIDERATIONS
Diuretics, potassium-sparing ■ Act directly on the distal renal tubules, inhibiting sodium reabsorption and potassium excretion	■ Edema ■ Hypertension ■ Diagnosis of primary hyperaldosteronism	■ An older patient may need a smaller dosage because of his susceptibility to drug-induced diuresis and hyperkalemia.
Diuretics, thiazide and thiazide-like ■ Interfere with sodium transport, thereby increasing renal excretion of sodium, chloride, water, potassium, and calcium	■ Edema ■ Hypertension ■ Diabetes insipidus	■ Age-related changes in cardiovascular and renal function make the elderly patient more susceptible to excessive diuresis, which may lead to dehydration, hypovolemia, hyponatremia, hypomagnesemia, and hypokalemia.
Estrogens ■ Promote development and maintenance of the female reproductive system and secondary sexual characteristics; inhibit release of pituitary gonadotropins	■ Moderate to severe vasomotor symptoms of menopause ■ Atrophic vaginitis ■ Carcinoma of the breast and prostate ■ Prophylaxis of postmenopausal osteoporosis	■ A postmenopausal woman on long-term estrogen therapy has an increased risk of developing endometrial cancer.
Histamine$_2$ receptor antagonists ■ Inhibit histamine's action at histamine$_2$ receptors in gastric parietal cells, reducing gastric acid output and concentration, regardless of the stimulatory agent or basal conditions	■ Duodenal ulcer ■ Gastric ulcer ■ Hypersecretory states ■ Reflux esophagitis ■ Stress ulcer prophylaxis	■ These drugs should be used cautiously in an elderly patient because of the increased risk of developing adverse reactions, particularly those affecting the CNS.

PHARMACOLOGY	INDICATIONS	SPECIAL CONSIDERATIONS
Insulin ■ Increases glucose transport across muscle and fat–cell membranes to reduce blood glucose levels ■ Promotes conversion of glucose to glycogen ■ Stimulates amino acid uptake and conversion to protein in muscle cells ■ Inhibits protein degradation ■ Stimulates triglyceride formation and lipoprotein lipase activity; inhibits free fatty acid release from adipose tissue	■ Diabetic ketoacidosis ■ Diabetes mellitus ■ Diabetes mellitus inadequately controlled by diet and oral antidiabetics ■ Hyperkalemia	■ Insulin is available in many forms that differ in onset, peak, and duration of action; the prescriber will specify the individual dosage and form. ■ Blood glucose measurement is an important guide to dosage and management. ■ The elderly patient's diet and ability to recognize hypoglycemia are important. ■ A source of diabetic teaching should be provided, especially for the elderly patient, who may need follow-up home care.
Iron supplements, oral ■ Needed in adequate amounts for erythropoiesis and efficient oxygen transport; essential component of hemoglobin	■ Iron deficiency anemia	■ Iron-induced constipation is common among elderly patients; stress proper diet to minimize constipation. ■ An elderly patient may also need higher doses because of reduced gastric secretions and because achlorhydria may lower the capacity for iron absorption.

(continued)

PREVENTING ADVERSE DRUG REACTIONS IN OLDER PATIENTS *(continued)*

PHARMACOLOGY	INDICATIONS	SPECIAL CONSIDERATIONS
Nitrates ■ Relax smooth muscle; typically used for vascular effects (vasodilatation)	■ Angina pectoris ■ Acute MI	■ Severe hypotension and cardiovascular collapse may occur if nitrates are combined with alcohol. ■ Transient dizziness, syncope, or other signs of cerebral ischemia may occur; instruct the elderly patient to take nitrates while sitting.
Nonsteroidal anti-inflammatory drugs (NSAIDs) ■ Interfere with prostaglandins involved with pain; anti-inflammatory action contributes to analgesic effect	■ Pain ■ Inflammation ■ Fever	■ A patient over age 60 may be more susceptible to the toxic effects of NSAIDs because of decreased renal function; these drugs' effects on renal prostaglandins may cause fluid retention and edema, a drawback for a patient with heart failure.
Opioid agonists ■ Act at specific opiate receptor–binding sites in the CNS and other tissues; alter pain perception without affecting other sensory functions	■ Analgesia ■ Pulmonary edema ■ Preoperative sedation ■ Anesthesia ■ Cough suppression ■ Diarrhea	■ Lower doses are usually indicated for elderly patients, who tend to be more sensitive to the therapeutic and adverse effects of these drugs.
Opioid agonist-antagonists ■ Act, in theory, on different opiate receptors in the CNS to a greater or lesser degree, thus yielding slightly different effects	■ Pain	■ Lower doses may be indicated in patients with renal or hepatic dysfunction to prevent drug accumulation.

PREVENTING ADVERSE DRUG REACTIONS IN OLDER PATIENTS (continued)

PHARMACOLOGY	INDICATIONS	SPECIAL CONSIDERATIONS
Opioid antagonists ■ Act differently depending on whether an opioid agonist has been administered previously, the actions of that opioid, and the extent of physical dependence on it	■ Opioid-induced respiratory depression ■ Adjunct in treating opiate addiction	■ These drugs are contraindicated for opioid addicts, in whom they may produce an acute abstinence syndrome.
Penicillins ■ Inhibit bacterial cell-wall synthesis, causing rapid cell lysis; most effective against fast-growing susceptible organisms	■ Infection caused by susceptible organisms	■ An elderly patient (and others with low resistance from immunosuppressants or radiation therapy) should be taught the signs and symptoms of bacterial and fungal superinfection.
Phenothiazines ■ Believed to function as dopamine antagonists, blocking postsynaptic dopamine receptors in various parts of the CNS; antiemetic effects resulting from blockage of the chemoreceptor trigger zones	■ Psychosis ■ Nausea and vomiting ■ Anxiety ■ Severe behavior problems ■ Tetanus ■ Porphyria ■ Intractable hiccups ■ Neurogenic pain ■ Allergies and pruritus	■ An older adult needs a lower dosage because he's more sensitive to these drugs' therapeutic and adverse effects, especially cardiac toxicity, tardive dyskinesia, and other extrapyramidal effects. ■ Dosage should be adjusted to patient response.

(continued)

PREVENTING ADVERSE DRUG REACTIONS
IN OLDER PATIENTS (continued)

PHARMACOLOGY	INDICATIONS	SPECIAL CONSIDERATIONS
Salicylates ■ Decrease formation of prostaglandins involved in pain and inflammation	■ Pain ■ Inflammation ■ Fever	■ A patient over age 60 with impaired renal function may be more susceptible to toxic effects. ■ The effect of salicylates on renal prostaglandins may cause fluid retention and edema, a significant disadvantage for a patient with heart failure.
Selective serotonin reuptake inhibitors ■ Inhibit reuptake of serotonin; have little or no effect on other neurotransmitters	■ Major depression ■ Obsessive compulsive disorder ■ Bulimia nervosa	■ These drugs should be used cautiously in a patient with hepatic impairment.
Sulfonamides ■ Inhibit folic acid biosynthesis needed for cell growth	■ Bacterial and parasitic infections ■ Inflammation	■ These drugs should be used cautiously in elderly patients, who are more susceptible to bacterial and fungal superinfection, folate deficiency anemia, and renal and hematologic effects because of diminished renal function.
Tetracyclines ■ Inhibit bacterial protein synthesis	■ Bacterial, protozoal, rickettsial, and fungal infections ■ Sclerosing agent	■ Some elderly patients have decreased esophageal motility; administer tetracyclines with caution, and watch for local irritation from slowly passing oral forms.

PREVENTING ADVERSE DRUG REACTIONS
IN OLDER PATIENTS (continued)

PHARMACOLOGY	INDICATIONS	SPECIAL CONSIDERATIONS
Thrombolytic enzymes ■ Convert plasminogen to plasmin for promotion of clot lysis	■ Thrombosis, thromboembolism	■ Patients age 75 and older are at greater risk for cerebral hemorrhage because they're more apt to have cerebrovascular disease.
Thyroid hormones ■ Have catabolic and anabolic effects ■ Influence normal metabolism, growth and development, and every organ system; vital to normal CNS function	■ Hypothyroidism ■ Nontoxic goiter ■ Thyrotoxicosis ■ Diagnostic use	■ In a patient over age 60, the initial hormone replacement dose should be 25% less than the recommended dose.
Thyroid hormone antagonists ■ Inhibit iodine oxidation in the thyroid gland through a block of iodine's ability to combine with tyrosine to form thyroxine	■ Hyperthyroidism ■ Preparation for thyroidectomy ■ Thyrotoxic crisis ■ Thyroid carcinoma	■ Serum thyroid-stimulating hormone should be monitored as a sensitive indicator of thyroid hormone levels. Dosage adjustment may be required.
Tricyclic antidepressants ■ Inhibit neurotransmitter reuptake, resulting in increased concentration and enhanced activity of neurotransmitters in the synaptic cleft	■ Depression ■ Obsessive compulsive disorder ■ Enuresis ■ Severe, chronic pain	■ Lower doses are indicated in elderly patients because they're more sensitive to both the therapeutic and adverse effects of tricyclic antidepressants.

ADVERSE REACTIONS MISINTERPRETED AS AGE-RELATED CHANGES

In elderly patients, adverse drug reactions can easily be misinterpreted as the typical signs and symptoms of aging. The table below, which shows possible adverse reactions for common drug classes, can help you avoid such misinterpretations.

DRUG CLASSES	Agitation	Anxiety	Arrhythmias	Ataxia	Changes in appetite	Confusion	Constipation	Depression	
ACE inhibitors						●	●	●	
Alpha₁ blockers		●					●	●	
Antianginals	●	●	●			●			
Antiarrhythmics			●				●		
Anticholinergics	●	●	●			●	●	●	
Anticonvulsants	●		●	●	●	●	●	●	
Antidepressants, tricyclic	●	●	●	●	●	●	●		
Antidiabetics, oral									
Antihistamines						●	●	●	
Antilipemics							●		
Antiparkinsonians	●	●		●	●	●	●	●	
Antipsychotics	●	●	●	●	●	●	●	●	
Barbiturates	●	●	●			●			
Benzodiazepines	●			●		●	●	●	
Beta blockers		●	●					●	
Calcium channel blockers		●	●				●		
Corticosteroids	●					●		●	
Diuretics						●			
Nonsteroidal anti-inflammatory drugs		●				●	●	●	
Opioids	●	●				●	●	●	
Skeletal muscle relaxants	●	●		●		●		●	
Thyroid hormones			●		●				

(Header: **ADVERSE REACTIONS**)

Difficulty breathing	Disorientation	Dizziness	Drowsiness	Edema	Fatigue	Hypotension	Insomnia	Memory loss	Muscle weakness	Restlessness	Sexual dysfunction	Tremors	Urinary dysfunction	Visual changes
		●			●	●	●				●			●
		●	●	●	●	●	●				●		●	●
		●		●	●	●	●			●	●		●	●
●		●		●	●									
	●	●	●		●	●		●	●	●			●	●
●		●	●	●	●	●	●					●	●	●
●	●	●	●		●	●	●			●	●	●	●	●
		●			●									
	●	●	●		●							●	●	●
		●			●		●		●		●		●	●
	●	●	●		●	●	●		●			●	●	●
		●	●		●	●	●			●	●	●	●	●
●	●		●		●	●				●				
●	●	●	●		●		●	●	●			●	●	●
●		●			●	●		●			●	●	●	●
●		●		●	●	●	●				●		●	●
				●	●		●		●					●
		●			●	●			●				●	
		●	●		●		●		●					●
●	●	●	●		●	●	●	●		●	●		●	●
		●	●		●	●	●					●		
							●					●		

diuretic. Reduced response to hypoglycemia may cause a geriatric patient to delay seeking treatment until the hypoglycemia worsens. Reduced thyroid function may decrease body metabolism, which can slow drug metabolism.

Age-related changes in the respiratory, GI, urinary, and musculoskeletal systems also may cause adverse reactions in a geriatric patient. For example, decreased respiratory function may lead to increased sensitivity to respiratory depressants, such as opioids and barbiturates. Decreased GI motility and activity may cause constipation and greater sensitivity to the effects of anticholinergic drugs.

Adverse reactions can easily be mistaken for signs and symptoms of aging. (See *Adverse drug reactions misinterpreted as age-related changes*, pages 128 and 129.) Be sure to ask your patient or his caregiver when such symptoms as confusion, fatigue, and urinary dysfunction began. If they first appeared *after* he started taking a particular drug, their cause may be the drug — not the aging process.

Several risk factors help identify geriatric patients who are prone to adverse reactions. These risk factors include ad-vanced age, small physique, multiple illnesses, use of multiple drugs, type of drugs prescribed (such as CNS depressants), previous adverse reactions, living alone, and malnutrition. By identifying high-risk geriatric patients, you can help protect them by monitoring them closely, preventing errors, identifying drug-related problems promptly, and intervening as needed.

ENGLISH–SPANISH DRUG PHRASE TRANSLATOR

MEDICATION HISTORY

Do you take any medications?
- Prescription?
- Over-the-counter?
- Other?

Which prescription medications do you take routinely?
- How often do you take them?
  Once daily?
  Twice daily?
  Three times daily?
  Four times daily?
  More often?

Which over-the-counter medications do you take routinely?
- How often do you take them?
- Once daily?
- Twice daily?
- Three times daily?
- Four times daily?
- More often?

¿Toma Ud. medicamentos?
- ¿De receta?
- ¿Sin necesidad de receta?
- ¿Otro?

¿Qué medicamentos de receta toma Ud. por rutina?
- ¿Con qué frecuencia los toma?
  ¿Una vez al día?
  ¿Dos veces al día?
  ¿Tres veces al día?
  ¿Cuátro veces al día?
  ¿Con más frecuencia?

¿Qué medicamentos que no necesitan receta toma Ud. por rutina?
- ¿Con que frecuencia los toma?
- ¿Una vez al día?
- ¿Dos veces al día?
- ¿Tres veces al día?
- ¿Cuatro veces al día?
- ¿Con más frecuencia?

Which medications do you take periodically?	¿Qué medicamentos toma Ud. periódicamente?
Why do you take these medications?	¿Por qué toma Ud. estos medicamentos?
What is the dosage for each medication?	¿Cuál es la dosis para cada uno de los medicamentos?
How does each medication make you feel?	¿Cómo le hace sentirse cada medicamento?
Are you allergic to any medications?	¿Está Ud. alérgico(a) a algúnos medicamentos?
– Which medications?	– ¿A qué medicamentos?
– What happens when you have an allergic reaction?	– ¿Qué pasa cuando Ud. tiene una reacción alérgica?

PATIENT TEACHING

PURPOSE OF THE MEDICATION

This medication will:	Este medicamento hará que:
– elevate your blood pressure.	– su presión sanguínea suba.
– improve circulation to your _____.	– la circulación por (la región del cuerpo) mejore.
– lower your blood pressure.	– su presión sanguínea baje.
– lower your blood sugar.	– el nivel de azucar en la sangre baje.
– make your heart rhythm more even.	– el ritmo del corazón sea más uniforme.
– raise your blood sugar.	– su nivel de azucar en la sangre suba.
– reduce or prevent the formation of blood clots.	– se reduzca o evite la formación de coágulos de sangre.
– remove fluid from your body.	– se le quite fluido en el cuerpo.

– remove fluid from your feet, ankles, or legs.

– remove fluid from your lungs so that they work better.

– remove fluid from your pancreas so that it works better.

This medication will help your body to:

– kill the bacteria in your _____.

– slow down your heart rate.

– soften your bowel movements.

– speed up your heart rate.

– use insulin more efficiently.

This medication will help you to:

– breathe better.

– fight infections.

– relax.

– sleep.

– think more clearly.

This medication will relieve or reduce:

– the acid production in your stomach.

– anxiety.

– bladder spasms.

– burning in your stomach or chest.

– burning when you urinate.

– diarrhea.

– muscle cramps.

– nausea.

– pain in your _____.

– se le quite fluido de los pies, tobillos o piernas.

– se le quite fluido de los pulmones para que funcionen mejor.

– se le quite fluido de la páncreas para que funcione mejor.

Este medicamento le ayudará a su cuerpo a:

– destruir la bacteria de la (región infectada).

– reducir el latir del corazón.

– ablandar sus evacuaciones.

– acelerar el latir del corazón.

– usar la insulina más eficazmente.

Este medicamento le ayudará a Ud. a:

– respirar con mayor facilidad.

– luchar contra infecciones.

– relajarse.

– dormir.

– pensar con mayor claridad.

Este medicamento le aliviará o disminuirá:

– la producción de acido en el estómago.

– la angustia.

– espasmos en la vejiga.

– sensación ardiente en el estómago o tórax.

– sensación ardiente al orinar.

– diarrea.

– espasmos en los músculos.

– nausea.

– dolor en la (el) _____.

This medication will help your body to produce more or less:
- antibodies.
- clotting factors.

- insulin.
- platelets.
- red blood cells.
- white blood cells.

Este medicamento le ayudará a su cuerpo a producir más o menos:
- anticuerpos.
- factores o agentes coagulantes.
- insulina.
- plaquetas.
- células rojas de sangre.
- células blancas de sangre.

This medication or treatment will destroy:
- antibodies.
- bacteria.
- cancer cells.
- clotting factors.

- platelets.
- red blood cells.
- white blood cells.

Este medicamento o tratamiento destruirá:
- anticuerpos.
- bacteria.
- células cancerosas.
- factores o agentes coagulantes.
- plaquetas.
- células rojas de sangre.
- células blancas de sangre.

MEDICATION ADMINISTRATION

I would like to give you:
- an injection.
- an I.V. medication.

- a liquid medication.

- a medicated cream or powder.
- a medication through your epidural catheter.
- a medication through your rectum.
- a medication through your _____ tube.
- a medication under your tongue.

Quisiera darle a Ud. un(a):
- inyección.
- medicamento por vía intravenosa.
- medicamento en forma líquida.
- medicamento en pomada o polvo.
- medicamento por el catéter epidural.
- medicamento por el recto.

- medicamento por su _____ tubo.
- medicamento debajo de la lengua.

– some pill(s).
– a suppository.

– píldoras.
– supositorio.

This is how you take this medication.

Así se toma este medicamento.

If you can't swallow this pill, I can crush it and mix it in some food or liquid such as:

Si Ud. no se puede tragar esta píldora, puedo aplastarla y mezclarla en un alimento/líquido, tal como:

– applesauce.
– pudding.
– yogurt.

– puré de manzana.
– pudín.
– yogur.

If you can't swallow this pill, I can get it in another form.

Si Ud. no puede tragarse esta píldora, puede obtenerla en otra forma.

If you can't swallow a pill, you can crush it and mix it in soft food.

Si Ud. no se puede tragar la píldora, la puede moler y mezclarla en un alimento blando.

I need to mix this medication in juice or water.

Tengo que mezclar este medicamento en jugo (zumo) o agua.

I need to give you this injection in your:
– abdomen.
– buttocks.
– hip.
– outer arm.
– thigh.

Tengo que ponerle esta inyección:
– en el abdomen.
– en las nalgas.
– en la cadera.
– en el brazo.
– en el muslo.

I need to give you this medication I.V.

Tengo que darle este medicamento por via intravenosa (I.V.).

Place it under your tongue.

Póngaselo debajo de la lengua.

You should feel some burning when it is under your tongue.

Ud. debiera sentir un ardor cuando se lo pone debajo de la lengua.

This indicates that it is working.

Esto indica que está tomando efecto.

Some medications are coated with a special substance to protect your stomach from getting upset.

Algunos medicamentos están cubiertos con una sustancia especial para protegerle contra un trastorno estomacal.

Do not chew:
  – enteric-coated pills.

  – long-acting pills.

  – capsules.
  – sublingual medication.

No masque Ud.:
  – píldoras con recubrimien-toentérico.
  – píldoras de efecto prolonga-do.
  – cápsulas.
  – medicamentos sublinguales.

Ask your doctor or pharmacist whether you can:
  – mix your medication with food or fluids.

  – take your medication with or without food.

Pregúntele Ud. a su doctor o farmacéutico si debiera:
  – mezclar su medicamento con un alimento o con líquidos.
  – tomar su medicamento con o sin alimento.

You need to take your medication:
  – after meals.
  – before meals.
  – on an empty stomach.
  – with meals or food.

Ud. tiene que tomarse el medicamento:
  – después de las comidas.
  – antes de las comidas.
  – con el estómago vacío.
  – con las comidas o con un alimento.

SKIPPING DOSES

If you skip or miss a dose:

  – Take it as soon as you remember it.

Si Ud. omite o se salta una dosis:

  – Tómesela encuanto se acuerde.

– Wait until the next dose.

– Call the doctor if you are not sure.

– Do not take an extra dose.

– Espérese hasta la siguiente dosis.

– Llame al doctor si Ud. no está seguro(a).

– No se tome una dosis extra.

Adverse effects

Some common adverse effects of _____ are:
- constipation
- diarrhea
- difficulty sleeping
- dry mouth
- fatigue
- headache
- itching
- light-headedness
- nausea
- poor appetite
- rash
- upset stomach
- weight loss or gain
- frequent urination.

Unos efectos adversos comunes a _____ son:
- estreñimiento
- diarrea
- dificultad en dormir
- boca seca
- fatiga
- dolor de cabeza
- comezón (picazón)
- mareo
- nausea
- poco apetito
- erupción
- trastorno estomacal
- perdida o aumento de peso
- orinar con frecuencia.

These adverse effects:
- will go away after your body gets used to the medication.
- may persist as long as you take the medication.

Estos efectos adversos:
- desaparecerán una vez que su cuerpo se acostumbre al medicamento.
- puede continuar mientras Ud. tome el medicamento.

If they bother you, speak to your doctor about changing your medication.

Si le molestan a Ud., hable con su doctor acerca de que le cambie el medicamento.

If you have an adverse reaction to your medication, call your doctor right away.

Si Ud. tiene una reacción adversa a su medicamento, llame a su doctor inmediatamente.

OTHER CONCERNS

Tell your doctor if you are pregnant or breast-feeding.

Dígale a su doctor si Ud. está ebarazada o si cría a los pechos.

While you are taking this medication, ask your doctor if:
- you can safely take other over-the-counter medications.
- you can drink alcoholic beverages.
- your medications interact with each other.

Mientras Ud. tome este medicamento, pregúntele a su doctor si:
- puede tomar otros medicamentos que no necesitan receta.
- puede tomar bebidas alcohólicas.
- sus medicamentos interaccionan uno con el otro.

STORING MEDICATION

You should keep your medication:
- in a cool, dry place.
- in the refrigerator.
- at room temperature.
- out of direct sunlight.
- away from heat.
- away from children.

Ud. debiera guardar sus medicamentos:
- en un lugar fresco, seco.
- en el refrigerador.
- al tiempo.
- fuera de la luz de sol.
- lejos de la calefacción.
- lejos del alcance de los niños.

Do not keep your medication:

- in a warm place or near heat.
- in the sun.
- in your pocket.
- in the bathroom medicine cabinet.

No guarde Ud. su medicamento:

- en un lugar caliente ni cerca de la calefacción.
- en el sol.
- en su bolsillo.
- en el botiquín del baño.

TEACHING A PATIENT TO GIVE A SUBCUTANEOUS INJECTION

To give yourself an injection, follow these steps:
- Draw up the medication.
- Replace the cap carefully.

- Decide where you are going to give the injection.
- Clean the skin area with alcohol.
- Gently pinch up a little skin over the area.
- Using a dartlike motion, stab the needle into your skin.
- Gently pull back on the plunger to see if there is any blood in the syringe.
- Steadily push the medication into your skin.

- Pull the needle out.
- Apply gentle pressure with the alcohol wipe.
- Dispose of the needle in a proper receptacle.

Así es como uno se pone una inyección a sí mismo(a):
- Saque el medicamento.
- Coloque de nuevo la tapa con cuidado.

- Decida Ud. donde va a ponerse la inyección.
- Limpie el área de la piel con alcohol.
- Suavemente pellizque un poco de piel sobre el área.
- Con un movimiento rápido, penetre la aguja en su piel.

- Con cuidado retire el émbolo para ver si hay sangre en la jeringa.
- Constantemente empuje el medicamento dentro de su piel.

- Saque la aguja.
- Ejerza presión suavemente con un limpión de alcohol.
- Deshagase de la aguja en un recipiente apropiado.

INSULIN PREPARATION AND ADMINISTRATION

The doctor has ordered insulin for you.

To draw up insulin, follow these steps:
- Wipe the rubber top of the insulin bottle with alcohol.

- Remove the needle cap.

El doctor ha recetado insulina para Ud.

Para extraer la insulina siga las siguientes pasos:
- Limpie la tapa de hule (goma) de la botella de la insulina con alcohol.
- Quítele el capuchón a la aguja.

– Pull out the plunger until the end of the plunger in the barrel aligns with the number of units of insulin that you need.

– Push the needle through the rubber top of the insulin bottle.

– Inject the air into the bottle.

– Without removing the needle from the bottle, turn it upside down.

– Withdraw the plunger until the end of the plunger aligns with the number of units you need.

– Gently pull the needle out of the bottle.

To mix insulin, follow these steps:

– Wipe the rubber tops of the insulin bottles with alcohol.

– Gently roll the cloudy insulin between your palms.

– Remove the needle cap.

– Pull out the plunger until the end of the plunger in the barrel aligns with the number of units of NPH or Lente insulin that you need.

– Saque el émbolo hasta el otro extremo del émbolo en la cuba esté al nivel de la dosis de insulina (número de unidades) que Ud. necesita.

– Empuje la aguja por la tapa de hule (goma) de la botella de insulina.

– Inyecte el aire dentro de la botella.

– Sin sacar la aguja de la botella, póngala al revés.

– Retire el émbolo hasta que llegue la insulina al número de unidades que Ud. necesita.

– Retire Ud. la aguja de la botella suavemente.

Para mezclar la insulina siga los siguientes pasos:

– Limpie la tapa de hule (goma) de las botellas de insulina con alcohol.

– Suavemente mueva la insulina turbia entre las palmas de la mano.

– Retire el capuchón de la aguja.

– Saque el émbolo hasta que el otro extremo del émbolo en el barril esté al nivel con la dosis de insulina turbia (NPH o insulina Lente) (número de unidades) que Ud. necesita.

- Push the needle through the rubber top of the cloudy insulin bottle.
- Inject the air into the bottle.
- Remove the needle.
- Pull out the plunger until the end of the plunger in the barrel aligns with the number of units of clear regular insulin that you need.
- Push the needle through the rubber top of the clear insulin bottle.
- Inject the air into the bottle.
- Without removing the needle, turn the bottle upside down.
- Withdraw the plunger until it aligns with the number of units of clear regular insulin that you need.
- Gently pull the needle out of the bottle.
- Push the needle into the cloudy (NPH or Lente) insulin without injecting it into the bottle.
- Withdraw the plunger until you reach your total dosage of insulin in units (regular combined with NPH or Lente).
- We will practice again.

- Empuje la aguja por la tapa de goma (hule) de la botella de insulina turbia.
- Inyecte el aire dentro de la botella.
- Saque la aguja.
- Retire el émbolo hasta que el otro extremo del émbolo en el barril esté al nivel con la dosis de insulina clara (regular) (número de unidades) que Ud. necesita.
- Empuje Ud. la aguja por la tapa de goma de la botella de insulna clara.
- Inyecte el aire dentro de la botella.
- Sin sacar la aguja, vuelva la botella al revés.

- Retire el émbolo hasta que llegue a la dosis de insulina (regular) clara (número de unidades) que Ud. necesita.
- Suavemente saque Ud. la aguja de la botella.
- Empuje la aguja en la insulina turbia (NPH o insulina Lente) sin inyectarla dentro de la botella.
- Retire el émbolo hasta que llegue a su dosis total de insulina en unidades (regular y NPH/Lente conbinadas).

- Practicaremos juntos(as) otra vez.

HOME CARE PHRASES

Wash your hands before touching medications.

Lávese Ud. las manos antes de tocar los medicamentos.

Check the medication bottle for name, dose, and frequency (how often it's supposed to be taken).

En el envase del medicamento verifique Ud. el nombre, la dosis, y la frecuencia (con que frequencia se debe tomar).

Check the expiration date on all medications.

Verifique Ud. la fecha en la que el medicamento expira.

Store medications according to pharmacy instructions.

Guarde Ud. los medicamentos según las instrucciones de la farmacia.

Under adequate lighting, read medication labels carefully before taking doses.

Bajo luz adecuada, lea Ud. la etiqueta del medicamento con mucho cuidado antes de tomar las dosis.

Don't crush medication without first asking the doctor or pharmacist.

No machaque Ud. el medicamento sin antes preguntárselo al doctor o al farmacéutico.

Contact your doctor if a new or unexpected symptom or another problem appears.

Póngase Ud. en contacto con su doctor si un síntoma nuevo o inesperado u otros problemas aparecen.

Do not stop taking medication unless instructed by your doctor.

No deje Ud. de tomar el medicamento sólo que se lo ordene su doctor.

Discard outdated medications.

Deshágase Ud. de medicamentos caducos.

Never take someone else's medications.

Nunca tome Ud. los medicamentos de otra persona.

Keep a record of your current medications.

Apunte Ud. (tome nota de) sus medicamentos actuales.

GENERAL DRUG THERAPY PHRASES

DRUG CLASSES

Analgesic	Analgésico
Anesthetic	Anestético
Antacid	Antiácido
Antianginal agent	Agente antianginal
Antianxiety agent	Agente ansiolítico
Antiarrhythmic agent	Agente antiarrítmico
Antibiotic	Antibiótico
Anticancer agent	Agente anticarcinógeno
Anticoagulant	Anticoagulante
Anticonvulsant	Anticonvulsivante
Antidepressant	Antidepresivo
Antidiarrheal	Antidiarreico
Antifungal agent	Agente antifúngico
Antigout agent	Agente antigota
Antihistamine	Antihistamínico
Antihyperlipemic agent	Agente hiperlipémico
Antihypertensive agent	Agente antihipertenso
Anti-inflammatory agent	Agente antiinflamatorio
Antimalarial agent	Agente antimalárico
Antiparkinsonian agent	Agente antiparkinsoniano
Antipsychotic agent	Agente antipsicótico
Antipyretic	Antipirético
Antiseptic	Antiséptico

Antispasmodic	Antiespasmódico
Antithyroid agent	Agente antitiroideo
Antituberculosis agent	Agente antituberculoso
Antitussive agent	Agente antitusígeno
Antiviral agent	Agente antiviral
Appetite stimulant	Estimulante para el apetito
Appetite suppressant	Supresor de apetito
Bronchodilator	Broncodilatador
Decongestant	Descongestivo
Digestant	Digestivo (agente que estimula la digestión)
Diuretic	Diurético
Emetic	Emético
Fertility agent	Agente para la fertilidad
Hypnotic	Hipnótico
Insulin	Insulina
Laxative	Laxante
Muscle relaxant	Relajante de músculos
Oral contraceptive	Anticonceptivo oral
Oral hypoglycemic agent	Agente hipoglucémico oral
Sedative	Sedante
Steroid	Esteroide
Thyroid hormone	Hormona de la glándula tiroides
Vaccine	Vacuna
Vasodilator	Vasodilatador
Vitamin	Vitamina

Routes

Intradermal	Intradérmica
Intramuscular	Intramuscular
Intravenous	Intravenosa
Oral	Oral
Rectal	Rectal
Subcutaneous	Subcutánea
Topical	Tópica
Vaginal	Vaginal

Preparations

Capsule	Cápsula
Cream	Pomada
Drops	Gotas
Elixir	Elixir
Inhaler	Inhalador
Injection	Inyección
Lotion	Loción
Lozenge	Pastilla
Powder	Polvo
Spray	Atomizador
Suppository	Supositorio
Suspension	Suspensión
Syrup	Jarabe
Tablet	Tableta

FREQUENCY

Once daily	Una vez al día
Twice daily	Dos veces al día
Three times daily	Tres veces al día
Four times daily	Cuatro veces al día
In the morning	Por la mañana
With meals	Con las comidas
Before meals	Antes de las comidas
After meals	Después de las comidas
Before bedtime	Antes de acostarse
When you have _____	Cuando Ud. tome _____
Only when you need it	Sólo cuando lo necesite
Every four hours	Cada cuatro horas
Every six hours	Cada seis horas
Every eight hours	Cada ocho horas

To perform drug and I.V. fluid calculations, you need to understand drug weights and measures and know how to convert between systems and measures, compute drug dosages, perform special calculations, and make dosage adjustments for children.

SYSTEMS OF DRUG WEIGHTS AND MEASURES

The two most common systems of measurement used to prescribe drugs are the metric and the household systems. These are so widely used that most brands of medication cups for liquid measurements are calibrated in both systems. A third system, the apothecaries' system, is no longer popular, but you may encounter it occasionally. Other special systems of measurement are used for selected drugs.

Metric system

The metric system is the international system of measurement, the most widely used system, and the system used by the U.S. Pharmacopeia. This system offers many advantages. It enables accurate calculations of small drug dosages. It uses Arabic numerals, which are commonly used by prescribers worldwide. Plus, it's used by most manufacturers to calibrate newly developed drugs.

The metric system includes units for liquid and solid measures. These measurements offer relative ease of conversion within the metric system. (See *Metric measures*, page 148.)

LIQUID MEASURES
In the metric system, 1 liter (L) is about equal to 1 quart in the household system. Liters commonly are used for ordering and administering I.V. solutions. Milliliters (ml) typically are used for parenteral and some oral drugs.

METRIC MEASURES

METRIC WEIGHT EQUIVALENTS

1 kilogram (kg or Kg)	=	1,000 grams (g)
1 gram	=	1,000 milligrams (mg)
1 milligram	=	1,000 micrograms (mcg)
0.6 g	=	600 mg
0.3 g	=	300 mg
0.1 g	=	100 mg
0.06 g	=	60 mg
0.03 g	=	30 mg
0.015 g	=	15 mg
0.001 g	=	1 mg

METRIC VOLUME EQUIVALENTS

1 liter (l or L)	=	1,000 milliliters (ml)
1 milliliter	=	1,000 microliters (mcl)

METRIC WEIGHT CONVERSIONS

Household		Metric
1 oz	=	30 grams
1 lb	=	453.6 grams
2.2 lb	=	1 kilogram

METRIC VOLUME CONVERSIONS

Household		Metric
1 teaspoon (tsp)	=	5 ml
1 tablespoon (T or tbs)	=	15 ml
2 tablespoons	=	30 ml
8 ounces	=	240 ml
1 pint (pt)	=	473 ml
1 quart (qt)	=	946 ml
1 gallon (gal)	=	3,785 ml

SOLID MEASURES

The gram (g) is the basis for solid measures or units of weight in the metric system. Drugs commonly are ordered in grams (g), milligrams (mg), or micrograms (mcg). One milligram equals 1/1000 of a gram; 1 microgram equals 1/1000 of a milligram. Body weight usually is recorded in kilograms (kg). One kilogram equals 1,000 grams.

The following sample drug orders use the metric system:

■ 30 ml milk of magnesia P.O. h.s.

■ Ancef 1 g I.V. q 6 hours

■ Lanoxin 0.125 mg P.O. daily.

Household system

Most foods, recipes, over-the-counter drugs, and home remedies use the household system. Prescribers use this system less commonly than the metric system for ordering drugs. However, your knowledge of household measures may be useful in some situations.

LIQUID MEASURES

Liquid measurements in the household system include the teaspoon (commonly abbreviated tsp) and the tablespoon (commonly abbreviated either tbs or T). For drug purposes, these measurements have been standardized to 5 ml and 15 ml, respectively. Using these standardized amounts, 3 teaspoons equal 1 tablespoon, and 6 teaspoons equal 1 ounce (oz). Patients who need to measure doses by teaspoon or tablespoon should use a calibrated device to make sure they receive exactly the prescribed amount. They shouldn't use an ordinary household teaspoon to measure a teaspoon of a drug because the amount is likely to be inaccurate. Household teaspoon sizes vary from 4 to 6 ml or more.

The following sample drug orders use the household system:

■ 2 tsp Bactrim P.O. b.i.d.
■ Riopan 2 tbs P.O. 1 hour a.c. and h.s.

Apothecaries' system

Two features distinguish the apothecaries' system from other systems: the use of Roman numerals and the placement of the unit of measurement before the Roman numeral. For example, a measurement of 5 grains would be written as *grains V*.

In the apothecaries' system, equivalents among the various units of measure are close approximations of one another. By contrast, equivalents in the metric system are exact. When using apothecaries' equivalents for

calculations and conversions, the calculations aren't precise but fall within acceptable standards.

The apothecaries' system is the only system of measurement that uses symbols and abbreviations to represent units of measure. Although this system is infrequently used in health care, you need to be able to read dosages that are written in it and convert them to the metric system.

LIQUID MEASURES

The smallest unit of liquid measurement in the apothecaries' system is the minim, which is about the size of a drop of water. Fifteen to sixteen minims equal about 1 ml.

SOLID MEASURES

The grain (gr) is the smallest solid measure or unit of weight in the apothecaries' system. It equals about 60 mg. One dram equals about 60 gr.

The following sample drug order uses the apothecaries' system: Tylenol gr X P.O. q 4 hours p.r.n. for headache.

Special systems

For some drugs, you'll need to use a special system of measurement developed by the drug manufacturer. Three of the most common special systems are units, international units, and milliequivalents.

UNITS

Insulin is one of several drugs measured in units. Once commonly abbreviated "U," units should no longer be abbreviated because doing so can contribute to serious medication errors. Although many types of insulin exist, all are measured in units. The international standard of U-100 insulin means that 1 ml of insulin solution contains 100 units of insulin, regardless of type. The anticoagulant heparin is also measured in units. So are several antibiotics, which are available in liquid, solid, and powder forms for oral or parenteral use.

The unit isn't a standard measure. That's why different drugs measured in units may have no relationship to one another in quality or activity. That's also why each drug manufacturer provides specific information about measuring each drug that's given in units.

The following sample drug orders use units:
- 14 units NPH insulin S.C. this a.m.
- heparin 5,000 units S.C. q 12 hours.

- nystatin 200,000 units P.O. q 6 hours.

INTERNATIONAL UNITS

International units are used to measure biologicals, such as vitamins, enzymes, and hormones. For instance, the activity of calcitonin, a synthetic hormone used to regulate calcium, is expressed in international units. Once commonly abbreviated "IU," international units should no longer be abbreviated so that the abbreviation is not mistaken for "I.V."

The following sample drug orders use international units:
- 100 international units calcitonin (salmon) S.C. daily
- 8 international units somatropin S.C. three times per week.

MILLIEQUIVALENTS

Electrolytes may be measured in milliequivalents (mEq). Drug manufacturers provide information about the number of metric units needed to provide a prescribed number of milliequivalents. Potassium chloride (KCl), for example, is usually ordered in milliequivalents.

The following sample drug orders use milliequivalents:
- 30 mEq KCl P.O. b.i.d.

■ 1 L dextrose 5% in normal saline solution with 40 mEq KCl to be run at 125 ml/hour.

CONVERSIONS BETWEEN MEASUREMENT SYSTEMS

Sometimes you need to convert from one measurement system to another, particularly when a drug is prescribed in one system but only available in another system. To perform conversion calculations, you need to know the equivalents for the different measurement systems.

For a simple conversion, you may be able to use the standard equivalent, as shown earlier in *Metric measures*. For a more complex conversion, you may employ the equivalent and the fraction method, which is the most commonly used technique for converting between measurement systems.

Fraction method

For measurement conversions, the fraction method involves an equation consisting of two fractions. Set up the first fraction by placing the ordered dosage over the unknown (x) units of the available dosage.

For example, say a prescriber orders 7.5 ml of acetaminophen elixir to be given by mouth. To find the equivalent in teaspoons, first set up a fraction in which the milliliter dosage represents the ordered dosage and the teaspoon dosage represents the unknown available dosage:

$$\frac{7.5 \text{ ml}}{x \text{ tsp}}$$

Then set up the second fraction, which appears on the right side of the equation. This fraction consists of the standard equivalents between the ordered and the available measures. Because milliliters must be converted to teaspoons, the right side of the equation appears as:

$$\frac{5 \text{ ml}}{1 \text{ tsp}}$$

The same unit of measure should appear in the numerator of both fractions. Likewise, the same unit of measure should appear in both denominators. The entire equation should appear as:

$$\frac{7.5 \text{ ml}}{x \text{ tsp}} \times \frac{5 \text{ ml}}{1 \text{ tsp}}$$

To solve for x, you'll need to cross multiply.

$$x \text{ tsp} \times 5 \text{ ml} = 7.5 \text{ ml} \times 1 \text{ tsp}$$

$$x \text{ tsp} = \frac{7.5 \text{ ml} \times 1 \text{ tsp}}{5 \text{ ml}}$$

$$x \text{ tsp} = \frac{7.5 \times 1 \text{ tsp}}{5}$$

$$x \text{ tsp} = 1.5 \text{ tsp}$$

The patient should receive 1.5 tsp of acetaminophen elixir.

COMPUTATION OF DRUG DOSAGES

After verifying a drug order, you can compute the drug dosage. In this two-step process, first determine whether the ordered drug is available in units of the same measurement system. If it's not, convert the ordered drug measurement to the system used for the available drug, as previously described.

If the ordered units of measurement are available, move to step two: Calculate how much of the available dosage form should be given. For example, if the prescribed dose is 250 mg, determine the quantity of tablets, powder, or liquid that equals 250 mg. To determine that quantity, use the fraction, ratio, or desired-available method or dimensional analysis.

Fraction method

When using the fraction method to compute a drug dosage, write an equation consisting of two fractions. First, set up a fraction showing the number of units to be given over x, which represents the quantity of the dosage form.

On the other side of the equation, set up a fraction showing the number of units of the drug in its dosage form over the quantity of dosage forms that supply that number of units. The number of units and the quantity of dosage forms are specific for each drug. In most cases, the stated quantity equals 1. Information on the drug label should supply the details you need to form the second fraction.

For example, if the number of units to be given equals 250 mg, the first fraction in the equation is:

$$\frac{250 \text{ mg}}{x \text{ tab}}$$

The drug label states that each tablet contains 125 mg. So the second fraction is:

$$\frac{125 \text{ mg}}{1 \text{ tab}}$$

Note that the same units of measure appear in the numerators and the same units appear in the denominators. However, the units of measure in the denominators differ from the units in the numerators.

The entire equation should appear as:

$$\frac{250 \text{ mg}}{x \text{ tab}} = \frac{125 \text{ mg}}{1 \text{ tab}}$$

Solving for x determines the quantity of the dosage form, which is 2 tablets in this example.

Ratio method

To use the ratio method, write the amount of the drug to be given and the quantity of the dose (x) as a ratio. Using the previous example, you'd write:

$$250 \text{ mg} : x \text{ tab}$$

Next, complete the equation by forming a second ratio with the number of units in each tablet (or appropriate dosage form), which is listed on the manufacturer's label. Again using the example from above, the entire equation is:

$$250 \text{ mg} : x \text{ tab} :: 125 \text{ mg} : 1 \text{ tab}$$

To solve for x, set up an equation in which the product of the means (inner portions of the ratio) equals the product of the extremes (outer portions).

$$x \text{ tab} \times 125 \text{ mg} = 250 \text{ mg} \times 1 \text{ tab}$$

$$x \text{ tab} = \frac{250 \text{ mg} \times 1 \text{ tab}}{125 \text{ mg}}$$

$$x = 2 \text{ tab}$$

The patient should receive 2 tablets.

Desired-available method

Also called the dose over on-hand (D/H) method, the desired-available method lets you convert ordered units into available units and compute the drug dosage all in one step. The desired-available equation appears as:

x quantity to give =

$$\frac{\dfrac{\text{ordered}}{\text{units}}}{1} \times \frac{\text{conversion}}{\text{fraction}} \times \frac{\text{quantity of dosage form}}{\text{stated quantity of drug within each dosage form}}$$

For example, suppose you receive an order for gr X (10 gr) of a drug. The drug is available only in 300-mg tablets. To determine the number of tablets to give the patient, substitute gr X (the ordered number of units) for the first element of the equation. Then use the conversion fraction as the second portion of the formula. The conversion factor is:

$$\frac{60 \text{ mg}}{1 \text{ gr}}$$

The measure in the denominator must be the same as the measure in the ordered units. Because the order specified gr X, grains appears in the denominator of the conversion fraction.

The third element of the equation shows the dosage form over the stated drug quantity for that dosage form. Because the drug is available in 300-mg tablets, the fraction is:

$$\frac{1 \text{ tab}}{300 \text{ mg}}$$

The dosage form (in this case, tablets) should always appear in the numerator, and the quantity of drug in each dosage form should always appear in the denominator. The completed equation is:

$$x \text{ tab} = 10 \text{ gr} \times \frac{60 \text{ mg}}{1 \text{ gr}} \times \frac{1 \text{ tab}}{300 \text{ mg}}$$

Solving for x shows that the patient should receive 2 tablets.

The desired-available method has the advantage of using only one equation. However, it requires you to memorize a more elaborate equation than the one used in the fraction or ratio methods. Relying on your

memory of a more complicated equation may increase the chance of error.

Dimensional analysis

A variation of the ratio method, dimensional analysis (also called factor analysis or factor labeling) eliminates the need to memorize formulas and requires only one equation to determine the answer. To compare the two methods at a glance, read the following problem and solutions.

Suppose a prescriber orders 0.25 g of streptomycin sulfate I.M. The vial reads 2 ml = 1 g. How many milliliters should you give?

Dimensional analysis

$$\frac{0.25 \text{ g}}{1} \times \frac{2 \text{ ml}}{1 \text{g}} = 0.5 \text{ ml}$$

Ratio method

$$1 \text{ g} : 2 \text{ ml} :: 0.25 \text{ g} : x \text{ ml}$$
$$x = 2 \times 0.25$$
$$x = 0.5 \text{ ml}$$

When using dimensional analysis, you arrange a series of ratios, called factors, in a single (although sometimes lengthy) fractional equation. Each factor, written as a fraction, consists of two quantities and their related units of measurement. For instance, if 1,000 ml of a drug should be given over 8 hours, the relationship between 1,000 and 8 hours is expressed by the fraction

$$\frac{1{,}000 \text{ ml}}{8 \text{ hours}}$$

When a problem includes a quantity and a unit of measurement that are unrelated to any other factor in the problem, they serve as the numerator of the fraction, and 1 (implied) becomes the denominator.

Some mathematical problems contain all of the information needed to identify the factors, set up the equation, and find the solution. Other problems require the use of a conversion factor. Conversion factors are equivalents (for example, 1 g = 1,000 mg) that you can memorize or obtain from a conversion chart, such as the *Metric measures* included earlier in the chapter. Because the two quantities and units of measurement are equivalent, they can serve as the numerator or the denominator; thus, the conversion factor 1 g = 1,000 mg can be written in fraction form as

$$\frac{1{,}000 \text{ mg}}{1 \text{ g}} \quad \text{or} \quad \frac{1 \text{ g}}{1{,}000 \text{ mg}}$$

The factors given in the problem plus the conversion factors needed to solve the problem are called *knowns*. The quantity of the answer, of course, is *unknown*. When setting up an equation in dimensional analysis, work backward, beginning with the unit of measurement of the answer. After plotting all the knowns, find the solution by following this sequence:

- Cancel similar quantities and units of measurement.
- Multiply the numerators.
- Multiply the denominators.
- Divide the numerator by the denominator.

Mastering dimensional analysis can take practice, but you may find your efforts well rewarded. To understand more fully how dimensional analysis works, review the following problem and the steps taken to solve it.

A prescriber orders gr X of a drug. The pharmacy supplies the drug in 300-mg tablets (tab). How many tablets should you administer?

- Write down the unit of measurement of the answer, followed by an "equal to" symbol.

$$\text{tab} =$$

- Search the problem for the quantity with the same unit of measurement (if one doesn't exist, use a conversion factor). Place this quantity in the numerator and its related quantity and unit of measurement in the denominator.

$$tab = \frac{1 \text{ tab}}{300 \text{ mg}}$$

■ Separate the first factor from the next with a multiplication symbol.

$$tab = \frac{1 \text{ tab}}{300 \text{ mg}} \times$$

■ Place the unit of measurement of the denominator of the first factor in the numerator of the second factor. Then search the problem for the quantity with the same unit of measurement (if one doesn't exist, as in this example, use a conversion factor). Now place this quantity in the numerator and its related quantity and unit of measurement in the denominator, and follow with a multiplication symbol. Repeat this step until all known factors are included in the equation.

$$tab = \frac{1 \text{ tab}}{300 \text{ mg}} \times \frac{60 \text{ mg}}{1 \text{ gr}} \times \frac{10 \text{ gr}}{1}$$

■ Treat the equation as a large fraction. First, cancel similar units of measurement in the numerator and the denominator. (What remains should be what you began with—the unit of measurement of the answer. If not, recheck your equation to find and correct the error.)

Next, multiply the numerators and then the denominators. Finally, divide the numerator by the denominator.

$$tab = \frac{1 \text{ tab}}{300 \text{ mg}} \times \frac{60 \text{ mg}}{1 \text{ gr}} \times \frac{10 \text{ gr}}{1}$$

$$= \frac{60 \times 10 \text{ tab}}{300}$$

$$= \frac{600 \text{ tab}}{300}$$

$$= 2 \text{ tab}$$

For more practice, study the following examples, which use dimensional analysis to solve various mathematical problems common to dosage calculations and drug administration.

1. A patient weighs 140 lb. What is his weight in kg?

Unit of measurement of the answer: kg

1st factor (conversion factor):

$$\frac{1 \text{ kg}}{2.2 \text{ lb}}$$

2nd factor: $\dfrac{140 \text{ lb}}{1}$

$$kg = \frac{1 \text{ kg} \times 140 \text{ lb}}{2.2 \text{ lb}}$$

$$kg = \frac{140}{2.2}$$

$$x = 63.6 \text{ kg}$$

2. A prescriber orders 75 mg of a drug. The pharmacy stocks a mul-

tidose vial containing 100 mg/ml. How many milliliters should you administer?

Unit of measurement of the answer: ml

1st factor: $\dfrac{1 \text{ ml}}{100 \text{ mg}}$

2nd factor: $\dfrac{75 \text{ mg}}{1}$

$$\text{ml} = \frac{1 \text{ ml}}{100 \text{ mg}} \times \frac{75 \text{ mg}}{1}$$

$$= \frac{75 \text{ ml}}{100}$$

$$= 0.75 \text{ ml}$$

3. A prescriber orders 1 tsp of a cough elixir. The pharmacist sends up a bottle whose label reads 1 ml = 50 mg. How many milligrams should you administer?

Unit of measurement of the answer: mg

1st factor: $\dfrac{50 \text{ mg}}{1 \text{ ml}}$

2nd factor (conversion factor): $\dfrac{5 \text{ ml}}{1 \text{ tsp}}$

3rd factor: $\dfrac{1 \text{ tsp}}{1}$

$$\text{mg} = \frac{50 \text{ mg}}{1 \text{ ml}} \times \frac{5 \text{ ml}}{1 \text{ tsp}} \times \frac{1 \text{ tsp}}{1}$$

$$= \frac{50 \text{ mg} \times 5}{1}$$

$$= 250 \text{ mg}$$

4. A prescriber orders 1,000 ml of an I.V. solution to be administered over 8 hours. The I.V. tubing delivers 15 drops (gtt)/ml/minute. What is the infusion rate in gtt/minute?

Unit of measurement of the answer: gtt/minute

1st factor: $\dfrac{15 \text{ gtt}}{\text{ml}}$

2nd factor: $\dfrac{1,000 \text{ ml}}{8 \text{ hr}}$

3rd factor (conversion factor): $\dfrac{1 \text{ hr}}{60 \text{ min}}$

$$\text{gtt/minute} = \frac{15 \text{ gtt}}{1 \text{ ml}} \times \frac{1,000 \text{ ml}}{8 \text{ hr}} \times \frac{1 \text{ hr}}{60 \text{ min}}$$

$$\text{gtt/minute} = \frac{15 \text{ gtt} \times 1,000 \times 1}{8 \times 60 \text{ min}}$$

$$= \frac{15,000 \text{ gtt}}{480 \text{ min}}$$

$$= 31.3 \text{ or } 31 \text{ gtt/min}$$

5. A prescriber orders 10,000 units of heparin added to 500 ml of D_5W at 1,200 units/hour. How many drops per minute should you administer if the I.V. tubing delivers 10 gtt/ml?

Unit of measurement of the answer: gtt/minute

1st factor: $\dfrac{10 \text{ gtt}}{1 \text{ ml}}$

2nd factor: $\dfrac{500 \text{ ml}}{10,000 \text{ units}}$

3rd factor: $\dfrac{1,200 \text{ units}}{1 \text{ hour}}$

4th factor (conversion factor):

$$\dfrac{1 \text{ hr}}{60 \text{ minutes}}$$

gtt/minute =

$$\dfrac{10 \text{ gtt}}{1 \text{ ml}} \times \dfrac{500 \text{ ml}}{10,000 \text{ units}} \times \dfrac{1,200 \text{ units}}{1 \text{ hr}} \times \dfrac{1 \text{ hr}}{60 \text{ min}}$$

gtt/minute = $\dfrac{10 \times 500 \times 1,200 \text{ gtt}}{10,000 \times 60 \text{ min}}$

$= \dfrac{6,000,000 \text{ gtt}}{600,000 \text{ min}}$

$= 10 \text{ gtt/min}$

Special computations

You can use the fraction, ratio, and desired-available methods and dimensional analysis to compute drug dosages when the ordered drug and the available form of the drug occur in the same units of measure. You can also use these methods when the quantity of a particular dosage form differs from the units in which the dosage form is given.

For example, if a patient is to receive 1,000 mg of a drug available in liquid form and measured in milligrams, with 100 mg contained in 6 ml, how many milliliters should the patient receive? Because the ordered and the available dosages are in milligrams, you don't need to make conversions first. Rather, you can simply use the fraction method to determine the number of milliliters the patient should receive, which is 60 ml in this case.

Because the drug is to be given in ounces, you should determine the number of ounces using a conversion method. For the fraction method of conversion, the equation would appear as:

$$\dfrac{60 \text{ ml}}{x \text{ oz}} = \dfrac{30 \text{ ml}}{1 \text{ oz}}$$

Solving for x shows that the patient should receive 2 oz of the drug.

To use the desired-available method, change the order of the elements in the equation to correspond with the situation. The revised equation is:

$$x \text{ quantity to give} =$$

$$\frac{\text{ordered units}}{1} \times \frac{\text{quantity of dosage form}}{\substack{\text{stated quantity of} \\ \text{drug within each} \\ \text{dosage form}}}$$

$$\times \text{ conversion fraction}$$

Placing the given information into the equation results in:

$$x \text{ oz} = \frac{1,000 \text{ mg}}{1} \times \frac{6 \text{ ml}}{100 \text{ mg}} \times \frac{1 \text{ oz}}{30 \text{ ml}}$$

Solving for x shows that the patient should receive 2 oz of the drug.

Inexact nature of dosage computations

Converting drug measurements from one system to another and then determining the amount of a dosage form to give can easily produce inexact dosages. A rounding error during computation or discrepancies in the dosage may occur, depending on the conversion standard used in calculation. Or, you may determine a precise amount to be given, only to find that administering that amount is impossible. For example, precise computations may indicate that a patient should receive 0.97 tablet. Administering such an amount is impossible.

To help avoid calculation errors and discrepancies between theoretical and real dosages, follow this general rule: *No more than a 10% variation should exist between the dosage ordered and the dosage to be given.* Following this simple rule, if your calculations show that a patient should receive 0.97 tablet, you can safely give 1 tablet.

Computing parenteral dosages

The methods for computing oral drug dosages can also be used for parenteral dosages. The following example shows how to determine a parenteral drug dosage. Suppose a prescriber orders 75 mg of Demerol. The package label reads: meperidine (Demerol), 100 mg/ml. Using the fraction method to determine the number of milliliters the patient should receive, the equation is:

$$\frac{75 \text{ mg}}{x \text{ ml}} = \frac{100 \text{ mg}}{1 \text{ ml}}$$

To solve for x, cross multiply:

$$x \text{ ml} \times 100 \text{ mg} = 75 \text{ mg} \times 1 \text{ ml}$$

$$x \text{ ml} = \frac{75 \text{ mg} \times 1 \text{ ml}}{100 \text{ mg}}$$

$$x \text{ ml} = \frac{75 \text{ ml}}{100}$$

$$x = 0.75 \text{ ml}$$

The patient should receive 0.75 ml.

Reconstituting powders for injection

Although a pharmacist usually reconstitutes powders for parenteral use, nurses sometimes perform this function by following the directions on the drug label. To do this, first consult the drug label. The label gives the total quantity of drug in the vial or ampule, the amount and type of diluent to be added to the powder, and the strength and expiration date of the resulting solution. When you add diluent to a powder, the powder increases the fluid volume. That's why the label calls for less diluent than the total volume of the prepared solution. For example, a label may say to add 1.7 ml of diluent to a vial of powdered drug to obtain a 2-ml total volume of prepared solution.

Next, determine the amount of solution to administer using the manufacturer's information about the concentration of the solution. For example, if you want to administer 500 mg of a drug and the concentration of the prepared solution is 1 g (1,000 mg)/10 ml, use the following equation:

$$\frac{500 \text{ mg}}{x \text{ ml}} = \frac{1,000 \text{ mg}}{10 \text{ ml}}$$

The patient should receive 5 ml of the prepared solution.

I.V. drip rates and flow rates

Before you can calculate I.V. drip rates and flow rates, make sure you know the difference between them. The drip rate refers to the number of drops of solution to be infused per minute. The flow rate refers to the number of milliliters of fluid to be infused over 1 hour.

To calculate an I.V. drip rate, first set up a fraction showing the volume of solution to be delivered over the number of minutes in which that volume should be infused. For example, if a patient should receive 100 ml of solution in 1 hour, the fraction is:

$$\frac{100 \text{ ml}}{60 \text{ min}}$$

Next, multiply the fraction by the drip factor (the number of drops contained in 1 ml) to determine the drip rate. The drip factor varies among different I.V. sets and should appear on the package that contains the I.V. tubing administration set. Following the manufacturer's directions for drip factor is a crucial step. Standard administration sets have drip factors of

10, 15, or 20 gtt/ml. A microdrip (minidrip) set has a drip factor of 60 gtt/ml.

Use the following equation to determine the drip rate of an I.V. solution:

$$\text{gtt/min} = \frac{\text{total no. of ml}}{\text{total no. of min}} \times \text{drip factor}$$

The equation applies to I.V. solutions that infuse over many hours or to small-volume infusions, such as those used for antibiotics, usually given in less than 1 hour. For example, if an order requires 1,000 ml of 5% dextrose in normal saline solution to infuse over 12 hours and if the administration set delivers 15 gtt/ml, what should the drip rate be?

$$x\,\text{gtt/min} = \frac{1,000\text{ ml} \times 15\text{ gtt/ml}}{720\text{ min}}$$

$$x\,\text{gtt/min} = 20.83\text{ gtt/min}$$

The drip rate can be rounded to 21 gtt/minute.

You'll calculate flow rates when working with I.V. infusion pumps to set the number of milliliters to be delivered in 1 hour. To perform this calculation, you need to know the total volume (in milliliters) to be infused and the amount of time required for the infusion. Use the following equation:

$$\text{flow rate} = \frac{\text{total volume ordered}}{\text{number of hours}}$$

QUICK METHODS FOR CALCULATING DRIP RATES

Quicker methods exist for computing I.V. solution administration rates. To administer an I.V. solution with a microdrip set, adjust the flow rate (number of milliliters per hour) to equal the drip rate (number of drops per minute). To do this, divide the flow rate by 60 minutes and then multiply by the drip factor, which also equals 60. Because the flow rate and the drip factor are equal, the two arithmetic operations cancel each other out. For example, if the ordered flow rate were 125 ml/hour, the equation would be:

$$\text{drip rate (125)} = \frac{125\text{ ml} \times 60}{60\text{ min}}$$

Rather than spend time calculating the equation, you can simply use the number assigned to the flow rate as the drip rate.

For I.V. administration sets that deliver 15 gtt/ml, divide the flow rate by 4 to get the drip rate. For sets with a drip factor of 10 gtt/ml, divide the flow rate by 6 to find the drip rate.

Critical care calculations

On the critical care unit, many drugs are used to treat acute, life-threatening problems. This means that you must be able to perform calculations swiftly and accurately, prepare and infuse the drug, and then observe the patient closely to evaluate its effectiveness. Before administering a critical care drug, you must calculate the drug's concentration in an I.V. solution, the flow rate needed to deliver the desired dose, and the required dosage.

CALCULATING CONCENTRATION

To calculate the drug's concentration, use the following formula:

$$\text{concentration in mg/ml} = \frac{\text{mg of drug}}{\text{ml of fluid}}$$

To express the concentration in mcg/ml, multiply the answer by 1,000.

CALCULATING FLOW RATE

To determine the I.V. flow rate per minute, use the following formula:

$$\frac{\text{dose/min}}{x \text{ ml/min}} = \frac{\text{concentration of solution}}{1 \text{ ml of fluid}}$$

To calculate the hourly flow rate, first multiply the ordered dose, given in milligrams or micrograms per minute, by 60 minutes to determine the hourly dose. Then use the following equation to compute the hourly flow rate:

$$\frac{\text{hourly dose}}{x \text{ ml/hr}} = \frac{\text{concentration of solution}}{1 \text{ ml of fluid}}$$

CALCULATING DOSAGE

To determine the dosage in milligrams per kilogram of body weight per minute, first determine the concentration of the solution in milligrams per milliliter. (If a drug is ordered in micrograms, convert milligrams to micrograms by multiplying by 1,000.) To determine the dose in milligrams per hour, multiply the hourly flow rate by the concentration, using this formula:

$$\text{dose in mg/hr} = \text{hourly flow rate} \times \text{concentration}$$

Then calculate the dose in milligrams per minute. Divide the hourly dose by 60 minutes:

$$\text{dose in mg/min} = \frac{\text{dose in mg/hr}}{60 \text{ min}}$$

Divide the dose per minute by the patient's weight, using the following formula:

$$mg/kg/min = \frac{mg/min}{\text{patient's weight in kg}}$$

Finally, make sure that the drug is being given within a safe and therapeutic range. Compare the amount in milligrams per kilogram per minute to the safe range shown in a drug reference book.

The following examples show how to calculate an I.V. flow rate using the different formulas.

Example 1
A patient has frequent runs of ventricular tachycardia that subside after 10 to 12 beats. The prescriber orders 2 g (2,000 mg) of lidocaine in 500 ml of D_5W to infuse at 2 mg/minute. What's the flow rate in milliliters per minute? In milliliters per hour?

First, find the concentration of the solution by setting up a proportion with the unknown concentration in one fraction and the ordered dose in the other fraction:

$$\frac{x \text{ mg}}{1 \text{ ml}} = \frac{2,000 \text{ mg}}{500 \text{ ml}}$$

Cross multiply the fractions:

x mg × 500 ml = 2,000 mg × 1 ml

Solve for x by dividing each side of the equation by 500 ml and canceling units that appear in both the numerator and denominator:

$$\frac{x \text{ mg} \times \cancel{500 \text{ ml}}}{\cancel{500 \text{ ml}}} = \frac{2,000 \text{ mg} \times 1 \cancel{\text{ ml}}}{500 \cancel{\text{ ml}}}$$

$$x = \frac{2,000 \text{ mg}}{500}$$

$$x = 4 \text{ mg}$$

The concentration of the solution is 4 mg/ml. Next, calculate the flow rate per minute needed to deliver the ordered dose of 2 mg/minute. To do this, set up a proportion with the unknown flow rate per minute in one fraction and the concentration of the solution in the other fraction:

$$\frac{2 \text{ mg}}{x \text{ ml}} = \frac{4 \text{ mg}}{1 \text{ ml}}$$

Cross multiply the fractions:

x ml × 4 mg = 1 ml × 2 mg

Solve for x by dividing each side of the equation by 4 mg and canceling units that appear in both the numerator and denominator:

$$\frac{x \text{ mg} \times \cancel{4 \text{ mg}}}{\cancel{4 \text{ mg}}} = \frac{1 \text{ ml} \times 2 \cancel{\text{ mg}}}{4 \cancel{\text{ mg}}}$$

$$x = \frac{2 \text{ ml}}{4}$$

$$x = 0.5 \text{ ml}$$

The patient should receive 0.5 ml/minute of lidocaine. Because lidocaine must be given with an infusion pump, compute the hourly flow rate. Set up a proportion with the unknown flow rate per hour in one fraction and the flow rate per minute in the other fraction:

$$\frac{x \text{ ml}}{60 \text{ min}} = \frac{0.5 \text{ ml}}{1 \text{ min}}$$

Cross multiply the fractions:

x ml × 1 min = 0.5 ml × 60 min

Solve for x by dividing each side of the equation by 1 minute and canceling units that appear in the numerator and denominator:

$$\frac{x \text{ ml} \times \cancel{1 \text{ min}}}{1 \cancel{\text{min}}} = \frac{0.5 \text{ ml} \times 60 \cancel{\text{min}}}{1 \cancel{\text{min}}}$$

$$x = 30 \text{ ml}$$

Set the infusion pump to deliver 30 ml/hour.

Example 2

A 200-lb patient is scheduled to receive an I.V. infusion of dobutamine at 10 mcg/kg/minute. The package insert says to dilute 250 mg of the drug in 50 ml of dextrose 5% in water. Because the drug vial contains 20 ml of solution, the total to be infused is 70 ml (50 ml of D_5W plus 20 ml of solution). How many micrograms of

the drug should the patient receive each minute? Each hour?

First, compute the patient's weight in kilograms. To do this, set up a proportion with the weight in pounds and the unknown weight in kilograms in one fraction and the number of pounds per kilogram in the other fraction:

$$\frac{200 \text{ lb}}{x \text{ kg}} = \frac{2.2 \text{ lb}}{1 \text{ kg}}$$

Cross multiply the fractions:

x kg × 2.2 lb = 1 kg × 200 lb

Solve for x by dividing each side of the equation by 2.2 lb and canceling units that appear in the numerator and denominator:

$$\frac{x \text{ kg} \times 2.2 \text{ lb}}{2.2 \text{ lb}} = \frac{1 \text{ kg} \times 200 \text{ lb}}{2.2 \text{ lb}}$$

$$x = \frac{200 \text{ kg}}{2.2}$$

$$x = 90.9 \text{ kg}$$

The patient weighs 90.9 kg. Next, determine the dose in micrograms per minute by setting up a proportion with the patient's weight in kilograms and the unknown dose in micrograms per minute in one fraction and the known dose in micrograms per kilogram per minute in the other fraction:

$$\frac{90.9 \text{ kg}}{x \text{ mcg/min}} = \frac{1 \text{ kg}}{10 \text{ mcg/min}}$$

Cross multiply the fractions:

$$x \text{ mcg/min} \times 1 \text{ kg} =$$
$$10 \text{ mcg/min} \times 90.9 \text{ kg}$$

Solve for x by dividing each side of the equation by 1 kg and canceling units that appear in the numerator and denominator:

$$\frac{x \text{ mcg/min} \times \cancel{1 \text{ kg}}}{\cancel{1 \text{ kg}}} = \frac{10 \text{ mcg/min} \times 90.9 \cancel{\text{ kg}}}{\cancel{1 \text{ kg}}}$$

$$x = 909 \text{ mcg/min}$$

The patient should receive 909 mcg of dobutamine every minute. Finally, determine the hourly dose by multiplying the dose per minute by 60:

$$909 \text{ mcg/min} \times 60 \text{ min/hr} = 54,540 \text{ mcg/hr}$$

The patient should receive 54,540 mcg of dobutamine every hour.

PEDIATRIC DOSAGE CONSIDERATIONS

To determine the correct pediatric dosage of a drug, prescribers, pharmacists, and nurses usually use two computation methods. One is based on weight in kilograms. The other uses the child's body surface area. Other methods are less accurate and not recommended.

Dosage range per kilogram of body weight

Many pharmaceutical companies provide information on the safe dosage ranges for drugs given to children. Usually, the companies provide the dosage ranges in milligrams per kilogram of body weight and, in many cases, give similar information for adult dosage ranges. The following example and explanation show how to calculate the safe pediatric dosage range for a drug, using the company's suggested safe dosage range provided in milligrams per kilogram.

For a child, the prescriber orders a drug with a suggested dosage range of 10 to 12 mg/kg of body weight daily. The child weighs 12 kg. What is the safe daily dosage range for the child?

You must calculate the lower and upper limits of the dosage range provided by the manufacturer. First, calculate the dosage based on 10 mg/kg of body weight. Then, calculate the dosage based on 12 mg/kg of body weight. The answers represent the lower and upper limits of the daily dosage range, expressed in mg/kg of the child's weight.

Body surface area

Dosage computations based on the child's body surface area (BSA) may provide a safer, more accurate calculation. That's because the child's BSA is thought to parallel organ growth and maturation and metabolic rate.

To determine a child's BSA, use a three-column chart called a nomogram. (See *Using a pediatric nomogram*.) Mark the child's height in the first column and weight in the last column. Then draw a line between the two marks. The point at which the line intersects the vertical scale in the surface area column is the child's estimated body surface area in square meters.

To calculate the child's approximate dose, use the BSA measurement in the following equation:

$$\frac{\text{BSA of child}}{\text{average adult dose BSA } (1.73 \text{ m}^2)} \times \begin{array}{c}\text{average} \\ \text{adult} \\ \text{dose}\end{array} = \begin{array}{c}\text{child's} \\ \text{dose}\end{array}$$

The following example illustrates how to use this equation. Suppose the nomogram shows that a 25-lb (11.3-kg) child who is 33 inches (84 cm) tall has a BSA of 0.52 m². To determine this child's dose of a drug with

USING A PEDIATRIC NOMOGRAM

Body surface area (BSA) is critical when calculating dosages for children and when using highly potent drugs that need to be given in precise amounts. The nomogram shown here lets you plot the patient's height and weight to determine BSA. Here's how it works:

■ Locate the patient's height in the left column of the nomogram and weight in the right column.

■ Use a ruler to draw a straight line connecting the two points. The point where the line intersects the surface area column indicates the patient's BSA in square meters.

■ For an average-sized child, use the simplified nomogram in the box. Just find the child's weight in pounds on the left side of the scale, and then read the corresponding BSA on the right side.

Reprinted from Behrman: Nelson Textbook of Pediatrics, 17th edition, © 2003, with permission from Elsevier.

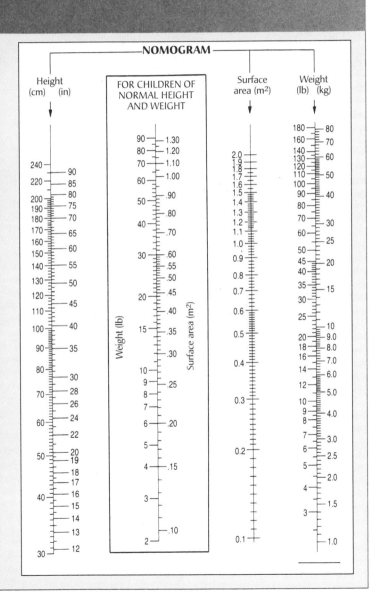

an average adult dose of 100 mg, the equation is:

$$\frac{0.52 \text{ mg}^2}{1.73 \text{ m}^2} \times 100 \text{ mg} = \begin{array}{c} 30.06 \text{ mg} \\ \text{(child's} \\ \text{dose)} \end{array}$$

The child should receive 30 mg of the drug.

Keep in mind that many facilities have guidelines that determine acceptable calculation methods for pediatric dosages. If you work with children, be sure to familiarize yourself with your facility's policies about pediatric dosages.

PART II

ADMINISTRATION AND MONITORING

5 / DRUG ADMINISTRATION

You may give drugs by many routes, including topical, oral, buccal, sublingual (S.L.), ophthalmic, otic, respiratory, nasogastric (NG), vaginal, rectal, subcutaneous (S.C.), intramuscular (I.M.), and intravenous (I.V.). No matter which route you use, you'll need to follow an established set of precautions to make sure you give the right drug in the right dose to the right patient at the right time and by the right route. These precautions include checking the order and medication administration record, checking the label, confirming the patient's identity, and responding to patient questions. Always follow standard safety procedures when giving drugs. (See *Drug safety procedures*, page 172.)

Check the order

Make sure you have a legible, written order for every drug you give and that the order makes sense for the patient and the drug. If you take a verbal order, make sure it's signed by the pre-

scriber within the time specified by your facility.

If your facility has a computerized ordering system, prescribers may be able to order drugs electronically. The computer indicates whether the pharmacy has the drug, and it triggers the pharmacy staff to fill the prescription. A computerized order may also generate a patient record on which you can document drug administration. In fact, you may be able to document the administration directly on the computer.

Computer systems offer several advantages over paper systems:

■ Drugs may arrive on the unit or floor more quickly.
■ Documentation is quicker and easier.
■ Prescribers can see at a glance which drugs have been given.
■ Errors no longer result from poor handwriting (although typing mistakes may occur).

DRUG SAFETY PROCEDURES

Whenever you give a drug, follow these safety procedures:

■ Never give a drug poured or prepared by someone other than you or the pharmacy.
■ Never allow the drug cart or tray out of your sight after you've prepared a dose.
■ Never leave a drug at a patient's bedside.

■ Never return unwrapped or prepared drugs to stock containers. Instead, dispose of them and notify the pharmacy.
■ Keep the drug cart locked at all times.
■ Follow standard precautions, as appropriate.

■ Computerized records are easier to store than paper records.

Check the medication record

Check the order on the patient's medication administration record against the prescriber's order.

Check the label

Before giving a drug, check its label three times to make sure you're giving the prescribed drug and the prescribed dose.
■ First, check the label when you take the container from the shelf or drawer.
■ Next, check the label just before pouring the drug into a cup or drawing it into a syringe.

■ Finally, check the label again before returning the container to the shelf or drawer.

For a unit-dose drug, open the container at the patient's bedside and check the label just after pouring the drug and again before discarding the wrapper.

ALERT *Don't give a drug from a poorly labeled or unlabeled container. Also, don't attempt to label a drug or to repair a label; a pharmacist must perform these actions.*

Confirm the patient's identity

Before giving a drug, ask the patient's full name, and confirm the patient's identity by checking the name and medical record number on his identification wristband against the medication administration record.

Don't rely on information that can vary during a hospital stay, such as a room or bed number. Check again that you have the correct drug, and make sure the patient has no allergy to it.

If the patient has drug allergies, check to make sure the chart and medication administration record are labeled accordingly and that the patient is wearing an allergy wristband identifying the allergen.

Respond to questions

If the patient questions you about a drug or dosage, check the medication administration record again. If the drug you're giving is correct, reassure the patient. Explain any changes in drugs or dosages. Also, as appropriate, explain possible adverse reactions and ask the patient to report anything that seems to be an adverse reaction.

TOPICAL ADMINISTRATION

Topical drugs, such as patches, lotions, and ointments, are applied directly to the skin. They're commonly used for local rather than systemic effects. Keep in mind, however, that certain types of topical drugs— known as transdermal drugs— are meant to enter the patient's bloodstream and exert a systemic effect after you apply them.

Equipment and preparation

Check the chart and the medication administration record. Gather the prescribed drug, sterile tongue blades, gloves, sterile gloves for open lesions, sterile 4″ × 4″ gauze pads, transparent semipermeable dressing, adhesive tape, normal saline solution, cotton-tipped applicators, cotton gloves, and linen savers, if needed.

Implementation

■ Confirm the patient's identity by asking his full name and checking the name and medical record number on his wristband.

■ Explain the procedure to the patient because, after discharge, he may have to apply the drug by himself.

■ Premedicate the patient with an analgesic if the procedure is uncomfortable. Give the analgesic time to take effect.

■ Wash your hands to reduce the risk of cross-contamination, and put on gloves.

■ Help the patient to a comfortable position, and expose the area to be treated. Make sure the skin or mucous membrane is intact (unless the drug has been prescribed to treat a skin lesion).

CLINICAL TIP *Applying a topical drug to broken or abraded skin may cause unwanted systemic absorption and further irritation.*

■ If needed, clean debris from the skin. Change your gloves if they become soiled.

TO APPLY PASTE, CREAM, OR OINTMENT

■ Open the container. Place the cap upside down to avoid contaminating its inner surface.

■ Remove a tongue blade from its sterile wrapper, and cover one end of it with the drug from the tube or jar. Then transfer the drug from the tongue blade to your gloved hand.

■ Apply the drug to the affected area as prescribed. (See *Applying pastes, creams, or ointments.*) Avoid excessive pressure when applying the drug because you could abrade the skin or cause the patient discomfort.

■ To prevent contamination of the drug, use a new sterile tongue blade each time you remove the drug from the container.

■ Remove and discard your gloves, and wash your hands.

TO APPLY TRANSDERMAL OINTMENT

■ Choose a site—usually a dry, hairless spot on the patient's chest or upper arm.

■ To promote absorption, wash the site with soap and warm water. Dry it thoroughly.

■ Put on gloves.

■ If the patient has a previously applied drug strip at another site, remove it and wash this area to clear away any drug residue.

■ If the area you choose is hairy, clip excess hair rather than shaving it; shaving causes irritation, which the drug may worsen.

■ Squeeze the prescribed amount of ointment onto the application strip or measuring paper. Don't get the ointment on your skin.

■ Apply the strip, drug side down, directly to the patient's skin.

■ Maneuver the strip slightly to spread a thin layer of ointment over a 3″ (8-cm) area, but don't rub the ointment into the skin.

■ Secure the application strip to the patient's skin by covering it with a semipermeable dressing or plastic wrap.

■ Tape the covering securely in place.

APPLYING PASTES, CREAMS, OR OINTMENTS

Apply the drug to the affected area with long, smooth strokes that follow the direction of hair growth, as shown. This technique avoids forcing drug into hair follicles, which can cause irritation and lead to folliculitis. If you'll be applying the drug to the patient's face, use cotton-tipped applicators for small areas, such as under the eyes. For larger areas, use a sterile gauze pad.

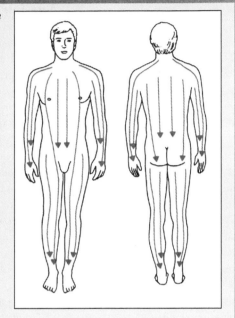

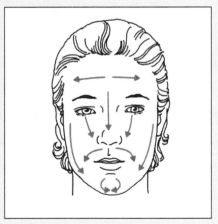

■ If required by your facility's policy, label the strip with the date, time, and your initials.

■ Remove your gloves and wash your hands.

TO APPLY A TRANSDERMAL PATCH

■ Wash your hands and put on gloves.

■ Remove the old patch.

■ Choose a dry and preferably hairless application site.

■ As with transdermal ointment, clip (don't shave) hair from the chosen site if needed. Wash the area with warm water and soap, and dry it thoroughly.

■ Open the drug package and remove the patch.

■ Without touching the adhesive surface, remove the clear plastic backing.

■ Apply the patch to the site without touching the adhesive.

■ If required by your facility's policy, label the patch with the date, time, and your initials.

TO REMOVE OINTMENT

■ Wash your hands and put on gloves.

■ Gently swab ointment from the patient's skin using a sterile 4″ × 4″ gauze pad saturated with normal saline solution.

■ Don't wipe too hard because you could irritate the skin.

■ Remove and discard your gloves, and wash your hands.

Nursing considerations

■ To prevent skin irritation from drug accumulation, never apply a drug without first removing previous applications.

■ Always wear gloves to prevent absorption by your skin.

■ Don't apply ointment to the eyelid or ear canal. The ointment may congeal and occlude the tear duct or ear canal.

■ Frequently inspect the treated area for allergic or other adverse reactions.

■ Don't apply a topical drug to scarred or callused skin because this type of skin may impair absorption.

ALERT *Don't place a defibrillator paddle on a transdermal patch. The aluminum on the patch can cause electrical arcing during defibrillation, resulting in smoke and thermal burns. If a patient has a patch on a standard paddle site, remove the patch before applying the paddle.*

ORAL ADMINISTRATION

Because oral drug administration is usually the safest, most convenient, and least expensive method, most drugs are given by this route. Drugs for oral administration come in many forms: tablets, enteric-coated tablets, capsules, syrups, elixirs, oils, liquids, suspensions, powders, and granules. Some require special preparation before administration, such as mixing with juice to make them more palatable.

Oral drugs sometimes are prescribed in higher dosages than their parenteral equivalents because, after absorption through the gastrointestinal (GI) system, they're broken down by the liver before they reach the systemic circulation.

Equipment and preparation

Check the chart and the medication administration record. Gather the prescribed drug and medication cup. If needed, gather a mortar and pestle for crushing pills and an appropriate vehicle, such as jelly or applesauce for crushed pills or juice, water, or milk for liquid drugs. These variations commonly are used for children or geriatric patients.

Implementation

■ Wash your hands.
■ Confirm the patient's identity by asking his full name and checking the name and medical record number on his wristband.
■ Assess the patient's condition, including level of consciousness and vital signs, as needed. Changes in the patient's condition may warrant withholding the drug.
■ Give the patient the drug. If appropriate, crush the drug to facilitate swallowing or mix it with an appropriate vehicle or liquid to aid swallowing, minimize adverse reactions, or promote absorption.
■ Stay with the patient until he has swallowed the drug. If he seems confused or disoriented, check his mouth to make sure he swallowed it. Return and reassess the patient's response within 1 hour after giving the drug.

Nursing considerations

■ Give acid or iron preparations through a straw to avoid damaging or staining the patient's teeth. Also, if a liquid drug has an unpleasant taste, give it through a straw; doing so makes the drug more palatable because it contacts fewer taste buds.
■ If the patient can't swallow a whole tablet or capsule, ask the pharmacist if the drug is available in liquid form or if it can be given by another route. If not,

GIVING BUCCAL AND SUBLINGUAL DRUGS

BUCCAL AND SUBLINGUAL ADMINISTRATION

Certain drugs are given buccally (between the cheek and teeth) or sublingually (under the tongue) to bypass the GI tract and promote absorption into the bloodstream. With either administration method, observe the patient carefully to make sure he doesn't swallow the drug or develop mucosal irritation.

Proper placement of buccal and sublingual (S.L.) tablets is the key to effective therapy with these drugs. For buccal administration, place the tablet in the patient's buccal pouch, between the cheek and teeth, as shown in the top illustration. For S.L. administration, place it under the tongue, as shown at the bottom.

Equipment and preparation

Check the chart and the medication administration record. Gather the prescribed drug, medication cup, and gloves.

Buccal drug placement

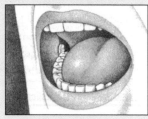

Implementation

■ Wash your hands. Put on gloves if you'll be placing the drug into the patient's mouth.

■ Confirm the patient's identity by asking his full name and checking the name and medical record number on his wristband.

S.L. drug placement

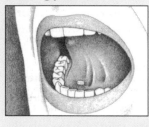

■ Place the tablet in the patient's mouth, as indicated. (See *Giving buccal and sublingual drugs*.)

■ Remove and discard your gloves, and wash your hands.

ask the pharmacist if the tablet can be crushed or if capsules can be opened and mixed with food.

■ Don't crush sustained-action drugs, buccal tablets, S.L. tablets, or enteric-coated drugs.

■ Instruct the patient to keep the drug in place until it dissolves completely to ensure absorption. Caution the patient against chewing the tablet or touching it with his tongue to prevent accidental swallowing.

■ Tell the patient not to smoke before the drug has dissolved because nicotine constricts vessels, which slows absorption.

Nursing considerations

■ Don't give the patient liquids until the buccal tablet is absorbed, which can take up to 1 hour.

■ If the patient has angina, tell him to wet the nitroglycerin tablet with saliva and keep it under his tongue until it's fully absorbed.

ALERT Make sure a patient with angina knows where in his mouth to place nitroglycerin tablets, how many doses to take, and when to call for emergency help.

OPHTHALMIC ADMINISTRATION

Ophthalmic drugs—drops or ointments—serve diagnostic and therapeutic purposes. During an ophthalmic examination, they can be used to anesthetize the eye, dilate the pupil, and stain the cornea to identify anom-

alies. Therapeutic uses include eye lubrication and treatment of conditions such as glaucoma and infections.

Equipment and preparation

Check the chart and the medication administration record. Gather the prescribed ophthalmic drug, sterile cotton balls, gloves, warm water or normal saline solution, sterile gauze pads, and facial tissue. An eye dressing also may be used.

Make sure the drug is labeled for ophthalmic use. Then check the expiration date. Remember to date the container after the first use.

Inspect the ocular solution for cloudiness, discoloration, and precipitation, although some drugs are suspensions and normally appear cloudy. Don't use a solution that appears abnormal.

Implementation

■ Make sure you know which eye to treat because different drugs or doses may be ordered for each eye.

■ Confirm the patient's identity by asking his full name and checking the name and medical record number on his wristband.

■ Put on gloves.

APPLYING EYE OINTMENT

To apply eye ointment, squeeze a small ribbon of drug onto the inside edge of the conjunctival sac from the inner to the outer canthus. Cut off the ribbon by turning the tube. Don't touch the eye with the tip of the tube.

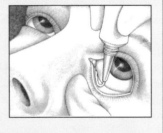

■ Have the patient sit or lie in the supine position. Instruct him to tilt his head back and toward his affected eye so that any excess drug can flow away from the tear duct, minimizing systemic absorption through the nasal mucosa.

■ Remove the dropper cap from the drug container, and draw the drug into the dropper. Or, if the bottle has a dropper tip, remove the cap and hold it or place it upside down to prevent contamination.

■ Before instilling eyedrops, instruct the patient to look up and away. This moves the cornea away from the lower lid and minimizes the risk of touching it with the dropper.

■ If the patient has an eye dressing, remove it by pulling it down and away from his forehead. Avoid contaminating your hands. Don't apply pressure to the area around the eyes.

■ To remove exudates or meibomian gland secretions, clean around the eye with sterile cotton balls or sterile gauze pads moistened with warm water or normal saline solution. Have the patient close his eye; then gently wipe the eyelids from the inner to the outer canthus. Use a fresh cotton ball or gauze pad for each stroke, and use a different cotton ball or pad for each eye.

TO INSTILL EYEDROPS

■ Steady the hand that's holding the dropper by resting it against the patient's forehead. With your other hand, gently pull down the lower lid of the affected eye, and instill the drops in the conjunctival sac. Never instill eyedrops directly onto the eyeball.

■ When teaching a geriatric patient how to instill eyedrops, keep in mind that he may have difficulty sensing drops in the eye. Suggest chilling the drug slightly because cold drops should be easier to feel when they enter the eye.

To apply eye ointment
■ Squeeze a small ribbon of drug into the conjunctival sac. (See *Applying eye ointment.*)

To complete ophthalmic administration
■ After instilling eyedrops or applying ointment, instruct the patient to close his eyes gently, without squeezing the lids shut. If you instilled drops, tell the patient to blink. If you applied ointment, tell him to roll his eyes behind closed lids to help distribute the drug over the eyeball.

■ Use a clean tissue to remove any excess drug that leaks from the eye. Use a fresh tissue for each eye to prevent cross-contamination.

■ Apply a new eye dressing, if needed.

■ Remove and discard your gloves. Wash your hands.

Nursing considerations
■ When giving an ophthalmic drug that may be absorbed systemically, gently press your thumb on the inner canthus for 1 to 2 minutes after instillation while the patient closes his eyes. Don't apply pressure around the eye.

■ To maintain the drug container's sterility, don't put the cap down after opening the container, and never touch the tip of the dropper or bottle to the eye area. Discard any solution remaining in the dropper before returning it to the bottle. If the dropper or bottle tip has become contaminated, discard it and use another sterile dropper. Never share eyedrops from patient to patient.

Otic Administration

Eardrops may be instilled to treat infection and inflammation, soften cerumen for later removal, produce local anesthesia, or facilitate removal of an insect trapped in the ear.

Equipment and preparation
Check the chart and the medication administration record. Gather the prescribed eardrops, gloves, a light, and facial tissue or cotton-tipped applicators. Cotton balls and a bowl of warm water may be needed as well.

First, warm the drug to body temperature in the bowl of warm water, or carry the drug in your pocket for 30 minutes before administration. If needed, test the temperature of the drug by placing a drop on your wrist. (If the drug is too hot, it may burn the patient's eardrum.) To avoid injuring the ear canal, check the dropper before use to make sure it's not chipped or cracked.

Implementation

■ Wash your hands and put on clean gloves.

■ Confirm the patient's identity by asking his full name and checking the name and medical record number on his wristband.

■ Have the patient lie on the side opposite the affected ear.

■ Straighten the patient's ear canal. (See *Eardrop administration for children*.)

■ Using a light, examine the ear canal. If you see drainage, gently clean the canal with the tissue or cotton-tipped applicators; drainage can reduce the drug's effectiveness.

■ Never insert an applicator into the ear canal past the point where you can see it.

■ Compare the label on the eardrops to the order on the patient's medication administration record. Check the label again while drawing the drug into the dropper. Check the label for the final time before re-

turning the eardrops to the shelf or drawer.

■ Straighten the patient's ear canal once again, and instill the ordered number of drops. To avoid patient discomfort, aim the dropper so that the drops fall against the sides of the ear canal, not on the eardrum. Hold the ear canal in position until you see the drug disappear down the canal. Then release the ear.

■ Instruct the patient to remain on his side for 5 to 10 minutes to allow the drug to run down into the ear canal.

■ Tuck a cotton ball with a small amount of petroleum jelly on it (if ordered) loosely into the opening of the ear canal to prevent the drug from leaking out. Be careful not to insert it too deeply into the canal because doing so may prevent drainage of secretions and increase pressure on the eardrum.

■ Clean and dry the outer ear.

■ If indicated, repeat the procedure in the other ear after 5 to 10 minutes.

■ Help the patient into a comfortable position.

■ Remove your gloves and wash your hands.

Nursing considerations

■ Be especially gentle because some conditions make the nor-

EARDROP ADMINISTRATION FOR CHILDREN

Although you need to straighten the ear canal when giving eardrops to any patient, adjust your technique based on the patient's age. For an adult or a child age 3 or older, pull the auricle up and back, as shown in the top illustration. For an infant or child younger than age 3, gently pull the auricle down and back, as shown in the bottom illustration. At this age, the ear canal is straighter and needs less manipulation.

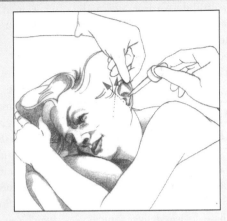

If the child struggles, gently rest the hand holding the dropper against his head to secure a safe position before giving the eardrops. This helps avoid damaging the ear canal with the dropper.

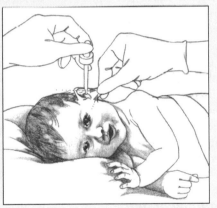

mally tender ear canal even more sensitive.

■ To prevent injury to the eardrum, never insert a cotton-tipped applicator into the ear canal past the point where you can see the tip.

■ After instilling eardrops to soften cerumen, irrigate the ear to promote its removal. If the patient has vertigo, keep the side rails of his bed up and assist him as needed during the procedure. Also, move slowly to avoid worsening his vertigo.

■ If needed, teach the patient to instill the eardrops correctly so that he can continue treatment at home. Review the procedure and let the patient try it himself while you observe.

RESPIRATORY ADMINISTRATION

Handheld oropharyngeal inhalers include the metered-dose inhaler and the turbo-inhaler. These devices deliver topical drugs to the respiratory tract, producing local and systemic effects. The mucosal lining of the respiratory tract absorbs the inhalant almost immediately. Examples of inhalants are bronchodilators, which improve airway patency and promote mucous drainage, and mucolytics, which liquefy tenacious bronchial secretions.

Equipment and preparation

Check the chart and the medication administration record. Gather the metered-dose inhaler or turbo-inhaler, prescribed drug, and normal saline solution.

Implementation

■ Confirm the patient's identity by asking his full name and checking the name and medical record number on his wristband.

TO USE A METERED-DOSE INHALER

■ Prepare the inhaler. (See *Preparing a metered-dose inhaler.*)

■ Place the inhaler about 1″ (2.5 cm) in front of the patient's open mouth.

■ Tell the patient to exhale.

■ If you're using a spacer, which can make the inhaler more effective, tell the patient to place the mouthpiece of the spacer in his mouth and to press his lips firmly around it.

■ As you push the bottle down against the mouthpiece, instruct the patient to inhale slowly through his mouth and to continue inhaling until his lungs feel full. Compress the bottle against the mouthpiece only once.

■ Remove the inhaler and tell the patient to hold his breath for several seconds. Then instruct him to exhale slowly through pursed lips to keep distal bronchioles open and allow increased drug absorption and diffusion.

■ Have the patient gargle with normal saline solution or water to remove the drug from his mouth and the back of his throat. This step helps prevent oral fungal infections. Warn the patient not to swallow after gargling, but rather to spit out the liquid.

To use a turbo-inhaler

■ Prepare the inhaler. (See *Preparing a turbo-inhaler*, page 186.)

■ Holding the inhaler with the mouthpiece at the bottom, slide the sleeve all the way down and then up again to puncture the capsule and release the drug. Do this only once.

■ Have the patient exhale completely and tilt his head back. Instruct him to place the mouthpiece in his mouth, close his lips around it, and inhale once. Tell him to hold his breath for several seconds.

■ Remove the inhaler from the patient's mouth, and tell him to exhale as much air as possible.

■ Repeat the procedure until the patient has inhaled all the drug in the device.

■ Have the patient gargle with normal saline solution, if desired.

Nursing considerations

■ Teach the patient how to use the inhaler so he can continue treatments after discharge, if

Preparing a metered-dose inhaler

Before using a metered-dose inhaler, shake the inhaler bottle. Then remove the cap and insert the stem of the bottle into the small hole on the flattened portion of the mouthpiece, as shown here.

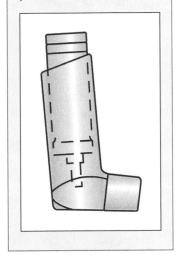

needed. Explain that overdosage can cause the drug to lose its effectiveness. Tell him to record the date and time of each inhalation and his response.

■ Some oral respiratory drugs may cause restlessness, palpitations, nervousness, and other systemic effects. They can also cause hypersensitivity reactions,

PREPARING A TURBO-INHALER

To prepare a turbo-inhaler, hold the mouthpiece in one hand. With the other hand, slide the sleeve away from the mouthpiece as far as possible, as shown here.

Next, unscrew the tip of the mouthpiece by turning it counterclockwise. Press the colored portion of the drug capsule into the propeller stem of the mouthpiece. Then screw the inhaler together again.

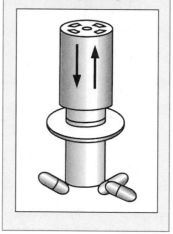

spasm occurs, discontinue the drug and call the prescriber to order another drug.

■ If the patient must receive a bronchodilator and a corticosteroid, give the bronchodilator first so his air passages can open fully before you give the corticosteroid.

■ Instruct the patient to keep an extra inhaler handy.

■ Instruct the patient to discard the inhaler after taking the prescribed number of doses and to then start a new inhaler.

NASOGASTRIC ADMINISTRATION

Besides providing an alternate means of nourishment for patients who can't eat normally, an NG tube allows direct instillation of drugs into the GI system.

Equipment and preparation

Check the chart and the medication administration record. Gather equipment for use at the bedside, including the prescribed drug, a towel or linen-saver pad, 50- or 60-ml piston-type catheter-tip syringe, feeding tubing, two 4″ × 4″ gauze pads, stethoscope, gloves, diluent (juice, water, or a nutritional

such as rash, urticaria, or bronchospasm.

■ Give oral respiratory drugs cautiously to patients with heart disease because these drugs may potentiate coronary insufficiency, arrhythmias, or hypertension. If paradoxical broncho-

supplement), cup for mixing drug and fluid, spoon, 50-ml cup of water, and rubber band. Pill-crushing equipment and a clamp (if not already attached to the tube) may also be needed.

Make sure that liquids are at room temperature to avoid abdominal cramping. Also ensure that the cup, syringe, spoon, and gauze are clean.

Implementation

■ Wash your hands and put on gloves.

■ Confirm the patient's identity by asking his full name and checking the name and medical record number on his wristband.

■ Unpin the tube from the patient's gown. To avoid soiling the sheets during the procedure, fold back the bed linens and drape the patient's chest with a towel or linen-saver pad.

■ Help the patient into Fowler's position, if his condition allows.

■ After unclamping the tube, auscultate the patient's abdomen about 3″ (7.5 cm) below the sternum as you gently insert 10 ml of air into the tube with the 50- or 60-ml syringe. You should hear the air bubble entering the stomach. Gently draw back on the piston of the syringe. The appearance of gastric

contents suggests that the tube is patent and in the stomach.

■ If no gastric contents appear or if you meet resistance, the tube may be lying against the gastric mucosa. Withdraw the tube slightly or turn the patient to free it.

■ Clamp the tube, detach the syringe, and lay the end of the tube on the 4″ × 4″ gauze pad.

■ If the drug is in tablet form, crush it before mixing it with the diluent. Make sure the particles are small enough to pass through the eyes at the distal end of the tube. Keep in mind that some drugs (extended-release, enteric-coated, or S.L. drugs, for example) shouldn't be crushed. If you aren't sure, ask the pharmacist. Also, check to see if the drug comes in liquid form or if a capsule form may be opened and the contents poured into a diluent. Pour liquid drugs into the diluent and stir well.

■ Reattach the syringe, without the piston, to the end of the tube. Then give the drug through the attached syringe. (See *Giving a drug by nasogastric tube*, page 188.)

■ If the drug flows smoothly, slowly give the entire dose. If it doesn't flow, it may be too thick. If so, dilute it with water. If you suspect that tube placement is inhibiting flow, stop the proce-

GIVING A DRUG BY NASOGASTRIC TUBE

To administer a drug by the naso-gastric (NG) route, hold the NG tube upright at a level slightly above the patient's nose. Then open the clamp and pour the drug in slowly and steadily, as shown here. To keep air from entering the patient's stomach, hold the tube at a slight angle and add more drug before the syringe empties.

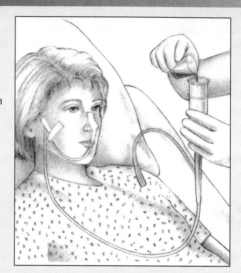

dure and reevaluate the placement.

■ Watch the patient's reaction. Stop immediately if you see signs of discomfort.

■ As the last of the drug flows out of the syringe, start to irrigate the tube by adding 30 to 50 ml of water (15 to 30 ml for a child). Irrigation clears the drug from the tube and reduces the risk of clogging.

■ When the water stops flowing, clamp the tube. Detach the syringe and discard it properly.

■ Fasten the tube to the patient's gown and make the patient comfortable.

■ Leave the patient in Fowler's position or on his right side with his head partially elevated for at least 30 minutes to promote flow and prevent esophageal reflux.

■ Remove and discard your gloves, and wash your hands.

Nursing considerations

■ If you must give a tube feeding as well as instill a drug, give the drug first to make sure the patient receives it all.

■ Certain drugs, such as Dilantin, bind with tube feedings, decreasing the drug's availability. Stop the tube feeding for 2 hours before and after giving the dose, according to your facility's policy.

■ If residual stomach contents exceed 150 ml, withhold the drug and feeding, and notify the prescriber. Excessive stomach contents may indicate intestinal obstruction or paralytic ileus.

■ Never crush enteric-coated, buccal, S.L., or sustained-release drugs.

■ If the NG tube is on suction, turn it off for 20 to 30 minutes after giving a drug.

VAGINAL ADMINISTRATION

Vaginal drugs can be inserted as topical treatment for infection—particularly *Trichomonas vaginalis* infection—and vaginal candidiasis or inflammation. Suppositories melt when they contact the vaginal mucosa, and the drug diffuses topically.

Vaginal drugs usually come with a disposable applicator that enables drug placement in the anterior and posterior fornices. Vaginal administration is most effective when the patient can remain lying down afterward to retain the drug.

Equipment and preparation

Check the chart and the medication administration record. Gather the prescribed drug and applicator (if needed), gloves, water-soluble lubricant, and a small sanitary pad.

Implementation

■ If possible, plan to give vaginal drugs at bedtime when the patient is recumbent.

■ Confirm the patient's identity by asking her full name and checking the name and medical record number on her wristband.

■ Wash your hands, explain the procedure to the patient, and provide privacy.

■ Ask the patient to void.

■ Ask the patient if she would rather insert the drug herself. If so, provide appropriate instructions. If not, proceed with the following steps.

■ Help the patient into the lithotomy position. Drape her, exposing only her perineum.

■ Remove the suppository from the wrapper and lubricate it with water-soluble lubricant.

■ Put on gloves, and expose the vagina by spreading the labia. If you see discharge, wash

GIVING A VAGINAL DRUG

After cleaning the perineum, keep the patient's labia separated. Then insert the suppository or vaginal applicator about 3″ to 4″ (7.5 to 10 cm) into her vagina, as shown here. Fully depress the plunger on the vaginal applicator to release the entire dose.

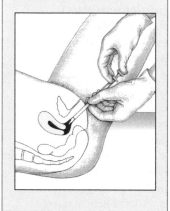

■ Remove and discard your gloves.
■ To keep the drug from soiling the patient's clothing and bedding, provide a sanitary pad.
■ Help the patient return to a comfortable position, and tell her to stay in bed as much as possible for the next several hours.
■ Wash your hands.

Nursing considerations

■ Refrigerate vaginal suppositories that melt at room temperature.
■ If possible, teach the patient how to insert the vaginal drug because she may have to give it to herself after discharge. Give her instructions in writing if possible.
■ Instruct the patient not to insert a tampon after inserting a vaginal drug because the tampon will absorb the drug and decrease its effectiveness.

the area with several cotton balls soaked in warm, soapy water. Clean each side of the perineum and then the center, using a fresh cotton ball for each stroke. Then insert the prescribed drug. (See *Giving a vaginal drug*.)
■ After insertion, wash the applicator with soap and warm water, and store or discard it, as appropriate. Label it so it will be used only for one patient.

RECTAL ADMINISTRATION

A rectal suppository is a small, solid, medicated mass, usually cone shaped, with a cocoa butter or glycerin base. It may be inserted to stimulate peristalsis and defecation or to relieve pain, vomiting, and local irritation. An ointment is a semisolid drug used to produce local effects. It may be applied externally to the anus or internally to the rectum.

Equipment and preparation

Check the chart and the medication administration record. Gather the rectal suppository or tube of ointment and applicator, 4″ × 4″ gauze pads, gloves, and a water-soluble lubricant. A bedpan also may be needed.

Store rectal suppositories in the refrigerator until needed to prevent softening and possibly decreased drug effectiveness. A softened suppository is also difficult to handle and insert. To harden it again, hold the suppository (in its wrapper) under cold running water.

Implementation

■ Confirm the patient's identity by asking his full name and checking the name and medical record number on his wristband.
■ Wash your hands.

TO INSERT A RECTAL SUPPOSITORY

■ Place the patient on his left side in Sims' position. Drape him with the bedcovers, exposing only his buttocks.

■ Put on gloves. Unwrap the suppository and lubricate it with water-soluble lubricant.
■ Lift the patient's upper buttock with your nondominant hand to expose the anus.
■ Instruct the patient to take several deep breaths through his mouth to relax the anal sphincter and reduce anxiety. When he's relatively relaxed, insert the suppository. (See *Inserting a rectal suppository*, page 192.)
■ Encourage the patient to lie quietly and, if applicable, to retain the suppository for the correct length of time. Press on his anus with a gauze pad, if needed, until the urge to defecate passes.
■ Remove and discard your gloves, and then wash your hands.

TO APPLY AN OINTMENT

■ Wash your hands.
■ For external application, don gloves and use a gauze pad to spread the drug over the anal area. For internal application, attach the applicator to the tube of ointment, and coat the applicator with water-soluble lubricant.
■ Expect to use about 1″ (2.5 cm) of ointment. To gauge how much pressure to use during application, try squeezing a

INSERTING A RECTAL SUPPOSITORY

Using the index finger of your dominant hand, insert the rectal suppository—tapered end first—about 3″ (7.5 cm) until you feel it pass the patient's internal anal sphincter, as shown. Direct the tapered end of the suppository toward the side of the rectum so it contacts the membranes.

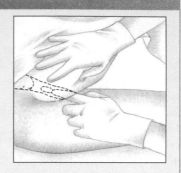

small amount from the tube before you attach the applicator.

■ Lift the patient's upper buttock with your nondominant hand to expose the anus.

■ Tell the patient to take several deep breaths through his mouth to relax the anal sphincter and reduce discomfort during insertion. Then gently insert the applicator, directing it toward the umbilicus.

■ Squeeze the tube to eject the drug.

■ Remove the applicator and place a folded 4″ × 4″ gauze pad between the patient's buttocks to absorb excess ointment.

■ Disassemble the tube and applicator and recap the tube. Clean the applicator with soap and warm water. Remove and discard your gloves. Then wash your hands thoroughly.

Nursing considerations

■ Because the intake of food and fluid stimulates peristalsis, a suppository for relieving constipation should be inserted about 30 minutes before mealtime to help soften the stool and promote defecation. A medicated retention suppository should be inserted between meals.

■ Tell the patient not to expel the suppository. If retaining it is difficult, put him on a bedpan.

■ Make sure that the patient's call button is handy, and watch for his signal because he may be unable to suppress the urge to defecate.

■ Inform the patient that the suppository may discolor his next bowel movement.

SUBCUTANEOUS ADMINISTRATION

Injection of a drug into S.C. tissue allows slower, more sustained administration than an I.M. injection. Drugs and solutions delivered by the S.C. route are injected through a relatively short needle using sterile technique.

Equipment and preparation

Check the chart and the medication administration record. Gather gloves, the prescribed drug, a needle of appropriate gauge and length, 1- to 3-ml syringe, and alcohol pads. Other materials may include an antiseptic cleanser, filter needle, insulin syringe, and insulin pump.

Inspect the drug to make sure it's not cloudy and is free of precipitates. Wash your hands and put on gloves.

FOR SINGLE-DOSE AMPULES

Wrap the neck of the ampule in an alcohol pad and snap off the top. If desired, attach a filter needle to the syringe and withdraw the drug. Tap the syringe to clear air from it. Cover the needle with the needle sheath by placing the sheath on the counter or drug cart and sliding the needle into the sheath. Before discarding the ampule, check the label against the patient's medication administration record. Discard the filter needle and the ampule. Attach the appropriate needle to the syringe.

FOR SINGLE-DOSE OR MULTIDOSE VIALS

Reconstitute powdered drugs according to the instructions on the label. Clean the rubber stopper on the vial with an alcohol pad. Pull the syringe plunger back until the volume of air in the syringe equals the volume of drug to be withdrawn from the vial. Insert the needle into the vial. Inject the air, invert the vial, and keep the bevel tip of the needle below the level of the solution as you withdraw the prescribed amount of drug.

Tap the syringe to clear air from it. Cover the needle with the needle sheath by placing the sheath on the counter or drug cart and sliding the needle into the sheath.

Check the drug label against the patient's medication administration record before returning the multidose vial to the shelf or drawer or before discarding the single-dose vial.

SELECTING A SUBCUTANEOUS INJECTION SITE

To select an appropriate site for subcutaneous (S.C.) injection, evaluate appropriate areas on the abdomen, upper arms, thighs, shoulders, and lower back, as shown. If the patient is receiving ongoing S.C. injections, establish a rotation pattern and use the next planned site. Rotating sites promotes drug absorption and helps prevent adverse reactions.

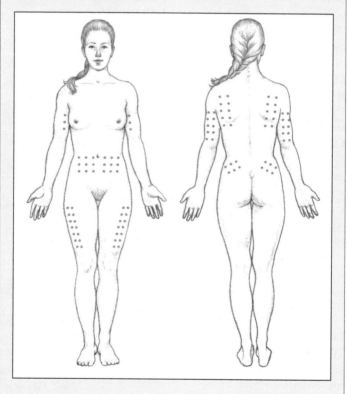

Implementation

■ Confirm the patient's identity by asking his full name and checking the name and medical record number on his wristband.

■ Choose an injection site and tell the patient where you'll be

INJECTING A SUBCUTANEOUS DRUG

To give a subcutaneous (S.C.) injection, hold the syringe in your dominant hand. Use the index finger and thumb of your nondominant hand to firmly pinch the skin around the injection site, elevating the S.C. tissue and forming a 1" (2.5-cm) fat fold, as shown at right.

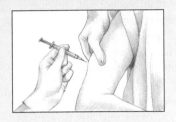

Now, using the free fingers of your nondominant hand, pull the needle sheath back to uncover the site. Some drugs, such as heparin, should always be injected at a 90-degree angle.

Release the skin to avoid injecting the drug into compressed tissue and irritating the nerves. Then pull the plunger back slightly to check for blood return. If blood appears, withdraw the needle, prepare another syringe, and repeat the procedure. If no blood appears, slowly inject the drug.

Tell the patient he'll feel a prick as you insert the needle. Then, insert it quickly, in one motion, at a 45- or 90-degree angle, as shown below. The needle length and the angle you use depend on the amount of S.C. tissue at

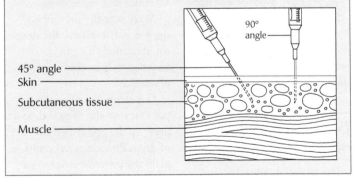

Release the skin to avoid injecting the drug into compressed tissue and irritating the nerves. Then pull the plunger back slightly to check for blood return. If blood appears, withdraw the needle, prepare another syringe, and repeat the procedure. If no blood appears, slowly inject the drug.

giving the injection. (See *Selecting a subcutaneous injection site*.)

■ Put on gloves. Position and drape the patient if needed.

■ Clean the injection site with an alcohol pad. Loosen the protective needle sheath.

■ Give the injection. (See *Injecting a subcutaneous drug*.)

■ After injection, remove the needle at the same angle you used to insert it. Cover the site with an alcohol pad, and massage the site gently.

■ Remove the alcohol pad and check the injection site for bleeding or bruising.

■ Don't recap the needle. Follow your facility's policy to dispose of the injection equipment.

■ Remove and discard your gloves. Wash your hands.

Nursing considerations

■ Don't aspirate for blood return when giving insulin or heparin. It's not necessary with insulin and may cause a hematoma with heparin.

■ Don't massage the site after giving heparin.

ALERT *Repeated injections in the same site can cause lipodystrophy, a natural immune response. This adverse reaction can be minimized by rotating injection sites.*

INTRAMUSCULAR ADMINISTRATION

You'll use I.M. injections to deposit up to 5 ml of a drug deep into well-vascularized muscle for rapid systemic action and absorption.

Equipment and preparation

Check the chart and the medication administration record. Gather the prescribed drug, diluent or filter needle (if needed), 3- to 5-ml syringe, 20G to 25G needle 1″ to 3″ in length, gloves, and alcohol pads.

Make sure the equipment is sterile. The needle may be packaged separately or already attached to the syringe. Needles used for I.M. injections are longer than those used for S.C. injections because they reach deep into the muscle. Needle length also depends on the injection site, the patient's size, and the amount of S.C. fat covering the muscle. A larger needle gauge accommodates viscous solutions and suspensions.

Make sure the prescribed drug is sterile. Check the drug for abnormal changes in color and clarity. If in doubt, ask the pharmacist.

Use alcohol to wipe the stopper that tops the drug vial, and draw up the prescribed amount of drug. Provide privacy and explain the procedure to the patient. Position and drape him appropriately, making sure that the site is well lit and exposed.

Implementation

- Wash your hands.
- Confirm the patient's identity by asking his full name and checking the name and medical record number on his wristband.
- Next, select an appropriate injection site. (See *Choosing an intramuscular injection site*, page 198.)
- Loosen, but don't remove, the needle sheath.
- Gently tap the site to stimulate nerve endings and minimize pain.
- Clean the site with an alcohol pad starting at the site and moving outward in expanding circles to about 2" (5 cm). Allow the skin to dry because wet alcohol stings in the puncture.
- Put on gloves.
- With the thumb and index finger of your nondominant hand, gently stretch the skin.
- With the syringe in your dominant hand, remove the needle sheath with the free fingers of the other hand.
- Position the syringe perpendicular to the skin surface and a few inches from the skin. Tell the patient that he'll feel a prick. Then quickly and firmly thrust the needle into the muscle.
- Pull back slightly on the plunger to aspirate for blood. If

blood appears, the needle is in a blood vessel. Withdraw it, prepare a fresh syringe, and inject into another site. If no blood appears, inject the drug slowly and steadily to let the muscle distend gradually. You should feel little or no resistance. Gently but quickly remove the needle at a 90-degree angle.

- Apply gentle pressure to the site with the alcohol pad. Massage the relaxed muscle, unless contraindicated, to distribute the drug and promote absorption.
- Inspect the site for bleeding or bruising. Apply pressure as needed.
- Discard all equipment properly. Don't recap needles; put them in an appropriate biohazard container to avoid needlestick injuries.
- Remove and discard your gloves. Wash your hands.

Nursing considerations

- To slow absorption, some drugs are dissolved in oil. Mix them well before use.
- If you must inject more than 5 ml, divide the solution and inject it in two sites.
- Rotate injection sites for a patient who needs repeated injections.

CHOOSING AN INTRAMUSCULAR INJECTION SITE

When choosing a site for an intramuscular (I.M.) injection, keep these guidelines in mind:

■ The dorsogluteal and ventrogluteal muscles are used most commonly for I.M. injections.

■ The deltoid muscle may be used for injecting 2 ml or less.

■ The vastus lateralis muscle is used most commonly in children.

■ The rectus femoris may be used in infants.

Avoid any site that looks inflamed, edematous, or irritated. Also, avoid using a site that contains moles, birthmarks, scar tissue, or other lesions.

Dorsogluteal muscle

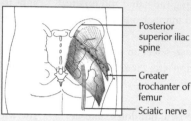

- Posterior superior iliac spine
- Greater trochanter of femur
- Sciatic nerve

Ventrogluteal muscle

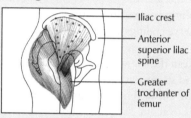

- Iliac crest
- Anterior superior iliac spine
- Greater trochanter of femur

Deltoid muscle

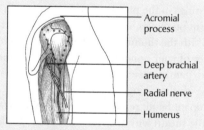

- Acromial process
- Deep brachial artery
- Radial nerve
- Humerus

Vastus lateralis and rectus femoris muscles

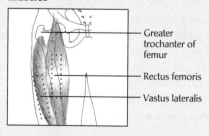

- Greater trochanter of femur
- Rectus femoris
- Vastus lateralis

■ Urge the patient to relax the muscle to reduce pain and bleeding.

■ Never inject into the gluteal muscles of a child who has been walking for less than 1 year.

ALERT Keep in mind that I.M. injections can damage local muscle cells and elevate the creatine kinase level, which can be confused with the elevated level caused by myocardial infarction. Diagnostic tests can be used to differentiate between them.

I.V. BOLUS ADMINISTRATION

In this method, rapid I.V. administration allows the drug level to peak quickly in the bloodstream. This method may also be used for drugs that can't be given I.M. because they're toxic or because the patient has a reduced ability to absorb them. In addition, I.V. bolus administration may be used to deliver drugs that can't be diluted. Bolus doses may be injected directly into a vein or through an existing I.V. line.

Equipment and preparation

Check the chart and the medication administration record. Gather the prescribed drug, 20G needle and syringe, diluent (if needed), tourniquet, alcohol pad, sterile 4″ × 4″ gauze pad, gloves, adhesive bandage, and tape. Other materials may include a winged device primed with normal saline solution and second syringe (and needle) filled with normal saline solution.

Draw the drug into the syringe and dilute it if needed.

Implementation

■ Confirm the patient's identity by asking his full name and checking the name and medical record number on his wristband.

■ Wash your hands and put on gloves.

TO GIVE A DIRECT INJECTION

■ Select the largest vein suitable to dilute the drug and minimize irritation.

■ Apply a tourniquet above the site to distend the vein. Clean the site with an alcohol pad working outward in a circle.

■ If you're using the needle of the drug syringe, insert it at a 30-degree angle with the bevel up. The bevel should reach ¼″ (0.6 cm) into the vein. Insert a winged device bevel-up at a 10- to 25-degree angle. Lower the angle once you get into the vein.

Advance the needle into the vein. Tape the wings in place when you see blood return, and attach the syringe containing the drug.

■ Check for blood backflow.

■ Remove the tourniquet and inject the drug at the prescribed rate.

■ Check for blood backflow to ensure that the needle remained in place and the entire injected drug entered the vein.

■ For a winged device, flush the line with normal saline solution from the second syringe to ensure complete delivery.

■ Withdraw the needle and apply pressure to the site with the sterile gauze pad for at least 3 minutes to prevent hematoma.

■ Apply an adhesive bandage when the bleeding stops.

■ Remove and discard your gloves. Wash your hands.

TO INJECT THROUGH AN EXISTING LINE

■ Wash your hands and put on gloves.

■ Check the compatibility of the drug.

■ Close the flow clamp, wipe the injection port with an alcohol pad, and inject the drug as you would a direct injection.

■ Open the flow clamp and readjust the flow rate.

■ Remove and discard your gloves. Wash your hands.

■ If the drug isn't compatible with the I.V. solution, flush the line with normal saline solution before and after the injection.

Nursing considerations

■ If the existing I.V. line is capped, making it an intermittent infusion device, verify patency and placement of the device before injecting the drug. Then flush the device with normal saline solution, give the drug, and follow with the appropriate flush.

ALERT *Immediately report signs of acute allergic reaction or anaphylaxis. If extravasation occurs, stop the injection, estimate the amount of infiltration, and notify the prescriber.*

■ When giving diazepam or chlordiazepoxide hydrochloride through a steel needle winged device or an I.V. line, flush with bacteriostatic water to prevent precipitation.

I.V. ADMINISTRATION THROUGH A SECONDARY LINE

A secondary I.V. line is a complete I.V. set connected to the lower Y-port (secondary port) of a primary line instead of to the

I.V. catheter or needle. It features an I.V. container, long tubing, and either a microdrip or macrodrip system. A secondary line can be used for continuous or intermittent drug infusion. When used continuously, it permits drug infusion and titration while the primary line maintains a constant total infusion rate.

A secondary I.V. line used only for intermittent drug administration is called a piggyback set. In this case, the primary line maintains venous access between drug doses. A piggyback set includes a small I.V. container, short tubing, and usually a macrodrip system. It connects to the primary line's upper Y-port (piggyback port).

Equipment and preparation

Check the chart and the medication administration record. Gather the prescribed I.V. drug, diluent (if needed), prescribed I.V. solution, administration set with secondary injection port, 22G needle 1″ in length or a needleless system, alcohol pads, 1″ (2.5-cm) adhesive tape, time tape, labels, infusion pump, extension hook, and solution for intermittent piggyback infusion.

Wash your hands. Inspect the I.V. container for cracks, leaks, or contamination. Check the

drug's expiration date and its compatibility with the primary solution. Determine whether the primary line has a secondary injection port.

If needed, add the drug to the secondary I.V. solution (usually 50- to 100-ml "mini-bags" of normal saline solution or D_5W). To do so, remove any seals from the secondary container and wipe the main port with an alcohol pad. Inject the prescribed drug and agitate the solution to mix the drug. Label the I.V. mixture.

Insert the administration set spike and attach the needle or needleless system. Open the flow clamp and prime the line. Then close the flow clamp.

Some drugs come in vials for hanging directly on an I.V. pole. In this case, inject the diluent directly into the drug vial. Then spike the vial, prime the tubing, and hang the set.

Implementation

■ If the drug is incompatible with the primary I.V. solution, replace the primary solution with a fluid that's compatible with both solutions. Then flush the line before starting the drug infusion.

■ Hang the container of the secondary set and wipe the injection port of the primary line with an alcohol pad.

■ Insert the needle or needle-less system from the secondary line into the injection port, and tape it securely to the primary line.

■ To run the container of the secondary set by itself, lower the primary set's container with an extension hook. To run both containers simultaneously, place them at the same height.

■ Open the clamp and adjust the drip rate.

■ For continuous infusion, set the secondary solution to the desired drip rate; then adjust the primary solution to the desired total infusion rate.

■ For intermittent infusion, wait until the secondary solution has completely infused; then adjust the primary drip rate, as required.

■ If the secondary solution tubing is being reused, close the clamp on the tubing and follow your facility's policy: Either remove the needle or needleless system and replace it with a new one, or leave it taped in the injection port and label it with the time it was first used.

■ Leave the empty container in place until you replace it with a new dose of drug at the prescribed time. If the tubing won't be reused, discard it appropriately with the I.V. container.

Nursing considerations

■ If facility policy allows, use a pump for drug infusion. Place a time tape on the secondary container to help prevent an inaccurate administration rate.

■ When reusing secondary tubing, change it according to your facility's policy, usually every 48 to 72 hours. Inspect the injection port for leakage with each use; change it more often if needed.

■ Except for lipids, don't piggyback a secondary I.V. line to a total parenteral nutrition line because it risks contamination.

6

I.V. THERAPY: TOOLS AND TROUBLESHOOTING

Intravenous (I.V.) therapy is a specialized and sometimes complex form of drug delivery that requires skill, training, and close monitoring of the patient and the delivery system. The resources in this chapter offer easy access to key information you can use to help establish, maintain, and troubleshoot I.V. therapy. These resources include the following:

■ Major electrolyte components of I.V. solutions

■ Understanding osmolality, osmolarity, and pH

■ Calculating drip rates

■ Preventing and treating extravasation

■ Infusion rates for selected drugs

■ Types of parenteral nutrition

■ Managing I.V. flow rate deviations

■ Risks of peripheral I.V. therapy

■ Risks of central venous therapy

■ How to avoid transfusion errors

■ Blood compatibility

■ Transfusing blood and selected components

MAJOR ELECTROLYTE COMPONENTS OF I.V. SOLUTIONS

SOLUTION	SODIUM (mEq/L)	POTASSIUM (mEq/L)	OSMOLARITY (mOsm/L)	TONICITY
Aminosyn 3.5% M	47	13	477	hypertonic
Aminosyn 7% with electrolytes	70	66	1,013	hypertonic
Aminosyn 8.5% with electrolytes	70	66	1,160	hypertonic
Dextrose 2.5% in half-strength lactated Ringer's injection	~65.5	2	265	isotonic
Dextrose 5% in electrolyte no. 48	25	20	348	isotonic
Dextrose 5% in electrolyte no. 75	40	35	402	hypertonic
Dextrose 5% in sodium chloride 0.11%	19	–	290	isotonic
Dextrose 5% in sodium chloride 0.2%	34 or 38.5	–	320–330	isotonic
Dextrose 5% in sodium chloride 0.33%	51 or 56	–	355–365	isotonic
Dextrose 5% in sodium chloride 0.45%	77	–	~405	hypertonic
Dextrose 5% in sodium chloride 0.9%	154	–	~560	hypertonic
Dextrose 50% with electrolyte pattern A	84	40	2,800	hypertonic

CALCIUM (mEq/L)	MAGNESIUM (mEq/L)	CHLORIDE (mEq/L)	ACETATE (mEq/L)	PHOSPHATE (MILLIMOLES)	OTHER
–	3	40	58	3.5	amino acids 3.5%
–	10	96	124	30	amino acids 7%
–	10	98	142	30	amino acids 8.5%
1.4–1.5	~55	–	–	lactate 14	–
–	3	24	–	3	lactate 23
–	–	48	–	15	lactate 20
–	–	19	–	–	–
–	–	34 or 38.5	–	–	–
–	–	51 or 56	–	–	–
–	–	77	–	–	–
–	–	154	–	–	–
10	16	115	–	–	gluconate 13 sulfate 16

(continued)

MAJOR ELECTROLYTE COMPONENTS
OF I.V SOLUTIONS *(continued)*

SOLUTION	SODIUM (mEq/L)	POTASSIUM (mEq/L)	OSMOLARITY (mOsm/L)	TONICITY
Dextrose 50% with electrolyte pattern N	90	80	2,875	hypertonic
Dextrose 50% with electrolyte no. 1	110	80	2,917	hypertonic
5% Travert and electrolyte no. 2	56	25	449	hypertonic
FreAmine III 3% with electrolytes	35	24.5	405	hypertonic
Ionosol B in dextrose 5% in water	57	25	426	hypertonic
Ionosol MB in dextrose 5% in water	25	20	352	hypotonic
Ionosol T in dextrose 5% in water	40	35	432	hypertonic
Isolyte E	140	10	310	isotonic
Isolyte G with dextrose 5%	65	17	555	hypertonic
Lactated Ringer's injection	130	4	~273	isotonic
Normosol-M in dextrose 5%	40	13	363	hypertonic
Plasma-Lyte A	140	5	294	isotonic
Plasma-Lyte R	140	10	312	isotonic
ProcalAmine	35	24	735	hypertonic

Calcium (mEq/L)	Magnesium (mEq/L)	Chloride (mEq/L)	Acetate (mEq/L)	Phosphate (millimoles)	Other
–	16	150	–	28	sulfate 16
–	16	140	36	24	–
–	6	56	–	12.5	lactate 25
–	5	41	44	3.5	amino acids 3%
–	5	49	–	7	lactate 25
–	3	22	–	3	lactate 23
–	–	40	–	15	lactate 20
5	3	103	49	–	citrate 8
–	–	149	–	–	ammonium 70
2.7–3	–	~109	–	–	lactate 28
–	3	40	16	–	–
–	3	98	27	–	gluconate 23
5	3	103	47	–	lactate 8
3	5	41	47	3.5	amino acids 3% glycerin 3%

(continued)

MAJOR ELECTROLYTE COMPONENTS OF I.V. SOLUTIONS (continued)

SOLUTION	SODIUM (mEq/L)	POTASSIUM (mEq/L)	OSMOLARITY (mOsm/L)	TONICITY
Ringer's injection	147 or 147.5	4	310	isotonic
Sodium bicarbonate 5%	595	–	1,190–1,203	hypertonic
Sodium chloride 0.45%	77	–	154	hypotonic
Sodium chloride 0.9%	154	–	308	isotonic
Sodium chloride 3%	513	–	1,030	hypertonic
Sodium chloride 5%	855	–	1,710	hypertonic
Sodium lactate 1/6 M	167	–	330	isotonic
Travasol 3.5% with electrolytes	25	15	450	hypertonic
Travasol 5.5% with electrolytes	70	60	850	hypertonic
Travasol 8.5% with electrolytes	70	60	1,160	hypertonic
Fat emulsion 10%, 20%, 30%	–	–	258–310	isotonic

Calcium (mEq/L)	Magnesium (mEq/L)	Chloride (mEq/L)	Acetate (mEq/L)	Phosphate (millimoles)	Other
4 or 4.5	–	155 or 156	–	–	–
–	–	–	–	–	HCO$_3$ 595
–	–	77	–	–	–
–	–	154	–	–	–
–	–	513	–	–	–
–	–	855	–	–	–
–	–	–	–	–	lactate 167
–	5	25	52	7.5	–
–	10	70	102	30	–
–	10	70	141	30	–
–	–	–	–	–	egg yolk phospho-lipids 1.2%

UNDERSTANDING OSMOLALITY, OSMOLARITY, AND pH

Osmolality, osmolarity, and pH can be used to identify potential infusion problems, such as phlebitis or fluid shift.

Osmolality

Osmolality is the measure of a solute concentration in kilograms of water and expresses the solution's osmotic pressure. It's measured in milliosmols/kilogram (mOsm/kg).

Osmolarity

Osmolarity is the measure of a solute concentration in liters of solution. It's measured in milliosmols/liter (mOsm/L). The osmolarity of plasma is 290 mOsm/L; of hypotonic solutions, less than 240 mOsm/L; of isotonic solutions,

CALCULATING DRIP RATES

When calculating the flow rate of I.V. solutions, remember that the number of drops needed to deliver 1 ml varies with the type of administration set you're using. To calculate the drip rate, you must know the calibration of the drip rate for each specific manufacturer's product. As a

	ORDERED VOLUME	
	500 ml/24 hour or 21 ml/hour	1,000 ml/24 hour or 42 ml/hour
Macrodrip (drops/ml)		
10	3	7
15	5	11
20	7	14
Microdrip (drops/ml)		
60	21	42

240 to 340 mOsm/L; and of hypertonic solutions, more than 340 mOsm/L. Hypotonic and hypertonic solutions cause vessel irritation or chemical phlebitis. Hypotonic solutions cause a vascular-to-cellular fluid shift; hypertonic solutions, cellular-to-vascular fluid shift.

pH

The pH is the degree of acidity or alkalinity of a solution. Normal range is 7.35 to 7.45. The pH of an acid is less than 7.35; the pH of a base, more than 7.45. Solutions that are mildly acidic or alkaline usually present no infusion risk, but when values fall outside the normal range, the patient is at risk for vein irritation, chemical phlebitis, or fluid shift.

quick guide, refer to the table below. Use this formula to calculate specific drip rates:

$$\frac{\text{volume of infusion (in ml)}}{\text{time of infusion (in minutes)}} \times \text{drip factor (in drops/ml)} = \text{drops/minute}$$

1,000 ml/20 hour or 50 ml/hour	1,000 ml/10 hour or 100 ml/hour	1,000 ml/8 hour or 125 ml/hour	1,000 ml/6 hour or 166 ml/hour
8	17	21	28
13	25	31	42
17	34	42	56
50	100	125	166

PREVENTING AND TREATING EXTRAVASATION

Extravasation—the escape of a vesicant into surrounding tissue—can result from a punctured vein or from leakage around a venipuncture site. Vesicants can cause blisters, severe local tissue damage, delayed healing, infection, disfigurement, and loss of function. The patient may need multiple debridements or amputation.

Preventing extravasation

To avoid extravasation when giving vesicants, use proper administration techniques and follow these guidelines:

■ Don't use an existing I.V. line unless you're sure it's patent. Perform a new venipuncture to ensure correct needle placement and vein patency.

■ Select the site carefully. Use a distal vein that allows successive proximal venipunctures. To avoid tendon and nerve damage, don't use the back of the hand. Also avoid the wrist and fingers (they're hard to immobilize), previously damaged areas, and areas with poor circulation.

■ Check for blood return before starting the infusion, and flush the needle to ensure patency. Palpate the vein and surrounding area while flushing; if swelling occurs, the solution is infiltrating.

■ Use a transparent film dressing to allow inspection.

■ Start the infusion with D_5W or normal saline solution.

■ Give vesicants after testing the I.V. line with normal saline solution and before any activities that could dislodge the needle.

■ Don't use an infusion pump because it could worsen infiltration.

■ Give the drug by slow I.V. push through a free-flowing I.V. line or by small-volume infusion (50 to 100 ml).

■ Check the infusion site for erythema or infiltration. Tell the patient to report burning, stinging, pruritus, or temperature changes.

■ After giving the drug, instill several milliliters of normal saline solution to flush the drug from the vein and avoid drug leakage when the needle is removed.

Treating extravasation

Extravasation of vesicants requires emergency treatment according to your facility's protocol. Essential steps include these:

■ Stop the infusion, aspirate the remaining drug in the catheter, and remove the I.V. line unless you need the needle to infiltrate the antidote.

■ Estimate the amount of extravasated solution, and tell the prescriber.

■ Instill the appropriate antidote according to facility protocol.

■ Have the patient elevate the affected arm or leg and avoid excessive pressure on the site.

■ Document the site, the patient's symptoms, the estimated amount of infiltrated solution, and the treatment. Include the prescriber's name and the time of notification. Continue documenting the site's appearance and patient's symptoms.

■ As appropriate, apply ice to the affected area for 15 to 20 minutes every 4 to 6 hours for about 3 days. (For etoposide and vinca alkaloids, apply warm compresses instead.)

■ Have the patient rest and elevate the site for 48 hours before resuming normal activity.

■ If skin breakdown occurs, apply silver sulfadiazine cream and gauze dressings or wet-to-dry povidone-iodine dressings.

■ If extravasation is severe, debridement, plastic surgery, and physical therapy may be needed.

INFUSION RATES FOR SELECTED DRUGS

These infusion rates are based on the concentrations shown at the top of each table. Be sure to check the label on the drug you're infusing to verify the correct infusion rate.

Epinephrine infusion rates
Mix 1 mg in 250 ml (4 mcg/ml).

DOSE (MCG/MIN)	INFUSION RATE (ML/HR)
1	15
2	30
3	45
4	60
5	75
6	90
7	105
8	120
9	135
10	150
15	225
20	300
25	375
30	450
35	525
40	600

Isoproterenol infusion rates
Mix 1 mg in 250 ml (4 mcg/ml).

DOSE (MCG/MIN)	INFUSION RATE (ML/HR)
0.5	8
1	15
2	30
3	45
4	60
5	75
6	90
7	105
8	120
9	135
10	150
15	225
20	300
25	375
30	450

Nitroglycerin infusion rates

Determine the infusion rate in ml/hr using the ordered dose and the concentration of the drug solution.

DOSE (MCG/MIN)	25 MG/ 250 ML (100 MCG/ML)	50 MG/ 250 ML (200 MCG/ML)	100 MG/ 250 ML (400 MCG/ML)
5	3	2	1
10	6	3	2
20	12	6	3
30	18	9	5
40	24	12	6
50	30	15	8
60	36	18	9
70	42	21	10
80	48	24	12
90	54	27	14
100	60	30	15
150	90	45	23
200	120	60	30

(continued)

INFUSION RATES FOR SELECTED DRUGS (continued)

Dobutamine infusion rates

Mix 250 mg in 250 ml of D_5W (1,000 mcg/ml). Determine the infusion rate in ml/hr using the ordered dose (shown in mcg/kg/minute below) and the patient's weight in pounds or kilograms.

DOSE (MCG/ KG/MIN)	lb 88 kg 40	99 45	110 50	121 55	132 60	143 65	154 70
2.5	6	7	8	8	9	10	11
5	12	14	15	17	18	20	21
7.5	18	20	23	25	27	29	32
10	24	27	30	33	36	39	42
12.5	30	34	38	41	45	49	53
15	36	41	45	50	54	59	63
20	48	54	60	66	72	78	84
25	60	68	75	83	90	98	105
30	72	81	90	99	108	117	126
35	84	95	105	116	126	137	147
40	96	108	120	132	144	156	168

165	176	187	198	209	220	231	242
75	80	85	90	95	100	105	110
11	12	13	14	14	15	16	17
23	24	26	27	29	30	32	33
34	36	38	41	43	45	47	50
45	48	51	54	57	60	63	66
56	60	64	68	71	75	79	83
68	72	77	81	86	90	95	99
90	96	102	108	114	120	126	132
113	120	128	135	143	150	158	165
135	144	153	162	171	180	189	198
158	168	179	189	200	210	221	231
180	192	204	216	228	240	252	264

(continued)

Dopamine infusion rates

Mix 400 mg in 250 ml of D_5W (1,600 mcg/ml). Determine the infusion rate in ml/hr using the ordered dose (shown in mcg/kg/minute below) and the patient's weight in pounds or kilograms.

DOSE (MCG/ KG/MIN)	lb 88 kg 40	99 45	110 50	121 55	132 60	143 65	154 70
2.5	4	4	5	5	6	6	7
5	8	8	9	10	11	12	13
7.5	11	13	14	15	17	18	20
10	15	17	19	21	23	24	26
12.5	19	21	23	26	28	30	33
15	23	25	28	31	34	37	39
20	30	34	38	41	45	49	53
25	38	42	47	52	56	61	66
30	45	51	56	62	67	73	79
35	53	59	66	72	79	85	92
40	60	68	75	83	90	98	105
45	68	76	84	93	101	110	118
50	75	84	94	103	113	122	131

165	176	187	198	209	220	231
75	80	85	90	95	100	105
7	8	8	8	9	9	10
14	15	16	17	18	19	20
21	23	24	25	27	28	30
28	30	32	34	36	38	39
35	38	40	42	45	47	49
42	45	48	51	53	56	59
56	60	64	68	71	75	79
70	75	80	84	89	94	98
84	90	96	101	107	113	118
98	105	112	118	125	131	138
113	120	128	135	143	150	158
127	135	143	152	160	169	177
141	150	159	169	178	188	197

(continued)

INFUSION RATES FOR SELECTED DRUGS (continued)

Nitroprusside infusion rates

Mix 50 mg in 250 ml of D_5W (200 mcg/ml). Determine the infusion rate in ml/hr using the ordered dose (shown in mcg/kg/minute below) and the patient's weight in pounds or kilograms.

DOSE (MCG/ KG/MIN)	lb 88 kg 40	99 45	110 50	121 55	132 60	143 65	154 70
0.3	4	4	5	5	5	6	6
0.5	6	7	8	8	9	10	11
1	12	14	15	17	18	20	21
1.5	18	20	23	25	27	29	32
2	24	27	30	33	36	39	42
3	36	41	45	50	54	59	63
4	48	54	60	66	72	78	84
5	60	68	75	83	90	98	105
6	72	81	90	99	108	117	126
7	84	95	105	116	126	137	147
8	96	108	120	132	144	156	168
9	108	122	135	149	162	176	189
10	120	135	150	165	180	195	210

165	176	187	198	209	220	231	242
75	80	85	90	95	100	105	110
7	7	8	8	9	9	9	10
11	12	13	14	14	15	16	17
23	24	26	27	29	30	32	33
34	36	38	41	43	45	47	50
45	48	51	54	57	60	63	66
68	72	77	81	86	90	95	99
90	96	102	108	114	120	126	132
113	120	128	135	143	150	158	165
135	144	153	162	171	180	189	198
158	168	179	189	200	210	221	231
180	192	204	216	228	240	252	264
203	216	230	243	257	270	284	297
225	240	255	270	285	300	315	330

TYPES OF PARENTERAL NUTRITION

TYPE	SOLUTION COMPONENTS/LITER	SPECIAL CONSIDERATIONS
Standard I.V. therapy	■ Dextrose, water, electrolytes in varying amounts, for example: – dextrose 5% in water (D_5W) = 170 calories/L – $D_{10}W$ = 340 calories/L – normal saline solution = 0 calories ■ Vitamins as ordered	■ Nutritionally incomplete; doesn't provide sufficient calories to maintain adequate nutritional status
Total parenteral nutrition (TPN) by central venous line	■ $D_{15}W$ to $D_{25}W$ (1 L dextrose 25% = 850 nonprotein calories) ■ Crystalline amino acids 2.5% to 8.5% ■ Electrolytes, vitamins, trace elements, and insulin as ordered ■ Lipid emulsion 10% to 20% (usually infused as a separate solution)	***Basic solution*** ■ Nutritionally complete ■ Requires minor surgical procedure for central venous line insertion (can be done at bedside by the physician) ■ Highly hypertonic solution ■ May cause metabolic complications (glucose intolerance, electrolyte imbalance, essential fatty acid deficiency) ***I.V. lipid emulsion*** ■ May not be used effectively in severely stressed patients (especially burn patients) ■ May interfere with immune mechanisms; in patients suffering respiratory compromise, reduces carbon dioxide buildup ■ Given by central venous line; irritates peripheral vein in long-term use

TYPES OF PARENTERAL NUTRITION (continued)

TYPE	SOLUTION COMPONENTS/LITER	SPECIAL CONSIDERATIONS
Protein-sparing therapy	■ Crystalline amino acids in same amounts as TPN ■ Electrolytes, vitamins, minerals, and trace elements as ordered	■ Nutritionally complete ■ Requires little mixing ■ May be started or stopped any time during the hospital stay ■ Other I.V. fluids, drugs, and blood by-products may be administered through the same I.V. line ■ Not as likely to cause phlebitis as peripheral parenteral nutrition ■ Adds a major expense; has limited benefits
Total nutrient admixture	■ One day's nutrients are contained in a single, 3-L bag (also called 3:1 solution) ■ Combines lipid emulsion with other parenteral solution components	■ See TPN (p. 222) ■ Reduces need to handle bag, cutting risk of contamination ■ Decreases nursing time and reduces need for infusion sets and electronic devices, lowering facility costs, increasing patient mobility, and allowing easier adjustment to home care ■ Has limited use because not all types and amounts of components are compatible ■ Precludes use of certain infusion pumps because they can't accurately deliver large volumes of solution; precludes use of standard I.V. tubing filters because a 0.22 micron filter blocks lipid and albumin molecules.

(continued)

TYPES OF PARENTERAL NUTRITION (continued)

TYPE	SOLUTION COMPONENTS/LITER	SPECIAL CONSIDERATIONS
Peripheral parenteral nutrition (PPN)	■ D_5W to $D_{10}W$ ■ Crystalline amino acids 2.5% to 5% ■ Electrolytes, minerals, vitamins, and trace elements as ordered ■ Lipid emulsion 10% or 20% (1 L of dextrose 10% and amino acids 3.5% infused at the same time as 1 L of lipid emulsion = 1,440 nonprotein calories) ■ Heparin or hydrocortisone as ordered	**Basic solution** ■ Nutritionally complete for a short time ■ Can't be used in nutritionally depleted patients ■ Can't be used in volume restricted patients because PPN requires large fluid volume ■ Doesn't cause weight gain ■ Avoids insertion and care of central venous line but needs adequate venous access; site must be changed every 72 hours ■ Delivers less hypertonic solutions than central venous line TPN ■ May cause phlebitis and increases risk of metabolic complications ■ Less chance of metabolic complications than with central venous line TPN **I.V. lipid emulsion** ■ As effective as dextrose as calorie source ■ Diminishes phlebitis if infused at the same time as basic nutrient solution ■ Irritates vein in long-term use ■ Reduces carbon dioxide buildup if patient has pulmonary compromise

MANAGING I.V. FLOW RATE DEVIATIONS

PROBLEM	CAUSE	NURSING INTERVENTIONS
Flow rate too slow	■ Venous spasm after insertion ■ Venous obstruction from bending arm ■ Pressure change (decreasing fluid in bottle causes solution to run slower because of decreasing pressure)	■ Apply warm soaks over site. ■ Secure with an arm board if necessary. ■ Readjust flow rate.
	■ Elevated blood pressure	■ Readjust flow rate. Use infusion pump or controller to ensure correct flow rate.
	■ Cold solution	■ Allow solution to warm to room temperature before hanging.
	■ Change in solution viscosity from added drug	■ Readjust flow rate.
	■ I.V. container too low or patient's arm or leg too high	■ Hang container higher or remind patient to keep his arm below heart level.
	■ Bevel against vein wall (positional cannulation)	■ Withdraw needle slightly, or place a folded $2'' \times 2''$ gauze pad over or under catheter hub to change angle.
	■ Excess tubing dangling below insertion site	■ Replace tubing with shorter piece, or tape excess tubing to I.V. pole, below flow clamp. (Make sure tubing isn't kinked.)
	■ Cannula too small	■ Remove cannula in use and insert a larger-bore cannula, or use an infusion pump.
	■ Infiltration or clotted cannula	■ Remove cannula in use and insert a new cannula.
	■ Kinked tubing	■ Check tubing over its entire length and unkink it.
	■ Clogged filter	■ Remove filter and replace with a new one.
	■ Tubing memory (tubing compressed at area clamped)	■ Massage or milk tubing by pinching and wrapping it around a pencil four or five times. Quickly pull pencil out of coiled tubing.

(continued)

MANAGING I.V. FLOW RATE DEVIATIONS (continued)

PROBLEM	CAUSE	NURSING INTERVENTIONS
Flow rate too fast	■ Patient or visitor manipulating clamp	■ Instruct patient not to touch clamp. Place tape over it. Administer I.V. solution with infusion pump or controller if needed.
	■ Tubing disconnected from catheter	■ Wipe distal end of tubing with alcohol, reinsert firmly into catheter hub, and tape at connection site. Consider using tubing with luer-lock connections.
	■ Change in patient position	■ Administer I.V. solution with infusion pump or controller to ensure correct flow rate.
	■ Flow clamp drifting because of patient movement	■ Place tape below clamp.

RISKS OF PERIPHERAL I.V. THERAPY

COMPLICATIONS AND FINDINGS	POSSIBLE CAUSES	NURSING INTERVENTIONS
Local complications		
Phlebitis ■ Tenderness at tip of and proximal to venous access device ■ Redness at tip of cannula and along vein ■ Puffy area over vein ■ Hard vein on palpation ■ Elevated temperature	■ Poor blood flow around venous access device ■ Friction from cannula movement in vein ■ Venous access device left in vein too long ■ Clotting at cannula tip (thrombophlebitis) ■ Drug or solution with high or low pH or high osmolarity	■ Remove venous access device. ■ Apply warm soaks. ■ Notify a physician if patient has a fever. ■ Document patient's condition and your interventions. *Prevention* ■ Restart infusion using larger vein for irritating solution, or restart with a smaller-gauge device to ensure adequate blood flow. ■ Use filter to reduce risk of phlebitis. ■ Tape device securely to prevent motion.
Infiltration ■ Swelling at and above I.V. site (may extend along entire limb) ■ Discomfort, burning, or pain at site (may be painless) ■ Tight feeling at site ■ Decreased skin temperature around site ■ Blanching at site ■ Continuing fluid infusion even when vein is occluded (although rate may decrease) ■ Absent backflow of blood	■ Venous access device dislodged from vein ■ Perforated vein	■ Stop infusion. If extravasation is likely, infiltrate the site with an antidote. ■ Apply warm soaks to aid absorption. Elevate limb. ■ Check for pulse and capillary refill periodically to assess circulation. ■ Restart infusion above infiltration site or in another limb. ■ Document patient's condition and your interventions. *Prevention* ■ Check I.V. site often. ■ Don't obscure area above site with tape. ■ Teach patient to observe I.V. site and report pain or swelling.

(continued)

RISKS OF PERIPHERAL I.V. THERAPY (continued)

COMPLICATIONS AND FINDINGS	POSSIBLE CAUSES	NURSING INTERVENTIONS

Local complications (continued)

Cannula dislodgment
- Loose tape
- Cannula partly backed out of vein
- Solution infiltrating

■ Loosened tape, or tubing snagged in bed linens, resulting in partial retraction of cannula
■ Cannula pulled out by confused patient

■ If no infiltration occurs, retape without pushing cannula back into vein. If pulled out, apply pressure to I.V. site with sterile dressing.
Prevention
■ Tape venipuncture device securely on insertion.

Occlusion
- No increase in flow rate when I.V. container is raised
- Blood backflow in line
- Discomfort at insertion site

■ I.V. flow interrupted
■ Heparin lock not flushed
■ Blood backflow in line when patient walks
■ Line clamped too long

■ Use mild flush injection. Don't force it. If unsuccessful, remove I.V. line and insert a new one.
Prevention
■ Maintain I.V. flow rate.
■ Flush promptly after intermittent piggyback administration.
■ Have patient walk with arm bent at the elbow to reduce the risk of blood backflow.

Vein irritation or pain at I.V. site
- Pain during infusion
- Possible blanching if vasospasm occurs
- Red skin over vein during infusion
- Rapidly developing signs of phlebitis

■ Solution with high or low pH or high osmolarity, such as 40 mEq/L of potassium chloride, phenytoin, and some antibiotics (vancomycin, erythromycin, and nafcillin)

■ Decrease the flow rate.
■ Try using an electronic flow device to achieve a steady flow.
Prevention
■ Dilute solutions before administration. For example, give antibiotics in 250-ml solution rather than 100-ml solution. If drug has low pH, ask pharmacist if drug can be buffered with sodium bicarbonate. (Check your facility's policy.)
■ If long-term therapy of irritating drug is planned, ask physician to use central I.V. line.

RISKS OF PERIPHERAL I.V. THERAPY (continued)

COMPLICATIONS AND FINDINGS	POSSIBLE CAUSES	NURSING INTERVENTIONS
Local complications (continued)		
Hematoma ■ Tenderness at venipuncture site ■ Bruised area around site ■ Inability to advance or flush I.V. line	■ Vein punctured through opposite wall at time of insertion ■ Leakage of blood from needle displacement ■ Inadequate pressure applied when cannula is discontinued	■ Remove venous access device. ■ Apply pressure and warm soaks to affected area. ■ Recheck for bleeding. ■ Document patient's condition and your interventions. *Prevention* ■ Choose a vein that can accommodate the size of venous access device. ■ Release tourniquet as soon as insertion is successful.
Severed cannula ■ Leakage from cannula shaft	■ Cannula inadvertently cut by scissors ■ Reinsertion of needle into cannula	■ If broken part is visible, try to retrieve it. If unsuccessful, notify a physician. ■ If portion of cannula enters bloodstream, place tourniquet above I.V. site to prevent progression of broken part. ■ Notify physician and radiology department. ■ Document patient's condition and your interventions. *Prevention* ■ Don't use scissors around I.V. site. ■ Never reinsert needle into cannula. ■ Remove unsuccessfully inserted cannula and needle together.

(continued)

RISKS OF PERIPHERAL I.V. THERAPY (continued)

COMPLICATIONS AND FINDINGS	POSSIBLE CAUSES	NURSING INTERVENTIONS
Local complications (continued)		
Venous spasm ■ Pain along vein ■ Flow rate sluggish when clamp completely open ■ Blanched skin over vein	■ Severe vein irritation from irritating drugs or fluids ■ Administration of cold fluids or blood ■ Very rapid flow rate (with fluids at room temperature)	■ Apply warm soaks over vein and surrounding area. ■ Decrease flow rate. *Prevention* ■ Use a blood warmer for blood or packed red blood cells.
Thrombosis ■ Painful, red, swollen vein ■ Sluggish or stopped I.V. flow	■ Injury to endothelial cells of vein wall, allowing platelets to adhere and thrombi to form	■ Remove venous access device; restart infusion in opposite limb if possible. ■ Apply warm soaks. ■ Watch for I.V. therapy–related infection; thrombi provide an excellent environment for bacterial growth. *Prevention* ■ Use proper venipuncture techniques to reduce injury to vein.
Thrombophlebitis ■ Severe discomfort ■ Red, swollen, hardened vein	■ Thrombosis and inflammation	■ Same as for thrombosis. *Prevention* ■ Check site frequently. Remove venous access device at first sign of redness and tenderness.
Nerve, tendon, or ligament damage		
■ Extreme pain (similar to electrical shock when nerve is punctured) ■ Numbness and muscle contraction ■ Delayed effects, including paralysis, numbness, and deformity	■ Improper venipuncture technique resulting in injury to surrounding nerves, tendons, or ligaments ■ Tight taping or improper splinting with arm board	■ Stop procedure. *Prevention* ■ Don't repeatedly penetrate tissues with venous access device. ■ Don't apply excessive pressure when taping; don't encircle limb with tape. ■ Pad arm boards and tape securing arm boards if possible.

RISKS OF PERIPHERAL I.V. THERAPY (continued)

COMPLICATIONS AND FINDINGS	POSSIBLE CAUSES	NURSING INTERVENTIONS
Systemic complications		
Systemic infection (septicemia or bacteremia) ■ Fever, chills, and malaise for no apparent reason ■ Contaminated I.V. site, usually with no visible signs of infection at site	■ Failure to maintain aseptic technique during insertion or site care ■ Severe phlebitis, which can set up ideal conditions for organism growth ■ Poor taping that permits venous access device to move, which can introduce organisms into bloodstream ■ Prolonged indwelling time of device ■ Weak immune system	■ Notify a physician. ■ Administer drugs as prescribed. ■ Culture the site and device. ■ Monitor vital signs. *Prevention* ■ Use scrupulous aseptic technique when handling solutions and tubing, inserting venous access device, and discontinuing infusion. ■ Secure all connections. ■ Change I.V. solutions, tubing, and venous access device at recommended times. ■ Use I.V. filters.
Vasovagal reaction ■ Sudden collapse of vein during venipuncture ■ Sudden pallor, sweating, faintness, dizziness, and nausea ■ Decreased blood pressure	■ Vasospasm from anxiety or pain	■ Lower the head of the bed. ■ Have patient take deep breaths. ■ Check vital signs. *Prevention* ■ Prepare patient for therapy to relieve his anxiety. ■ Use local anesthetic to prevent pain.

(continued)

RISKS OF PERIPHERAL I.V. THERAPY (continued)

COMPLICATIONS AND FINDINGS	POSSIBLE CAUSES	NURSING INTERVENTIONS
Systemic complications (continued)		
Allergic reaction ■ Itching ■ Watery eyes and nose ■ Bronchospasm ■ Wheezing ■ Urticarial rash ■ Edema at I.V. site ■ Anaphylactic reaction (flushing, chills, anxiety, itching, palpitations, paresthesia, wheezing, seizures, cardiac arrest) up to 1 hour after exposure	■ Allergens such as medications	■ If reaction occurs, stop infusion immediately. ■ Maintain a patent airway. ■ Notify a physician. ■ Administer antihistamine, corticosteroid, and antipyretic drugs, as prescribed. ■ Give aqueous epinephrine subcutaneously, as prescribed. Repeat as needed and prescribed. *Prevention* ■ Obtain patient's allergy history. Be aware of cross-allergies. ■ Assist with test dosing and document any new allergies. ■ Monitor patient carefully during first 15 minutes of administration of a new drug.
Circulatory overload ■ Discomfort ■ Engorged neck veins ■ Respiratory distress ■ Increased blood pressure ■ Crackles ■ Increased difference between fluid intake and output	■ Roller clamp loosened to allow run-on infusion ■ Flow rate too rapid ■ Miscalculation of fluid requirements	■ Raise the head of the bed. ■ Administer oxygen as needed. ■ Notify a physician. ■ Give drugs (probably furosemide) as prescribed. *Prevention* ■ Use pump, controller, or rate minder for elderly or compromised patients. ■ Recheck calculations of fluid requirements. ■ Monitor infusion frequently.

RISKS OF PERIPHERAL I.V. THERAPY (continued)

COMPLICATIONS AND FINDINGS	POSSIBLE CAUSES	NURSING INTERVENTIONS

Systemic complications (continued)

Air embolism
- Respiratory distress
- Unequal breath sounds
- Weak pulse
- Increased central venous pressure
- Decreased blood pressure
- Loss of consciousness

Possible causes:
- Solution container empty
- Solution container empties, and added container pushes air down the line (if line not purged first)

Nursing interventions:
- Discontinue infusion.
- Place patient on left side in Trendelenburg's position to allow air to enter right atrium.
- Administer oxygen.
- Notify a physician.
- Document patient's condition and your interventions.

Prevention
- Purge tubing of air completely before starting infusion.
- Use air-detection device on pump or air-eliminating filter proximal to I.V. site.
- Secure connections.

RISKS OF CENTRAL VENOUS THERAPY

COMPLICATIONS AND FINDINGS	POSSIBLE CAUSES	NURSING INTERVENTIONS
Infection ■ Redness, warmth, tenderness, swelling at insertion or exit site ■ Possible exudate of purulent material ■ Local rash or pustules ■ Fever, chills, malaise ■ Leukocytosis ■ Nausea and vomiting ■ Elevated urine glucose level	■ Failure to maintain aseptic technique during catheter insertion or care ■ Failure to comply with dressing change protocol ■ Wet or soiled dressing remaining on site ■ Immunosuppression ■ Irritated suture line ■ Contaminated catheter or solution ■ Frequent opening of catheter or long-term use of single I.V. access site	■ Monitor temperature frequently. ■ Watch vital signs closely. ■ Culture the site. ■ Redress aseptically. ■ Possibly use antibiotic ointment locally. ■ Treat systemically with antibiotics or antifungals, depending on culture results and physician order. ■ Catheter may be removed. ■ Draw central and peripheral blood cultures; if the same organism appears in both, then catheter is primary source and should be removed. ■ If cultures don't match but are positive, the catheter may be removed or the infection may be treated through the catheter. ■ If the catheter is removed, culture its tip. ■ Document interventions. ***Prevention*** ■ Maintain sterile technique. Use sterile gloves, masks, and gowns when appropriate. ■ Observe dressing-change protocols. ■ Teach about restrictions on swimming, bathing, and so on. (With adequate white blood cell count, a physician may allow these activities.) ■ Change wet or soiled dressing immediately. ■ Change dressing more often if catheter is in femoral area or near tracheostomy.

RISKS OF CENTRAL VENOUS THERAPY *(continued)*

COMPLICATIONS AND FINDINGS	POSSIBLE CAUSES	NURSING INTERVENTIONS
Infection *(continued)*		Provide tracheostomy care after catheter care. ■ Examine solution for cloudiness and turbidity before infusing; check fluid container for leaks. ■ Monitor urine glucose level in patients receiving total parenteral nutrition (TPN); if greater than 2+, suspect early sepsis. ■ Use a 0.22-micron filter (or a 1.2-micron filter for 3-in-1 TPN solutions). ■ Catheter may be changed frequently. ■ Keep the system closed as much as possible.

Pneumothorax, hemothorax, chylothorax, hydrothorax

■ Decreased breath sounds on affected side ■ With hemothorax, decreased hemoglobin level because of blood pooling ■ Abnormal chest X-ray	■ Repeated or long-term use of same vein ■ Cardiovascular disease ■ Lung puncture by catheter during insertion or exchange over a guidewire ■ Large blood vessel puncture with bleeding inside or outside the lung ■ Lymph node puncture with leakage of lymph fluid ■ Infusion of solution into chest area through infiltrated catheter	■ Notify a physician. ■ Remove catheter or assist with removal. ■ Give oxygen. ■ Set up and assist with chest tube insertion. ■ Document interventions. ***Prevention*** ■ Position patient head down with a rolled towel between his scapulae to dilate and expose the internal jugular or subclavian vein as much as possible during catheter insertion. ■ Look for early signs of fluid infiltration (swelling in the shoulder, neck, chest, and arm). ■ Make sure the patient is immobilized and prepared for insertion. Active patients may need to be sedated or taken to the operating room.

(continued)

RISKS OF CENTRAL VENOUS THERAPY *(continued)*

COMPLICATIONS AND FINDINGS	POSSIBLE CAUSES	NURSING INTERVENTIONS
Air embolism ■ Respiratory distress ■ Unequal breath sounds ■ Weak pulse ■ Increased central venous pressure ■ Decreased blood pressure ■ Alteration or loss of consciousness	■ Intake of air into the central venous system during catheter insertion or tubing changes, or inadvertent opening, cutting, or breaking of catheter	■ Clamp catheter immediately. ■ Turn patient on the left side, head down, so that air can enter the right atrium. Maintain this position for 20 to 30 minutes. ■ Give oxygen. ■ Notify a physician. ■ Document interventions. *Prevention* ■ Purge all air from tubing before hookup. ■ Teach patient to perform Valsalva's maneuver during catheter insertion and tubing changes. ■ Use air-eliminating filters. ■ Use an infusion device with air detection capability. ■ Use luer-lock tubing, tape the connections, or use locking devices for all connections.
Thrombosis ■ Edema at puncture site ■ Erythema ■ Ipsilateral swelling of arm, neck, and face ■ Pain along vein ■ Fever, malaise ■ Chest pain ■ Dyspnea ■ Cyanosis	■ Sluggish flow rate ■ Composition of catheter material (polyvinyl chloride catheters are more thrombogenic) ■ Hematopoietic status of patient ■ Limb edema ■ Infusion of irritating solutions	■ Notify a physician. ■ Possibly remove catheter. ■ Possibly infuse anticoagulant doses of heparin. ■ Verify thrombosis with diagnostic studies. ■ Apply warm, wet compresses locally. ■ Don't use limb on affected side for subsequent venipuncture. ■ Document interventions. *Prevention* ■ Maintain steady flow rate with infusion pump, or flush catheter at regular intervals. ■ Use catheters made of less thrombogenic materials or catheters coated to prevent thrombosis. ■ Dilute irritating solutions. ■ Use a 0.22-micron filter for infusions.

HOW TO AVOID TRANSFUSION ERRORS

Proper identification of the patient and the ordered blood product is essential, as is following your facility's policy and taking these precautions:

■ Match the patient's name, medical record number, ABO and Rh status, and blood bank identification numbers with the label on the blood bag.

■ Check the expiration date.

■ Have another nurse verify the information.

■ On the blood slip, fill in the required data and sign your name. The blood slip will prove useful if the patient develops an adverse reaction.

■ Double-check the physician's order to make sure you're transfusing the correct product.

■ Make sure the blood was typed and crossmatched within 48 hours—a Food and Drug Administration requirement for transfusions.

BLOOD COMPATIBILITY

Precise typing and crossmatching of donor and recipient blood can avoid transfusions of incompatible blood, which can be fatal. Red blood cells (RBCs) are classified as type A, B, or AB, depending on the antigen detected on the cell, or type O, which has no detectable A or B antigens. Similarly, blood plasma has or lacks anti-A or anti-B antibodies.

A person with type O blood is a universal donor. Because this blood lacks A or B antigens, it can be transfused in an emergency in limited amounts to any patient regardless of blood type and with little risk of reaction. A person with AB blood is a universal recipient. Because his blood lacks A and B antibodies, he can receive types A, B, or O blood (given as packed RBCs). This table shows ABO compatibility at a glance.

BLOOD GROUP	ANTIBODIES IN PLASMA	COMPATIBLE RBCs	COMPATIBLE PLASMA
Recipient			
O	Anti-A and anti-B	O	O, A, B, AB
A	Anti-B	A, O	A, AB
B	Anti-A	B, O	B, AB
AB	Neither anti-A nor anti-B	AB, A, B, O	AB
Donor			
O	Anti-A and anti-B	O, A, B, AB	O
A	Anti-B	A, AB	A, O
B	Anti-A	B, AB	B, O
AB	Neither anti-A nor anti-B	AB	AB, A, B, O

TRANSFUSING BLOOD AND SELECTED COMPONENTS

BLOOD COMPONENT	INDICATIONS	CROSSMATCHING
Whole blood Complete (pure) blood Volume: 450 or 500 ml	■ To restore blood volume lost from hemorrhaging, trauma, or burns	■ ABO identical: Type A receives A; type B receives B; type AB receives AB; type O receives O ■ Rh match needed
Packed red blood cells (RBCs) Same RBC mass as whole blood but with 80% of the plasma removed Volume: 250 ml	■ To restore or maintain oxygen-carrying capacity ■ To correct anemia and blood loss that occurs during surgery ■ To increase RBC mass	■ Type A receives A or O ■ Type B receives B or O ■ Type AB receives AB, A, B, or O ■ Type O receives O ■ Rh match needed
Platelets Platelet sediment from RBCs or plasma Volume: 35–50 ml/unit	■ To treat thrombocytopenia caused by decreased platelet production, increased platelet destruction, or massive transfusion of stored blood ■ To treat acute leukemia and marrow aplasia ■ To improve platelet count preoperatively in a patient whose count is 100,000/mm^3 or less	■ ABO compatibility not needed but preferable with repeated platelet transfusions ■ Rh match preferred
Fresh frozen plasma (FFP) Uncoagulated plasma separated from RBCs and rich in coagulation factors V, VIII, and IX Volume: 180–300 ml	■ To expand plasma volume ■ To treat postoperative hemorrhage or shock ■ To correct an undetermined coagulation factor deficiency ■ To replace a specific factor when that factor alone isn't available ■ To correct factor deficiencies resulting from hepatic disease	■ ABO compatibility not needed but preferable with repeated platelet transfusions ■ Rh match preferred

Nursing considerations

- Use a straightline or Y-type I.V. set to infuse blood over 2–4 hours.
- Avoid giving whole blood when the patient can't tolerate the circulatory volume.
- Reduce the risk of a transfusion reaction by adding a microfilter to the administration set to remove platelets.
- Warm blood if giving a large quantity.

- Use a straightline or Y-type I.V. set to infuse blood over 2–4 hours.
- Bear in mind that packed RBCs provide the same oxygen–carrying capacity as whole blood with less risk of volume overload.
- Give packed RBCs, as ordered, to prevent potassium and ammonia buildup, which may occur in stored plasma.
- Avoid giving packed RBCs for anemic conditions correctable by nutritional or drug therapy.

- Use a component drip administration set to infuse 100 ml over 15 minutes.
- As prescribed, premedicate with antipyretics and antihistamines if the patient's history includes a platelet transfusion reaction.
- Avoid giving platelets when the patient has a fever.
- Prepare to draw blood for a platelet count, as ordered, 1 hour after the platelet transfusion to determine platelet transfusion increments.
- Keep in mind that a physician seldom orders a platelet transfusion for conditions in which platelet destruction is accelerated, such as idiopathic thrombocytopenic purpura and drug–induced thrombocytopenia.

- Use a straightline I.V. set and administer the infusion rapidly.
- Keep in mind that large-volume transfusions of FFP may require correction for hypocalcemia because citric acid in FFP binds calcium.

(continued)

BLOOD COMPONENT	INDICATIONS	CROSSMATCHING
Albumin 5% (buffered saline); albumin 25% (salt poor)		
A small plasma protein prepared by fractionating pooled plasma Volume: 5% = 12.5 g/250 ml 25% = 12.5 g/50 ml	■ To replace volume lost because of shock from burns, trauma, surgery, or infections ■ To replace volume and prevent marked hemoconcentration ■ To treat hypoproteinemia (with or without edema)	■ Not needed
Factor VIII (cryoprecipitate)		
Insoluble portion of plasma recovered from FFP Volume: about 30 ml (freeze dried)	■ To treat a patient with hemophilia A ■ To control bleeding from factor VIII deficiency ■ To replace fibrinogen or deficient factor VIII	■ ABO compatibility not needed but preferable

NURSING CONSIDERATIONS

■ Use a straight-line I.V. set with rate and volume dictated by the patient's condition and response.
■ Remember that reactions to albumin (fever, chills, nausea) are rare.
■ Avoid mixing albumin with protein hydrolysates and alcohol solutions.
■ Consider delivering albumin as a volume expander until the laboratory completes crossmatching for a whole blood transfusion.
■ Keep in mind that albumin is contraindicated in severe anemia and given cautiously in cardiac and pulmonary disease because heart failure may result from circulatory overload.

■ Use the administration set supplied by the manufacturer. Administer factor VIII with a filter. Standard dose recommended for treatment of acute bleeding episodes in hemophilia is 15–20 units/kg.
■ Half-life of factor VIII (8–10 hours) warrants repeated transfusions at specified intervals to maintain normal levels.

GUIDE TO TRANSFUSION REACTIONS

Any patient receiving a transfusion of processed blood products can experience a transfusion reaction. Transfusion reactions typically result from antigen–antibody reactions; they also may result from bacterial contamination.

REACTIONS AND CAUSES	SIGNS AND SYMPTOMS
Allergic ■ Allergen in donor blood ■ Donor blood hypersensitive to certain drugs	■ Anaphylaxis (chills, facial swelling, laryngeal edema, pruritus, urticaria, wheezing), fever, nausea, and vomiting
Bacterial contamination ■ Organisms that can survive cold, such as *Pseudomonas* and *Staphylococcus*	■ Chills, fever, vomiting, abdominal cramping, diarrhea, shock, signs of renal failure
Febrile ■ Bacterial lipopolysaccharides ■ Antileukocyte recipient antibodies directed against donor white blood cells	■ Temperature up to 104° F (40° C), chills, headache, facial flushing, palpitations, cough, chest tightness, increased pulse rate, flank pain
Hemolytic ■ ABO or Rh incompatibility ■ Intradonor incompatibility ■ Improper crossmatching ■ Improperly stored blood	■ Chest pain, dyspnea, facial flushing, fever, chills, shaking, hypotension, flank pain, hemoglobinuria, oliguria, bloody oozing at the infusion site or surgical incision site, burning sensation along vein receiving blood, shock, renal failure
Plasma protein incompatibility ■ Immunoglobulin-A incompatibility	■ Abdominal pain, diarrhea, dyspnea, chills, fever, flushing, hypotension

Nursing Interventions

■ Give antihistamines as prescribed.
■ Monitor patient for anaphylactic reaction and give epinephrine and corticosteroids if indicated.

■ Provide broad–spectrum antibiotics, corticosteroids, or epinephrine.
■ Maintain strict blood storage control.
■ Change blood administration set and filter every 4 hours or after every 2 units.
■ Infuse each unit of blood over 2–4 hours; stop the infusion if the time span exceeds 4 hours.
■ Maintain sterile technique when giving blood products.

■ Relieve symptoms with an antipyretic, an antihistamine, or meperidine, as prescribed.
■ If the patient needs further transfusions, use frozen RBCs, add a leukocyte-removal filter to the blood line, or premedicate the patient with acetaminophen, as prescribed, before starting another transfusion.

■ Monitor blood pressure.
■ Manage shock with I.V. fluids, oxygen, epinephrine, a diuretic, and a vasopressor, as indicated.
■ Obtain post–transfusion-reaction blood samples and urine specimens for analysis.
■ Watch for evidence of hemorrhage from disseminated intravascular coagulation.

■ Give oxygen, fluids, epinephrine, or a corticosteroid as prescribed.

THERAPEUTIC DRUG MONITORING GUIDELINES

DRUG	LABORATORY TEST MONITORED	THERAPEUTIC RANGES OF TEST
aminoglycoside antibiotics (amikacin, gentamicin, tobra- mycin)	Amikacin peak trough Gentamicin/tobramycin peak trough Creatinine	20–30 mcg/ml 1–8 mcg/ml 4–8 mcg/ml 2 mcg/ml 0.6–1.3 mg/dl
angiotensin- converting enzyme (ACE) inhibitors (be- nazepril, captopril, enalapril, enalaprilat, fosinopril, lisinopril, moexipril, quinapril, ramipril, trandolapril)	WBC with differential Creatinine BUN Potassium	***** 0.6–1.3 mg/dl 5–20 mg/dl 3.5–5 mEq/L
amphotericin B	Creatinine BUN Electrolytes (especially potassium and magnesium) Liver function CBC with differential and platelets	0.6–1.3 mg/dl 5–20 mg/dl Potassium: 3.5–5 mEq/L Magnesium: 1.5–2.5 mEq/L Sodium: 135–145 mEq/L Chloride: 98–106 mEq/L * *****
antibiotics	WBC with differential Cultures and sensitivities	*****
biguanides (metformin)	Creatinine Fasting glucose Glycosylated hemoglobin CBC	0.6–1.3 mg/dl 70–110 mg/dl 5.5%–8.5% of total hemoglobin *****

Note: *****For those areas marked with asterisks, the following values can be used:

Hemoglobin: Women: 12–16 g/dl
  Men: 14–18 g/dl
Hematocrit: Women: 37%–48%
  Men: 42%–52%
RBCs: 4–5.5 million/mm³
WBCs: 5–10 thousand/mm³

Differential: Neutrophils: 45%–74%
  Bands: 0%–8%
  Lymphocytes: 16%–45%
  Monocytes: 4%–10%
  Eosinophils: 0%–7%
  Basophils: 0%–2%

MONITORING GUIDELINES

Wait until giving third dose to check drug levels. Obtain blood for peak level 30 minutes after I.V. infusion ends or 60 minutes after I.M. administration. For trough levels, draw blood just before next dose. Dosage may need to be adjusted accordingly. Recheck after three doses. Monitor creatinine and BUN levels and urine output for signs of decreasing renal function. Monitor urine for increased proteins, cells, casts.

Monitor WBC with differential before therapy, monthly during the first 3 – 6 months, and then periodically for the first year. Monitor renal function and potassium level periodically.

Monitor creatinine, BUN, and electrolyte levels at least weekly during therapy. Also, regularly monitor blood counts and liver function test results during therapy.

Specimen cultures and sensitivities will determine the cause of the infection and the best treatment. Monitor WBC with differential weekly during therapy.

Check renal function and hematologic values before starting therapy and at least annually thereafter. If the patient has impaired renal function, don't use metformin because it may cause lactic acidosis. Monitor response to therapy by periodically evaluating fasting glucose and glycosylated hemoglobin levels. A patient's home monitoring of glucose levels helps monitor compliance and response.

(continued)

*For those areas marked with one asterisk, the following values can be used:

ALT: 7–56 units/L
AST: 5–40 units/L
Alkaline phosphatase: 17–142 units/L
LDH: 60–220 units/L
GGT: < 40 units/L
Total bilirubin: 0.2–1 mg/dl

THERAPEUTIC DRUG MONITORING GUIDELINES (continued)

Drug	Laboratory test monitored	Therapeutic ranges of test
carbamazepine	Carbamazepine CBC with differential Liver function BUN Platelet count	4–12 mcg/ml ***** * 5–20 mg/dl 150–450 x 10^3/mm^3
clozapine	WBC with differential	*****
corticosteroids (cortisone, hydrocortisone, prednisone, prednisolone, triamcinolone, methylprednisolone, dexamethasone, betamethasone)	Electrolytes (especially potassium) Fasting glucose	Potassium: 3.5–5 mEq/L Magnesium: 1.7–2.1 mEq/L Sodium: 135–145 mEq/L Chloride: 98–106 mEq/L Calcium: 8.6–10 mg/dl 70–110 mg/dl
digoxin	Digoxin Electrolytes (especially potassium, magnesium, and calcium) Creatinine	0.8–2 ng/ml Potassium: 3.5–5 mEq/L Magnesium: 1.7–2.1 mEq/L Sodium: 135–145 mEq/L Chloride: 98–106 mEq/L Calcium: 8.6–10 mg/dl 0.6–1.3 mg/dl
diuretics	Electrolytes Creatinine BUN Uric acid Fasting glucose	Potassium: 3.5–5 mEq/L Magnesium: 1.7–2.1 mEq/L Sodium: 135–145 mEq/L Chloride: 98–106 mEq/L Calcium: 8.6–10 mg/dl 0.6–1.3 mg/dl 5–20 mg/dl 2–7 mg/dl 70–110 mg/dl

Note: *****For those areas marked with asterisks, the following values can be used:

Hemoglobin: Women: 12–16 g/dl
  Men: 14–18 g/dl
Hematocrit: Women: 37%–48%
  Men: 42%–52%
RBCs: 4–5.5 million/mm^3
WBCs: 5–10 thousand/mm^3

Differential: Neutrophils: 45%–74%
  Bands: 0%–8%
  Lymphocytes: 16%–45%
  Monocytes: 4%–10%
  Eosinophils: 0%–7%
  Basophils: 0%–2%

MONITORING GUIDELINES

Monitor blood counts and platelets before therapy, monthly during the first 2 months, and then yearly. Liver function, BUN level, and urinalysis should be checked before and periodically during therapy.

Obtain WBC with differential before starting therapy, weekly during therapy, and 4 weeks after stopping the drug.

Monitor electrolyte and glucose levels regularly during long-term therapy.

Check digoxin levels just before the next dose or at least 6 hours after the last dose. To monitor maintenance therapy, check drug levels at least 1–2 weeks after therapy starts or changes. Make any adjustments in therapy based on entire clinical picture, not solely on drug levels. Also, check electrolyte levels and renal function periodically during therapy.

To monitor fluid and electrolyte balance, perform baseline and periodic determinations of electrolyte, calcium, BUN, uric acid, and glucose levels.

(continued)

*For those areas marked with one asterisk, the following values can be used:

ALT: 7–56 units/L
AST: 5–40 units/L
Alkaline phosphatase: 17–142 units/L
LDH: 60–220 units/L
GGT: < 40 units/L
Total bilirubin: 0.2–1 mg/dl

THERAPEUTIC DRUG MONITORING GUIDELINES (continued)

DRUG	LABORATORY TEST MONITORED	THERAPEUTIC RANGES OF TEST
erythropoietin	Hematocrit	Women: 36%–48% Men: 42%–52%
	Serum ferritin	10–83 mg/ml
	Transferrin saturation	220–400 mg/dl
ethosuximide	Ethosuximide	40–100 mcg/ml
	Liver function	*
	CBC with differential	*****
gemfibrozil	Lipids	Total cholesterol: < 200 mg/dl LDL: < 130 mg/dl HDL: Women: 40–75 mg/dl Men: 37–70 mg/dl Triglycerides: 10–160 mg/dl
	Liver function	*
	Serum glucose	70–100 mg/dl
heparin	Activated partial thromboplastin time (aPTT)	1.5–2.5 times control
HMG-CoA reductase inhibitors (fluvastatin, lovastatin, pravastatin, simvastatin)	Lipids	Total cholesterol: < 200 mg/dl LDL: < 130 mg/dl HDL: Women: 40–75 mg/dl Men: 37–70 mg/dl Triglycerides: 10–160 mg/dl
	Liver function	*
insulin	Fasting glucose	70–110 mg/dl
	Glycosylated hemoglobin	5.5%–8.5% of total hemoglobin

Note: *****For those areas marked with asterisks, the following values can be used:

Hemoglobin: Women: 12–16 g/dl
   Men: 14–18 g/dl
Hematocrit: Women: 37%–48%
   Men: 42%–52%
RBCs: 4–5.5 million/mm³
WBCs: 5–10 thousand/mm³

Differential: Neutrophils: 45%–74%
   Bands: 0%–8%
   Lymphocytes: 16%–45%
   Monocytes: 4%–10%
   Eosinophils: 0%–7%
   Basophils: 0%–2%

Monitoring guidelines

After therapy starts or changes, monitor hematocrit twice weekly for 2–6 weeks until stabilized in the target range and a maintenance dose determined. Monitor hematocrit regularly thereafter.

Check drug level 8–10 days after therapy starts or changes. Periodically monitor CBC with differential, liver function tests, and urinalysis.

Therapy is usually withdrawn after 3 months if response is inadequate. Patient must be fasting to measure triglyceride levels. Periodically obtain blood counts during the first 12 months.

When drug is given by continuous I.V. infusion, check aPTT every 4 hours in the early stages of therapy, and daily thereafter. When drug is given by deep S.C. injection, check aPTT 4–6 hours after injection, and daily thereafter.

Perform liver function tests at baseline, 6–12 weeks after therapy starts or changes, and about every 6 months thereafter. If response is inadequate in 6 weeks, consider changing the therapy.

Monitor response to therapy by evaluating glucose and glycosylated hemoglobin levels. Glycosylated hemoglobin level is a good measure of long-term control. A patient's home monitoring of glucose levels helps measure compliance and response.

(continued)

*For those areas marked with one asterisk, the following values can be used:

ALT: 7–56 units/L
AST: 5–40 units/L
Alkaline phosphatase: 17–142 units/L
LDH: 60–220 units/L
GGT: < 40 units/L
Total bilirubin: 0.2–1 mg/dl

THERAPEUTIC DRUG MONITORING GUIDELINES (continued)

DRUG	LABORATORY TEST MONITORED	THERAPEUTIC RANGES OF TEST
isotretinoin	Pregnancy test	Negative
	Liver function	*
	Lipids	Total cholesterol: < 200 mg/dl
		LDL: < 130 mg/dl
		HDL:
		Women: 40–75 mg/dl
		Men: 37–70 mg/dl
		Triglycerides: 10–160 mg/dl
	CBC with differential	*****
	Platelet count	150–450 x 10^3/mm^3
linezolid	CBC with differential and platelets	*****
	Cultures and sensitivities	
	Platelet count	150–450 x 10^3/mm^3
	Liver function	*
	Amylase	35–118 international units/L
	Lipase	10–150 units/L
lithium	Lithium	0.6–1.2 mEq/L
	Creatinine	0.6–1.3 mg/dl
	CBC	*****
	Electrolytes (especially potassium and sodium)	Potassium: 3.5–5 mEq/L
		Magnesium: 1.7–2.1 mEq/L
		Sodium: 135–145 mEq/L
		Chloride: 98–106 mEq/L
	Fasting glucose	70–110 mg/dl
	Thyroid function tests	TSH: 0.2–5.4 micro-units/ml
		T_3: 80–200 ng/dl
		T_4: 5.4–11.5 mcg/dl

Note: *****For those areas marked with asterisks, the following values can be used:

Hemoglobin: Women: 12–16 g/dl
  Men: 14–18 g/dl
Hematocrit: Women: 37%–48%
  Men: 42%–52%
RBCs: 4–5.5 million/mm^3
WBCs: 5–10 thousand/mm^3

Differential: Neutrophils: 45%–74%
  Bands: 0%–8%
  Lymphocytes: 16%–45%
  Monocytes: 4%–10%
  Eosinophils: 0%–7%
  Basophils: 0%–2%

MONITORING GUIDELINES

Use a serum or urine pregnancy test with a sensitivity of at least 25 mIU/ml. Perform one test before therapy and a second test during the second day of the menstrual cycle before therapy begins or at least 11 days after the last unprotected act of sexual intercourse, whichever is later. Repeat pregnancy tests monthly. Obtain baseline liver function tests and lipid levels; repeat every 1–2 weeks until a response is established (usually 4 weeks).

Obtain baseline CBC with differential and platelet count. Repeat weekly, especially if more than 2 weeks of therapy are received. Monitor liver function tests and amylase and lipase levels during therapy.

Checking lithium levels is crucial to safe use of the drug. Obtain lithium levels immediately before next dose. Monitor levels twice weekly until stable. Once at steady state, levels should be checked weekly; when the patient is on the appropriate maintenance dose, levels should be checked every 2–3 months. Monitor creatinine, electrolyte, and fasting glucose levels; CBC; and thyroid function test results before therapy starts and periodically during therapy.

(continued)

*For those areas marked with one asterisk, the following values can be used:

ALT: 7–56 units/L
AST: 5–40 units/L
Alkaline phosphatase: 17–142 units/L
LDH: 60–220 units/L
GGT: < 40 units/L
Total bilirubin: 0.2–1 mg/dl

THERAPEUTIC DRUG MONITORING GUIDELINES (continued)

DRUG	LABORATORY TEST MONITORED	THERAPEUTIC RANGES OF TEST
methotrexate	Methotrexate	Normal elimination: ~ 10 micromol 24 hours postdose; ~ 1 micromol 48 hours postdose; < 0.2 micromol 72 hours postdose
	CBC with differential	*****
	Platelet count	150–450 x 10³/mm³
	Liver function	*
	Creatinine	0.6–1.3 mg/dl
nonnucleoside reverse transcriptase inhibitors (nevirapine, delavirdine, efavirenz)	Liver function	*
	CBC with differential and platelets	*****
	Lipids	Total cholesterol: < 200 mg/dl LDL: < 130 mg/dl HDL: Women: 40–75 mg/dl Men: 37–70 mg/dl Triglycerides: 10–160 mg/dl
	Amylase	35–118 international units/L
phenytoin	Phenytoin	10–20 mcg/ml
	CBC	*****
potassium chloride	Potassium	3.5–5 mEq/L
procainamide	Procainamide	3–10 mcg/ml (procainamide)
	N-acetylprocainamide (NAPA)	10–30 mcg/ml (combined procainamide and NAPA)
	CBC	*****

Note: *****For those areas marked with asterisks, the following values can be used:

Hemoglobin: Women: 12–16 g/dl
  Men: 14–18 g/dl
Hematocrit: Women: 37%–48%
  Men: 42%–52%
RBCs: 4–5.5 million/mm³
WBCs: 5–10 thousand/mm³

Differential: Neutrophils: 45%–74%
  Bands: 0%–8%
  Lymphocytes: 16%–45%
  Monocytes: 4%–10%
  Eosinophils: 0%–7%
  Basophils: 0%–2%

MONITORING GUIDELINES

Monitor methotrexate levels according to dosing protocol. Monitor CBC with differential, platelet count, and liver and renal function test results more frequently when therapy starts or changes and when methotrexate levels may be elevated, such as when the patient is dehydrated.

Obtain baseline liver function tests and monitor closely during the first 12 weeks of therapy. Continue to monitor regularly during therapy. Check CBC with differential and platelet count before therapy and periodically during therapy. Monitor lipid levels during efavirenz therapy. Monitor amylase level during efavirenz and delavirdine therapy.

Monitor phenytoin levels immediately before next dose and 7–10 days after therapy starts or changes. Obtain a CBC at baseline and monthly early in therapy. Watch for toxic effects at therapeutic levels. Adjust the measured level for hypoalbuminemia or renal impairment, which can increase free drug levels.

Check level weekly after oral replacement therapy starts until stable and every 3–6 months thereafter.

Measure procainamide levels 6–12 hours after a continuous infusion is started or immediately before the next oral dose. Combined (procainamide and NAPA) levels can be used as an index of toxicity when renal impairment exists. Obtain CBC periodically during longer-term therapy.

(continued)

*For those areas marked with one asterisk, the following values can be used:

ALT: 7–56 units/L
AST: 5–40 units/L
Alkaline phosphatase: 17–142 units/L
LDH: 60–220 units/L
GGT: < 40 units/L
Total bilirubin: 0.2–1 mg/dl

THERAPEUTIC DRUG MONITORING GUIDELINES (continued)

DRUG	LABORATORY TEST MONITORED	THERAPEUTIC RANGES OF TEST
protease inhibitors (amprenavir, indinavir, lopinavir, nelfinavir, ritonavir, saquinavir)	Fasting glucose	70–110 mg/dl
	Liver function	*
	CBC with differential	*****
	Lipids	Total cholesterol: < 200 mg/dl
		LDL: < 130 mg/dl
		HDL:
		Women: 40–75 mg/dl
		Men: 37–70 mg/dl
		Triglycerides: 10–160 mg/dl
	Amylase	35–118 international units/L
	CK	Women: 20–170 international units/L
		Men: 30–220 international units/L
quinidine	Quinidine	2–6 mcg/ml
	CBC	*****
	Liver function	*
	Creatinine	0.6–1.3 mg/dl
	Electrolytes (especially potassium)	Potassium: 3.5–5 mEq/L
		Magnesium: 1.7–2.1 mEq/L
		Sodium: 135–145 mEq/L
		Chloride: 98–106 mEq/L
sulfonylureas	Fasting glucose	70–110 mg/dl
	Glycosylated hemoglobin	4%–7% of total hemoglobin
theophylline	Theophylline	10–20 mcg/ml

Note: *****For those areas marked with asterisks, the following values can be used:

Hemoglobin: Women: 12–16 g/dl
  Men: 14–18 g/dl
Hematocrit: Women: 37%–48%
  Men: 42%–52%
RBCs: 4–5.5 million/mm^3
WBCs: 5–10 thousand/mm^3

Differential: Neutrophils: 45%–74%
  Bands: 0%–8%
  Lymphocytes: 16%–45%
  Monocytes: 4%–10%
  Eosinophils: 0%–7%
  Basophils: 0%–2%

MONITORING GUIDELINES

Obtain baseline glucose level, liver function test results, CBC with differential, and lipid, CK, and amylase levels. Monitor them during therapy.

Obtain levels immediately before next oral dose and 30–35 hours after therapy starts or changes. Periodically obtain blood counts, liver and kidney function test results, and electrolyte levels. With more specific assays, therapeutic levels are < 1 mcg/1 ml.

Monitor response to therapy by periodically evaluating fasting glucose and glycosylated hemoglobin levels. Patient should monitor glucose levels at home to help measure compliance and response.

Obtain theophylline levels immediately before next dose of sustained release oral product and at least 2 days after therapy starts or changes.

(continued)

*For those areas marked with one asterisk, the following values can be used:

ALT: 7–56 units/L
AST: 5–40 units/L
Alkaline phosphatase: 17–142 units/L
LDH: 60–220 units/L
GGT: < 40 units/L
Total bilirubin: 0.2–1 mg/dl

THERAPEUTIC DRUG MONITORING GUIDELINES (continued)

DRUG	LABORATORY TEST MONITORED	THERAPEUTIC RANGES OF TEST
thiazolidinediones (rosiglitazone, pioglitazone)	Fasting glucose Glycosylated hemoglobin Liver function	70–110 mg/dl 4%–7% of total hemoglobin *
thyroid hormone	Thyroid function tests	TSH: 0.2–5.4 micro-units/ml T_3: 80–200 ng/dl T_4: 5.4–11.5 mcg/dl
valproate sodium, valproic acid, divalproex sodium	Valproic acid Liver function Ammonia Fibrinogen BUN Creatinine CBC with differential Platelet count	50–100 mcg/ml * 15–45 mcg/dl 150–360 mg/dl 5–20 mg/dl 0.6–1.3 mg/dl ***** 150–450 x 10^3/mm³
vancomycin	Vancomycin Creatinine	20–40 mcg/ml (peak) 5–15 mcg/ml (trough) 0.6–1.3 mg/dl
warfarin	INR	2 to 3: For an acute MI, atrial fibrillation, treatment of pulmonary embolism, prevention of systemic embolism, tissue heart valves, valvular heart disease, or prophylaxis or treatment of venous thrombosis. 2.5 to 3.5: For mechanical prosthetic valves or recurrent systemic embolism.

Note: *****For those areas marked with asterisks, the following values can be used:

Hemoglobin: Women: 12–16 g/dl
   Men: 14–18 g/dl
Hematocrit: Women: 37%–48%
   Men: 42%–52%
RBCs: 4–5.5 million/mm³
WBCs: 5–10 thousand/mm³

Differential: Neutrophils: 45%–74%
   Bands: 0%–8%
   Lymphocytes: 16%–45%
   Monocytes: 4%–10%
   Eosinophils: 0%–7%
   Basophils: 0%–2%

Monitoring guidelines

Monitor response by evaluating fasting glucose and hemoglobin A1c levels. Obtain baseline liver function test results, and repeat tests periodically during therapy.

Monitor thyroid function test results every 2–3 weeks until appropriate maintenance dose is determined, and annually thereafter.

Monitor liver function test results, ammonia level, coagulation test results, renal function test results, CBC, and platelet count at baseline and periodically during therapy. Liver function test results should be closely monitored during the first 6 months.

Vancomycin levels may be checked with third dose, at the earliest. Draw peak levels 1.5–2.5 hours after a 1–hour infusion or I.V. infusion is complete. Draw trough levels within 1 hour of next dose. Renal function can be used to adjust dosage.

Check INR daily, beginning 3 days after therapy starts. Continue checking it until therapeutic goal is achieved, and monitor it periodically thereafter. Also, check levels 7 days after any change in warfarin dose or concomitant, potentially interacting therapy.

*For those areas marked with one asterisk, the following values can be used:

ALT: 7–56 units/L
AST: 5–40 units/L
Alkaline phosphatase: 17–142 units/L
LDH: 60–220 units/L
GGT: < 40 units/L
Total bilirubin: 0.2–1 mg/dl

NORMAL LABORATORY TEST VALUES

Normal values may differ from laboratory to laboratory. SI indicates Standard International Units.

Hematology
Bleeding time
Template: 3–6 minutes
  (SI, 3–6 minutes)
Ivy: 3–6 minutes
  (SI, 3–6 minutes)
Duke: 1–3 minutes
  (SI, 1–3 minutes)

Fibrinogen, plasma
200–400 mg/dl (SI, 2–4 g/L)

Hematocrit
Men: 42%–52%
  (SI, 0.42–0.52)
Women: 36%–48%
  (SI, 0.36–0.48)

Hemoglobin, total
Men: 14–17.4 g/dl
  (SI, 140–174 g/L)
Women: 12–16 g/dl
  (SI, 120–160 g/L)

Activated partial thromboplastin time
21–35 seconds
  (SI, 21–35 seconds)

Platelet aggregation
3–5 minutes (SI, 3–5 minutes)

Platelet count
140,000–400,000/mm^3
  (SI, 140–400 × 10^9/L)

Prothrombin time
10–14 seconds (SI, 10–14 seconds); INR for patients on warfarin therapy, 2–3 (SI, 2–3); those with prosthetic heart valve, 2.5–3.5 (SI, 2.5–3.5)

Red blood cell count
Men: 4.5–5.5 million/mm^3
  venous blood
  (SI, 4.5–5.5 × 10^{12}/L)
Women: 4–5 million/mm^3
  venous blood
  (SI, 4–5 × 10^{12}/L)

Red cell indices
Mean corpuscular volume:
  82–98 femtoliters
Mean corpuscular hemoglobin:
  26–34 picograms/cell
Mean corpuscular hemoglobin concentration: 31–37 g/dl

Reticulocyte count
0.5%–1.5% of total red blood cell count (SI, 0.005–0.025)

White blood cell count
4,500–10,500 cells/mm^3

White blood cell differential, blood
Neutrophils: 54%–75%
  (SI, 0.54–0.75)
Lymphocytes: 25%–40%
  (SI, 0.25–0.40)
Monocytes: 2%–8%
  (SI, 0.02–0.08)
Eosinophils: up to 4%
  (SI, up to 0.04)
Basophils: up to 1%
  (SI, up to 0.01)

NORMAL LABORATORY TEST VALUES *(continued)*

Blood chemistry

Alanine aminotransferase
Adults: 10–35 units/L
  (SI, 0.17–0.6 mukat/L)
Newborns: 13–45 units/L
  (SI, 0.22–0.77 mukat/L)

Amylase, serum
≥ *age 18:* 25–85 units/L
  (SI, 0.39–1.45 mukat/L)

Arterial blood gases
pH: 7.35–7.45 (SI, 7.35–7.45)
Paco$_2$: 35–45 mm Hg
  (SI, 4.7–5.3 kPa)
Pao$_2$: 80–100 mm Hg
  (SI, 10.6–13.3 kPa)
HCO$_3^-$: 22–26 mEq/L
  (SI, 22–25 mmol/L)
Sao$_2$: 94%–100%
  (SI, 0.94–1.00)

Aspartate transaminase
Men: 14–20 units/L
  (SI, 0.23–0.33 mukat/L)
Women: 7–34 units/L
  (SI, 0.12–0.58 mukat/L)

Bilirubin, serum
Adults, total: 0.2–1 mg/dl
  (SI, 3.5–17 micromol/L)
Neonates, total: 1–10 mg/dl
  (SI, 17–170 micromol/L)
Neonates, unconjugated indirect:
  0–10 mg/dl
  (SI, 0–170 micromol/L)

Blood urea nitrogen
8–20 mg/dl
  (SI, 2.9–7.5 mmol/L)

Calcium, serum
Adults: 8.2–10.2 mg/dl
  (SI, 2.05–2.54 mmol/L)
Children: 8.6–11.2 mg/dl
  (SI, 2.15–2.79 mmol/L)

Carbon dioxide, total, blood
22–26 mEq/L
  (SI, 22–26 mmol/L)

Cholesterol, total, serum
Men: ≤ 205 mg/dl (desirable)
  (SI, ≤ 5.30 mmol/L)
Women: ≤ 190 mg/dl (desirable)
  (SI, ≤ 4.90 mmol/L)

Creatine kinase, isoenzymes
CK-BB: none
CK-MB: 0–7%
CK-MM: 96–100%

Creatinine, serum
Adults: 0.6–1.3 mg/dl
  (SI, 53–115 micromol/L)

Glucose, plasma, fasting
70–110 mg/dl
  (SI, 3.9–6.1 mmol/L)

Glucose, plasma, 2-hour postprandial
≤ 145 mg/dl (SI, ≤ 8 mmol/L)

Lactate dehydrogenase
Total: 71–207 units/L in adults
  (SI, 1.2–3.52 mukat/L)
LD$_1$: 14%–26% (SI, 0.14–0.26)
LD$_2$: 29%–39% (SI, 0.29–0.39)
LD$_3$: 20%–26% (SI, 0.20–0.26)
LD$_4$: 8%–16% (SI, 0.08–0.16)
LD$_5$: 6%–16% (SI, 0.06–0.16)

(continued)

NORMAL LABORATORY TEST VALUES *(continued)*

Lipase
≤160 units/L (SI, ≤2.72 mukat/L)

Magnesium, serum
1.8–2 6 mg/dl
   (SI, 0.74–1.07 mmol/L)

Phosphates, serum
2.7–4.5 mg/dl
   (SI, 0.87–1.45 mmol/L)

Potassium, serum
3.8–5 mEq/L
   (SI, 3.5–5 mmol/L)

Protein, serum
Total: 6.3–8.3 g/dl
   (SI, 64–83 g/L)
Albumin fraction: 3.5–5 g/dl
   (SI, 35–50 g/L)

Sodium, serum
135–145 mEq/L
   (SI, 135–145 mmol/L)

Triglycerides, serum
Men ≥ age *20:* 40–180 mg/dl
   (SI, 0.11–2.01 mmol/L)
Women ≥ age *20:*
   10–190 mg/dl
   (SI, 0.11–2.21 mmol/L)

Uric acid, serum
Men: 3.4–7 mg/dl
   (SI, 202–416 micromol/L)
Women: 2.3–6 mg/dl
   (SI, 143–357 micromol/L)

PART III

COMPLICATIONS

8 / MEDICATION ERRORS

In the state where you practice nursing, many types of health care professionals, including doctors, nurse practitioners, dentists, podiatrists, and optometrists, may be legally permitted to prescribe, dispense, and administer drugs. Most often, however, doctors prescribe drugs, pharmacists dispense them, and nurses give them.

That means you're almost always on the front line when it comes to patients and their drugs. It also means you bear a major share of the responsibility for avoiding medication errors. Besides following your facility's administration policies, you can help prevent medication errors by reviewing the common ones outlined here and taking steps to prevent them.

Also, don't forget the importance of sound patient teaching in minimizing medication errors. You'll find a review of this important topic at the end of the chapter, plus several key resources to help you administer drugs safely.

DRUG ORDERS

Drug orders must be prepared and filled carefully to avoid problems such as the ones described here.

Pharmacy computer systems

The Institute for Safe Medication Practices (ISMP) performed a field test on 307 pharmacy computer systems and found that only 4 detected all of the unsafe orders in the test. Many system missed potentially lethal orders, doses that exceeded safe limits, duplicated drug ingredients, and orders to give oral solutions by the I.V. route.

CLINICAL TIP *Don't rely on the pharmacy computer system to detect unsafe orders. Before you give a drug, make sure you understand the indications, correct* *dosage, and adverse effects. If necessary, check a current drug reference.*

Confusing drug names

Many drug names have a similar enough sound or spelling to be confused with one another. For instance, Lantus (insulin glargine [rDNA origin]) could be confused with Lente insulin. Cardene could be confused with Cardura, Avinza with Invanz, and Amikin with Amicar. These mix-ups could easily happen with either verbal or written orders.

CLINICAL TIP Be aware of the drugs your patient takes regularly, and question any deviations from his regular routine. As with any drug, take your time and read the label carefully. And stay ahead of the curve by reviewing the list of look-alike and sound-alike drugs at the end of this chapter.

Abbreviations

Abbreviating drug names is risky and increases the chance of error. Here's just one example. A doctor wrote "May take own supply of EPO" on the chart of a cancer patient being admitted to the hospital. On the surface, this seems like a reasonable statement, since a cancer patient with anemia may receive epoetin alfa, commonly abbreviated EPO, to stimulate production of red blood cells. But this patient wasn't anemic. Sensing that something was wrong, the pharmacist interviewed the patient, who confirmed that he was indeed taking EPO—evening primrose oil—to lower his cholesterol level.

CLINICAL TIP Ask prescribers to spell out all drug names.

Unclear orders

A patient was supposed to receive one dose of the antineoplastic lomustine to treat brain cancer. Typically, this drug is given as a single oral dose once every 6 weeks. The doctor's order read "Administer h.s." Because the order was misinterpreted to mean every night, the patient received nine daily doses, developed severe thrombocytopenia and leukopenia, and died.

CLINICAL TIP If you're unfamiliar with a drug, check a drug reference before giving it. If a prescriber specifies an administration time but not the frequency, clarify the order. When documenting orders, note "h.s. nightly" or "h.s.– one dose today."

Unit dangers

Several reports to the ISMP involved errors related to drugs ordered in units. In one case, an order was written as "add 10U of regular insulin to each TPN bag." The pharmacist preparing the solution misread the dose to be 100 units. In another case, a pharmacy technician entering orders misinterpreted a sliding scale when the insulin order used "U" as an abbreviation for units, an error that could have caused a 10-fold overdose if a nurse hadn't caught it. Yet another report involved a nurse who received a verbal order to resume an insulin drip but wrote "resume heparin drip." Fortunately, the pharmacist caught the error.

CLINICAL TIP *Before you give a drug such as insulin or heparin, which are ordered in units, always check the prescriber's written order against the provided dose. And never abbreviate "units." If you must accept a verbal drug order, have another nurse listen in; then transcribe that order directly onto an order form and repeat it to ensure that you've transcribed it correctly.*

Inadvertent overdose

The inadvertent prescribing of harmful acetaminophen doses has become a disturbing trend. Prescribers may write orders for combined acetaminophen and opioid analgesic tablets (Lortab, Tylox, Darvocet-N) for patients who need pain relief without realizing that the total acetaminophen dose could be toxic.

Consider this order: "Tylox, 1 to 2 tablets every 4 hours, as needed, for pain." By taking the higher dose, the patient would receive 1,000 mg of acetaminophen every 4 hours, exceeding the maximum recommended dose of 4 g/day.

CLINICAL TIP *To prevent an acetaminophen overdose from combined analgesics, note the amount of acetaminophen in each drug. Beware of substitutions by the pharmacy because the amount of acetaminophen may vary.*

Lipid-based drugs

Serious medication errors, some fatal, have occurred because of confusion between certain lipid-based (liposomal) drugs and their conventional counterparts. The drugs involved include:

- lipid-based amphotericin B (Abelcet, Amphotec, AmBisome) and conventional amphotericin B for injection (available generically and as Fungizone)
- the pegylated liposomal form of doxorubicin (Doxil) and its conventional form, doxorubicin hydrochloride (Adriamycin, Rubex)

■ a liposomal form of daunorubicin (DaunoXome, daunorubicin citrate liposomal) and conventional daunorubicin hydrochloride (Cerubidine).

🍀 *CLINICAL TIP* *Lipid-based products have different dosages than their conventional counterparts. Check the original order and labels carefully to avoid confusion.*

DRUG PREPARATION

Drug preparation is another key point where errors may occur. Whether you prepare a drug yourself or the pharmacy prepares it for you, be alert for possible problems.

Injectable solution color changes

In two cases, alert nurses noticed that antineoplastics prepared in the pharmacy didn't look the way they should. In the first error, a 6-year-old child was to receive 12 mg of methotrexate intrathecally. In the pharmacy, a 1-g vial was mistakenly selected instead of a 20-mg vial, and the drug was reconstituted with 10 ml of normal saline solution. The vial containing 100 mg/ml was incorrectly labeled as containing 2 mg/ml, and 6 ml of the solution was drawn into a syringe. Although the syringe label indicated 12 mg of drug, the syringe actually contained 600 mg of drug.

When the nurse received the syringe and noted that the drug's color didn't seem right, she returned it to the pharmacy for verification. The pharmacist retrieved the vial used to prepare the dose and drew the remaining solution into another syringe. The solutions in both syringes matched, and no one noticed the vial's 1-g label. The pharmacist concluded that a manufacturing change caused the color difference.

The child received the 600-mg dose and experienced seizures 45 minutes later. A pharmacist responding to the emergency detected the error. The child received an antidote and recovered.

In the second error, a 20-year-old patient with leukemia received mitomycin instead of mitoxantrone. The nurse had questioned the drug's unusual bluish tint, but the pharmacist had assured her that the color difference was the result of a change in manufacturer. Fortunately, the patient didn't suffer any harm.

🍀 *CLINICAL TIP* *If a familiar drug has an unfamiliar*

appearance, find out why. If the pharmacist cites a manufacturing change, ask him to double-check whether he has received verification from the manufacturer. Document the appearance discrepancy, your actions, and the pharmacist's response in the patient record.

Inattentiveness

When a hospital pharmacy received an order for Fludara (fludarabine), a pharmacy technician asked the pharmacist if Navelbine (vinorelbine) was the same as Fludara (both are antineoplastics). The preoccupied pharmacist said "yes," and the technician prepared the Navelbine, but labeled it as Fludara. The pharmacist checked the preparation but didn't notice the error, and the patient received the wrong drug.

CLINICAL TIP *To prevent errors of this type, the hospital posted tables of antineoplastics and their dosing guidelines in the pharmacy. As an added safeguard, the pharmacy now sends the empty drug vial or box top with the prepared solution so the nurse can double-check it before infusing the drug.*

Incorrect allergy history

After a patient was admitted to the hospital, a nurse faxed a list of the patient's allergies to the pharmacy. The pharmacist couldn't read it, so he accessed the files from the patient's previous admission. However, these records didn't reflect an allergy to the anti-infective cefazolin that the patient had recently developed.

A consulting doctor ordered cefazolin, and the pharmacy processed the order. The medication administration record (MAR) generated by the pharmacy's database didn't indicate the allergy, and the nurse didn't know about it either.

The patient received cefazolin and became hypotensive and unresponsive. The nurse immediately notified the doctor and gave the antihistamine diphenhydramine. The patient recovered and was discharged the next day.

CLINICAL TIP *Obtain a new allergy history with each admission. If the patient's history must be faxed, name the drugs, note how many are included, and follow the facility's faxing safeguards. If the pharmacy also adheres to strict guidelines, the computer-generated MAR should be accurate.*

Dropper confusion

Ordering drugs such as liquid ferrous sulfate by the dropperful is a dangerous practice. One person might correctly consider the dropper full when the liquid meets the upper calibration mark; another might incorrectly fill the entire length of the dropper. Also, parents giving the drug at home may use a different dropper, which could significantly change the dose given.

CLINICAL TIP *Dosing directions for liquid drugs should always be expressed as weight per volume, such as 15 mg/0.6 ml. Verify the correct dose and teach parents to use only the dropper provided. Show them the mark on the dropper that indicates a full dose, and ask them to demonstrate the proper technique.*

Syringe tip caps and children

Syringe tip caps pose several dangers for children. The cap is a potential choking hazard to a small child. If you forget to remove the cap from an oral syringe before you give a drug, the cap could blow off into the child's mouth when you press the plunger. If a cap from an oral or a hypodermic syringe gets lost in the linens, the child may find it later and swallow or aspirate it.

CLINICAL TIP *Remove and discard the cap in a secure sharps container before you give the drug; don't place the cap in a trash can where the child may find it later. Also, teach parents about the potential danger of syringe tip caps. Tell them to store a capped syringe where children can't reach it and to remove the cap and dispose of it properly before giving the drug.*

GIVING DRUGS

Another major time for medication errors is during administration. Make sure you follow all of your facility's administration requirements, and be careful to avoid the following potential problems.

Misidentifying patients

Two common administration errors are failing to check the patient's identification and confusing patients with similar names. Using a tactic that helps prevent wrong-site surgery—involving the patient in the identification process—could also help prevent these medication errors.

CLINICAL TIP *Urge the patient to clearly state his full name, even without being asked, at admission and before accepting drugs, procedures, or treatments. Teach him to offer his identification bracelet for inspection when anyone arrives with drugs and to insist on having it replaced if it's removed.*

Herbal remedies

Surveys suggest that one-third of Americans or more use herbal supplements as medicine. Some people take them with conventional drugs; others use them as replacements. Herbal supplements are available without a prescription and, consequently, can't be tracked on a pharmacy computer. Plus, because government quality assurance standards don't apply to herbal supplements, their ingredients may be misrepresented or contaminated.

Research on the effects of herbs is limited. Because these products may contain a mixture of chemicals, their use carries risks.

CLINICAL TIP Ask the patient about his use of alternative therapies, including herbs, and record your findings in his medical record. Monitor the patient carefully, and report unusual events. Ask the patient to keep a diary of all therapies he uses and to take the diary for review each time he visits a health care professional.

Calculation errors

A physician assistant wrote the following order for a woman being admitted to the hospital for neck surgery: "methylprednisolone 10.6 g (30 mg/kg) over 1 hour IVPB before surgery" to minimize inflammation. The patient weighed 154 lb (70 kg), so the dose should have been 2.1 g, and not 10.6 g. Because neither the pharmacist nor the nurse independently checked the calculation, the patient received an overdose. She developed significant hyperglycemia and hypokalemia but recovered without injury.

CLINICAL TIP Writing the mg/kg or mg/m² dose and the calculated dose provides a safeguard against calculation errors. Whenever a prescriber provides the calculation, double-check it and document that the dose was verified.

Eyedrops for two or more

Using one bottle of eyedrops to treat several patients may seem like a good way to prevent waste, control cost, and save time. Some facilities, for example, give shared eyedrops to multiple patients undergoing outpatient cataract surgery. But this practice has risks.

Eyedrops contain preservatives to prevent bacterial growth, but contaminants may remain on the bottle top's inner surfaces or outer grooves. The dropper can also become contaminated if it accidentally touches an infected eye. Indeed, cross-infections have been reported.

Further, giving the wrong drug or wrong concentration is more likely when containers are shared because patient names don't appear on the containers. A patient may receive the wrong drops because the nurse can't check the bottle label against the patient's identification.

CLINICAL TIP Just as sharing any drug is poor practice, eyedrops shouldn't be used for more than one patient. If unit doses aren't available for surgical patients, each patient should fill his prescriptions before admission and bring his drugs with him.

Trouble with liquids

Liquid drugs may be more error-prone than solid drugs because of the calculations and dosage measurements needed. Here are a few examples: A 5-year-old boy who was receiving imipramine to treat his enuresis was given a 5-fold overdose because of an incorrectly compounded suspension. In another case, a prescription of Augmentin was dispensed with the instruction to take 2½ tsp instead of 2½ ml. In yet another, a mother who misunderstood the written directions

gave her child 7 ml instead of 0.7 ml of a liquid drug.

CLINICAL TIP Don't assume that liquid drugs are less likely to cause harm than other forms, including parenteral ones. Pediatric and geriatric patients commonly receive liquid drugs and may be especially sensitive to the effects of an inaccurate dose. If a unit-dose form isn't available, calculate carefully, and double-check your math and the drug label.

Celexa, Celebrex, and Cerebyx confusion

An 80-year-old woman mistakenly received 20 mg of Celexa (citalopram), a selective serotonin reuptake inhibitor (SSRI), b.i.d. for 1 month for arthritis pain. She should have received 100 mg of Celebrex (celecoxib), a nonsteroidal anti-inflammatory drug. A member of the pharmacy staff had confused the drug names when pulling the product from the shelf. The patient wasn't harmed, but the potential for harm was great because she was already taking an SSRI.

CLINICAL TIP Help prevent errors related to Celebrex, Celexa, and the anticonvulsant Cerebyx (fosphenytoin) by asking prescribers to use the generic name and by confirming the drug's indication if the order doesn't clearly state it. For verbal orders, repeat the drug name and your understanding of its indication to the prescriber.

Labels and toxicity

A container of 5% acetic acid, used to clean tracheostomy tubing, was left near nebulization equipment in the room of a 10-month-old infant. A respiratory therapist mistook the liquid for normal saline solution and used it to dilute albuterol for the child's nebulizer treatment. During treatment, the child experienced bronchospasm, hypercapnic dyspnea, tachypnea, and tachycardia.

CLINICAL TIP Leaving potentially dangerous chemicals near patients is extremely risky, especially when the container labels don't indicate toxicity. To prevent such problems, never leave dangerous unlabeled substances near a patient, read the label on every drug you prepare, and never give anything that isn't labeled.

Dosage equations

A 13-month study at Albany (NY) Medical Center examined 200 prescribing errors arising from the use of dosage equations. Almost 70% involved pediatric patients, for whom dosage equations are commonly used. Mistakes in decimal point

placement, mathematical calculation, or expression of the regimen accounted for more than 50% of the errors. Examples include prescribing the entire day's drug as a single dose instead of at intervals and using an entire day's dose at each interval. Use of dosage equations invites medication errors.

CLINICAL TIP Alternatives to dosage equations include using established ranges or tables, incorporating a calculator into a computer order entry system, and requiring both the calculated dose and dosage equation on orders to facilitate independent checks.

After you calculate a drug dosage, always have another nurse calculate it independently to double-check your results. If doubts or questions remain or if the calculations don't match, ask a pharmacist to calculate the dose before you give the drug.

Misreading orders

Two reports concerned incorrect dosing of the tricyclic antidepressant nortriptyline (Pamelor or Aventyl) when ordered for neuropathic pain syndromes. The cases involved 10-mg and 20-mg orders that were misread as 100 mg and 200 mg, respectively. One patient who received an incorrect dose required hospitalization; the other developed sedation and orthostatic hypotension after two doses, which led to recognition of the error.

🍀 CLINICAL TIP *Nortriptyline and other tricyclic antidepressants aren't prescribed as frequently as they once were. To make sure you're familiar with recommended dosages, refer to a drug reference and then ask a pharmacist.*

Air bubbles in pump tubing

After starting an I.V. drip to give insulin, 2 units/hour, to a 9-year-old patient, a nurse noted air bubbles in the tubing and pump chamber. To remove the bubbles and promote proper flow, she disconnected the tubing and increased the pump rate to 200 ml/hour. When the bubbles were cleared, she reconnected the tubing and restarted the infusion without resetting the rate. The child received about 50 units of insulin before the error was detected. Fortunately, the child wasn't harmed.

🍀 CLINICAL TIP *To clear bubbles from I.V. tubing, never increase the flow rate to flush the line. Instead, remove the tubing from the pump, disconnect it from the patient, and use the flow-control clamp to establish gravity flow. When the bubbles have been removed, return the tubing to the pump, restart the infusion, and recheck the flow rate.*

Misplacing decimals

A patient in the intensive care unit was to receive the opioid fentanyl, 12.5 to 25 mcg I.V. every 4 to 6 hours, as needed, for pain. Unit stock consisted of 5-ml ampules of fentanyl at 0.05 mg/ml, so each ampule contained 0.25 mg (250 mcg). A nurse preparing a dose confused the volume needed when she converted from milligrams to micrograms and gave 5 ml, thinking it contained 25 mcg. The patient suffered respiratory arrest but was resuscitated.

🍀 CLINICAL TIP *Numerous serious fentanyl errors have been reported, and a misplaced decimal point caused many of them. A safer alternative for intermittent dosing is I.V. morphine. Fentanyl doses are best prepared in the pharmacy rather than on the unit. If a fentanyl dose must be prepared, refer to dosing charts, follow the facility's protocols, and ask another nurse to check your calculations.*

Incorrect administration route

A nurse was caring for a patient who had a jejunostomy tube for oral drugs and a central I.V. line for hyperalimentation and I.V. drugs. At the bedside was a stock bottle of digoxin elixir. After checking the concentration, the nurse used a syringe to withdraw 2.5 ml of elixir for a 0.125-mg dose. She then mistakenly gave the elixir through the central line rather than the jejunostomy tube.

Using an incorrect route put the patient at risk for overdose and secondary infection from unsterile I.V. administration. Fortunately, he was receiving antibiotics for an infection and suffered no adverse reactions.

CLINICAL TIP *This case emphasizes the need to ensure that the right route is being used to give any drug. When the patient has multiple lines, label the distal end of each line. Using a parenteral syringe to prepare oral liquid drugs increases the chance for error because the syringe tip fits easily into I.V. ports. To safely give an oral drug through a feeding tube, use a dose prepared by the pharmacy and a syringe with the appropriate tip.*

Stress

A nurse-anesthetist gave the sedative midazolam (Versed) to the wrong patient. When she discovered the error, she grabbed what she thought was a vial of the antidote flumazenil (Romazicon), withdrew 2.5 ml, and gave it. When the patient didn't respond, she realized she'd grabbed a vial of ondansetron (Zofran), an antiemetic, instead. Another practitioner assisted with proper I.V. administration of flumazenil, and the patient recovered without harm.

CLINICAL TIP *Committing a serious error can cause enormous stress and cloud your judgment. If you're involved in a medication error, ask another professional to give the antidote.*

PATIENT TEACHING

Patients being discharged from an acute care setting may be at a greater risk for adverse drug reactions arising from drug-drug interactions. Changes are commonly made to patients' previous drug regimens before discharge, either by altering a previous dose or adding one or more new drugs. Adverse effects may go unnoticed by the prescriber or unreported when the patient is at home. Carefully review the patient's drugs upon discharge, inform him of any potential adverse drug effects to be aware of, and tell him to call the prescriber if adverse effects become bothersome.

The following general guidelines will help you make sure the patient receives the maximum benefits from drug therapy while minimizing the risk of adverse reactions, accidental overdose, and harmful changes in effectiveness.

■ Instruct the patient to learn the brand and generic names of all drugs he takes and to inform his regular prescriber about them.

■ Before you give a patient a drug, ask him to report unusual reactions experienced in the past, allergies to foods and other substances, special medical problems, and drugs taken over the last few weeks, including over-the-counter (OTC) drugs or herbs. If you detect potential problems from interactions, educate the patient about them and, as needed, tell the patient to consult his prescriber.

■ Advise the patient to always read the label before taking a drug, to take it exactly as prescribed, and never to share prescription drugs.

■ Warn the patient not to change brands of a drug without consulting the prescriber, to avoid harmful changes in effectiveness. Certain generic preparations aren't equivalent in effect to brand-name preparations of the same drug.

■ Tell the patient to check the expiration date before taking a drug.

■ Instruct the patient to place drugs that are outdated or no longer needed in a sealed container before discarding them. Explain that some pharmacies accept such drugs for safe disposal. Also, tell the patient to keep such drugs out of the reach of children and pets.

■ Tell the patient to store each drug in its original container, at room temperature (unless directed otherwise), and in places that aren't accessible to children or exposed to sunlight. Advise against storing drugs in the bathroom medicine cabinet, in the kitchen close to heat, or in the glove compartment or trunk of an automobile, where extremes of temperature and humidity will cause deterioration.

■ Caution the patient about mixing different drugs in a single container, removing a drug from its original container, or removing the label. Relying on memory to identify a drug and specific directions for its use is dangerous.

■ If the patient must remove pills from their original container to use a daily or weekly "medication planner" as a reminder, tell him to attach an index card to the planner with the drug's name, strength, dosing instructions, and physical description written on the card. This is particularly important when the patient takes more than one prescription drug.

■ Stress the importance of telling the prescriber about adverse reactions.

■ Encourage the patient to have all prescriptions filled at the same pharmacy so the pharmacist can identify and warn against potentially harmful drug interactions. Also, tell the patient to inform the pharmacist and prescriber about any OTC drugs or herbs he takes.

■ Instruct the patient to call the emergency medical service or poison control center immediately if he or someone else has taken an overdose. Tell the patient to keep these telephone numbers handy at all times.

■ Advise the patient to inform medical personnel about use of drugs before undergoing surgery (including dental surgery).

■ Tell the patient to have a sufficient supply of drugs when traveling. He should carry them with him and not pack them in his luggage.

LOOK-ALIKE AND SOUND-ALIKE DRUG NAMES

Watch out for the following drug names that resemble other drug names either in the way they're spelled or the way they sound. Don't confuse antivirals that use abbreviations for identification. Also, don't mix up different iron salts because their elemental content may vary.

abciximab and infliximab

acetazolamide and acetohexamide

acetylcholine and acetylcysteine

acetylcysteine and acetylcholine

Aciphex and Aricept

Aggrastat and argatroban

albuterol and atenolol or Albutein

Aldactone and Aldactazide

Aldomet and Aldoril or Anzemet

alitretinoin and tretinoin

alprazolam and alprostadil

amantadine and rimantadine

Ambien and Amen

Amicar and Amikin

Amikin and Amicar

amiloride and amiodarone

aminophylline and amitriptyline or ampicillin

Aminosyn and Amikacin

amiodarone and amiloride

amitriptyline and nortriptyline or aminophylline

amlodipine and amiloride

Anafranil and enalapril, nafarelin, or alfentanil

anakinra and amikacin

Antabuse and Anturane

Anturane and Accutane or Artane

Anzemet and Aldomet

Apresoline and Apresazide

Aquasol A and AquaMEPHYTON

Aricept and Ascriptin

Artane and Anturane or Altace

Asacol and Os-Cal

atenolol and timolol or albuterol

Atrovent and Alupent

Avinza and Invanz

azathioprine and azidothymidine, Azulfidine, or azatadine

bacitracin and Bactroban

baclofen and Bactroban

BCG intravesical and BCG vaccine

Benadryl and Bentyl or Benylin

Benemid and Beminal

Bentyl and Aventyl or Benadryl

benztropine and bromocriptine or brimonidine

Betagan and BetaGen or Betapen

Bumex and Buprenex

bupropion and buspirone

calcifediol and calcitriol

Carbatrol and carvedilol

carboplatin and cisplatin

Cardene and Cardura or codeine

Cardizem SR and Cardene SR

Cardura and Coumadin, K-Dur, Cardene, or Cordarone

Catapres and Cetapred or Combipres

Celebrex and Cerebyx or Celexa

Celexa and Celebrex or Cerebyx

Cerebyx and Cerezyme, Celexa, or Celebrex

Chloromycetin and chlorambucil

chlorpromazine and chlorpropamide

Ciloxan and Cytoxan or cinoxacin

cimetidine and simethicone

Citrucel and Citracal

clomiphene and clomipramine or clonidine

clonidine and quinidine or clomiphene

clorazepate and clofibrate

clotrimazole and co-trimoxazole

clozapine and Cloxapen, clofazimine, or Klonopin

codeine and Cardene, Lodine, or Cordran

corticotropin and cosyntropin

Cozaar and Zocor

cyclosporine and cycloserine

cyproheptadine and cyclobenzaprine

dacarbazine and Dicarbosil or procarbazine

Dantrium and Daraprim

Demerol and Demulen, Dymelor, or Temaril

desipramine and disopyramide or imipramine

desmopressin and vasopressin

desonide and Desogen or Desoxyn

Desoxyn and digoxin or digitoxin

dexamethasone and desoximetasone

Dexedrine and dextran or Excedrin

Diamox and Diabinese

diazepam and diazoxide

diazoxide and Dyazide

diclofenac and Diflucan or Duphalac

dicyclomine and dyclonine or doxycycline

digoxin and doxepin, Desoxyn, or digitoxin

Dilantin and Dilaudid

dimenhydrinate and diphenhydramine

Diprivan and Ditropan

dipyridamole and disopyramide

disopyramide and desipramine or dipyridamole

Ditropan and Diazepam

dobutamine and dopamine

doxapram and doxorubicin, doxepin, or doxazosin

doxepin and doxazosin, digoxin, doxapram, or Doxidan

doxycycline and doxylamine or dicyclomine

d-penicillamine and penicillin

dronabinol and droperidol

droperidol and dronabinol

DynaCirc and Dynacin

Elavil and Equanil or Mellaril

Eldepryl and enalapril

enalapril and Anafranil or Eldepryl

Endep and Depen

ephedrine and epinephrine

epinephrine and ephedrine or norepinephrine

Epogen and Neupogen

Estratab and Estratest

Ethmozine and Erythrocin

ethosuximide and methsuximide

etidronate and etretinate, etidocaine, or etomidate

Eurax and Serax or Urex

Femara and FemHRT

fentanyl and alfentanil

Flexeril and Floxin or Flaxedil

Flomax and Fosamax or Volmax

floxuridine and fludarabine or flucytosine

flunisolide and fluocinonide

fluorouracil and fludarabine, flucytosine, or floxuridine

fluoxetine and fluvoxamine or fluvastatin

(continued)

LOOK-ALIKE AND SOUND-ALIKE DRUG NAMES (continued)

fluticasone and fluconazole

fluvastatin and fluoxetine

folic acid and folinic acid

fosinopril and lisinopril

furosemide and torsemide

glimepiride and glyburide or glipizide

guanabenz and guanadrel or guanfacine

guaifenesin and guanfacine

Haldol and Halcion or Halog

hydralazine and hydroxyzine

hydrocortisone and hydroxychloroquine

hydromorphone and morphine

hydroxyzine and hydroxyurea or hydralazine

HyperHep and Hyperstat or Hyper-Tet

Hyperstat and Nitrostat

idarubicin and daunorubicin or doxorubicin

ifosfamide and cyclophosphamide

imipramine and desipramine

Imodium and Ionamin

Imuran and Inderal

Inderal and Inderide, Isordil, Adderall, or Imuran

Isoptin and Intropin

Isordil and Isuprel or Inderal

K-Phos-Neutral and Neutra-Phos-K

Lamictal and Lamisil

lamotrigine and lamivudine

Lanoxin and Levoxyl or levothyroxine

Lantus and Lente

Leukeran and leucovorin

Levatol or Lipitor

levothyroxine and liothyronine or liotrix

Lithobid and Levbid

Lithonate and Lithostat

Lithotabs and Lithobid or Lithostat

Lodine and codeine, iodine, or Iopidine

Lorabid and Lortab

lorazepam and alprazolam

Lotensin and Loniten or lovastatin

Luvox and Lasix

magnesium sulfate and manganese sulfate

Maxidex and Maxzide

Mellaril and Elavil

melphalan and Mephyton

Mestinon and Mesantoin or Metatensin

metaproterenol and metoprolol or metipranolol

methicillin and mezlocillin

methimazole and mebendazole or methazolamide

methocarbamol and mephobarbital

methylprednisolone and medroxyprogesterone

methyltestosterone and medroxyprogesterone

metoprolol and metaproterenol or metolazone

Mevacor and Mivacron

Micronor and Micro-K or Micronase

Minocin and niacin or Mithracin

mitomycin and mithramycin

Monopril and Monurol

Nalfon and Naldecon

naloxone and naltrexone

Navane and Nubain or Norvasc

nelfinavir and nevirapine

Nicoderm and Nitro-Dur

Nicorette and Nordette

nifedipine and nimodipine or nicardipine

Nitro-Bid and Nicobid

LOOK-ALIKE AND SOUND-ALIKE DRUG NAMES (continued)

nitroglycerine and nitroprusside

norepinephrine and epinephrine

Noroxin and Neurontin

nortriptyline and amitriptyline

Nubain and Navane

nystatin and Nitrostat

Ocuflox and Ocufen

olsalazine and olanzapine

opium tincture and camphorated opium tincture

oxaprozin and oxazepam

oxymorphone and oxymetholone

pancuronium and pipecuronium

Parlodel and pindolol

paroxetine and paclitaxel

Paxil and Doxil, paclitaxel, or Taxol

pemoline and Pelamine

penicillin G benzathine and Polycillin, penicillamine, or other types of penicillin

penicillin G potassium and Polycillin, penicillamine, or other types of penicillin

penicillin G procaine and Polycillin, penicillamine, or other types of penicillin

penicillin G sodium and Polycillin, penicillamine, or other types of penicillin

penicillin V potassium and Polycillin, penicillamine, or other types of penicillin

pentobarbital and phenobarbital

pentostatin and pentosan

Persantine and Periactin

phentermine and phentolamine

phenytoin and mephenytoin

pindolol and Parlodel, Panadol, or Plendil

Pitocin and Pitressin

Plendil and pindolol

pralidoxime and pramoxine or pyridoxine

Pravachol and Prevacid or propranolol

prednisolone and prednisone

Premarin and Primaxin

Prilosec and Prozac, Prinivil, or Plendil

primidone and prednisone

Prinivil and Proventil or Prilosec

ProAmatine and protamine

probenecid and Procanbid

procainamide and probenecid

promethazine and promazine

propranolol and Pravachol

ProSom and Proscar or Prozac

protamine and Protopam or Protropin

Prozac and Proscar, Prilosec, or ProSom

pyridoxine and pralidoxime or Pyridium

Questran and Quarzan

quinidine and quinine or clonidine

ranitidine and ritodrine or rimantadine

Reminyl and Robinul

Restoril and Vistaril

riboflavin and ribavirin

rifabutin and rifampin or rifapentine

Rifater and Rifadin or Rifamate

risperidone and reserpine or Risperdal

Ritalin and Rifadin

ritodrine and ranitidine

ritonavir and Retrovir

Sandimmune and Sandoglobulin or Sandostatin

saquinavir and saquinavir mesylate (the dosages are different)

(continued)

LOOK–ALIKE AND SOUND–ALIKE DRUG NAMES *(continued)*

Sarafem and Serophene

selegiline and Stelazine or Sertraline

Serentil and Serevent or Aventyl

Serzone and Seroquel

simethicone and cimetidine

Sinequan and saquinavir

Solu-Cortef and Solu-Medrol

somatropin and somatrem or sumatriptan

sotalol and Stadol

streptozocin and streptomycin

sufentanil and alfentanil or fentanyl

sulfadiazine and sulfasalazine

sulfamethoxazole and sulfamethizole

sulfamethoxazole alone and combination products

sulfasalazine and sulfisoxazole, salsalate, or sulfadiazine

sulfisoxazole and sulfasalazine

sulfisoxazole alone and combination products

sulfonamide drugs

sumatriptan and somatropin

Survanta and Sufenta

Tegretol and Toradol

Tenex and Xanax, Entex, or Ten-K

terbinafine and terbutaline

terbutaline and tolbutamide or terbinafine

terconazole and tioconazole

Testoderm and Estraderm

testosterone and testolactone

thiamine and Thorazine

thioridazine and Thorazine

Tigan and Ticar

timolol and atenolol

Timoptic and Viroptic

tobramycin and Trobicin

Tobrex and Tobradex

tolnaftate and Tornalate

Toradol and Tegretol

Trandate and Trental

Trental and Trendar or Trandate

triamcinolone and Triaminicin or Triaminicol

triamterene and trimipramine

trifluoperazine and triflupromazine

trimipramine and triamterene or trimeprazine

Ultracet and Ultracef

Urispas and Urised

valacyclovir and valganciclovir

Vancenase and Vanceril

Vanceril and Vansil

Verelan and Vivarin, Ferralyn, or Virilon

Versed and VePesid

vidarabine and cytarabine

vinblastine and vincristine, vindesine, or vinorelbine

Visine and Visken

Volmax and Flomax

Voltaren and Ventolin or Verelan

Wellbutrin and Wellcovorin or Wellferon

Xanax and Zantac, Tenex, or Zyrtec

Xenical and Xeloda

Zarontin and Zaroxolyn

Zaroxolyn and Zarontin

Zebeta and DiaBeta

Zestril and Zostrix

Zocor and Zoloft

Zofran and Zosyn, Zantac, or Zoloft

Zyprexa and Zyrtec

Zyrtec and Zyprexa

DRUGS THAT SHOULDN'T BE CRUSHED

Many drug forms, such as slow-release, enteric-coated, encapsulated beads, wax-matrix, sublingual, and buccal forms, are made to release their active ingredients over a certain period of time or at preset points after administration. The disruptions caused by crushing these drug forms can dramatically affect the absorption rate and increase the risk of adverse reactions.

Other reasons not to crush these drug forms include such considerations as taste, tissue irritation, and unusual formulation—for example, a capsule within a capsule, a liquid within a capsule, or a multiple-compressed tablet. Avoid crushing the following drugs, listed by brand name, for the reasons noted beside them.

Accutane (irritant)

Aciphex (delayed release)

Adalat CC (sustained release)

Advicor (extended release)

Aggrenox (extended release)

Allegra D (extended release)

Altocor (extended release)

Amnesteem (irritant)

Arthrotec (delayed release)

Asacol (delayed release)

Augmentin XR (extended release)

Avinza (extended release)

Azulfidine EN-tabs (enteric coated)

Bellergal-S (slow release)

Biaxin XL (extended release)

Bisacodyl (enteric coated)

Bontril Slow-Release (slow release)

Breonesin (liquid filled)

Brexin L.A. (slow release)

Bromfed (slow release)

Bromfed-PD (slow release)

Calan SR (sustained release)

Carbatrol (extended release)

Cardizem CD, LA, SR (slow release)

Cartia XT (extended release)

Ceclor CD (slow release)

Ceftin (strong, persistent taste)

Charcoal Plus DS (enteric coated)

Chloral Hydrate (liquid within a capsule, taste)

Chlor-Trimeton Allergy 8-hour and 12-hour (slow release)

Choledyl SA (slow release)

Cipro XR (extended release)

Claritin-D 12-hour (slow release)

Claritin-D 24-hour (slow release)

Colace (liquid within a capsule)

Colazal (granules within capsules must reach colon intact)

Colestid (protective coating)

Compazine Spansules (slow release)

Concerta (extended release)

Congess SR (sustained release)

Contac 12 Hour, Maximum Strength 12 Hour (slow release)

Cotazym-S (enteric coated)

Covera-HS (extended release)

Creon (enteric coated)

Cytovene (irritant)

Dallergy, Dallergy-Jr (slow release)

Deconamine SR (slow release)

Depakene (slow release, mucous membrane irritant)

(continued)

DRUGS THAT SHOULDN'T BE CRUSHED (continued)

Depakote (enteric coated)

Depakote ER (extended release)

Desyrel (taste)

Dexedrine Spansule (slow release)

Diamox Sequels (slow release)

Dilacor XR (extended release)

Dilatrate-SR (slow release)

Diltia XT (extended release)

Dimetapp Extentabs (slow release)

Ditropan XL (slow release)

Dolobid (irritant)

Drisdol (liquid filled)

Dristan (protective coating)

Drixoral (slow release)

Dulcolax (enteric coated)

DynaCirc CR (slow release)

Easprin (enteric coated)

Ecotrin (enteric coated)

Ecotrin Maximum Strength (enteric coated)

E.E.S. 400 Filmtab (enteric coated)

Effexor XR (extended release)

Emend (hard gelatin capsule)

E-Mycin (enteric coated)

Entex LA (slow release)

Entex PSE (slow release)

Eryc (enteric coated)

Ery-Tab (enteric coated)

Erythrocin Stearate (enteric coated)

Erythromycin Base (enteric coated)

Eskalith CR (slow release)

Extendryl JR, SR (slow release)

Feldene (mucous membrane irritant)

Feosol (enteric coated)

Feratab (enteric coated)

Fergon (slow release)

Fero-Folic 500 (slow release)

Fero-Grad-500 (slow release)

Ferro-Sequel (slow release)

Feverall Children's Capsules, Sprinkle (taste)

Flomax (slow release)

Furnatinic (slow release)

Geocillin (taste)

Glucophage XR (extended release)

Glucotrol XL (slow release)

Guaifed (slow release)

Guaifed-PD (slow release)

Guaifenex LA (slow release)

Guaifenex PSE (slow release)

Humibid DM, LA, Pediatric (slow release)

Hydergine LC (liquid within a capsule)

Hytakerol (liquid filled)

Iberet (slow release)

ICAPS Plus (slow release)

ICAPS Time Release (slow release)

Imdur (slow release)

Inderal LA (slow release)

Indocin SR (slow release)

InnoPran XL (extended release)

Ionamin (slow release)

Isoptin SR (sustained release)

Isordil Sublingual (sublingual)

Isordil Tembids (slow release)

Isosorbide Dinitrate Sublingual (sublingual)

Kaon-Cl (slow release)

K-Dur (slow release)

Klor-Con (slow release)

Klotrix (slow release)

K-Tab (slow release)

Levbid (slow release)

Levsinex Timecaps (slow release)

Lithobid (slow release)

Macrobid (slow release)

DRUGS THAT SHOULDN'T BE CRUSHED (continued)

Mestinon Timespans (slow release)
Metadate CD, ER (extended release)
Methylin ER (extended release)
Micro-K Extencaps (slow release)
Motrin (taste)
MS Contin (slow release)
Mucinex (extended release)
Naprelan (slow release)
Nexium (sustained release)
Niaspan (extended release)
Nitroglyn (slow release)
Nitrong (slow release)
Nitrostat (sublingual)
Norflex (slow release)
Norpace CR (slow release)
Oramorph SR (slow release)
Oruvail (extended release)
OxyContin (slow release)
Pancrease (enteric coated)
Pancrease MT (enteric coated)
Paxil CR (controlled release)
PCE (slow release)
Pentasa (controlled release)
Phazyme (slow release)
Phazyme 95 (slow release)
Phenytex (extended release)
Plendil (slow release)
Prelu-2 (slow release)
Prevacid, Prevacid SoluTab (delayed release)
Prilosec (slow release)
Prilosec OTC (delayed release)
Pro-Banthine (taste)
Procanbid (slow release)
Procardia (delayed absorption)
Procardia XL (slow release)
Protonix (delayed release)

Proventil Repetabs (slow release)
Prozac Weekly (slow release)
Quibron-T/SR (slow release)
Quinidex Extentabs (slow release)
Respaire SR (slow release)
Respbid (slow release)
Risperdal M-Tab (delayed release)
Ritalin-LA, -SR (slow release)
Rondec-TR (slow release)
Sinemet CR (slow release)
Slo-bid Gyrocaps (slow release)
Slo-Niacin (slow release)
Slo-Phyllin GG, Gyrocaps (slow release)
Slow FE (slow release)
Slow-K (slow release)
Slow-Mag (slow release)
Sorbitrate (sublingual)
Sotret (irritant)
Sudafed 12 Hour (slow release)
Sustaire (slow release)
Tegretol-XR (extended release)
Ten-K (slow release)
Tenuate Dospan (slow release)
Tessalon Perles (slow release)
Theobid Duracaps (slow release)
Theochron (slow release)
Theoclear LA (slow release)
Theolair-SR (slow release)
Theo-Sav (slow release)
Theospan-SR (slow release)
Theo-24 (slow release)
Theovent (slow release)
Theo-X (slow release)
Thorazine Spansules (slow release)
Tiazac (sustained release)
Topamax (taste)

(continued)

DRUGS THAT SHOULDN'T BE CRUSHED (continued)

Toprol XL (extended release)
T-Phyl (slow release)
Trental (slow release)
Trinalin Repetabs (slow release)
Tylenol Extended Relief (slow release)
Uniphyl (slow release)
Vantin (taste)
Verelan, Verelan PM (slow release)
Volmax (slow release)

Voltaren (enteric coated)
Voltaren-XR (extended release)
Wellbutrin SR (sustained release)
Xanax XR (extended release)
Zerit XR (extended release)
Zomig-ZMT (delayed release)
ZORprin (slow release)
Zyban (slow release)
Zyrtec-D 12 hour (extended release)

DIALYZABLE DRUGS

The amount of a drug removed by dialysis differs among patients and depends on several factors, including the patient's condition, drug's properties, length of dialysis, dialysate used, rate of blood flow or dwell time, and purpose of dialysis. This table shows the general effect of hemodialysis on selected drugs.

Drug	Level Reduced by Hemodialysis	Drug	Level Reduced by Hemodialysis
acetaminophen	Yes (may not influence toxicity)	cefaclor	Yes
		cefadroxil	Yes
acetazolamide	No	cefamandole	Yes
acyclovir	Yes	cefazolin	Yes
allopurinol	Yes	cefepime	Yes
alprazolam	No	cefonicid	Yes (only by 20%)
amikacin	Yes	cefoperazone	Yes
amiodarone	No	cefotaxime	Yes
amitriptyline	No	cefotetan	Yes (only by 20%)
amlodipine	No	cefoxitin	Yes
amoxicillin	Yes	cefpodoxime	Yes
amoxicillin and clavulanate potassium	Yes	ceftazidime	Yes
		ceftibuten	Yes
		ceftizoxime	Yes
amphotericin B	No	ceftriaxone	No
ampicillin	Yes	cefuroxime	Yes
ampicillin and sulbactam sodium	Yes	cephalexin	Yes
		cephalothin	Yes
		cephradine	Yes
aspirin	Yes	chloral hydrate	Yes
atenolol	Yes	chlorambucil	No
azathioprine	Yes	chloramphenicol	Yes (very small amount)
aztreonam	Yes		
captopril	Yes	chlordiazepoxide	No
carbamazepine	No		
		chloroquine	No
carbenicillin	Yes	chlorpheniramine	No
carmustine	No		

(continued)

DIALYZABLE DRUGS *(continued)*

DRUG	LEVEL REDUCED BY HEMODIALYSIS	DRUG	LEVEL REDUCED BY HEMODIALYSIS
chlorpromazine	No	doxycycline	No
chlorthalidone	No	enalapril	Yes
cimetidine	Yes	erythromycin	Yes (only by 20%)
ciprofloxacin	Yes (only by 20%)	ethacrynic acid	No
cisplatin	No	ethambutol	Yes (only by 20%)
clindamycin	No	ethchlorvynol	Yes
clofibrate	No	ethosuximide	Yes
clonazepam	No	famciclovir	Yes
clonidine	No	famotidine	No
clorazepate	No	fenoprofen	No
cloxacillin	No	flecainide	No
codeine	No	fluconazole	Yes
colchicine	No	flucytosine	Yes
cortisone	No	fluorouracil	Yes
co-trimoxazole	Yes	fluoxetine	No
cyclophosphamide	Yes	flurazepam	No
diazepam	No	foscarnet	Yes
diazoxide	No	fosinopril	No
diclofenac	No	furosemide	No
dicloxacillin	No	gabapentin	Yes
didanosine	Yes	ganciclovir	Yes
digoxin	No	gemfibrozil	No
diltiazem	No	gentamicin	Yes
diphenhydramine	No	glipizide	No
dipyridamole	No	glutethimide	Yes
disopyramide	Yes	glyburide	No
doxazosin	No	guanfacine	Yes
doxepin	No	haloperidol	No
doxorubicin	No	heparin	No
		hydralazine	No
		hydrochlorothiazide	No
		hydroxyzine	No

DIALYZABLE DRUGS *(continued)*

DRUG	LEVEL REDUCED BY HEMODIALYSIS	DRUG	LEVEL REDUCED BY HEMODIALYSIS
ibuprofen	No	methadone	Yes
imipenem and cilastatin	No	methicillin	Yes
		methotrexate	No
imipramine	No	methyldopa	No
indapamide	Yes	methylpred-nisolone	Yes
indomethacin	No		
insulin	No	metoclopra-mide	Yes
irbesartan	No		
iron dextran	No	metolazone	No
isoniazid	No	metoprolol	No
isosorbide	No	metronidazole	Yes
isradipine	Yes	mexiletine	Yes
kanamycin	No	mezlocillin	Yes
ketoconazole	No	miconazole	No
ketoprofen	Yes	midazolam	No
labetalol	No	minocycline	No
levofloxacin	Yes	minoxidil	Yes
lidocaine	No	misoprostol	No
lisinopril	No	morphine	No
lithium	No	nabumetone	No
lomefloxacin	Yes	nadolol	Yes
lomustine	Yes	nafcillin	No
loracarbef	No	naproxen	No
loratadine	No	nelfinavir	Yes
lorazepam	Yes	netilmicin	Yes
mechloaretha-mine	No	nifedipine	No
		nimodipine	No
mefenamic acid	No	nitrofurantoin	Yes
		nitroglycerin	No
meperidine	No	nitroprusside	Yes
mercaptop-urine	No	nizatidine	No
		norfloxacin	No
meropenem	No	nortriptyline	No

(continued)

DIALYZABLE DRUGS (continued)

Drug	Level Reduced By Hemodialysis	Drug	Level Reduced By Hemodialysis
ofloxacin	Yes	rofecoxib	No
olanzapine	No	sertraline	No
omeprazole	No	sotalol	Yes
oxacillin	No	stavudine	Yes
oxazepam	No	streptomycin	Yes
paroxetine	No	sucralfate	Yes
penicillin G	Yes	sulbactam	No
pentamidine	No	sulfamethoxazole	Yes
pentazocine	Yes		
perindopril	Yes	sulindac	No
phenobarbital	Yes	temazepam	No
phenylbutazone	No	theophylline	Yes
		ticarcillin	Yes
phenytoin	No	ticarcillin and clavulanate	Yes
piperacillin	Yes		
piperacillin and tazobactam	Yes	timolol	No
		tobramycin	Yes
piroxicam	No	tocainide	Yes
prazosin	No	tolbutamide	No
prednisone	No	topiramate	Yes
primidone	Yes	trazodone	No
procainamide	Yes	triazolam	No
promethazine	No	trimethoprim	Yes
propoxyphene	No	valacyclovir	Yes
propranolol	No	valproic acid	No
protriptyline	No	valsartan	No
pyridoxine	Yes	vancomycin	No
quinapril	No	verapamil	No
quinidine	Yes	warfarin	No
quinine	Yes		
ranitidine	Yes		
rifampin	No		

DRUGS THAT PROLONG THE QTc INTERVAL

Changes in a patient's heart rate can affect the QT interval of his electrocardiogram. To account for variations in the degree to which the QT interval is affected, you can use a formula such as the one below. Such formulas let you determine the QTc interval, also called the corrected QT interval.

$$\frac{QT \text{ interval}}{\sqrt{R\text{-}R \text{ interval}}} = QTc \text{ interval}$$

For men under age 55, a normal QTc interval is 350 to 430 milliseconds (msec). For women under age 55, a normal QTc interval is 350 to 450 msec.

A prolonged QTc interval may cause fatal arrhythmias, including ventricular tachycardia and torsades de pointes. The causes of a prolonged QTc interval include disorders, such as hypokalemia, hypomagneseima, renal failure, and heart failure. An abnormal QTc interval also may result from the following drugs.

amantadine	gatifloxacin	ondansetron
amiodarone	gemifloxacin	pentamidine
aripiprazole	granisetron	pimozide
arsenic trioxide	halofantrine	procainamide
azithromycin	haloperidol	quetiapine
chloral hydrate	ibutilide	quinidine
chlorpromazine	indapamide	risperidone
cisapride	isradipine	salmeterol
clarithromycin	levofloxacin	sotalol
disopyramide	levomethadyl	sparfloxacin
dofetilide	lithium	sumatriptan
dolasetron	mesoridazine	tacrolimus
domperidone	methadone	tamoxifen
droperidol	moexipril and hydrochlorothiazide	thioridazine
erythromycin		tizanidine
felbamate	moxifloxacin	venlafaxine
flecainide	naratriptan	voriconazole
foscarnet	nicardipine	ziprasidone
fosphenytoin	octreotide	zolmitriptan

CYTOCHROME P-450 ENZYMES AND COMMON DRUG INTERACTIONS

Cytochrome P-450 enzymes, identified by "CYP" followed by numbers and letters identifying the enzyme families and subfamilies, are found throughout the body (mainly in the liver), and are important in the metabolism of many drugs. The following table lists potential drug-drug

CYP ENZYME	SUBSTRATES
1A2	Amitriptyline, caffeine, chlordiazepoxide, clomipramine, clozapine, cyclobenzaprine, desipramine, diazepam, haloperidol, imipramine, olanzapine, tacrine, theophylline, warfarin, zileuton
2C9	Amitriptyline, carvedilol, clomipramine, dapsone, diazepam, diclofenac, flurbiprofen, fluvastatin, glimepiride, ibuprofen, imipramine, indomethacin, losartan, mirtazapine, naproxen, omeprazole, phenytoin, piroxicam, ritonavir, sildenafil, tolbutamide, torsemide, S-warfarin, zafirlukast, zileuton
2C19	Amitriptyline, carisoprodol, clomipramine, diazepam, imipramine, lansoprazole, mephenytoin, omeprazole, pentamidine, R-warfarin
2D6	Amitriptyline, carvedilol, chlorpheniramine, chlorpromazine, clomipramine, clozapine, codeine, cyclobenzaprine, desipramine, dextromethorphan, donepezil, doxepin, fentanyl, flecainide, fluoxetine, fluphenazine, fluvoxamine, haloperidol, hydrocodone, imipramine, loratadine, maprotiline, meperidine, methadone, metoprolol, mexiletine, morphine, methamphetamine, nortriptyline, oxycodone, paroxetine, perphenazine, propafenone, propoxyphene, propranolol, risperidone, thioridazine, timolol, tramadol, trazodone, venlafaxine
3A4	Alfentanil, alprazolam, amiodarone, amitriptyline, amlodipine, atorvastatin, bromocriptine, buspirone, carbamazepine, clarithromycin, clomipramine, clonazepam, cocaine, corticosteroids, cyclophosphamide, cyclosporine, dapsone, delavirdine, doxorubicin, dexamethasone, diazepam, diltiazem, disopyramide, ergotamine, erythromycin, ethosuximide, etoposide, felodipine, fentanyl, fexofenadine, finasteride, flutamide, fluvastatin, ifosfamide, imipramine, indinavir, isradipine, itraconazole, ketoconazole, lidocaine, loratadine, losartan, lovastatin, midazolam, methadone, methylprednisolone, miconazole, nefazodone, nicardipine, nifedipine, nimodipine, nisoldipine, paclitaxel, pravastatin, prednisone, quinidine, quinine, rifabutin, ritonavir, saquinavir, sertraline, sildenafil, simvastatin, tacrolimus, tamoxifen, teniposide, testosterone, triazolam, troleandomycin, verapamil, vinca alkaloids, warfarin, zileuton, zolpidem

interactions based on the substrates, inducers, and inhibitors that can influence drug metabolism. This table includes common drug interactions; keep in mind that drugs not included in this table may be metabolized by one of the CYP enzymes as well.

INDUCERS	INHIBITORS
Cigarette smoking, phenobarbital, phenytoin, primidone, rifampin, ritonavir	Ciprofloxacin, cimetidine, clarithromycin, enoxacin, erythromycin, fluvoxamine, grapefruit juice, isoniazid, ketoconazole, levofloxacin, mexiletine, norethindrone, norfloxacin, omeprazole, paroxetine, tacrine, zileuton
Carbamazepine, phenobarbital, phenytoin, primidone, rifampin	Amiodarone, chloramphenicol, cimetidine, co-trimoxazole, disulfiram, fluconazole, fluoxetine, fluvastatin, fluvoxamine, isoniazid, itraconazole, ketoconazole, metronidazole, omeprazole, ritonavir, sulfinpyrazone, ticlopidine, zafirlukast
No information available.	Felbamate, fluconazole, fluoxetine, fluvoxamine, omeprazole, ticlopidine
Carbamazepine, phenobarbital, phenytoin, primidone	Amiodarone, chloroquine, cimetidine, fluoxetine, fluphenazine, fluvoxamine, haloperidol, paroxetine, perphenazine, propafenone, propoxyphene, quinidine, ritonavir, sertraline, thioridazine
Barbiturates, carbamazepine, glucocorticoids, griseofulvin, nafcillin, phenytoin, primidone, rifabutin, rifampin	Clarithromycin, cyclosporine, danazol, delavirdine, diltiazem, erythromycin, fluconazole, fluoxetine, fluvoxamine, grapefruit juice, indinavir, isoniazid, itraconazole, ketoconazole, metronidazole, miconazole, nefazodone, nelfinavir, nicardipine, nifedipine, norfloxacin, omeprazole, prednisone, quinidine, quinine, rifabutin, ritonavir, saquinavir, sertraline, troleandomycin, verapamil, zafirlukast

ADVERSE AND ALLERGIC REACTIONS

A drug that produces desired or expected effects also can cause undesirable or even harmful effects. The resulting adverse reactions may range from mild discomforts that decline over time or disappear when therapy ends to debilitating diseases that become chronic or even to life-threatening allergic or toxic reactions.

Adverse reactions may be related to dose or to patient sensitivity. Most result from a drug's known pharmacologic effects and are dose-related. In most cases, these reactions can be predicted. Reactions that result from a patient's unusual sensitivity to a drug or its components are less common and more difficult to predict.

ALERT *Many common adverse reactions, such as nausea, diarrhea, dizziness, and dry mouth, don't endanger a patient's health. However, they can threaten compliance with drug therapy. To help prevent this problem, teach your patient about potential adverse effects and ways to cope with them. Also, urge the patient to consult the prescriber rather than stopping therapy or self-treating bothersome adverse effects.*

DOSE-RELATED REACTIONS

Dose-related reactions include secondary effects, hypersusceptibility, iatrogenic effects, and toxicity.

SECONDARY EFFECTS

A drug typically produces not only therapeutic effects but also secondary effects that may be adverse or beneficial. For example, the analgesic morphine has the primary effect of relieving pain. However, it also has two adverse secondary effects: constipation and respiratory depression. The drug diphenhydramine, which has primary effects as an antihistamine, also has a secondary effect: sedation. In this case, the secondary effect may be beneficial, because the drug can be used as a sleep aid.

HYPERSUSCEPTIBILITY

A patient can be hypersusceptible to a drug's pharmacologic actions. Even when receiving the usual therapeutic dose of a drug, a hypersusceptible patient may experience an excessive therapeutic response or enhanced secondary effects. Hypersusceptibility typically results from altered pharmacokinetics, which leads to a higher-than-expected drug level. It also may stem from increased receptor sensitivity, which can increase therapeutic or adverse drug effects.

IATROGENIC EFFECTS

Iatrogenic effects can mimic disorders. For example, such drugs as antineoplastics, aspirin, corticosteroids, and indomethacin commonly cause gastrointestinal (GI) irritation and bleeding, which can be mistaken for signs of peptic ulcer disease or GI tumor. Other iatrogenic effects include propranolol-induced asthma, methicillin-induced nephritis, and gentamicin-induced deafness.

TOXICITY

When a patient intentionally or accidentally takes an excessive dose of a drug, a toxic drug reaction may result. The patient may have an exaggerated response to the drug, which can lead to transient, minor changes or to more serious, sometimes irreversible reactions, such as respiratory depression, cardiovascular collapse, or death. To help minimize toxic reactions, give lower doses to chronically ill or geriatric patients, whose reduced renal clearance may predispose them to toxicity.

The key to resolving serious drug reactions successfully is quickly and accurately identifying the drug involved and then immediately beginning appropriate treatment. (See *Managing selected drug reactions*.) You'll find more information to help you manage the toxic effects of drug overdose in the next chapter.

PATIENT SENSITIVITY

Less common than dose-related reactions, patient sensitivity–related adverse reactions result from a patient's unusual and extreme sensitivity to a drug. These reactions arise from a unique tissue response rather than from an exaggerated pharmacologic action. Extreme patient sensitivity can take the form of a drug allergy, an idio-

(Text continues on page 304.)

Managing selected drug reactions

Reactions and effects	Interventions	Selected causative drugs
Anemia, aplastic ■ Bleeding from mucous membranes, ecchymoses, petechiae ■ Fatigue, pallor, progressive weakness, shortness of breath, tachycardia progressing to heart failure ■ Fever, oral and rectal ulcers, sore throat without characteristic inflammation	■ Stop drug, if possible. ■ Provide vigorous supportive care, including transfusions, neutropenic isolation, antibiotics, and oxygen. ■ Give colony-stimulating factors if needed. ■ In severe cases, a bone marrow transplant may be needed.	■ altretamine ■ aspirin (long-term) ■ carbamazepine ■ chloramphenicol ■ co-trimoxazole ■ ganciclovir ■ gold salts ■ hydrochloro-thiazide ■ mephenytoin ■ methimazole ■ penicillamine ■ phenothiazines ■ propylthiouracil ■ triamterene ■ zidovudine
Anemia, hemolytic ■ Chills, fever, back and abdominal pain (hemolytic crisis) ■ Jaundice, malaise, splenomegaly ■ Signs of shock	■ Stop drug. ■ Provide supportive care, including transfusions and oxygen. ■ As needed, obtain a blood sample for Coombs' tests.	■ levodopa ■ levodopa-carbidopa ■ mefenamic acid ■ methyldopa ■ penicillins ■ phenazopyridine ■ primaquine ■ quinidine ■ quinine ■ sulfonamides
Bone marrow toxicity (agranulocytosis) ■ Enlarged lymph nodes, spleen, and tonsils ■ Septicemia, shock ■ Progressive fatigue and weakness, then sudden overwhelming infection with chills, fever, headache, and tachycardia	■ Stop drug. ■ Begin antibiotic therapy while awaiting blood culture and sensitivity results. ■ Provide supportive therapy, including neutropenic isolation, warm saline gargles, and oral hygiene.	■ angiotensin-converting enzyme inhibitors ■ aminoglutethimide ■ carbamazepine ■ chloramphenicol ■ clomipramine ■ cotrimoxazole

(continued)

MANAGING SELECTED DRUG REACTIONS *(continued)*

REACTIONS AND EFFECTS	INTERVENTIONS	SELECTED CAUSATIVE DRUGS
Bone marrow toxicity (agranulocytosis) *(continued)*		
■ Pneumonia ■ Ulcers in the colon, mouth, and pharynx		■ flucytosine ■ gold salts ■ penicillamine ■ phenothiazines ■ phenytoin ■ procainamide ■ propylthiouracil ■ sulfonylureas
Bone marrow toxicity (thrombocytopenia)		
■ Fatigue, weakness, lethargy, malaise ■ Hemorrhage, loss of consciousness, shortness of breath, tachycardia ■ Sudden onset of ecchymoses or petechiae; large blood-filled bullae in the mouth	■ Stop drug or reduce dosage. ■ Administer corticosteroids and platelet transfusions. ■ As needed, provide platelet-stimulating factors.	■ ciprofloxacin ■ cisplatin ■ floxuridine ■ flucytosine ■ ganciclovir ■ gold salts ■ heparin ■ interferons alfa-2a and alpha-2b ■ lymphocyte immune globulin ■ methotrexate ■ penicillamine ■ procarbazine ■ quinidine ■ quinine ■ tetracyclines ■ valproic acid
Cardiomyopathy		
■ Acute hypertensive reaction ■ Atrial and ventricular arrhythmias ■ Chest pain ■ Heart failure ■ Chronic cardiomyopathy ■ Pericarditis-myocarditis syndrome	■ Discontinue drug, if possible. ■ Closely monitor patients also receiving radiation therapy. ■ Institute cardiac monitoring at earliest sign of problems. ■ If patient is receiving doxorubicin, limit cumulative dose to less than 500 mg/m^2.	■ cyclophosphamide ■ cytarabine ■ daunorubicin ■ doxorubicin ■ idarubicin ■ mitoxantrone

MANAGING SELECTED DRUG REACTIONS (continued)

REACTIONS AND EFFECTS	INTERVENTIONS	SELECTED CAUSATIVE DRUGS
Dermatologic toxicity ■ May vary from phototoxicity to acneiform eruptions, alopecia, exfoliative dermatitis, lupus erythematosus-like reactions, toxic epidermal necrolysis	■ Stop drug. ■ Give topical antihistamines and analgesics.	■ androgens ■ barbiturates ■ corticosteroids ■ cephalosporins ■ gold salts ■ hydralazine ■ interferons ■ iodides ■ penicillins ■ pentamidine ■ phenothiazines ■ procainamide ■ psoralens ■ quinolones ■ sulfonamides ■ sulfonylureas ■ tetracyclines ■ thiazides
Hepatotoxicity ■ Abdominal pain, hepatomegaly ■ Abnormal levels of alanine aminotransferase, aspartate aminotransferase, serum bilirubin, and lactate dehydrogenase ■ Bleeding, low-grade fever, mental changes, weight loss ■ Dry skin, pruritus, rash ■ Jaundice	■ Reduce dosage or stop drug. ■ Monitor vital signs, blood levels, weight, intake and output, and fluids and electrolytes. ■ Promote rest. ■ Perform hemodialysis, if needed. ■ Provide symptomatic care: vitamins A, B complex, D, and K; potassium for alkalosis; salt-poor albumin for fluid and electrolyte balance; neomycin for GI flora; stomach aspiration for blood; reduced dietary protein; and lactulose for blood ammonia.	■ amiodarone ■ asparaginase ■ carbamazepine ■ chlorpromazine ■ chlorpropamide ■ cytarabine ■ dantrolene ■ erythromycin estolate ■ ifosfamide ■ isoniazid ■ ketoconazole ■ leuprolide ■ methotrexate ■ methyldopa ■ mitoxantrone ■ niacin ■ phenobarbital ■ plicamycin ■ quinolones ■ sulindac

(continued)

MANAGING SELECTED DRUG REACTIONS (continued)

REACTIONS AND EFFECTS	INTERVENTIONS	SELECTED CAUSATIVE DRUGS
Nephrotoxicity ■ Altered creatinine clearance (decreased or increased) ■ Blurred vision, dehydration (depending on part of kidney affected), edema, mild headache, pallor ■ Casts, albumin, or red or white blood cells in urine ■ Dizziness, fatigue, irritability, slowed mental processes ■ Electrolyte imbalance ■ Elevated blood urea nitrogen level ■ Oliguria	■ Reduce dosage or stop drug. ■ Perform hemodialysis, if needed. ■ Monitor vital signs, weight changes, and urine volume. ■ Give symptomatic care: fluid restriction and loop diuretics to reduce fluid retention, I.V. solutions to correct electrolyte imbalance.	■ aminoglycosides ■ cephalosporins ■ cisplatin ■ contrast media ■ corticosteroids ■ cyclosporine ■ gallium ■ gold salts (parenteral) ■ nitrosoureas ■ nonsteroidal anti-inflammatory drugs ■ penicillin ■ pentamidine isethionate ■ plicamycin ■ vasopressors or vasoconstrictors
Neurotoxicity ■ Akathisia ■ Bilateral or unilateral palsies ■ Muscle twitching, tremor ■ Paresthesia ■ Seizures ■ Strokelike syndrome ■ Unsteady gait ■ Weakness	■ Notify prescriber as soon as changes appear. ■ Reduce dosage or stop drug. ■ Watch closely for changes in the patient's condition. ■ Provide symptomatic care: Stay with the patient, reassure him, and protect him during seizures. Provide a quiet environment, draw shades, and speak in soft tones. Maintain the airway, and ventilate the patient as needed.	■ aminoglycosides ■ cisplatin ■ cytarabine ■ isoniazid ■ nitroprusside ■ polymyxin B injection ■ vinca alkaloids

MANAGING SELECTED DRUG REACTIONS (continued)

REACTIONS AND EFFECTS	INTERVENTIONS	SELECTED CAUSATIVE DRUGS
Ocular toxicity ■ Acute glaucoma ■ Blurred, colored, or flickering vision ■ Cataracts ■ Corneal deposits ■ Diplopia ■ Miosis ■ Mydriasis ■ Optic neuritis ■ Scotomata ■ Vision loss	■ Notify prescriber as soon as changes appear. ■ Stop drug if possible. (Some oculotoxic drugs used to treat serious conditions may be restarted at a reduced dosage after the eyes are rested and have returned to near normal.) ■ Watch carefully for changes in symptoms. ■ Provide treatment for symptoms.	■ amiodarone ■ antibiotics such as chloramphenicol ■ anticholinergics ■ chloroquine ■ clomiphene ■ corticosteroids ■ cyclophosphamide ■ cytarabine ■ cardiac glycosides ■ ethambutol ■ hydroxychloroquine ■ lithium carbonate ■ methotrexate ■ phenothiazines ■ quinidine ■ quinine ■ rifampin ■ tamoxifen ■ vinca alkaloids
Ototoxicity ■ Alaxia ■ Hearing loss ■ Tinnitus ■ Vertigo	■ Notify prescriber as soon as changes appear. ■ Stop drug or reduce dosage. ■ Watch carefully for symptomatic changes.	■ aminoglycosides ■ antibiotics, such as colistimethate sodium, erythromycin, gentamicin, kanamycin, and streptomycin ■ chloroquine ■ cisplatin ■ loop diuretics ■ minocycline ■ quinidine ■ quinine ■ salicylates ■ vancomycin

(continued)

MANAGING SELECTED DRUG REACTIONS *(continued)*

REACTIONS AND EFFECTS	INTERVENTIONS	SELECTED CAUSATIVE DRUGS
Pseudomembranous colitis ■ Abdominal pain ■ Colonic perforation ■ Fever ■ Hypotension ■ Severe dehydration ■ Shock ■ Sudden, copious diarrhea (watery or bloody)	■ Stop drug and give another antibiotic, such as vancomycin or metronidazole. ■ Maintain fluid and electrolyte balance. ■ Check serum electrolyte levels daily. If pseudomembranous colitis is mild, order an ion exchange resin. ■ Monitor vital signs and hydration status. ■ Immediately report signs of shock to physician. ■ Observe for signs of hypokalemia, especially malaise and weak, rapid, irregular pulse.	■ antibiotics

syncratic response, or an allergy to latex in a drug's packaging or delivery equipment.

A drug allergy develops when a patient's immune system identifies a drug, metabolite, or contaminant as a dangerous foreign substance that must be neutralized or destroyed. Previous exposure to the drug or to one with a similar chemical makeup sensitizes the patient's immune system. Then, reexposure causes an allergic reaction. Such a reaction directly injures cells and tissues. It also produces broader systemic damage by triggering cells to release vasoactive and inflammatory substances.

An allergic reaction can vary in intensity from a mild itchy rash to an immediate, life-threatening anaphylactic reac-

IDENTIFYING ALLERGIC REACTIONS

Allergies to drugs and other allergens are categorized into four basic types.

TYPE	RESPONSE	EXAMPLES
I	Immediate reactions to stings and drugs	Anaphylaxis, urticaria, angio-edema
II	Drug-induced autoimmune disorders	Sulfonamide-induced granulocy-topenia, quinidine-induced thrombocytopenic purpura, hydralazine-induced systemic lupus erythematosus
III	Reactions to penicillins, sul-fonamides, iodides; anti-body targeted against tissue antigens	Urticarial skin eruptions, arthral-gia, lymphadenopathy, fever
IV	Reexposure to an antigen	Poison ivy and its resulting con-tact dermatitis

tion with circulatory collapse and swelling of the larynx and bronchioles. (See *Identifying allergic reactions*.)

Some sensitivity-related reactions don't result from a drug's pharmacologic properties or an allergic response. Instead, they're specific to the individual. The cause of these distinctive responses isn't fully understood, but experts believe genetics play an important role.

Keep in mind that an allergic reaction may stem not from the drug itself but from packaging and administration materials that contain latex. Latex allergy is a reaction to certain proteins in latex rubber. The amount of latex exposure needed to cause an allergic reaction isn't known, but increasing exposure to latex proteins increases the risk of an allergic reaction. By using an appropriate screening procedure, you can help find out whether your patient is at risk. (See *Screening for latex allergy*, page 306.)

People sensitive to latex may experience symptoms within minutes, or they may take hours. Mild reactions cause red skin, rash, hives, or itching. More severe reactions cause

SCREENING FOR LATEX ALLERGY

To determine whether your patient has a latex sensitivity or allergy, ask the following screening questions:

Allergies

■ Do you have a history of hay fever, asthma, eczema, allergies, or rashes? If so, what type of reaction do you have?

■ Have you experienced an allergic reaction, local sensitivity, or itching after being exposed to any latex products, such as balloons or condoms?

■ If you experience shortness of breath or wheezing when blowing up latex balloons, describe your reaction.

■ Do you have shortness of breath or wheezing after blowing up balloons or after a dental visit? Do you have itching in or around your mouth after eating a banana?

■ Are you allergic to any foods, especially bananas, avocados, kiwi, or chestnuts? If so, describe your reaction.

Occupation

■ What's your occupation?
■ Are you exposed to latex in your occupation?

■ Have you had a reaction to latex products at work? If so, describe your reaction.

■ If you've developed a rash on your hands after wearing latex gloves, how long after putting on the gloves did it take for the rash to develop?

■ What did the rash look like?

Personal history

■ Do you have any birth defects? If yes, explain.

■ Have you ever had itching, swelling, hives, cough, shortness of breath, or other allergic symptoms during or after using a condom, using a diaphragm, or having a vaginal or rectal examination?

Surgical history

■ Have you had any previous surgical procedures? Did you have any complications? If so, describe them.

■ Have you had previous dental procedures? Did you have any complications? If so, describe them.

■ Do you have spina bifida or a urinary tract problem that requires surgery or catheterization?

MANAGING A LATEX ALLERGY REACTION

If your patient is having an allergic reaction to latex, act immediately. If the latex product that caused the reaction is known, remove it and perform the following measures using latex-free equipment:

■ If the allergic reaction develops during drug administration or a procedure, stop it immediately.

■ Assess airway, breathing, and circulation.

■ Administer 100% oxygen, and monitor oxygen saturation.

■ Start an I.V. with lactated Ringer's solution or normal saline solution.

■ Give epinephrine according to the patient's symptoms.

■ Give famotidine I.V.

■ If the patient has evident bronchospasm, give nebulized albuterol.

■ Secondary treatment for latex allergy reaction is aimed at treating the swelling and tissue reaction to the latex as well as breaking the chain of events involved in the allergic reaction. It includes:

– diphenhydramine I.V.

– methylprednisolone I.V.

■ Document the event and the exact cause, if known. If latex particles have entered the I.V. line, insert a new I.V. line with a new catheter, new tubing, and new infusion attachments as soon as possible.

runny nose, sneezing, itchy eyes, scratchy throat, difficulty breathing, and rarely, shock. Recognizing the signs and symptoms and knowing how to quickly manage a latex reaction will help control the situation. (See *Managing a latex allergy reaction*.)

10 / OVERDOSE

If your patient has signs of acute drug toxicity resulting from overdose, start advanced life support measures as needed. Give the prescribed antidote, if available, and take steps to block absorption and speed elimination of the drug. Consult with a poison control center for additional information about treatment of specific toxins.

Because early intervention can help prevent serious toxicity, review the signs and symptoms of selected drug overdoses, as outlined below.

Acetaminophen overdose

In an acute acetaminophen overdose, hepatotoxicity can result if plasma levels reach 300 mcg/ml 4 hours after ingestion or 50 mcg/ml 12 hours after ingestion. Signs and symptoms include cyanosis, anemia, jaundice, skin eruptions, fever, emesis, central nervous system (CNS) stimulation, delirium, and methemoglobinemia progressing to CNS depression,

coma, vascular collapse, seizures, and death.

Acetaminophen poisoning develops in stages:
- *Stage 1 (12 to 24 hours after ingestion):* nausea, vomiting, diaphoresis, anorexia
- *Stage 2 (24 to 48 hours after ingestion):* clinically improved but elevated liver function test results
- *Stage 3 (72 to 96 hours after ingestion):* peak hepatotoxicity
- *Stage 4 (7 to 8 days after ingestion):* recovery.

Analeptic overdose

Individual responses to overdose with analeptic drugs, such as amphetamines or cocaine, vary widely. Toxic doses also vary, depending on the drug and the route of ingestion.

Signs and symptoms of analeptic overdose include restlessness, tremor, hyperreflexia, tachypnea, confusion, aggressiveness, hallucinations, and panic; fatigue and depression usually follow the excitement stage. Other effects may include arrhythmias, shock, altered blood pressure, nausea, vomiting, diarrhea, and abdominal cramps; death is usually preceded by seizures and coma.

Anticholinergic overdose

Effects of an anticholinergic overdose include such peripheral effects as blurred vision; dilated, nonreactive pupils; decreased or absent bowel sounds; dry mucous membranes; dysphagia; flushed, hot, dry skin; hypertension; hyperthermia; increased respiratory rate; urine retention; and tachycardia.

Anticoagulant overdose

Effects of an oral anticoagulant overdose vary with severity. They may include internal or external bleeding or skin necrosis, but the most common sign is hematuria. Excessively prolonged prothrombin time or minor bleeding mandates withdrawal of therapy; withholding one or two doses may be adequate in some cases.

Antihistamine overdose

Drowsiness is the usual symptom of antihistamine overdose. Seizures, coma, and respiratory depression may occur with severe overdose. Certain histamine antagonists—such as diphenhydramine—also block cholinergic receptors and produce modest anticholinergic symptoms, such as dry mouth, flushed skin, fixed and dilated pupils, and gastrointestinal (GI) symptoms, especially in children. Phenothiazine-type antihistamines such as promethazine also block dopamine receptors. Movement disorders mimicking Parkinson's disease may occur.

Barbiturate overdose

A barbiturate overdose causes an unsteady gait, slurred speech, sustained nystagmus, somnolence, confusion, respiratory depression, pulmonary edema, areflexia, and coma. Typical shock syndrome with tachycardia and hypotension, jaundice, hypothermia followed by fever, and oliguria may occur.

Benzodiazepine overdose

An overdose of benzodiazepines produces somnolence, confusion, coma, hypoactive reflexes, dyspnea, labored breathing, hypotension, bradycardia, slurred speech, and unsteady gait or impaired coordination.

Digoxin overdose

Digoxin overdose mainly causes GI, cardiovascular, and CNS

effects. With severe overdose, hyperkalemia may develop rapidly and result in life-threatening cardiac effects.

Digoxin has caused almost every kind of arrhythmia; various combinations of arrhythmias may occur in the same patient. Patients with chronic digoxin toxicity commonly have ventricular arrhythmias, atrioventricular conduction disturbances, or both. Patients with digoxin-induced ventricular tachycardia have a high risk of death because ventricular fibrillation or asystole may result.

ALERT Cardiac evidence of digoxin toxicity may occur with or without other evidence of toxicity and commonly precedes other toxic effects. Because cardiotoxic effects can also occur in heart disease, determining whether these effects result from an underlying heart disease or digoxin toxicity may be difficult.

CNS depressant overdose

Signs of CNS depressant overdose include prolonged coma, hypotension, hypothermia followed by fever, and inadequate ventilation even without significant respiratory depression. Absence of pupillary reflexes, dilated pupils, loss of deep tendon reflexes, tonic muscle spasms, and apnea may occur as well.

Iron supplement overdose

ALERT Symptoms of poisoning result from iron's acute corrosive effects on the GI mucosa as well as the adverse metabolic effects caused by iron overload. Iron supplements represent a major source of poisoning, especially in small children. In fact, as little as 1 g of ferrous sulfate can kill an infant.

Four stages of acute iron poisoning have been identified. Signs and symptoms may occur within the first 10 to 60 minutes of ingestion, or they may be delayed several hours.

The first findings reflect acute GI irritation and include epigastric pain, nausea, and vomiting. The patient may have green diarrhea, then tarry stools, then melena. Hematemesis may be accompanied by drowsiness, lassitude, shock, and coma. Local erosion of the stomach and small intestine may further enhance the absorption of iron. If the patient doesn't die in the first phase, a second phase of apparent recovery may last 24 hours.

A third phase, which can occur 4 to 48 hours after ingestion, is marked by CNS abnormalities, metabolic acidosis, hepatic dysfunction, renal failure, and bleeding diathesis. This phase may progress to circulatory failure, coma, and death.

If the patient survives, the fourth phase consists of late complications of acute iron intoxication and may occur 2 to 6 weeks after overdose. Pyloric and duodenal stenosis may cause gastric outlet obstruction resulting in persistent vomiting.

Patients who develop vomiting, diarrhea, leukocytosis, or hyperglycemia and have an abdominal X-ray positive for iron within 6 hours of ingestion are likely to be at risk for serious toxicity.

Nonsteroidal anti-inflammatory drug overdose

Clinical manifestations of overdose with nonsteroidal antiinflammatory drugs include dizziness, drowsiness, paresthesia, vomiting, nausea, abdominal pain, headache, sweating, nystagmus, apnea, and cyanosis.

Opiate overdose

Rapid I.V. administration of opiates may result in overdose because of the delay in maximum CNS effect (30 minutes). The most common signs of morphine overdose are respiratory depression with or without CNS depression and miosis (pinpoint pupils). Other acute toxic effects include hypotension, bradycardia, hypothermia, shock, apnea, cardiopulmonary arrest, circulatory collapse, pulmonary edema, and seizures.

Phenothiazine overdose

CNS depression from a phenothiazine overdose is characterized by deep, unarousable sleep, possible coma, hypotension or hypertension, extrapyramidal symptoms, abnormal involuntary muscle movements, agitation, seizures, arrhythmias, electrocardiogram changes, hypothermia or hyperthermia, and autonomic nervous system dysfunction.

Salicylate overdose

Effects of salicylate overdose include metabolic acidosis with respiratory alkalosis, hyperpnea, tachypnea, seizures, tetany, and cardiovascular, respiratory, and renal collapse.

Tricyclic antidepressant overdose

An overdose of tricyclic antidepressants is commonly life-threatening, particularly when combined with alcohol. The first 12 hours after ingestion are a stimulatory phase characterized by excessive anticholinergic activity (agitation, irritation, confusion, hallucinations, hyperthermia, parkinsonian symptoms, seizures, urine retention, dry mucous membranes, pupillary dilation, constipation, and ileus). This phase precedes CNS depressant effects, including hypothermia, decreased or absent reflexes, sedation, hypotension, cyanosis, and cardiac irregularities, including tachycardia, conduction disturbances, and quinidine-like effects on the electrocardiogram.

CLINICAL TIP The severity of an overdose is best indicated by a widening of the QRS complex, which usually represents severe toxicity. Obtaining serum measurements usually isn't helpful. Metabolic acidosis may follow hypotension, hypoventilation, and seizures.

TREATMENT FOR POISONING AND OVERDOSE

Institute advanced life support measures, including the following, as indicated for acute drug toxicity.

■ Establish and maintain an airway. This usually involves inserting an oropharyngeal or endotracheal airway.

■ If the patient isn't breathing, start ventilation with a bag-valve mask until a mechanical ventilator is available. Give oxygen based on readings from pulse oximetry or arterial blood gas levels.

■ Maintain circulation. Start an I.V. infusion, and obtain laboratory specimens to assess for toxic drug levels, electrolytes, and glucose levels as indicated.

■ If the patient is hypotensive, give fluids and vasopressors such as dopamine. If the patient is hypertensive, prepare to give an antihypertensive (usually beta blockers if catecholamines were ingested).

■ Prepare to treat arrhythmias as indicated for the specific toxin.

■ Protect the patient from injury, and watch for seizures. Observe the patient, and provide supportive care.

Consult a poison control center for information about treating ingestion of a specific toxin. (See *Managing poisoning and overdose*, pages 314 to 319.) If the patient has a substance abuse problem, recognize that treatment will be long-term and probably will include relapses. Make sure you understand the signs and symptoms of toxicity, so you can help the patient recover from the addiction. (See *Managing acute toxicity*, pages 320 to 326.)

MANAGING POISONING AND OVERDOSE

ANTIDOTE AND INDICATIONS	NURSING CONSIDERATIONS
acetylcysteine (Mucomyst, Mucosil) ■ Treatment of acetaminophen toxicity	■ Use cautiously in elderly or debilitated patients and in patients with asthma or severe respiratory insufficiency. ■ Don't use with activated charcoal. ■ Don't combine with amphotericin B, ampicillin, chymotrypsin, erythromycin lactobionate, hydrogen peroxide, oxytetracycline, tetracycline, iodized oil, or trypsin. Administer separately.
activated charcoal (Actidose-Aqua, CharcoAid, Liqui-Char) ■ Treatment of poisoning or overdose with most oral drugs, except caustic agents and hydrocarbons	■ Don't give to semiconscious or unconscious patients. ■ If possible, administer within 30 minutes of poisoning. Administer larger dose if patient has food in his stomach. ■ Don't give with syrup of ipecac because charcoal inactivates ipecac. If a patient received syrup of ipecac, give charcoal after he has finished vomiting. ■ Don't give in ice cream, milk, or sherbet because they reduce adsorption capacity of charcoal. ■ Powder form is most effective. Mix with tap water to form a thick syrup. You may add a small amount of fruit juice or flavoring to make the syrup more palatable. ■ You may need to repeat the dose if the patient vomits shortly after administration.
aminocaproic acid (Amicar) ■ Antidote for alteplase, streptokinase, or urokinase toxicity	■ Use cautiously with hormonal contraceptives and estrogens because they may increase the risk of hypercoagulability. ■ For infusion, dilute solution with sterile water for injection, normal saline solution, dextrose 5% in water (D_5W), or Ringer's solution. ■ Monitor coagulation studies, heart rhythm, and blood pressure.

MANAGING POISONING AND OVERDOSE (continued)

ANTIDOTE AND INDICATIONS	NURSING CONSIDERATIONS
amyl nitrite ■ Antidote for cyanide poisoning	■ Amyl nitrite is effective within 30 seconds, but its effects last only 3 to 5 minutes. ■ To administer, wrap ampule in cloth and crush. Hold near the patient's nose and mouth so he can inhale vapor. ■ Monitor the patient for orthostatic hypotension. ■ The patient may experience headache after administration.
atropine sulfate ■ Antidote for anti-cholinesterase toxicity	■ Atropine sulfate is contraindicated for patients with glaucoma, myasthenia gravis, obstructive uropathy, or unstable cardiovascular status. ■ Monitor intake and output to detect urine retention.
botulism antitoxin, trivalent equine ■ Treatment of botulism	■ Obtain an accurate patient history of allergies, especially to horses, and of reactions to immunizations. ■ Test the patient for sensitivity (against a control of normal saline solution in the opposing limb) before administration. Read results after 5 to 30 minutes. A wheal indicates a positive reaction, requiring patient desensitization. ■ Keep epinephrine 1:1,000 available in case of allergic reaction.
deferoxamine mesylate (Desferal) ■ Adjunctive treatment of acute iron intoxication	■ Don't give to patients with severe renal disease or anuria. Use cautiously in patients with impaired renal function. ■ Keep epinephrine 1:1,000 available in case of allergic reaction. ■ Use I.M. route if possible. Use I.V. route only when the patient is in shock. ■ To reconstitute for I.M. administration, add 2 ml of sterile water for injection to each ampule. Make sure the drug dissolves completely. To reconstitute for I.V. administration, dissolve as for I.M. use but in normal saline solution, D_5W, or lactated Ringer's solution.

(continued)

MANAGING POISONING AND OVERDOSE (continued)

ANTIDOTE AND INDICATIONS	NURSING CONSIDERATIONS

deferoxamine mesylate (Desferal) *(continued)*

- Monitor intake and output carefully. Warn patient that his urine may turn red.
- Reconstituted solution can be stored for up to 1 week at room temperature. Protect from light.

digoxin immune Fab (ovine) (Digibind, DigiFab)

- Treatment of potentially life-threatening digoxin intoxication

- Use cautiously in patients allergic to sheep proteins, papaya extracts, or the pineapple enzyme bromelain. Performing a skin test before administering the drug to a high-risk patient may be appropriate, but such testing isn't routine.
- Use only in patients in shock or cardiac arrest with ventricular arrhythmias such as ventricular tachycardia or fibrillation; with progressive bradycardia, such as severe sinus bradycardia; or with second- or third-degree atrioventricular block unresponsive to atropine.
- Infuse through a 0.22-micron membrane filter, if possible.
- Refrigerate powder for reconstitution. If possible, use reconstituted drug immediately, although you may refrigerate it for up to 4 hours.
- Drug interferes with digoxin immunoassay measurements, resulting in misleading standard serum digoxin levels until the drug is cleared from the body (about 2 days).
- Total serum digoxin levels may rise after administration of this drug, reflecting fat-bound (inactive) digoxin.
- Monitor potassium levels closely.

edetate calcium disodium (Calcium Disodium Versenate)

- Treatment of lead poisoning in patients with blood levels >50 mcg/dl

- Don't give to patients with severe renal disease or anuria.
- Avoid using I.V. route in patients with lead encephalopathy because intracranial pressure may increase; use I.M. route.
- Avoid rapid infusion; I.M. route is preferred, especially for children.
- If giving a large dose, give with dimercaprol to avoid toxicity.

MANAGING POISONING AND OVERDOSE *(continued)*

ANTIDOTE AND INDICATIONS	NURSING CONSIDERATIONS
edetate calcium disodium (Calcium Disodium Versenate) *(continued)*	■ Force fluids to facilitate lead excretion except in patients with lead encephalopathy. ■ Before giving, obtain baseline intake and output, urinalysis, blood urea nitrogen, and serum alkaline phosphatase, calcium, creatinine, and phosphorus levels. Then monitor these values on first, third, and fifth days of treatment. Monitor electrocardiogram periodically. ■ If procaine hydrochloride has been added to I.M. solution to minimize pain, watch for local reaction.
methylene blue ■ Treatment of cyanide poisoning	■ Don't give to patients with severe renal impairment or hypersensitivity to drug. ■ Use with caution in glucose-6-phosphate dehydrogenase deficiency; may cause hemolysis. ■ Avoid extravasation; S.C. injection may cause necrotic abscesses. ■ Warn the patient that methylene blue will discolor his urine and stools and stain his skin. Hypochlorite solution rubbed on skin will remove stains.
naloxone hydrochloride (Narcan) ■ Treatment of respiratory depression caused by opioid drugs ■ Treatment of postoperative opioid depression ■ Treatment of asphyxia neonatorum caused by administration of opioid analgesics to a mother in late labor	■ Use cautiously in patients with cardiac irritability or opioid addiction. ■ Monitor respiratory depth and rate. Be prepared to provide oxygen, ventilation, and other resuscitative measures. ■ Duration of opioid may exceed that of naloxone, causing the patient to relapse into respiratory depression and requiring repeated administration. ■ You may administer drug by continuous I.V. infusion to control adverse effects of epidurally administered morphine. ■ You may see "overshoot" effect—the patient's respiratory rate after receiving drug exceeds his rate before respiratory depression occurred. ■ Naloxone is the safest drug to use when the cause of respiratory depression is uncertain.

(continued)

MANAGING POISONING AND OVERDOSE *(continued)*

ANTIDOTE AND INDICATIONS	NURSING CONSIDERATIONS

naloxone hydrochloride (Narcan) *(continued)*

- This drug doesn't reverse respiratory depression caused by diazepam. The reversal agent for benzodiazepines is flumazenil.
- Although generally believed ineffective in treating respiratory depression caused by nonopioid drugs, naloxone may reverse coma induced by alcohol intoxication.

pralidoxime chloride (Protopam Chloride)

- Antidote for organophosphate poisoning and cholinergic drug overdose

- Don't give to patients poisoned with carbaryl (Sevin), a carbamate insecticide, because it increases Sevin's toxicity.
- Use cautiously in patients with renal insufficiency, myasthenia gravis, asthma, or peptic ulcer.
- Use in hospitalized patients only; have respiratory and other supportive equipment available.
- Administer antidote as soon as possible after poisoning. Treatment is most effective if started within 24 hours of exposure.
- Before administering, suction secretions and make sure airway is patent.
- Dilute drug with sterile water containing no preservatives. Give atropine with pralidoxime.
- If the patient's skin was exposed, remove his clothing and wash his skin and hair with sodium bicarbonate, soap, water, and alcohol as soon as possible. He may need a second washing. When washing the patient, wear gloves and protective clothes to avoid exposure.
- Observe the patient for 48 to 72 hours after he ingested poison. Delayed absorption may occur. Watch for signs of rapid weakening in the patient with myasthenia gravis being treated for overdose of cholinergic drugs. He may pass quickly from cholinergic crisis to myasthenic crisis and require more cholinergic drugs to treat the myasthenia. Keep edrophonium available.

MANAGING POISONING AND OVERDOSE (continued)

ANTIDOTE AND INDICATIONS	NURSING CONSIDERATIONS
protamine sulfate ■ Treatment of heparin overdose	■ Use cautiously after cardiac surgery. ■ Administer slowly to reduce adverse reactions. Have equipment available to treat shock. ■ Monitor the patient continuously, and check vital signs frequently. ■ Watch for spontaneous bleeding (heparin "rebound"), especially in patients undergoing dialysis and in those who have had cardiac surgery. ■ Protamine sulfate may act as an anticoagulant in extremely high doses.
syrup of ipecac (ipecac syrup) ■ Induction of vomiting in acute poisoning, when advisable	■ Syrup of ipecac is contraindicated for semicomatose, unconscious, and severely inebriated patients and for those with seizures, shock, or absent gag reflex. ■ Don't give after ingestion of petroleum distillates or volatile oils because of the risk of aspiration pneumonitis. Don't give after ingestion of caustic substances, such as lye, because further injury can result. ■ Before giving, make sure you have ipecac syrup, not ipecac fluid extract (14 times more concentrated, and deadly). ■ If two doses don't induce vomiting, consider gastric lavage. ■ If the patient also needs activated charcoal, give charcoal after he has vomited, or charcoal will neutralize the emetic effect. ■ The American Academy of Pediatrics (AAP) no longer recommends that parents keep a bottle of syrup of ipecac in the home because it can be improperly administered and has been abused by persons with eating disorders such as bulimia. AAP recommends that parents keep the universal poison control telephone number (1-800-222-1222) posted by their telephone.

MANAGING ACUTE TOXICITY

SUBSTANCE	SIGNS AND SYMPTOMS	INTERVENTIONS
Alcohol ■ Beer and wine ■ Distilled spirits ■ Other products, such as cough syrup, aftershave, or mouthwash	■ Alcohol breath odor ■ Ataxia ■ Bradycardia ■ Coma ■ Hypotension ■ Hypothermia ■ Nausea and vomiting ■ Respiratory depression ■ Seizures	■ Give activated charcoal and a saline cathartic. Induce vomiting or perform gastric lavage according to your facility's protocol. ■ Start I.V. fluid replacement and give D_5W, thiamine, B-complex vitamins, and vitamin C to prevent dehydration and hypoglycemia and to correct nutritional deficiencies. ■ Take steps to protect the patient from injury. ■ Give an anticonvulsant, such as diazepam, to control seizures. ■ Watch the patient for evidence of withdrawal, such as hallucinations and alcohol withdrawal delirium. ■ Auscultate the patient's lungs often to detect crackles or rhonchi, possibly indicating aspiration pneumonia. If you note these breath sounds, consider antibiotics. ■ Monitor the patient's neurologic status and vital signs every 15 minutes until he's stable. Assist with dialysis if vital functions are severely depressed.
Amphetamines ■ Amphetamine sulfate ■ Dextroamphetamine sulfate ■ Methamphetamine	■ Altered mental status (from confusion to paranoia) ■ Coma ■ Diaphoresis ■ Dilated reactive pupils ■ Dry mouth ■ Exhaustion ■ Hallucinations ■ Hyperactive deep tendon reflexes ■ Hypertension	■ If the drug was taken orally, give activated charcoal and a sodium or magnesium sulfate cathartic. ■ Lower the patient's urine pH to 5 by adding ammonium chloride or ascorbic acid to his I.V. solution. ■ Force diuresis using mannitol. ■ Give a short-acting barbiturate, such as pentobarbital, to control stimulant-induced seizures. ■ Take steps to protect the patient from injury, especially if he's paranoid or having hallucinations. ■ Give haloperidol to treat agitation or assaultive behavior.

MANAGING ACUTE TOXICITY (continued)

SUBSTANCE	SIGNS AND SYMPTOMS	INTERVENTIONS
Amphetamines (continued)	■ Hyperthermia ■ Shallow respirations ■ Tachycardia ■ Tremors and seizure activity	■ Give an alpha-adrenergic blocker, such as phentolamine, for hypertension. ■ Watch for cardiac arrhythmias. If these develop, consider propranolol to treat tachyarrhythmias or lidocaine to treat ventricular arrhythmias. ■ Treat hyperthermia with tepid sponge baths or a hypothermia blanket. ■ Provide a quiet environment to avoid overstimulation. ■ Be alert for evidence of withdrawal, such as abdominal tenderness, muscle aches, and long periods of sleep. ■ Observe suicide precautions, especially if the patient shows signs of withdrawal.
Antipsychotics ■ Chlorpromazine ■ Phenothiazines ■ Thioridazine	■ Constricted pupils ■ Decreased deep tendon reflexes ■ Decreased level of consciousness (LOC) ■ Dry mouth ■ Dysphagia ■ Extrapyramidal effects (dyskinesia, opisthotonos, muscle rigidity, ocular deviation) ■ Hypotension ■ Hypothermia or hyperthermia ■ Photosensitivity ■ Respiratory depression ■ Seizures ■ Tachycardia	■ Consider activated charcoal and a cathartic. Don't induce vomiting because phenothiazines have an antiemetic effect. ■ Give diphenhydramine to treat extrapyramidal effects. ■ In severe cases, give physostigmine salicylate to reverse anticholinergic effects. ■ Replace fluids I.V. to correct hypotension; monitor the patient's vital signs frequently. ■ Monitor respiratory rate, and give oxygen if needed. ■ Give an anticonvulsant such as diazepam or a short-acting barbiturate such as pentobarbital sodium to control seizures. ■ Keep the patient's room dark to avoid worsening his photosensitivity.

(continued)

MANAGING ACUTE TOXICITY (continued)

SUBSTANCE	SIGNS AND SYMPTOMS	INTERVENTIONS
Anxiolytic sedative-hypnotics ■ Benzo- diazepines	■ Coma ■ Confusion ■ Decreased reflexes ■ Drowsiness ■ Hypotension ■ Seizures ■ Shallow respirations ■ Stupor	■ Consider activated charcoal and a cathartic. Induce vomiting or perform gastric lavage according to your facility's protocol. ■ Give supplemental oxygen to correct hypoxia-induced seizures. ■ Replace fluids I.V. to correct hypotension; monitor vital signs frequently. ■ For benzodiazepine overdose, or to reverse the effect of benzodiazepine–induced sedation or respiratory depression, give flumazenil.
Barbiturate sedative-hypnotics ■ Amobarbital sodium ■ Phenobarbital ■ Secobarbital sodium	■ Blisters or bullous lesions ■ Cyanosis ■ Depressed LOC (from confusion to coma) ■ Flaccid muscles and absent reflexes ■ Hyperthermia or hypothermia ■ Hypotension ■ Nystagmus ■ Poor pupil reaction to light ■ Respiratory depression	■ Consider activated charcoal and a saline cathartic. Induce vomiting or perform gastric lavage according to your facility's protocol. ■ Maintain the patient's blood pressure with I.V. fluid challenges and vasopressors. ■ If the patient has taken a phenobarbital overdose, give sodium bicarbonate I.V. to alkalinize the urine and speed the drug's elimination. ■ Apply a hyperthermia or hypothermia blanket to help return the patient's temperature to normal. ■ Prepare the patient for hemodialysis or hemoperfusion if toxicity is severe. ■ Perform frequent neurologic assessments, and check the patient's pulse rate, temperature, skin color, and reflexes frequently. ■ Notify a physician if you see signs of respiratory distress or pulmonary edema. ■ Watch for evidence of withdrawal, such as hyperreflexia, tonic-clonic seizures, and hallucinations. Provide symptomatic relief of withdrawal symptoms. ■ Institute safety measures to protect the patient from injury.

MANAGING ACUTE TOXICITY *(continued)*

SUBSTANCE	SIGNS AND SYMPTOMS	INTERVENTIONS
Cocaine	■ Abdominal pain ■ Alternating euphoria and apprehension ■ Coma ■ Confusion ■ Dilated pupils ■ Fever ■ Hyperexcitability ■ Hyperpnea ■ Hypertension or hypotension ■ Nausea and vomiting ■ Pallor or cyanosis ■ Perforated nasal septum or mouth sores ■ Respiratory arrest ■ Spasms and seizures ■ Tachycardia ■ Tachypnea ■ Visual, auditory, and olfactory hallucinations	■ Calm the patient by talking to him in a quiet room. ■ If cocaine was ingested, induce vomiting or perform gastric lavage; give activated charcoal followed by a saline cathartic. ■ Give the patient a tepid sponge bath, and give an antipyretic to reduce fever. ■ Monitor the patient's blood pressure and heart rate. Expect to give propranolol for symptomatic tachycardia. ■ Give an anticonvulsant, such as diazepam, to control seizures. ■ Scrape the inside of the patient's nose to remove residual bits of the drug. ■ Monitor cardiac rate and rhythm. Cocaine use may cause ventricular fibrillation and cardiac standstill. Defibrillate the patient, and begin cardiopulmonary resuscitation, if indicated.
Glutethimide	■ Apnea ■ CNS depression (from unresponsiveness to deep coma) ■ Drowsiness ■ Hypotension ■ Hypothermia ■ Impaired thought processes (memory, judgment, attention span)	■ If the drug was taken orally, induce vomiting or perform gastric lavage according to your facility's protocol; give activated charcoal and a cathartic. ■ Maintain the patient's blood pressure with I.V. fluid challenges and vasopressors. ■ Assist with hemodialysis or hemoperfusion if the patient has hepatic or renal failure or is in a prolonged coma. *(continued)*

MANAGING ACUTE TOXICITY (continued)

SUBSTANCE	SIGNS AND SYMPTOMS	INTERVENTIONS
Glutethimide (continued)	■ Irritability ■ Nystagmus ■ Paralytic ileus ■ Poor bladder control ■ Respiratory depression ■ Slurred speech ■ Small, reactive pupils ■ Twitching, spasms, and seizures	■ Give an anticonvulsant, such as diazepam, for seizures. ■ Perform hourly neurologic assessments: Coma may recur because of the drug's slow release from fat deposits. ■ Be alert for signs of increased intracranial pressure, such as decreasing LOC and widening pulse pressure. Consider mannitol. ■ Watch for evidence of withdrawal, such as hyperreflexia, tonic–clonic seizures, and hallucinations, and provide symptomatic relief of withdrawal symptoms. ■ Institute safety measures to protect the patient from injury.
Hallucinogens ■ Lysergic acid diethylamide (LSD) ■ Mescaline (peyote)	■ Agitation and anxiety ■ Depersonalization ■ Dilated pupils ■ Fever ■ Flashback experiences ■ Hallucinations ■ Hyperactive movement ■ Intensified perceptions ■ Impaired judgment ■ Increased heart rate ■ Moderately increased blood pressure ■ Synesthesia	■ Reorient the patient repeatedly to time, place, and person. ■ Take steps to protect the patient from injury. ■ Calm the patient by talking to him in a quiet room. ■ If the drug was taken orally, induce vomiting or perform gastric lavage according to your facility's protocol; give activated charcoal and a cathartic. ■ Give diazepam I.V. to control seizures.

MANAGING ACUTE TOXICITY (continued)

SUBSTANCE	SIGNS AND SYMPTOMS	INTERVENTIONS
Opioids ■ Codeine ■ Heroin ■ Hydromor- phone hydrochloride ■ Morphine	■ Bradycardia ■ Constricted pupils ■ Depressed LOC ■ Hypotension ■ Hypothermia ■ Seizures ■ Skin changes (pruritus, urti- caria, flushed skin) ■ Slow, deep respirations	■ Give naloxone until the drug's CNS depressant effects are reversed. ■ Replace fluids I.V. to increase circulatory volume. ■ Correct hypothermia by applying extra blankets; if the patient's body temperature doesn't increase, use a hyperthermia blanket. ■ Reorient the patient frequently. ■ Auscultate the lungs often for crackles, possibly indicating pulmonary edema. (Onset may be delayed.) ■ Give oxygen via nasal cannula, mask, or mechanical ventilation to correct hypoxemia from hypoventilation. ■ Monitor cardiac rate and rhythm, being alert for atrial fibrillation. (This should resolve when hypoxemia is corrected.) ■ Be alert for signs of withdrawal, such as piloerection (goose flesh), diaphoresis, and hyperactive bowel sounds. ■ Take steps to protect the patient from injury.
Phencyclidine (PCP)	■ Amnesia ■ Blank stare ■ Cardiac arrest ■ Decreased awareness of sur- roundings ■ Drooling ■ Gait ataxia ■ Hyperactivity ■ Hypertensive crisis ■ Hyperthermia ■ Muscle rigidity	■ If the drug was taken orally, induce vomiting or perform gastric lavage according to your facility's protocol; instill and remove activated charcoal repeatedly. ■ Acidify the patient's urine with ascorbic acid to increase drug excretion. ■ Expect to continue to acidify urine for 2 weeks because signs and symptoms may recur when fat cells release PCP stores.

(continued)

MANAGING ACUTE TOXICITY (continued)

SUBSTANCE	SIGNS AND SYMPTOMS	INTERVENTIONS
Phencyclidine (PCP) (continued)	■ Nystagmus ■ Recurrent coma ■ Seizures ■ Violent behavior	■ Give diazepam and haloperidol to control agitation or psychotic behavior. ■ Take steps to protect the patient from injury. ■ Give diazepam to control seizures. ■ Institute seizure precautions. ■ Provide a quiet environment and dimmed light. ■ Give propranolol for hypertension and tachycardia, and give nitroprusside for severe hypertension. ■ Closely monitor urine output and serial renal function tests. Rhabdomyolysis, myoglobinuria, and renal failure may occur in severe intoxication. ■ If renal failure develops, prepare the patient for hemodialysis.

11 / INTERACTIONS

Interactions can occur between two drugs or between a drug and a food, herbal supplement, or lifestyle factor. Interactions may alter drug effects, skew laboratory test results, or produce physical or chemical incompatibilities. The more drugs a patient takes, the greater the chances are that a drug interaction will occur. Remember, however, that not all drug interactions have a negative effect; in fact, they may be used purposefully to achieve a therapeutic benefit.

DRUG-DRUG INTERACTIONS

Interactions between drugs can cause additive effects, synergistic effects, antagonistic effects, and altered absorption, metabolism, or excretion. Drugs also may be physically incompatible. (See *Compatibility of drugs combined in a syringe*, pages 328 and 329.)

ADDITIVE EFFECTS

An additive effect occurs when a patient receives two drugs with similar actions equal to the effect of a higher dose of either drug given alone. Causing an additive effect, such as by giving two different analgesics, allows the use of lower doses of each drug, which decreases the risk of adverse reactions. It also provides greater pain control than could be produced by one drug, probably because of differing mechanisms of action.

SYNERGISTIC EFFECTS

A synergistic effect, or potentiation, happens if two drugs with the same effect produce a greater response when taken together than when taken alone. In this type of interaction, one drug enhances the effect of the other.

ANTAGONISTIC EFFECTS

An antagonistic effect develops when the combined response of *(Text continues on page 330.)*

COMPATIBILITY OF DRUGS COMBINED IN A SYRINGE

KEY

Y = compatible for at least 30 minutes

P = provisionally compatible; administer within 15 minutes

P(5) = provisionally compatible; administer within 5 minutes

N = not compatible

* = conflicting data

(A blank space indicates no available data.)

	atropine sulfate	butorphanol tartrate	chlorpromazine HCl	cimetidine HCl	codeine phosphate	dexamethasone sodium phosphate	dimenhydrinate	diphenhydramine HCl	droperidol	fentanyl citrate	glycopyrrolate	heparin Na	hydromorphone HCl	hydroxyzine HCl	meperidine HCl	metoclopramide HCl
atropine sulfate		Y	P	Y			P	P	P	P	Y	P(5)	Y	P*	P	P
butorphanol tartrate	Y		Y	Y			N	Y	Y	Y				Y	Y	Y
chlorpromazine HCl	P	Y		N			N	P	P	P	Y	N	Y	P	P	P
cimetidine HCl	Y	Y	N					Y	Y	Y	Y	P(5)*	Y	Y	Y	
codeine phosphate											Y			Y		
dexamethasone sodium phosphate								N*			N		N*			Y
dimenhydrinate	P	N	N					P	P	P	N	P(5)	Y	N	P	P
diphenhydramine HCl	P	Y	P	Y		N*	P		P	P	Y		Y	P	P	Y
droperidol	P	Y	P	Y			P	P		P	Y	N		P	P	P
fentanyl citrate	P	Y	P	Y			P	P	P			P(5)	Y	P	P	P
glycopyrrolate	Y		Y	Y	Y	N	N	Y	Y				Y	Y	Y	
heparin Na	P(5)		N	P(5)*			P(5)		N	P(5)					N	P(5)*
hydromorphone HCl	Y		Y	Y		N*	Y	Y		Y	Y			Y		
hydroxyzine HCl	P*	Y	P	Y	Y		N	P	P	P	Y		Y		P	P
meperidine HCl	P	Y	P	Y			P	P	P	P	Y	N		P		P
metoclopramide HCl	P	Y	P			Y	P	Y	P	P		P(5)*		P	P	
midazolam HCl	Y	Y	Y	Y			N	Y	Y	Y	Y		Y	Y	Y	Y
morphine sulfate	P	Y	P	Y			P	P	P	P	Y	N*		P	N	P
nalbuphine HCl	Y			Y				Y	Y		Y			Y		
pentazocine lactate	P	Y	P	Y			P	P	P	P	N	N	Y	P	P	P
pentobarbital Na	P	N	N	N			N	N	N	N	N		Y	N	N	
perphenazine	Y	Y	Y	Y			Y	Y	Y	Y				Y	Y	P*
phenobarbital Na												P(5)	N			
prochlorperazine edisylate	P	Y	P	Y			N	P	P	P	Y		N*	P	P	P
promazine HCl	P		P	Y			N	P	P	P	Y			P	P	P
promethazine HCl	P	Y	P	Y			N	P	P	P	Y	N	Y	P	P	P*
ranitidine HCl	Y		N*			Y	Y	Y		Y	Y		Y	N	Y	Y
scopolamine HBr	P	Y	P	Y			P	P	P	P	Y		Y	P	P	P
secobarbital Na			N								N					
sodium bicarbonate											N					N
thiethylperazine maleate		Y												Y		
thiopental Na			N				N	N			N				N	

	midazolam HCl	morphine sulfate	nalbuphine HCl	pentazocine lactate	pentobarbital Na	perphenazine	phenobarbital Na	prochlorperazine edisylate	promazine HCl	promethazine HCl	ranitidine HCl	scopolamine HBr	secobarbital Na	sodium bicarbonate	thiethylperazine maleate	thiopental Na
atropine sulfate	Y	P	Y	P	P	Y		P	P	P	Y	P				
butorphanol tartrate	Y	Y		Y	N	Y		Y		Y		Y			Y	
chlorpromazine HCl	Y	P		P	N	Y		P	P	P	N*	P				N
cimetidine HCl	Y	Y	Y	Y	N	Y		Y	Y	Y		Y	N			
codeine phosphate																
dexamethasone sodium phosphate											Y					
dimenhydrinate	N	P		P	N	Y		N	N	N	Y	P				N
diphenhydramine HCl	Y	P	Y	P	N	Y		P	P	P	Y	P				N
droperidol	Y	P	Y	P	N	Y		P	P	P		P				
fentanyl citrate	Y	P		P	N	Y		P	P	P	Y	P				
glycopyrrolate	Y	Y	Y	N	N			Y	Y	Y	Y	Y	N	N		N
heparin Na		N*		N			P(5)		N							
hydromorphone HCl	Y			Y	Y		N	N*		Y	Y	Y			Y	
hydroxyzine HCl	Y	P	Y	P	N	Y		P	P	P	N	P				
meperidine HCl	Y	N		P	N	Y		P	P	P	Y	P				N
metoclopramide HCl	Y	P		P		P*		P	P	P*	Y	P		N		
midazolam HCl		Y	Y		N	N		N	Y	Y	N	Y			Y	
morphine sulfate	Y			P	N*	Y		P*	P	P*	Y	P				N
nalbuphine HCl	Y				N			Y		N*	Y	Y			Y	
pentazocine lactate		P			N	Y		P	P*	P*	Y	P				
pentobarbital Na	N	N*	N	N			N		N	N	N	P		Y		Y
perphenazine	N	Y		Y	N			Y		Y	Y	Y			N	
phenobarbital Na											N					
prochlorperazine edisylate	N	P*	Y	P	N	Y			P	P	Y	P				N
promazine HCl	Y	P		P*	N			P		P		P				
promethazine HCl	Y	P*	N*	P*	N	Y		P	P		Y	P				N
ranitidine HCl	N	Y	Y	Y	N	Y	N	Y		Y		Y			Y	
scopolamine HBr	Y	P	Y	P	P	Y		P	P	P	Y					Y
secobarbital Na																
sodium bicarbonate					Y											N
thiethylperazine maleate	Y		Y			N					Y					
thiopental Na		N			Y			N		N		Y		N		

two drugs is less than the response produced by either drug alone. For example, if levodopa is prescribed to decrease a patient's stiffness, rigidity, and other symptoms of Parkinson's disease, pyridoxine (vitamin B_6) can interfere with (or antagonize) levodopa's effects.

ALTERED ABSORPTION

Two drugs given together can change the absorption of one or both drugs. A drug that alters stomach acidity can affect a second drug's ability to dissolve in the stomach. Some drugs can interact to form an insoluble compound that can't be absorbed. After a drug is absorbed, the blood distributes it throughout the body as a free drug or protein-bound drug. When given together, two drugs can compete for protein-binding sites. This may increase the effects of one drug if it's displaced from the protein and becomes free, or unbound. For example, the oral anticoagulant warfarin is more than 97% protein-bound, and the anticonvulsant drug phenytoin successfully competes with warfarin for protein-binding sites. Combining these two drugs increases the amount of free warfarin,

which significantly increases the risk of bleeding.

ALTERED METABOLISM AND EXCRETION

Toxic drug levels can occur when one drug inhibits another's metabolism and excretion. For example, the antibiotic erythromycin may decrease hepatic metabolism of cyclosporine, resulting in a high cyclosporine level and nephrotoxicity.

Changes in hepatic blood flow from drug interactions or disease also may affect drug metabolism and excretion. Decreased hepatic blood flow affects drugs whose metabolism and excretion depend more on blood flow than on enzyme activity. Conversely, drugs whose metabolism and excretion depend on intrinsic enzyme activity typically aren't affected by changes in hepatic blood flow.

Some drug interactions affect only excretion. For example, the interaction between penicillin and the uricosuric drug probenecid can produce therapeutic effects. Probenecid decreases renal excretion of penicillin, which increases its half-life and level.

INCOMPATIBILITY

Drugs may be physically incompatible when combined together. A precipitate or particulate matter may form, the drug's color may change, or the drug may become hazy. In some cases, the incompatibility may not be visually noticeable. Make sure to consult a pharmacist or drug reference before mixing drugs, either in an I.V. line, a syringe, or a piggyback setup if you aren't familiar with their compatibility status.

DRUG–FOOD INTERACTIONS

Interactions with food can alter a drug's therapeutic effect and impair vitamin and mineral absorption in several ways. For one thing, food can alter the rate and amount of drug absorbed from the gastrointestinal tract, affecting bioavailability (the amount of a dose available to systemic circulation). For example, a high-fat meal can increase the bioavailability of the antifungal griseofulvin. A low-protein, high-carbohydrate diet can increase the bioavailability of theophylline.

Here's another interaction. Some drugs can stimulate enzyme production, increasing the metabolic rate and the demand for vitamins that are enzyme cofactors (substances that unite with the enzyme and allow it to function).

Other dangerous interactions can happen as well. For instance, when a patient eats tyramine-rich foods while taking a monoamine oxidase inhibitor, hypertensive crisis can occur. (See *Avoiding food interactions with MAO inhibitors*, page 332.)

Grapefruit juice can cause interactions with many drugs. For instance, when a patient drinks grapefruit juice with a 3-hydroxy-3-methylglutaryl coenzyme A (HMG-CoA) reductase inhibitor, cyclosporine, or amprenavir, drug toxicity may occur. Grapefruit juice also may delay the onset, decrease the absorption, or have other adverse effects on a drug. (See *Interactions between drugs and grapefruit juice*, page 333.)

AVOIDING FOOD INTERACTIONS WITH MAO INHIBITORS

In a patient taking a monoamine oxidase (MAO) inhibitor, foods that contain tyramine may produce a hypertensive crisis, which is characterized by a sudden severe increase in blood pressure, severe headache, sudden vision changes, and dizziness. To prevent this dangerous drug-food interaction, teach the patient which foods to avoid during treatment. Foods with a high tyramine content should be avoided completely, those with a moderate content may be eaten occasionally, and those with a low tyramine content are allowable in limited quantities.

Foods with a high tyramine content
- Aged cheese, such as blue, cheddar, and Swiss
- Aged or smoked meats, such as corned beef, herring, and sausage
- Beer
- Fava or broad beans such as Italian green beans
- Liver, such as chicken and beef liver
- Red wines, such as burgundy and Chianti
- Yeast extracts such as brewer's yeast

Foods with a moderate tyramine content
- Meat extracts such as bouillon
- Ripe avocados
- Ripe bananas
- Sour cream
- Yogurt

Foods with a low tyramine content
- American, mozzarella, cottage, and cream cheese
- Chocolate
- Distilled spirits, such as gin, vodka, and scotch
- Figs
- White wines

DRUG-HERB INTERACTIONS

Drug-herb interactions are a growing concern as more patients buy and use herbal supplements, often without reporting them to their prescriber. Many herbal supplements can interact with drug therapy. Here are just a few examples:
- Evening primrose oil can lower the seizure threshold and shouldn't be taken during anticonvulsant therapy.
- When taken with warfarin, gingko may increase the risk of bleeding.

INTERACTIONS BETWEEN DRUGS AND GRAPEFRUIT JUICE

When taken with certain drugs, grapefruit juice can significantly alter absorption, onset, blood level, excretion, and effects. To prevent these drug–food interactions, explain them to your patient and recommend that he avoid grapefruit juice during therapy.

Delayed absorption
- indinavir
- itraconazole
- quinidine

Delayed onset or increased effects
- midazolam
- triazolam

Increased blood levels
- amlodipine
- buspirone
- carbamazepine
- cyclosporine
- dextromethorphan
- diltiazem
- erythromycin
- felodipine
- lovastatin
- nicardipine
- nisoldipine
- saquinavir
- sildenafil
- simvastatin
- verapamil

Decreased levels in blood
- etoposide
- fexofenadine

Delayed excretion
- atorvastatin

- Ginseng may decrease warfarin's anticoagulant effect.

- St. John's wort may decrease the effects of protease inhibitors such as indinavir, nonnucleoside reverse transcriptase inhibitors such as nevirapine, digoxin, and cyclosporine.

- St. John's wort also may cause additive effects when taken with a selective serotonin reuptake inhibitor or other antidepressant, which could lead to serotonin syndrome, a serious, sometimes fatal reaction that causes myoclonus rigidity, mental status changes, hyperthermia, autonomic nervous system instability, rapid fluctuations in vital signs, delirium, and coma.

ALERT Although herbal supplements may be "natural" products, they can be harmful. To help avoid dangerous interactions, always ask your patient whether he takes any herbal or dietary supplements.

DRUG-LIFESTYLE INTERACTIONS

Lifestyle factors may interfere with a drug's therapeutic effects. For example, alcohol depresses the central nervous system (CNS), leading to sedation and drowsiness. If a patient combines alcohol with a drug that also depresses the CNS, the interaction enhances the drug's sedative effect and impairs the patient's psychomotor skills. That's why you should caution a patient to avoid alcohol during therapy with a barbiturate, benzodiazepine, or other drug that causes drowsiness or sedation.

Smoking may increase corticosteroid release, requiring higher dosages of these drugs. Heavy smoking can increase haloperidol metabolism, possibly necessitating a dosage adjustment. It also increases theophylline elimination, which decreases the drug's therapeutic effects.

ALERT   A smoker who is stable on a dose of theophylline may risk serious adverse reactions if he quits smoking without informing his prescriber. The former smoker may be receiving a higher-than-needed dose of theophylline, which may lead to toxicity.

EFFECTS ON DIAGNOSTIC TESTS

Drug interactions can alter laboratory tests. For example, a patient may undergo a test that measures creatinine level by using a colorimetric method. Many cephalosporins, such as cefazolin and cefoxitin, contain chromogens that aren't creatinine but can't be differentiated by the colorimetric method. As a result, the laboratory test may overestimate the patient's creatinine level, possibly leading to inadequate drug dosages.

Guaiac tests of feces to detect occult blood can show false-positive results in a patient who takes large amounts of iron supplements.

Blood glucose testing is the preferred method of monitoring diabetes. However, some diabetic patients monitor their glucose level with a urine test. Drugs that interfere with urine glucose testing include cephalothin, isoniazid, levodopa, probenecid, and large amounts (1 to 2 g daily) of ascorbic acid. False-positive results indicating a high glucose level could cause a patient to decrease his food intake or to increase his insulin doses when, in fact, the glucose level is stable.

Some drugs affect electrocardiogram tracings. For example, class Ia and III antiarrhythmics can prolong the QT interval, as can antihistamines, antibiotics, antifungals, antidepressants, and antipsychotics. Prolonging the QT interval can lead to torsades de pointes, ventricular fibrillation, and death. No one knows why these drugs prolong the QT interval; nevertheless, you should ask about a history of syncope or cardiac arrest before giving these drugs. Also obtain a detailed family history of syncope, sudden death at a young age, or congenital deafness because a family history of these disorders suggests a predisposition for prolonged QT interval.

PART IV

DRUG THERAPY IN COMMON DISEASES AND DISORDERS

12 / DRUGS FOR CARDIOVASCULAR DISORDERS

ANGINA PECTORIS

When the heart muscle needs more oxygenated blood than the coronary arteries can supply, the resulting myocardial ischemia produces a set of symptoms known as angina pectoris. The hallmark symptom is chest pain; often, the pain radiates into the jaw, neck, shoulder, between the shoulder blades, or down one arm, usually the left. Other symptoms that may accompany the pain include nausea, dyspnea, and diaphoresis.

Typically, angina arises when physical exertion or emotional stress places an increased demand on the heart, which in turn requires an increased supply of blood. If the coronary arteries are narrowed from plaque deposits, however, they may be unable to deliver the needed supply. A less common form of angina—Prinzmetal's angina—results from vasospasm and may occur with or without accompanying atherosclerotic changes.

Angina usually is diagnosed by physical examination and a careful medical history. Diagnostic tests may include an electrocardiogram, an exercise or thallium stress test, or a coronary angiogram. A complete blood count can rule out angina induced by anemia.

Treatment initially focuses on modifying the risk factors for coronary artery disease, including high blood pressure, cigarette smoking, high blood cholesterol levels, and excess weight. Drugs may be prescribed as well. Nitroglycerin relieves pain by relaxing blood vessels. Other drugs can reduce the workload of the heart. Beta blockers slow the heart rate and lessen the force of the heart muscle contraction. Calcium channel blockers are also effective in reducing the frequency and severity of angina attacks.

amlodipine
CONTRAINDICATIONS AND CAUTIONS

■ Contraindicated in patients hypersensitive to drug.

■ Use cautiously in patients with heart failure and patients receiving other peripheral vasodilators, especially those with severe aortic stenosis.

■ Because drug is metabolized by the liver, use cautiously and in reduced dosage in patients with severe hepatic disease.

KEY POINTS

■ Grapefruit juice increases amlodipine levels. Discourage use together.

■ Some patients, especially those with severe obstructive coronary artery disease, may have increased frequency, duration, or severity of angina or acute myocardial infarction (MI) at start of therapy or increase in dosage.

■ Monitor patient for evidence of heart failure, such as shortness of breath or swelling of hands and feet.

atenolol
CONTRAINDICATIONS AND CAUTIONS

■ Contraindicated in patients with cardiogenic shock, overt cardiac failure, or sinus bradycardia and greater than first-degree heart block.

■ Use cautiously in patients at risk for heart failure and in those with bronchospastic disease, diabetes, hyperthyroidism, or impaired renal or hepatic function.

KEY POINTS

■ Check apical pulse before giving drug; if slower than 60 beats/minute, withhold drug and call prescriber.

ALERT Withdraw drug gradually over 2 weeks to avoid serious adverse reactions.

■ Drug may alter dosage requirements of antidiabetic drugs in previously stabilized diabetic patients. Monitor blood glucose levels closely.

diltiazem
CONTRAINDICATIONS AND CAUTIONS

■ Contraindicated in patients hypersensitive to drug, patients with sick sinus syndrome or second- or third-degree atrioventricular (AV) block without an artificial pacemaker, and patients with acute MI, pulmonary congestion (documented by X-ray), systolic blood pressure below 90 mm Hg, or ventricular tachycardia.

■ I.V. forms are contraindicated in patients who have atrial fibrillation or flutter with an accessory bypass tract, as in Wolff-Parkinson-White syndrome or short–PR-interval syndrome.

■ Use cautiously in elderly patients and in those with heart failure or impaired hepatic or renal function.

KEY POINTS

■ Monitor blood pressure and heart rate when starting therapy and adjusting dosage.

■ Maximum antihypertensive effect may not occur for 14 days.

■ If systolic blood pressure is below 90 mm Hg or heart rate is below 60 beats/minute, withhold dose and notify prescriber.

isosorbide
CONTRAINDICATIONS AND CAUTIONS

■ Contraindicated in patients hypersensitive to nitrates, patients with idiosyncratic reactions to nitrates, and patients with acute MI with low left ventricular filling pressure, angle-closure glaucoma, increased intracranial pressure, severe hypotension, or shock.

■ Use cautiously in patients with blood volume depletion (as from diuretic therapy) or mild hypotension.

KEY POINTS

■ To prevent tolerance, patient should maintain a nitrate-free interval of 8 to 12 hours daily. The regimen for isosorbide mononitrate (one tablet on awakening and a second dose in 7 hours, or one extended-release tablet daily) aims to minimize nitrate tolerance by providing a substantial nitrate-free interval.

■ Drug may cause headaches, especially at the start of therapy. Dosage may be reduced temporarily, but tolerance usually develops. Treat headache with aspirin or acetaminophen.

■ Caution patient that stopping drug abruptly may cause coronary arteries to spasm, increasing anginal symptoms and the risk of MI.

metoprolol
CONTRAINDICATIONS AND CAUTIONS

■ Contraindicated in patients hypersensitive to drug or other beta blockers and in patients with cardiogenic shock, overt cardiac failure, or sinus bradycardia and greater than first-degree heart block.

■ Use cautiously in patients with diabetes, heart failure, or respiratory or hepatic disease.

KEY POINTS

🌀 *ALERT Always check patient's apical pulse rate before giving drug. If it's slower than 60 beats/minute, withhold drug and call prescriber immediately.*

■ When therapy is stopped, reduce dose gradually over 1 to 2 weeks.

■ Drug may alter dosage requirements of antidiabetic drugs in previously stabilized diabetic patients. Monitor blood glucose levels closely.

nadolol

CONTRAINDICATIONS AND CAUTIONS

■ Contraindicated in patients with bronchial asthma, cardiogenic shock, overt heart failure, and sinus bradycardia and greater than first-degree heart block.

■ Use cautiously in diabetic patients (because beta blockers may mask certain evidence of hypoglycemia), patients undergoing major surgery involving general anesthesia, and patients with chronic bronchitis, emphysema, heart failure, or renal or hepatic impairment.

KEY POINTS

🌀 *ALERT Check apical pulse before giving drug. If slower than 60 beats/minute, withhold drug and call prescriber.*

■ Monitor blood pressure often. If patient develops severe hypotension, give a vasopressor, as prescribed.

■ Abrupt discontinuation can worsen angina and cause MI. Dosage should be reduced gradually over 1 to 2 weeks.

nicardipine

CONTRAINDICATIONS AND CAUTIONS

■ Contraindicated in patients hypersensitive to drug and in those with advanced aortic stenosis.

■ Use cautiously in patients with heart failure, hypotension, or impaired hepatic or renal function.

KEY POINTS

■ Measure blood pressure often in early therapy to check for orthostatic hypotension. Maximum blood pressure response occurs about 1 hour after taking the immediate-release form, about 2 to 4 hours after the sustained-release form. Because blood pressure may vary widely based on blood level of drug, assess adequacy of antihypertensive effect 8 hours after dosing.

🌀 *ALERT Urge patient to report chest pain immediately. Some patients have increased frequency, severity, or duration of chest pain when therapy starts or dosage changes.*

■ Urge patient to rise from a sitting or lying position slowly to avoid dizziness from decreased blood pressure.

nifedipine

CONTRAINDICATIONS AND CAUTIONS

■ Contraindicated in patients hypersensitive to drug.

■ Use cautiously in elderly patients and patients with heart failure or hypotension. Give extended-release tablets cautiously to patients with severe GI narrowing.

KEY POINTS

■ Avoid the once-widespread sublingual use of nifedipine capsules (the "bite and swallow" method). Excessive hypotension, MI, and death may result.

■ Although rebound effect hasn't been observed when drug is stopped, dosage should be reduced slowly under prescriber's supervision.

■ Tell patient that chest pain may worsen briefly when therapy starts or dosage increases.

nitroglycerin

CONTRAINDICATIONS AND CAUTIONS

■ Contraindicated in patients hypersensitive to nitrates, patients allergic to adhesives (transdermal), and patients with angle-closure glaucoma, early MI, increased intracranial pressure, orthostatic hypotension, or severe anemia.

■ I.V. nitroglycerin is contraindicated in patients hypersensitive to it and in patients with cardiac tamponade, constrictive pericarditis, or restrictive cardiomyopathy.

■ Use cautiously in patients with hypotension or volume depletion.

KEY POINTS

■ Drug may cause headaches, especially at start of therapy. Dosage may be reduced temporarily, but tolerance usually develops. Treat headache with aspirin or acetaminophen.

■ Tolerance to drug can be minimized with a 10- to 12-hour nitrate-free interval. To achieve this, remove the transdermal system in the early evening and apply a new system the next morning or omit the last daily dose of a buccal, sustained-release, or ointment form. Check with the prescriber for changes in dosage regimen if tolerance is suspected.

■ Caution patient that stopping drug abruptly may cause coronary arteries to spasm.

propranolol

CONTRAINDICATIONS AND CAUTIONS

■ Contraindicated in patients with bronchial asthma, cardiogenic shock, heart failure (unless caused by a tachyarrhythmia responsive to propranolol), or sinus bradycardia and heart block greater than first-degree.

■ Use cautiously in elderly patients, patients with diabetes mellitus (because drug blocks some hypoglycemia symptoms), patients with thyrotoxicosis (because drug may mask its symptoms), patients taking other antihypertensives, and patients with hepatic disease, hepatic or renal impairment, or nonallergic bronchospastic diseases.

KEY POINTS

■ Always check patient's apical pulse before giving drug. If extremes in pulse rates occur, withhold drug and notify prescriber immediately.

■ Drug masks common signs and symptoms of shock and hypoglycemia.

🌀 **ALERT** *Tell patient not to stop drug suddenly because doing so can worsen chest pain and trigger an MI.*

verapamil

CONTRAINDICATIONS AND CAUTIONS

■ Contraindicated in patients hypersensitive to drug and patients with atrial flutter or fibrillation with an accessory bypass tract syndrome, cardiogenic shock, second- or third-degree AV block or sick sinus syndrome (except with a functioning pacemaker), severe heart failure (unless caused by verapamil therapy), severe hypotension, or severe left ventricular dysfunction.

■ I.V. verapamil is contraindicated in patients receiving I.V. beta blockers and patients with ventricular tachycardia.

■ Use cautiously in elderly patients and patients with hepatic disease, increased intracranial pressure, or renal disease.

KEY POINTS

■ Monitor blood pressure at the start of therapy and during dosage adjustments. Help patient walk because dizziness may occur.

■ Notify prescriber about evidence of heart failure, such as swelling of hands and feet and shortness of breath.

■ Caution patient against abruptly stopping drug.

CEREBROVASCULAR ACCIDENT

Commonly called a *stroke*, a cerebrovascular accident (CVA) is a sudden impairment of cerebral circulation in one or more blood vessels supplying the brain. The impairment interrupts or diminishes oxygen supply and commonly causes serious damage or necrosis in brain tissues.

The sooner circulation returns to normal, the better the chances of a complete recovery. However, about half of those who survive a CVA remain permanently disabled and experience a recurrence within weeks, months, or years.

CVA is the third most common cause of death in the United States and the most common cause of neurologic disability. It affects 500,000 people each year, half of whom die as a result. The major causes of CVA are thrombosis, embolism, and hemorrhage.

Factors that increase the risk of CVA include arrhythmias, atherosclerosis, cigarette smoking, diabetes mellitus, electrocardiogram changes, gout, high serum triglyceride levels, hypertension, lack of exercise, myocardial enlargement, postural hypotension, rheumatic heart disease, and use of hormonal contraceptives. A family history of CVA and a history of transient ischemic attacks (TIAs) indicate an increased risk as well.

CVAs are classified according to their course of progression. The least severe is the TIA, or *little stroke*, which results from a temporary interruption of blood flow, usually in the carotid and vertebrobasilar arteries. A progressive stroke, or *stroke-in-evolution (thrombus-in-evolution)*, begins with slight neurologic deficit and worsens in a day or two. In a completed stroke, neurologic deficits are maximal at onset and don't progress.

alteplase
CONTRAINDICATIONS AND CAUTIONS
■ Contraindicated in patients with a history of CVA, patients who had intraspinal or intracranial trauma or surgery within 2 months, and patients with active internal bleeding, aneurysm, arteriovenous malformation, bleeding diathesis, intracranial hemorrhage (current or previous), intracranial neoplasm, severe uncontrolled hypertension, seizure at onset of CVA (when used for acute ischemic CVA),

or suspicion of subarachnoid hemorrhage.

■ Use cautiously in patients age 75 or older, pregnant patients, patients who gave birth within the previous 10 days, patients having major surgery within 10 days (when bleeding is difficult to control because of its location), patients receiving anticoagulants, patients undergoing organ biopsy, and patients with acute pericarditis; cerebrovascular disease; diabetic hemorrhagic retinopathy; diastolic pressure of 110 mm Hg or higher; gastrointestinal (GI) or genitourinary (GU) bleeding; hemostatic defects caused by hepatic or renal impairment; mitral stenosis, atrial fibrillation, or other conditions that may lead to left heart thrombus; septic thrombophlebitis; subacute bacterial endocarditis; systolic pressure of 180 mm Hg or higher; or trauma (including cardiopulmonary resuscitation).

KEY POINTS

■ When used for acute ischemic CVA, drug should be given within 3 hours after symptoms begin and only when intracranial bleeding has been ruled out.

■ Avoid invasive procedures during thrombolytic therapy because bleeding is the most common adverse effect. Closely monitor patient for evidence of internal bleeding, and frequently check all puncture sites.

■ If uncontrollable bleeding occurs, stop infusion (and heparin) and notify prescriber.

aspirin

CONTRAINDICATIONS AND CAUTIONS

■ Contraindicated in patients hypersensitive to drug and in those with sensitivity reactions to nonsteroidal anti-inflammatory drugs; G6PD deficiency; or bleeding disorders, such as hemophilia, von Willebrand's disease, or telangiectasia.

■ Use cautiously in patients with GI lesions, hypoprothrombinemia, impaired renal function, severe hepatic impairment, thrombocytopenia, thrombotic thrombocytopenic purpura, or vitamin K deficiency.

KEY POINTS

■ During prolonged therapy, hematocrit, hemoglobin, prothrombin time, international normalized ratio, and renal function should be assessed periodically.

■ Aspirin irreversibly inhibits platelet aggregation. It should be discontinued 5 to 7 days before elective surgery to allow time for production and release of new platelets.

■ Advise patient to take drug with food, milk, antacid, or a large glass of water to reduce adverse GI reactions.

ticlopidine
CONTRAINDICATIONS AND CAUTIONS

■ Contraindicated in patients hypersensitive to drug and in those with active bleeding from peptic ulceration, active intracranial bleeding, hematopoietic disorders, or severe hepatic impairment.

■ Use cautiously and with close monitoring of complete blood count (CBC) and white blood cell (WBC) differentials. Moderate to severe neutropenia and agranulocytosis may occur in patients taking ticlopidine.

KEY POINTS

■ Because of life-threatening adverse reactions, give drug only to patients who are allergic to, can't tolerate, or have failed aspirin therapy.

■ Determine CBC and WBC differentials at second week of therapy and repeat every 2 weeks until end of third month. Stop drug in patients with platelet count of 80,000/mm^3 or less. If needed, give methylprednisolone 20 mg I.V. to nor-

malize bleeding time within 2 hours.

■ Warn patient to avoid aspirin and aspirin-containing products and to check with prescriber or pharmacist before taking over-the-counter drugs.

CORONARY ARTERY DISEASE

The dominant effect of coronary artery disease (CAD) is the loss of oxygen and nutrients to myocardial tissue because of reduced coronary blood flow. A near epidemic in the Western world, CAD occurs most often among older white people.

CLINICAL TIP *Although authorities once believed that hormone replacement therapy helped protect postmenopausal women from the effects of CAD, this belief may be mistaken. Indeed, hormone replacement therapy may increase the risk of certain cardiovascular problems.*

Atherosclerosis is the usual cause of CAD. In this form of arteriosclerosis, fatty, fibrous plaques narrow the lumen of the coronary arteries, reduce the volume of blood that can flow through them, and lead to myocardial ischemia. Plaque formation also predisposes to thrombosis, which can provoke an MI.

Atherosclerosis usually develops in high-flow, high-pressure arteries, such as those in the heart, brain, kidneys, and aorta, especially at bifurcation points. It has been linked to many risk factors: family history, hypertension, obesity, smoking, diabetes mellitus, stress, a sedentary lifestyle, and high serum cholesterol and triglyceride levels.

Uncommon causes of reduced coronary artery blood flow include dissecting aneurysms, infectious vasculitis, syphilis, and congenital defects in the coronary vascular system. Coronary artery spasms also may impede blood flow.

fluvastatin

CONTRAINDICATIONS AND CAUTIONS

■ Contraindicated in women of childbearing potential, pregnant women, breast-feeding women, patients hypersensitive to drug, and patients with active liver disease or unexplained persistently elevated transaminase levels.

■ Use cautiously in patients with severe renal impairment and a history of liver disease or heavy alcohol use.

KEY POINTS

■ Drug should be started only after diet and other nondrug therapies have proven ineffective. Patient should follow a standard low-cholesterol diet during therapy.

■ Liver function tests should be obtained at the start of therapy, 12 weeks after the start of therapy, at dose increases, and periodically during therapy.

■ Advise patient that it may take up to 4 weeks for the drug to be fully effective.

gemfibrozil

CONTRAINDICATIONS AND CAUTIONS

■ Contraindicated in patients hypersensitive to drug and in those with gallbladder disease, hepatic dysfunction, or severe renal dysfunction (including primary biliary cirrhosis).

KEY POINTS

■ Check complete blood count and liver function test results periodically during the first 12 months of therapy.

■ If drug has no beneficial effects after 3 months, expect prescriber to stop it.

■ Teach patient about proper dietary management of cholesterol and triglycerides. As appropriate, recommend weight-control, exercise, and smoking cessation programs.

lovastatin

CONTRAINDICATIONS AND CAUTIONS

■ Contraindicated in women of childbearing potential, pregnant women, breast-feeding women, patients hypersensitive to drug, and patients with active liver disease or unexplained persistently elevated transaminase levels.

■ Use cautiously in patients who consume large amounts of alcohol or have a history of liver disease.

KEY POINTS

■ Obtain liver function tests at the start of therapy, at 6 and 12 weeks after the start of therapy, at dose increases, and periodically during therapy.

🌀 *ALERT Urge patient to promptly report unexplained muscle pain, tenderness, or weakness, particularly when accompanied by malaise or fever.*

■ Tell patient to stop drug and notify prescriber immediately if she is or could be pregnant or if she wishes to breast-feed.

pravastatin

CONTRAINDICATIONS AND CAUTIONS

■ Contraindicated in women of childbearing potential, pregnant women, breast-feeding women, patients hypersensitive to drug, and patients with active liver disease or conditions that cause unexplained, persistently elevated transaminase levels.

■ Use cautiously in patients who consume large amounts of alcohol or have a history of liver disease.

KEY POINTS

■ Liver function tests should be performed at start of therapy and then periodically. A liver biopsy may be performed if elevated liver enzyme levels persist.

■ Inform patient that it will take up to 4 weeks for drug to achieve full therapeutic effect.

■ Tell patient to stop drug and notify prescriber immediately if she is or could be pregnant or she wishes to breast-feed.

simvastatin

CONTRAINDICATIONS AND CAUTIONS

■ Contraindicated in women of childbearing potential, pregnant women, breast-feeding women, patients hypersensitive to drug, and patients with active liver disease or conditions that cause unexplained, persistently elevated transaminase levels.

■ Use cautiously in patients who consume large amounts of alcohol or have a history of liver disease.

KEY POINTS

■ Liver function tests should be performed at start of therapy and then periodically. A liver biopsy may be performed if elevated liver enzyme levels persist.

■ Grapefruit juice increases drug levels and may increase the risk of adverse effects, including myopathy and rhabdomyolysis. Warn patient not to take drug with grapefruit juice.

■ Tell patient to stop drug and notify prescriber immediately if she is or could be pregnant or she wishes to breast-feed.

DEEP VEIN THROMBOSIS

An acute condition characterized by inflammation and thrombus formation, deep vein thrombosis (DVT) affects small or large veins, typically in the legs. This disorder commonly progresses to pulmonary embolism, a life-threatening complication.

Usually, a thrombus develops when damage to the epithelial lining of a vein causes platelets to aggregate, fibrin to form, and red blood cells, white blood cells, and additional platelets to become trapped in the fibrin. The enlarging clot may occlude the vessel lumen partially or totally, or it may detach and float in the circulation, only to lodge elsewhere in the systemic circulation. Thrombi form more rapidly in areas of slower blood flow because of the greater contact between platelets and thrombin accumulation.

DVT may be idiopathic, but it usually results from endothelial damage, accelerated blood clotting, and reduced blood flow. Predisposing factors are prolonged bed rest, trauma, surgery, childbirth, and use of hormonal contraceptives such as estrogens.

dalteparin
CONTRAINDICATIONS AND CAUTIONS

■ Contraindicated in patients hypersensitive to drug, heparin, or pork products; patients with active major bleeding; and patients with thrombocytopenia and antiplatelet antibodies in presence of drug.

■ Use with extreme caution in patients with a history of

heparin-induced thrombocytopenia; patients who have had recent brain, spinal, or ocular surgery; and patients at increased risk for hemorrhage, such as those with active ulceration, angiodysplastic gastrointestinal (GI) disease, bacterial endocarditis, congenital or acquired bleeding disorders, hemorrhagic cerebrovascular accident (CVA), or severe uncontrolled hypertension.

■ Use cautiously in patients with bleeding diathesis, hypertensive or diabetic retinopathy, platelet defects, recent GI bleeding, severe hepatic or renal insufficiency, or thrombocytopenia.

KEY POINTS

ALERT Patients receiving low–molecular-weight heparins or heparinoids who have epidural or spinal anesthesia or spinal puncture are at risk for developing epidural or spinal hematoma that can result in long-term paralysis. Risk increases with use of epidural catheters, drugs affecting hemostasis, or traumatic or repeated epidural or spinal punctures. Monitor these patients often for signs of neurologic impairment. Urgent treatment is needed.

■ DVT is a risk factor in patients who are candidates for prophylactic therapy, including those older than age 40, those who are obese, those undergoing surgery under general anesthesia lasting longer than 30 minutes, and those who have additional risk factors (such as malignancy or history of DVT or pulmonary embolism).

■ Drug isn't interchangeable (unit for unit) with unfractionated heparin or other low–molecular-weight heparin.

enoxaparin
CONTRAINDICATIONS AND CAUTIONS

■ Contraindicated in patients hypersensitive to drug, heparin, or pork products; patients with active major bleeding; and patients with thrombocytopenia and antiplatelet antibodies in presence of drug.

■ Use with extreme caution in patients with aneurysm, cerebrovascular hemorrhage, history of heparin-induced thrombocytopenia, spinal or epidural punctures (as with anesthesia), threatened abortion, or uncontrolled hypertension.

■ Use cautiously in elderly patients; patients with regional or lumbar block anesthesia; patients with blood dyscrasias, recent childbirth, pericarditis, pericardial effusion, renal insufficiency, or severe central nervous system trauma; and patients with conditions that place them at increased risk for hemorrhage, such as angiodysplastic GI disease, bacterial endocarditis, congenital or acquired bleeding disorders, hemorrhagic CVA, ulcer disease, or recent spinal, ocular, or brain surgery.

KEY POINTS

■ Patients receiving low–molecular-weight heparins or heparinoids who have epidural or spinal anesthesia or spinal puncture are at risk for epidural or spinal hematoma that can cause long-term paralysis. Risk increases with use of epidural catheters, drugs affecting hemostasis, or traumatic or repeated epidural or spinal punctures. Monitor these patients often for evidence of neurologic impairment. Urgent treatment is needed.

🌀 *ALERT Infants born to women who received enoxaparin during pregnancy may have an increased risk of congenital anomalies, including cerebral and limb anomalies, hypospadias, peripheral vascular malformation, fibrotic dysplasia, and cardiac defect.*

■ Enoxaparin isn't recommended for thromboprophylaxis in patients with prosthetic heart valves because they may be at higher risk for thromboembolism.

fondaparinux
CONTRAINDICATIONS AND CAUTIONS

■ Contraindicated in patients hypersensitive to drug, patients who weigh less than 50 kg (110 lb), patients with a creatinine clearance less than 30 ml/minute, and patients with active major bleeding, bacterial endocarditis, or thrombocytopenia with a positive test result for antiplatelet antibody in the presence of fondaparinux.

■ Use with extreme caution in patients being treated with platelet inhibitors and patients with conditions that increase the risk of bleeding, such as active ulcerative and angiodysplastic GI disease, congenital or acquired bleeding disorders, hemorrhagic CVA, or recent brain, spinal, or ocular surgery.

■ Use cautiously in elderly patients, patients who have had epidural or spinal anesthesia or spinal puncture (because epidural or spinal hematoma could cause paralysis), patients with a creatinine clearance of 30 to 50 ml/minute, patients with a history of heparin-induced thrombocytopenia, and patients with bleeding diathesis, uncontrolled arterial hypertension, or a history of recent GI ulceration, diabetic retinopathy, or hemorrhage.

KEY POINTS

■ Patients who have received epidural or spinal anesthesia are at increased risk for epidural or spinal hematoma, which may cause permanent paralysis. Monitor these patients closely for neurologic impairment.

■ Routinely assess patient for evidence of bleeding, and regularly monitor complete blood count (CBC), platelet count, creatinine level, and stool tests for occult blood. Stop drug if platelet count is less than 100,000/mm^3.

■ Anticoagulant effects may last 2 to 4 days after stopping drug in patients with normal renal function.

heparin
CONTRAINDICATIONS AND CAUTIONS

■ Contraindicated in patients hypersensitive to drug.

■ Conditionally contraindicated in patients with active bleeding, advanced renal disease, ascorbic acid deficiency and other conditions that increase capillary permeability, blood dyscrasia, bleeding tendencies (such as hemophilia, thrombocytopenia, or hepatic disease with hypoprothrombinemia), extensive areas of denuded skin, inaccessible ulcerative lesions (especially of GI tract) and open ulcerative wounds, severe hypertension, shock, subacute bacterial endocarditis, suppurative thrombophlebitis, suspected intracranial hemorrhage, or threatened abortion.

■ Also conditionally contraindicated during spinal tap or spinal anesthesia, during continuous tube drainage of stomach or small intestine, and during or after brain, ocular, or spinal cord surgery.

■ Although heparin use is clearly hazardous in these conditions, its risks and benefits must be evaluated.

■ Use cautiously in patients immediately postpartum, during menses, and in patients with alcoholism, asthma, GI ulcerations, history of allergies, mild hepatic or renal disease, or occupations with a high risk of physical injury.

KEY POINTS

■ Check order and vial carefully; heparin comes in various concentrations. USP units and international units aren't equivalent for heparin.

■ Abrupt withdrawal may cause increased coagulability; warfarin therapy usually overlaps heparin therapy to continue prophylaxis or treatment.

■ Measure partial thromboplastin time (PTT) carefully

and regularly. Anticoagulation is present when PTT values are 1½ to 2 times the control values. Monitor platelet count regularly. When new thrombosis accompanies thrombocytopenia (white clot syndrome), discontinue heparin.

tinzaparin
CONTRAINDICATIONS AND CAUTIONS

■ Contraindicated in patients hypersensitive to tinzaparin sodium or other low–molecular-weight heparins, heparin, sulfites, benzyl alcohol, or pork products. Also contraindicated in patients with active major bleeding and in those with history of heparin-induced thrombocytopenia.

■ Use cautiously in patients with increased risk of hemorrhage, such as those with bacterial endocarditis, and patients with congenital or acquired bleeding disorders (including hepatic failure and amyloidosis), diabetic retinopathy, GI ulceration, hemorrhagic stroke, and uncontrolled hypertension.

■ Use cautiously in breast-feeding patients; patients receiving platelet inhibitors; patients who recently had brain, spinal, or ocular surgery; and patients who may have reduced elimination of the drug, such as

elderly patients and those with renal insufficiency.

KEY POINTS

🌀 *ALERT When neuraxial anesthesia (epidural or spinal anesthesia) or spinal puncture is used, patient is at risk for spinal hematoma, which can cause permanent paralysis. Watch for evidence of neurologic impairment. Consider risks and benefits of neuraxial intervention if patient is receiving low–molecular-weight heparins or heparinoids.*

■ Warn women of possible hazards to fetus. Gasping syndrome may occur in premature infants when large amounts of benzyl alcohol are given.

■ Monitor platelet count during therapy, and stop drug if platelet count falls below 100,000/mm^3. Periodically monitor CBC and stool tests for occult blood during treatment.

warfarin
CONTRAINDICATIONS AND CAUTIONS

■ Contraindicated in pregnant patients, patients hypersensitive to drug, and patients with aneurysm; bleeding from the GI, genitourinary, or respiratory tract; blood dyscrasias; cerebrovascular hemorrhage; hemorrhagic tendencies; recent major regional lumbar block anesthesia, spinal puncture, or invasive diagnostic or therapeutic procedure; recent prostatectomy; recent surgery involving eye, brain, spinal cord, or a large open area; severe or malignant hypertension; severe renal or hepatic disease; subacute bacterial endocarditis, pericarditis, or pericardial effusion; or threatened abortion, eclampsia, or preeclampsia.

■ Avoid using drug in unsupervised patients, patients who live in areas without adequate laboratory facilities for coagulation testing, and patients with alcoholism, psychosis, senility, or a history of warfarin-induced necrosis.

■ Use cautiously in breast-feeding women, patients with drainage tubes in any orifice, patients at increased risk of hemorrhage, patients with regional or lumbar block anesthesia; and patients with colitis, diverticulitis, mild or moderate hypertension, or mild or moderate hepatic or renal disease.

KEY POINTS

■ Withhold drug and call prescriber at once in the event of fever or rash (signs of severe adverse reactions).

■ Prothrombin time and international normalized ratio (INR) determinations are essential for proper control. For chronic atrial fibrillation, INR ranges from 2 to 3.

■ Give warfarin at the same time daily.

ENDOCARDITIS

Endocarditis is a bacterial or fungal infection of the endocardium, heart valves, or a cardiac prosthesis. The infection causes fibrin and platelets to aggregate on the valve tissue and engulf circulating bacteria or fungi, which produces friable verrucous vegetations on the heart valves, the endocardial lining of a heart chamber, or the endothelium of a blood vessel. Vegetations may cover the valve surfaces, causing ulceration and necrosis. They also may extend to the chordae tendineae, leading to rupture and subsequent valvular insufficiency. Or they may embolize to the spleen, kidneys, central nervous system, and lungs.

Endocarditis occurs most often in I.V. drug abusers, patients with prosthetic heart valves, and those with mitral valve prolapse (especially men with a systolic murmur). These conditions have surpassed rheumatic heart disease as the leading risk factor. Other predisposing conditions include coarctation of the aorta, degenerative heart disease (especially calcific aortic stenosis), Marfan syndrome, pulmonary stenosis, subaortic and valvular aortic stenosis, tetralogy of Fallot, ventricular septal defects, and, rarely, syphilitic aortic valve. Some patients with endocarditis have no underlying heart disease.

Infecting organisms differ among patient groups. In patients with native valve endocarditis who aren't I.V. drug abusers, causative organisms usually include, in order of frequency, streptococci (especially *Streptococcus viridans*), staphylococci, and enterococci. Although many other bacteria occasionally cause the disorder, fungal causes are rare in this group. The mitral valve is involved most often, followed by the aortic valve.

In patients who are I.V. drug abusers, *Staphylococcus aureus* is the most common infecting organism. Less often, streptococci, enterococci, gram-negative bacilli, or fungi cause the disorder. Most often the tricuspid valve is involved, followed by the aortic valve and then the mitral valve.

In patients with prosthetic valve endocarditis, "early" cases (those that develop within 60 days of valve insertion) are usually from staphylococcal infection. Gram-negative aerobic organisms, fungi, streptococci, enterococci, or diphtheroids may also cause the disorder. This infection is commonly fulminating and life-threatening. "Late" cases (those that develop after 60 days) are similar to those of native valve endocarditis.

Untreated endocarditis is commonly fatal but, with proper treatment, about 70% of patients recover. The prognosis is worst when endocarditis causes severe valve damage, insufficiency, and heart failure, or when it involves a prosthetic valve.

cefazolin

CONTRAINDICATIONS AND CAUTIONS

■ Contraindicated in patients hypersensitive to drug or other cephalosporins.

■ Use cautiously in patients hypersensitive to penicillin because of possible cross-sensitivity with other beta-lactam antibiotics. Also use cautiously in breast-feeding women and patients with a history of colitis or renal insufficiency.

KEY POINTS

■ Expect to adjust dose and dosing interval if creatinine

clearance falls below 55 ml/
minute.

■ After reconstitution, inject
drug I.M. without further dilution. This drug isn't as painful
as other cephalosporins. Give
injection deep into a large muscle, such as the gluteus maximus
or lateral aspect of the thigh.

■ If large doses are given, therapy is prolonged, or patient is at
high risk, watch for evidence of
superinfection.

cephradine
CONTRAINDICATIONS AND
CAUTIONS

■ Contraindicated in patients
hypersensitive to drug or to
other cephalosporins.

■ Use cautiously in patients
hypersensitive to penicillin
because of possible cross-
sensitivity with other beta-
lactam antibiotics. Also use cautiously in breast-feeding women
and patients with a history of
colitis or renal insufficiency.

KEY POINTS

■ If large doses are given, therapy is prolonged, or patient is at
high risk, watch for evidence of
superinfection.

■ Instruct patient to take all of
the drug as prescribed, even if
he feels better before all of the
drug is gone.

■ Advise patient to take drug
with food or milk to lessen gas-
trointesinal (GI) discomfort. If
patient is taking suspension
form, tell him to shake it well
before measuring the dose.

flucytosine
CONTRAINDICATIONS AND
CAUTIONS

■ Contraindicated in patients
hypersensitive to drug.

■ Use with extreme caution in
patients with impaired hepatic
or renal function or bone marrow suppression.

KEY POINTS

■ Give capsules over 15 minutes to reduce adverse GI reactions.

■ Monitor blood, liver, and renal function studies frequently
during therapy; obtain susceptibility tests weekly to monitor
drug resistance.

■ If possible, assess blood drug
levels regularly to maintain
flucytosine at therapeutic level
of 40 to 60 mcg/ml. Blood levels above 100 mcg/ml may be
toxic.

imipenem and cilastatin
CONTRAINDICATIONS AND
CAUTIONS

■ Contraindicated in patients
hypersensitive to drug, patients
with a history of hypersensitivi-

ty to local anesthetics of the amide type, and patients with severe shock or heart block.

■ Use cautiously in infants younger than age 3 months, patients allergic to penicillins or cephalosporins because drug has similar properties, and patients with a history of seizure disorders, especially if they also have compromised renal function.

KEY POINTS

■ Monitor patient for bacterial or fungal superinfections and resistant infections during and after therapy.

■ Don't give I.M. solution by I.V. route.

■ Urge patient to notify prescriber about loose stools or diarrhea.

streptomycin
CONTRAINDICATIONS AND CAUTIONS

■ Contraindicated in patients hypersensitive to drug or other aminoglycosides.

■ Use cautiously in elderly patients and patients with impaired renal function or neuromuscular disorders.

KEY POINTS

■ Evaluate patient's hearing before therapy and for 6 months afterward. Notify pre-

scriber if patient complains of hearing loss, roaring noises, or fullness in ears.

■ Obtain blood for peak streptomycin level 1 to 2 hours after I.M. injection; for trough levels, draw blood just before next dose. Don't use a heparinized tube because heparin is incompatible with aminoglycosides.

■ Watch for evidence of superinfection, such as continued fever, chills, and increased pulse rate.

HEART FAILURE

A syndrome characterized by myocardial dysfunction, heart failure leads to impaired pump performance (reduced cardiac output) or to frank heart failure and abnormal circulatory congestion. Congestion of systemic venous circulation may result in peripheral edema or hepatomegaly; congestion of pulmonary circulation may cause pulmonary edema, an acute, life-threatening emergency.

Pump failure usually occurs in a damaged left ventricle (left-sided heart failure) but may occur in the right ventricle (right-sided heart failure) either as a primary disorder or secondary to left-sided heart failure. Sometimes left- and right-sided heart failure develop simultaneously.

Heart failure may result from a primary abnormality of the heart muscle (such as infarction) or from coronary artery disease, cardiomyopathy, a condition that reduces ventricular filling during diastole (such as mitral stenosis, constrictive pericarditis, or atrial fibrillation), or a condition that causes volume overloading or increased resistance to ventricular emptying (such as aortic stenosis or systemic hypertension).

Reduced cardiac output triggers three compensatory mechanisms: cardiac dilation, hypertrophy, and increased sympathetic activity. These mechanisms improve cardiac output at the expense of increased ventricular work. Chronic heart failure may worsen as a result of respiratory tract infections, pulmonary embolism, stress, increased sodium or water intake, and failure to comply with the prescribed treatment regimen.

Although heart failure may be acute (as a direct result of myocardial infarction [MI]), it's usually a chronic disorder that includes sodium and water retention by the kidneys. Advances in diagnostic and therapeutic techniques have greatly improved the outlook for patients with heart failure, but the prognosis still depends on the underlying cause and its response to treatment.

digoxin
CONTRAINDICATIONS AND CAUTIONS
■ Contraindicated in patients hypersensitive to drug and in those with digitalis-induced toxicity, ventricular fibrillation, or ventricular tachycardia unless caused by heart failure.

■ Use with extreme caution in elderly patients and those with acute MI, incomplete atrioventricular (AV) block, sinus bradycardia, premature ventricular contractions, chronic constrictive pericarditis, hypertrophic cardiomyopathy, renal insufficiency, severe pulmonary disease, or hypothyroidism.

KEY POINTS
■ Before giving drug, take and document apical pulse for 1 minute. Notify prescriber of significant changes (sudden increase or decrease in pulse rate, pulse deficit, irregular beats and, particularly, regularization of a previously irregular rhythm). If these occur, check blood pressure and obtain a 12-lead electrocardiogram (ECG).

■ Monitor digoxin levels. Therapeutic levels range from 0.8 to 2 nanograms/ml. Obtain blood for digoxin levels at least 6 to 8 hours after the last oral dose, preferably just before the next scheduled dose.

ALERT Excessive slowing of the pulse rate (60 beats/ minute or less) may signal digitalis toxicity. Withhold drug and notify prescriber.

dobutamine

CONTRAINDICATIONS AND CAUTIONS

■ Contraindicated in patients hypersensitive to drug or its components and in those with idiopathic hypertrophic subaortic stenosis.

■ Use cautiously in patients with a history of sulfite sensitivity and patients with a history of hypertension. Drug may cause exaggerated pressor response.

KEY POINTS

■ Before starting therapy with dobutamine, correct hypovolemia with plasma volume expanders.

■ Give a cardiac glycoside before dobutamine. Because drug increases AV node conduction, patients with atrial fibrillation may develop a rapid ventricular rate.

■ Continuously monitor ECG, blood pressure, pulmonary artery wedge pressure, cardiac output, and urine output.

enalaprilat

CONTRAINDICATIONS AND CAUTIONS

■ Contraindicated in patients hypersensitive to drug and in those with a history of angioedema related to previous treatment with an angiotensin-converting enzyme (ACE) inhibitor.

■ Use cautiously in patients with renal impairment, aortic stenosis, or hypertrophic cardiomyopathy.

KEY POINTS

■ Monitor complete blood count (CBC) with differential before and during therapy.

ALERT Instruct patient to report trouble breathing or swelling of the face, eyes, lips, or tongue. Although rare, death may result from a blocked airway.

■ Caution patient that drug may cause light-headedness, especially during the first few days of therapy. Tell him to rise slowly to minimize this effect and to notify prescriber if symptoms develop.

fosinopril
CONTRAINDICATIONS AND CAUTIONS
■ Contraindicated in breast-feeding women and patients hypersensitive to drug or to other ACE inhibitors.
■ Use cautiously in patients with impaired renal or hepatic function.

KEY POINTS
■ Assess renal and hepatic function before and periodically throughout therapy.
■ Instruct patient to contact prescriber about light-headedness or fainting.
■ Tell patient to notify prescriber immediately if she is or may be pregnant. Drug will need to be stopped.

inamrinone
CONTRAINDICATIONS AND CAUTIONS
■ Contraindicated in patients hypersensitive to inamrinone or bisulfites. Drug shouldn't be used during the acute phase of MI or in patients with severe aortic or pulmonic valvular disease in place of surgical correction of the obstruction.
■ Use cautiously in patients with hypertrophic cardiomyopathy.

■ Safety and effectiveness haven't been established in children younger than age 18.

KEY POINTS
■ Inamrinone is prescribed mainly for patients who haven't responded to cardiac glycosides, diuretics, and vasodilators.
■ Monitor platelet count. If it falls below 150,000/mm^3, decrease dosage.
■ Assess patient for hypersensitivity reactions, such as pericarditis, ascites, myositis vasculitis, and pleuritis.

milrinone
CONTRAINDICATIONS AND CAUTIONS
■ Contraindicated in patients hypersensitive to drug. Drug shouldn't be used during the acute phase of MI or in patients with severe aortic or pulmonic valvular disease in place of surgical correction of the obstruction.
■ Use cautiously in patients with atrial flutter or fibrillation because drug slightly shortens AV node conduction time and may increase ventricular response rate. Give a cardiac glycoside, if ordered, before starting milrinone.

KEY POINTS

■ Drug typically is given with digoxin and diuretics.

■ Improved cardiac output may increase urine output. Expect to reduce diuretic dosage as heart failure improves. Potassium loss may predispose patient to digitalis toxicity.

■ Monitor fluid and electrolyte status, blood pressure, heart rate, and renal function during therapy. Excessive decrease in blood pressure requires stopping the infusion or slowing the rate. Correct hypoxemia if it occurs during treatment.

nesiritide

CONTRAINDICATIONS AND CAUTIONS

■ Contraindicated in patients hypersensitive to drug or its components and in patients with cardiogenic shock, systolic blood pressure below 90 mm Hg, low cardiac filling pressures, conditions in which cardiac output depends on venous return, or conditions that make vasodilators inappropriate, such as valvular stenosis, restrictive or obstructive cardiomyopathy, constrictive pericarditis, or pericardial tamponade.

KEY POINTS

■ Drug may cause hypotension. Monitor patient's blood pressure closely, particularly if he also takes an ACE inhibitor.

■ Results of giving this drug for longer than 48 hours are unknown.

■ Urge patient to report symptoms of hypotension, such as dizziness, light-headedness, blurred vision, or sweating.

quinapril

CONTRAINDICATIONS AND CAUTIONS

■ Contraindicated in patients hypersensitive to ACE inhibitors and in those with a history of angioedema related to ACE inhibitor treatment.

■ Use cautiously in patients with impaired renal function.

KEY POINTS

🌀 ALERT *Urge patient to report trouble breathing or swelling of the face, eyes, lips, or tongue. Although rare, death may result from a blocked airway.*

■ Monitor renal and hepatic function, blood pressure, potassium levels, and CBC with differential.

■ Urge patient to notify prescriber if she is or may be pregnant. Drug will need to be stopped.

ramipril
CONTRAINDICATIONS AND CAUTIONS
■ Contraindicated in patients hypersensitive to ACE inhibitors and in those with a history of angioedema related to treatment with an ACE inhibitor.
■ Use cautiously in patients with renal impairment.

KEY POINTS
■ Assess renal function closely during the first few weeks of therapy and regularly thereafter. Patients with severe heart failure whose renal function depends on the renin-angiotensin-aldosterone system may develop acute renal failure during ACE inhibitor therapy. Hypertensive patients with renal artery stenosis also may show signs of worsening renal function during the first few days of therapy.

ALERT Rarely, swelling of the face, throat, and larynx may occur, especially the after first dose. Urge patient to report trouble breathing or swelling of the face, eyes, lips, or tongue.

■ Advise patient to notify prescriber if she is or may be pregnant. Drug will need to be stopped.

HYPERLIPIDEMIA

Hyperlipidemia is an elevation of lipids (fats) in the bloodstream. These lipids include cholesterol, cholesterol esters (compounds), phospholipids, and triglycerides. Increased serum lipid and cholesterol levels are linked to the development of atherosclerotic heart disease, although hyperlipidemia causes no symptoms until the atherosclerotic plaque obstructs blood flow.

Causes of hyperlipidemia may include genetic predisposition, excessive intake of dietary fats and cholesterol, obesity, diabetes mellitus, hypothyroidism, excessive alcohol use, and estrogen therapy. Use of certain drugs may raise serum lipid levels as well.

A diagnosis of hyperlipidemia is made based on a serum lipid profile that includes values for serum low-density lipoprotein cholesterol, high-density lipoprotein cholesterol, total cholesterol, and triglycerides.

Prevention and treatment of hyperlipidemia includes diet modification, a regular exercise regimen, cessation of smoking and excessive alcohol intake, the addition of antioxidants to the diet, and lipid-lowering drugs, if necessary.

atorvastatin
CONTRAINDICATIONS AND CAUTIONS
■ Contraindicated in women of childbearing potential, pregnant women, breast-feeding women, patients hypersensitive to drug, and patients with active liver disease or unexplained persistently elevated transaminase levels.

■ Use cautiously in patients with history of liver disease or heavy alcohol use.

KEY POINTS
■ Start drug therapy only after diet and other nondrug treatments prove ineffective. Patient should follow a standard low-cholesterol diet before and during therapy.

■ Obtain liver function tests and lipid levels before starting treatment, at 6 and 12 weeks after therapy starts, after dosage increases, and periodically during therapy.

■ Tell patient to stop drug and notify prescriber immediately if she is or could be pregnant or she wishes to breast-feed.

cholestyramine
CONTRAINDICATIONS AND CAUTIONS
■ Contraindicated in patients hypersensitive to bile-acid sequestering resins and patients with complete biliary obstruction.

■ Use cautiously in patients predisposed to constipation and patients with conditions aggravated by constipation, such as severe, symptomatic coronary artery disease.

KEY POINTS
■ Assess cholesterol and triglyceride levels regularly during therapy.

■ Monitor the patient's bowel habits. Encourage a diet high in fiber and fluids. If severe constipation occurs, decrease dosage, add a stool softener, or stop drug.

■ Long-term use may lead to deficiencies of vitamins A, D, E, and K, and folic acid.

fenofibrate
CONTRAINDICATIONS AND CAUTIONS
■ Contraindicated in patients hypersensitive to drug and in patients with gallbladder disease, hepatic dysfunction, primary biliary cirrhosis, severe renal dysfunction, or unexplained

persistent liver function abnormalities.

■ Use cautiously in patients with a history of pancreatitis.

KEY POINTS

■ Obtain baseline lipid levels and liver function test results before starting therapy.

■ Monitor liver function periodically throughout therapy. Stop drug if enzyme levels persist above three times the normal limit.

■ Watch for evidence of cholelithiasis, pancreatitis, myositis, rhabdomyolysis, and renal failure. Assess patient for muscle pain, tenderness, or weakness, especially with malaise or fever.

■ If the response is inadequate after 2 months of treatment at the maximum daily dose, therapy must be stopped.

fluvastatin
CONTRAINDICATIONS AND CAUTIONS

■ Contraindicated in women of childbearing potential, pregnant women, breast-feeding women, patients hypersensitive to drug, and patients with active liver disease or unexplained persistently elevated transaminase levels.

■ Use cautiously in patients with severe renal impairment or a history of liver disease or heavy alcohol use.

KEY POINTS

■ Drug should be started only after diet and other nondrug therapies have proven ineffective. Patient should follow a standard low-cholesterol diet during therapy.

■ Liver function tests should be performed at the start of therapy, after 12 weeks of therapy, after dose increases, and periodically during therapy.

■ Advise patient that it may take up to 4 weeks for the drug to be fully effective.

gemfibrozil
CONTRAINDICATIONS AND CAUTIONS

■ Contraindicated in patients hypersensitive to drug and patients with gallbladder disease, hepatic dysfunction (including primary biliary cirrhosis), or severe renal dysfunction.

KEY POINTS

■ Check complete blood count and liver function tests periodically during the first 12 months of therapy.

■ If drug has no beneficial effects after 3 months, expect prescriber to stop it.

■ Teach patient about proper dietary management of cholesterol and triglycerides. As appropriate, recommend weight-control, exercise, and smoking cessation programs.

lovastatin

CONTRAINDICATIONS AND CAUTIONS

■ Contraindicated in women of childbearing potential, pregnant women, breast-feeding women, patients hypersensitive to drug, and patients with active liver disease or unexplained persistently elevated transaminase levels.

■ Use cautiously in patients who consume large amounts of alcohol or have a history of liver disease.

KEY POINTS

■ Obtain liver function tests at the start of therapy, after 6 and 12 weeks, when doses increase, and periodically during therapy.

■ Advise patient to promptly report unexplained muscle pain, tenderness, or weakness, particularly when accompanied by malaise or fever.

■ Tell patient to stop drug and notify prescriber immediately if she is or may be pregnant or she wishes to breast-feed.

niacin

CONTRAINDICATIONS AND CAUTIONS

■ Contraindicated in patients hypersensitive to drug and in those with active peptic ulcers, arterial hemorrhage, hepatic dysfunction, or severe hypotension.

■ Use cautiously in patients with diabetes mellitus, gallbladder disease, or unstable angina and in patients with a history of allergy, gout, liver disease, peptic ulcer, or significant alcohol intake.

KEY POINTS

■ Check hepatic function and glucose level early in therapy.

■ Stress that niacin is a potent drug (not just a vitamin) that may cause serious adverse effects. Explain the importance of adhering to therapy.

■ Tell patient that flushing and warmth may subside with continued use and that alcohol consumption may increase flushing.

pravastatin

CONTRAINDICATIONS AND CAUTIONS

■ Contraindicated in women of childbearing potential, pregnant women, breast-feeding women, patients hypersensitive to drug, and patients with active liver disease or conditions that cause unexplained, persistently elevated transaminase levels.

- Use cautiously in patients who consume large amounts of alcohol or have a history of liver disease.

KEY POINTS

- Liver function tests should be performed at start of therapy and then periodically. A liver biopsy may be done if elevated liver enzyme levels persist.
- Inform patient that it will take up to 4 weeks for the drug to reach full therapeutic effect.
- Tell patient to stop drug and notify prescriber immediately if she is or may be pregnant or she wishes to breast-feed.

simvastatin
CONTRAINDICATIONS AND CAUTIONS

- Contraindicated in women of childbearing potential, pregnant women, breast-feeding women, patients hypersensitive to drug, and patients with active liver disease or conditions that cause unexplained, persistently elevated transaminase levels.
- Use cautiously in patients who consume large amounts of alcohol or have a history of liver disease.

KEY POINTS

- Liver function tests should be performed at start of therapy and then periodically. A liver biopsy may be performed if elevated liver enzyme levels persist.
- Grapefruit juice increases drug levels and may increase the risk of adverse effects, including myopathy and rhabdomyolysis. Warn patient not to take drug with grapefruit juice.
- Tell patient to stop drug and notify prescriber immediately if she is or may be pregnant or she wishes to breast-feed.

HYPERTENSION

An intermittent or a sustained elevation in diastolic or systolic blood pressure, hypertension occurs as two major types: essential (idiopathic) hypertension, the most common, and secondary hypertension, which results from kidney disease or another identifiable cause. Malignant hypertension is a severe, fulminant form of hypertension that may occur with both types.

Hypertension affects 15% to 20% of adults in the United States. If untreated, it carries a high mortality. Before age 55, a larger percentage of men than women have high blood pressure. This changes after age 55. Family history, race (most common in blacks), stress, obesity, a high intake of saturated fats or sodium, use of tobacco, sedentary lifestyle, and aging are risk factors for essential hypertension. Insulin resistance has also been implicated in some patients.

Secondary hypertension may result from renovascular disease; pheochromocytoma; primary hyperaldosteronism; Cushing's syndrome; thyroid, pituitary, or parathyroid dysfunction; coarctation of the aorta; pregnancy; neurologic disorders; and use of hormonal contraceptives or other drugs, such as cocaine, epoetin alfa, and cyclosporine. Stress can also stimulate the sympathetic nervous system to increase cardiac output and peripheral vascular resistance.

CLINICAL TIP *Systolic hypertension poses a risk that's equal to or greater than diastolic elevations. It's commonly seen in elderly people and presents a risk for cerebrovascular accident (CVA) or myocardial infarction.*

Hypertension is a major cause of CVA, heart disease, and renal failure. The prognosis is good if this disorder is detected early and if treatment begins before complications develop.

Severely elevated blood pressure (hypertensive crisis) may be fatal.

atenolol

CONTRAINDICATIONS AND CAUTIONS

■ Contraindicated in patients with sinus bradycardia, greater than first-degree heart block, overt cardiac failure, or cardiogenic shock.

■ Use cautiously in patients at risk for heart failure and in patients with bronchospastic disease, diabetes, hyperthyroidism, and impaired renal or hepatic function.

KEY POINTS

■ Check the patient's apical pulse before giving drug; if slower than 60 beats/minute, withhold drug and call prescriber.

■ Withdraw drug gradually over 2 weeks to avoid serious adverse reactions from abrupt withdrawal.

■ Drug may alter the dosage requirements of antidiabetics in previously stabilized diabetic patients. Monitor blood glucose levels closely.

benazepril

CONTRAINDICATIONS AND CAUTIONS

■ Contraindicated in patients hypersensitive to angiotensin-converting enzyme (ACE) inhibitors.

■ Use cautiously in patients with impaired hepatic or renal function.

KEY POINTS

■ Assess renal and hepatic function before and periodically throughout therapy, and monitor potassium levels.

■ Measure blood pressure when drug levels are at peak (2 to 6 hours after administration) and at trough (just before a dose) to verify adequate blood pressure control.

■ Inform patient that lightheadedness can occur, especially during the first few days of therapy. Advise rising slowly to minimize this effect, and urge patient to report dizziness to the prescriber.

doxazosin

CONTRAINDICATIONS AND CAUTIONS

■ Contraindicated in patients hypersensitive to drug or to quinazoline derivatives (including prazosin and terazosin)

■ Use cautiously in patients with impaired hepatic function.

KEY POINTS

■ Monitor blood pressure closely.

■ If syncope occurs, place patient in a recumbent position and treat supportively. A transient hypotensive response doesn't contraindicate continued therapy.

■ Warn patient about a possible first-dose effect (marked low blood pressure on standing up, with dizziness or fainting) similar to that produced by other alpha blockers. This is most common after the first dose but also can occur when dosage is adjusted or therapy interrupted.

enalaprilat

CONTRAINDICATIONS AND CAUTIONS

■ Contraindicated in patients hypersensitive to drug and patients with a history of angioedema from previous ACE inhibitor treatment.

■ Use cautiously in patients with aortic stenosis, hypertrophic cardiomyopathy, or renal impairment.

KEY POINTS

■ Monitor complete blood count (CBC) with differential before and during therapy.

■ Instruct patient to report trouble breathing or swelling of the face, eyes, lips, or tongue.

Although rare, death may result from a blocked airway.

■ Inform patient that light-headedness can occur, especially during the first few days of therapy. Advise rising slowly to minimize this effect, and urge patient to notify prescriber if symptoms develop.

eplerenone
CONTRAINDICATIONS AND CAUTIONS

■ Contraindicated in patients who have type 2 diabetes and microalbuminuria; patients with a potassium level that's above 5.5 mEq/L, a creatinine level above 2 mg/dl (in men) or 1.8 mg/dl (in women), or creatinine clearance less than 50 ml/minute; and patients taking potassium supplements, potassium-sparing diuretics (amiloride, spironolactone or triamterene), or strong CYP 3A4 inhibitors, such as ketoconazole and itraconazole.

■ Use cautiously in breast-feeding patients and patients with mild or moderate hepatic impairment. Use in pregnant women only if potential benefits justify risks to the fetus.

KEY POINTS

■ Drug reaches full therapeutic effect within 4 weeks.

■ Monitor patient for evidence of hyperkalemia.

■ Drug may be used alone or with other antihypertensives.

fenoldopam
CONTRAINDICATIONS AND CAUTIONS

■ No known contraindications.

■ Use cautiously in pregnant women (and only if clearly needed), breast-feeding women, patients with an acute cerebral infarction or hemorrhage (because drug may cause symptomatic hypotension), and patients with glaucoma or ocular hypertension (because drug can cause dose-dependent increases in intraocular pressure).

KEY POINTS

■ Drug causes dose-related tachycardia that diminishes over time but remains substantial at higher doses.

■ Monitor electrolyte levels, and watch for hypokalemia.

■ Tell patient that drug causes dose-related decreases in blood pressure and increases in heart rate. Advise patient to change positions slowly to avoid dizziness.

fosinopril

CONTRAINDICATIONS AND CAUTIONS

■ Contraindicated in breast-feeding women and patients hypersensitive to drug or other ACE inhibitors.

■ Use cautiously in patients with impaired renal or hepatic function.

KEY POINTS

■ Assess renal and hepatic function before and periodically during therapy.

■ Instruct patient to contact prescriber about light-headedness or fainting.

■ Tell patient to notify prescriber immediately if she is or may be pregnant. Drug will need to be stopped.

labetalol

CONTRAINDICATIONS AND CAUTIONS

■ Contraindicated in patients hypersensitive to drug and in those with bronchial asthma, cardiogenic shock, greater than first-degree heart block, overt cardiac failure, severe bradycardia, and other conditions that may cause severe and prolonged hypotension.

■ Use cautiously in patients with chronic bronchitis, emphysema, heart failure, hepatic fail-

ure, peripheral vascular disease, and pheochromocytoma.

KEY POINTS

■ Advise patient that dizziness is the most troublesome adverse reaction and tends to occur early in treatment, in patients who take diuretics, and in higher doses.

■ Monitor blood pressure frequently. Drug masks common signs and symptoms of shock.

■ Monitor glucose levels in diabetic patients closely because beta blockers may mask certain signs and symptoms of hypoglycemia.

olmesartan

CONTRAINDICATIONS AND CAUTIONS

■ Contraindicated in pregnant women and patients hypersensitive to the drug or its components.

■ Use cautiously in patients who are volume- or sodium-depleted, those whose renal function depends on the renin-angiotensin-aldosterone system (such as patients with severe heart failure), and those with unilateral or bilateral renal-artery stenosis.

KEY POINTS

■ Drug must be stopped immediately if patient becomes

pregnant; because it acts on the renin-angiotensin system, it may cause fetal and neonatal complications and death when given to pregnant women after the first trimester.

■ Symptomatic hypotension may occur in patients who are volume- or sodium-depleted, especially those being treated with high doses of a diuretic. If hypotension occurs, place patient supine and treat supportively. Treatment may continue once blood pressure is stabilized.

■ Monitor patient with heart failure for oliguria, azotemia, and acute renal failure.

quinapril
CONTRAINDICATIONS AND CAUTIONS

■ Contraindicated in patients hypersensitive to ACE inhibitors and in those with a history of angioedema from an ACE inhibitor.

■ Use cautiously in patients with impaired renal function.

KEY POINTS

ALERT *Urge patient to report trouble breathing and swelling of the face, throat, eyes, lips, or tongue. The risk is particularly high after the first dose.*

■ Monitor renal and hepatic function, blood pressure, potassium levels, and CBC with differential.

■ Advise patient to notify prescriber if she is or may be pregnant. Drug will need to be stopped.

MYOCARDIAL INFARCTION

With myocardial infarction (MI), also known as a *heart attack*, reduced blood flow through one of the coronary arteries results in myocardial ischemia and necrosis. Risk factors for MI include advanced age; diabetes mellitus; drug use, especially cocaine; elevated levels of serum triglycerides, total cholesterol, and low-density lipoproteins; family history; hypertension; obesity or excessive intake of saturated fats, carbohydrates, or salt; sedentary lifestyle; smoking; and stress or a "type A" personality (aggressive, ambitious, competitive, addicted to work, chronically impatient).

Men and postmenopausal women are more at risk for MI than premenopausal women, although it's becoming more common among younger women, especially those who smoke and take a hormonal contraceptive.

The site of an infarction depends on the vessels involved. Occlusion of the circumflex branch of the left coronary artery causes a lateral wall infarction; occlusion of the anterior descending branch of the left coronary artery, an anterior wall infarction. True posterior or inferior wall infarctions usually result from occlusion of the right coronary artery or one of its branches. Right ventricular infarctions can also result from right coronary artery occlusion, can accompany inferior infarctions, and may cause right-sided heart failure. With a transmural MI, tissue damage extends through all myocardial layers; with a subendocardial MI, damage is only in the innermost and possibly the middle layers.

Mortality is high when treatment is delayed; almost half of all sudden deaths from MI occur before hospitalization, within 1 hour of symptom onset. The prognosis improves if vigorous treatment begins immediately.

alteplase

CONTRAINDICATIONS AND CAUTIONS

■ Contraindicated in patients with a history of cerebrovascular accident (CVA) or intraspinal or intracranial trauma or surgery within 2 months and in patients with active internal bleeding, aneurysm, arteriovenous malformation, bleeding diathesis, intracranial neoplasm, intracranial hemorrhage (current or previous), seizure at onset of CVA when used for acute ischemic CVA, severe uncontrolled hypertension, or suspicion of subarachnoid hemorrhage.

■ Use cautiously in pregnant patients, patients within 10 days after giving birth, patients age 75 and older, patients receiving anticoagulants, patients scheduled for major surgery within 10 days (when bleeding is difficult to control because of its location), and patients having an organ biopsy.

■ Also use cautiously in patients with acute pericarditis or subacute bacterial endocarditis; cerebrovascular disease; diabetic hemorrhagic retinopathy; diastolic pressure of 110 mm Hg or higher; gastrointestinal (GI) or genitourinary (GU) bleeding; hemostatic defects caused by hepatic or renal impairment; mitral stenosis, atrial fibrillation, or other conditions that may lead to left-heart thrombus; septic thrombophlebitis; systolic pressure of 180 mm Hg or higher; or trauma (including cardiopulmonary resuscitation).

KEY POINTS

■ Have antiarrhythmics readily available, and carefully monitor patient's electrocardiogram (ECG). Coronary thrombolysis is linked with arrhythmias caused by reperfusion of ischemic myocardium. Such arrhythmias don't differ from those commonly linked with MI.

■ Avoid invasive procedures during thrombolytic therapy. Closely monitor patient for signs of internal bleeding, and frequently check all puncture sites. Bleeding is the most common adverse effect and may occur internally and at external puncture sites.

■ If uncontrollable bleeding occurs, stop infusion (and heparin) and notify prescriber.

aspirin

CONTRAINDICATIONS AND CAUTIONS

■ Contraindicated in patients hypersensitive to drug, patients with sensitivity reactions to nonsteroidal anti-inflammatory drugs, patients with G6PD deficiency, and patients with bleeding disorders, such as hemophilia, von Willebrand's disease, or telangiectasia.

■ Use cautiously in patients with GI lesions, hypoprothrombinemia, impaired renal func-

tion, thrombocytopenia, thrombotic thrombocytopenic purpura, severe hepatic impairment, or vitamin K deficiency.

KEY POINTS

■ During prolonged therapy, assess hematocrit, hemoglobin, prothrombin time (PT), international normalized ratio (INR), and renal function periodically.

■ Aspirin irreversibly inhibits platelet aggregation. It should be stopped 5 to 7 days before elective surgery to allow time for production and release of new platelets.

■ Advise patient to take drug with food, milk, antacid, or large glass of water to reduce adverse GI reactions.

dalteparin

CONTRAINDICATIONS AND CAUTIONS

■ Contraindicated in patients hypersensitive to drug, heparin, or pork products; patients with active major bleeding; and patients with thrombocytopenia and antiplatelet antibodies in presence of drug.

■ Use with extreme caution in patients with history of heparin-induced thrombocytopenia; patients at increased risk for hemorrhage, such as those with severe uncontrolled hypertension, bacterial endocarditis, congenital or acquired bleeding disorders, active ulceration, angiodysplastic GI disease, or hemorrhagic CVA; and patients who have had brain, spinal, or ocular surgery. Monitor vital signs.

■ Use cautiously in patients with bleeding diathesis, hypertensive or diabetic retinopathy, platelet defects, recent GI bleeding, severe hepatic or renal insufficiency, or thrombocytopenia.

KEY POINTS

■ Patients receiving low–molecular-weight heparins or heparinoids who have epidural or spinal anesthesia or spinal puncture risk epidural or spinal hematoma and long-term paralysis. The risk increases with use of epidural catheters, drugs affecting hemostasis, or traumatic or repeated epidural or spinal punctures. Monitor patient often for neurologic impairment. Urgent treatment is needed.

■ Monitor patient closely for thrombocytopenia.

■ For non–Q-wave MI, give with aspirin unless contraindicated.

heparin

CONTRAINDICATIONS AND CAUTIONS

■ Contraindicated in patients hypersensitive to drug.

■ Conditionally contraindicated in patients who have had brain, ocular, or spinal cord surgery and patients with active bleeding, blood dyscrasia, or bleeding tendencies, such as hemophilia, thrombocytopenia, or hepatic disease with hypoprothrombinemia; suspected intracranial hemorrhage; suppurative thrombophlebitis; inaccessible ulcerative lesions (especially of the GI tract) and open ulcerative wounds; extensive denuded skin; or ascorbic acid deficiency and other conditions that increase capillary permeability.

■ Also conditionally contraindicated during spinal tap or spinal anesthesia; during continuous tube drainage of stomach or small intestine; and in subacute bacterial endocarditis, shock, advanced renal disease, threatened abortion, or severe hypertension.

■ Although heparin use is clearly hazardous in these conditions, its risks and benefits must be evaluated.

■ Use cautiously in patients who are menstruating or just gave birth and in patients with alcoholism, mild hepatic or renal disease, occupations with a high risk of physical injury, or a history of allergies, asthma, or GI ulcerations.

KEY POINTS

■ Check order and vial carefully; heparin comes in various concentrations. USP units and international units aren't equivalent.

■ Abrupt withdrawal may cause increased coagulability; warfarin therapy usually overlaps heparin therapy for continued prophylaxis or treatment.

■ Measure partial thromboplastin time (PTT) carefully and regularly. Anticoagulation is present when PTT values are 1½ to 2 times the control values. Monitor platelet count regularly. When new thrombosis accompanies thrombocytopenia (white clot syndrome), discontinue heparin.

metoprolol

CONTRAINDICATIONS AND CAUTIONS

■ Contraindicated in patients hypersensitive to drug or other beta blockers and patients with cardiogenic shock, greater than first-degree heart block, overt cardiac failure, or sinus bradycardia.

■ Use cautiously in patients with diabetes, heart failure, or respiratory or hepatic disease.

KEY POINTS

ALERT *Always check patient's apical pulse rate before giving drug. If it's slower than 60 beats/minute, withhold drug and call prescriber immediately.*

■ When therapy is stopped, reduce dose gradually over 1 to 2 weeks.

■ Drug may alter dosage requirements of antidiabetic drugs in previously stabilized diabetic patients. Monitor blood glucose levels closely.

reteplase

CONTRAINDICATIONS AND CAUTIONS

■ Contraindicated in patients with active internal bleeding, aneurysm, arteriovenous malformation, bleeding diathesis, history of CVA, intracranial neoplasm, recent intracranial or intraspinal surgery or trauma, or severe uncontrolled hypertension.

■ Use cautiously in breast-feeding women; patients age 75 and older; patients with previous puncture of noncompressible vessels; patients with recent (within 10 days) major surgery, obstetric delivery, organ biopsy, GI or GU bleeding, or trauma;

patients with cerebrovascular disease, hypertension (systolic pressure 180 mm Hg or higher, diastolic pressure 110 mm Hg or higher), and conditions that may lead to left heart thrombus, including mitral stenosis, acute pericarditis, subacute bacterial endocarditis, and hemostatic defects; and patients with diabetic hemorrhagic retinopathy, septic thrombophlebitis, and other conditions in which bleeding would be difficult to manage.

KEY POINTS

■ Potency is expressed in units specific to reteplase and isn't comparable with other thrombolytic drugs.

■ Monitor ECG carefully during treatment. Coronary thrombolysis may cause arrhythmias linked with reperfusion. Be prepared to treat bradycardia or ventricular irritability.

■ Assess patient closely for bleeding. Avoid I.M. injections, invasive procedures, and nonessential handling of patient. Bleeding is the most common adverse reaction and may occur internally or at external puncture sites. If local measures don't control serious bleeding, stop anticoagulation therapy and notify prescriber. Withhold second bolus of reteplase.

streptokinase
CONTRAINDICATIONS AND CAUTIONS

■ Contraindicated in patients with active internal bleeding, acute or chronic hepatic or renal insufficiency, chronic pulmonary disease with cavitation, diverticulitis, previous severe allergic reaction to streptokinase, recent CVA, recent trauma with possible internal injuries, severe hypertension, subacute bacterial endocarditis or rheumatic valvular disease, ulcerative colitis, ulcerative wounds, visceral or intracranial malignant neoplasms, uncontrolled hypocoagulation, or recent cerebral embolism, thrombosis, or hemorrhage.

■ Also contraindicated within 10 days after intra-arterial diagnostic procedure or any surgery, including liver or kidney biopsy, lumbar puncture, thoracentesis, paracentesis, or extensive or multiple cutdowns.

■ I.M. injections and other invasive procedures are contraindicated during streptokinase therapy.

■ Use cautiously when treating arterial embolism that originates from the left side of the heart because of the danger of cerebral infarction.

KEY POINTS

■ Only prescribers with wide experience in thrombotic disease management should use streptokinase. Drug should be given only where clinical and laboratory monitoring can be performed.

■ Thrombolytic therapy in patients with acute MI may decrease infarct size, improve ventricular function, and decrease the risk of heart failure. For optimal effect, streptokinase must be given within 6 hours after symptoms start.

■ Monitor patient for excessive bleeding every 15 minutes for first hour, every 30 minutes for second through eighth hours, and then every 4 hours. If bleeding is evident, stop therapy and notify prescriber. Pretreatment with heparin or drugs that affect platelets causes a high risk of bleeding but may improve long-term results.

tenecteplase

CONTRAINDICATIONS AND CAUTIONS

■ Contraindicated in patients with an active internal bleed; bleeding diathesis; history of CVA; intracranial or intraspinal surgery or trauma during previous 2 months; intracranial neoplasm, aneurysm, or arteriovenous malformation; or severe uncontrolled hypertension.

■ Use cautiously in pregnant women; patients age 75 and older; patients who have had recent major surgery (such as coronary artery bypass graft), organ biopsy, obstetric delivery, or previous puncture of noncompressible vessels; and patients with acute pericarditis, cerebrovascular disease, diabetic hemorrhagic retinopathy, hemostatic defects, high risk of left ventricular thrombus, hypertension (systolic pressure 180 mm Hg or higher, or diastolic pressure 110 mm Hg or higher), recent GI or GU bleeding, recent trauma, septic thrombophlebitis, severe hepatic dysfunction, or subacute bacterial endocarditis.

KEY POINTS

■ Begin therapy as soon as possible after onset of MI symptoms.

■ Give heparin with tenecteplase but not in the same I.V. line.

■ Assess patient for bleeding. If serious bleeding occurs, stop heparin and antiplatelet drugs immediately.

■ Monitor ECG for reperfusion arrhythmias.

warfarin

CONTRAINDICATIONS AND CAUTIONS

■ Contraindicated in pregnant patients, patients hypersensitive to drug, and patients having major regional lumbar block anesthesia, spinal puncture, or diagnostic or therapeutic invasive procedures.

■ Also contraindicated in patients with aneurysm; bleeding from the GI, GU, or respiratory tract; blood dyscrasias; cerebrovascular hemorrhage; eclampsia or preeclampsia; hemorrhagic tendencies; recent prostatectomy; recent surgery involving the eye, brain, spinal cord, or large open areas; severe or malignant hypertension; severe renal or hepatic disease; subacute bacterial endocarditis, pericarditis, or pericardial effusion; or threatened abortion.

■ Avoid using drug in patients with a history of warfarin-induced necrosis; in unsupervised patients with senility, alcoholism, or psychosis; and in situations in which laboratory facilities are inadequate for coagulation testing.

■ Use cautiously in breast-feeding women and in patients with colitis, diverticulitis, mild or moderate hepatic or renal disease, or mild or moderate hypertension; patients with drainage tubes in any orifice; patients with regional or lumbar block anesthesia; and patients with conditions that increase the risk of hemorrhage.

KEY POINTS

■ Draw blood to establish baseline coagulation parameters before therapy. PT and INR determinations are essential for proper control.

■ Give warfarin at the same time daily.

■ Withhold drug and call prescriber at once if fever or rash (signs of severe adverse reactions) develop.

13 / DRUGS FOR ENDOCRINE DISORDERS

ADRENAL HYPOFUNCTION

Adrenal hypofunction may be either primary or secondary. Primary adrenal hypofunction is known as Addison's disease. It originates in the adrenal glands and is characterized by decreased mineralocorticoid, glucocorticoid, and androgen secretion. Addison's disease occurs when more than 90% of both adrenal glands is destroyed. This destruction usually results from an autoimmune process in which circulating antibodies react against the adrenal tissue. Other causes include tuberculosis, bilateral adrenalectomy, hemorrhage into the adrenal gland, neoplasms, and infections (histoplasmosis, cytomegalovirus). Rarely, a family history of autoimmune disease predisposes the patient to Addison's disease and other endocrinopathies. Addison's disease is relatively uncommon, although it can occur at any age and in either sex.

🍀 *CLINICAL TIP Suspect adrenal insufficiency in patients who have acquired immunodeficiency syndrome. Although symptoms may not be present, testing commonly reveals abnormal results.*

Secondary adrenal hypofunction results from impaired secretion of corticotropin by the pituitary gland and is characterized by glucocorticoid deficiency. Aldosterone secretion commonly is unaffected. The usual causes of secondary adrenal hypofunction include the abrupt halt of long-term steroid therapy, hypopituitarism, or the removal of a corticotropin-secreting tumor.

With early diagnosis and adequate replacement therapy, the prognosis for adrenal hypofunction is good. However, adrenal (addisonian) crisis is a medical emergency that requires immediate, vigorous treatment. This critical deficiency of mineralocorticoids and glucocorticoids usually follows acute stress, sepsis, trauma, surgery, or removal of steroid therapy in patients with chronic adrenal insufficiency. Adrenal crisis exhausts the body's stores of glucocorticoids in a person with adrenal hypofunction.

cortisone

CONTRAINDICATIONS AND CAUTIONS

■ Contraindicated in patients hypersensitive to drug or its ingredients, those with systemic fungal infections, and those receiving immunosuppressive doses with live-virus vaccines.

■ Use with extreme caution if patient had a recent myocardial infarction (MI).

■ Use cautiously in breastfeeding patients and patients with active hepatitis, cirrhosis, diabetes mellitus, diverticulitis, emotional instability, gastrointestinal (GI) ulcer, heart failure, hypertension, hypothyroidism, myasthenia gravis, nonspecific ulcerative colitis, ocular herpes simplex, osteoporosis, psychotic tendencies, recent intestinal anastomoses, renal disease, seizures, thromboembolic disorders, or tuberculosis.

KEY POINTS

■ Monitor patient for cushingoid effects, including moon face, buffalo hump, central obesity, thinning hair, hypertension, and infection.

■ Warn patient not to stop drug abruptly or without prescriber's consent.

■ Assess glucose levels. A patient with diabetes may need an adjustment in insulin dosage.

■ Watch for fluid and electrolyte imbalances. Patient may need a low-sodium diet and potassium supplements.

dexamethasone

CONTRAINDICATIONS AND CAUTIONS

■ Contraindicated in patients hypersensitive to drug or its ingredients, those with systemic fungal infections, and those receiving immunosuppressive doses with live-virus vaccines.

■ Use with extreme caution if patient had a recent MI.

■ Use cautiously in breastfeeding patients and patients with active hepatitis, cirrhosis, diabetes mellitus, diverticulitis, emotional instability, GI ulcer, heart failure, hypertension, hypothyroidism, myasthenia gravis, nonspecific ulcerative colitis, ocular herpes simplex, osteoporosis, psychotic tendencies, recent intestinal anastomoses, renal disease, seizures, thromboembolic disorders, or tuberculosis.

■ Because some formulations contain sulfite preservatives, use cautiously in patients sensitive to sulfites.

KEY POINTS

■ Monitor patient for cushingoid effects, including moon face, buffalo hump, central obesity, thinning hair, hypertension, and infection.

■ Warn patient not to stop drug abruptly or without prescriber's consent.

■ Explain the signs and symptoms of early adrenal insufficiency, including fatigue, muscle weakness, joint pain, fever, anorexia, nausea, shortness of breath, dizziness, and fainting.

fludrocortisone
CONTRAINDICATIONS AND CAUTIONS

■ Contraindicated in patients hypersensitive to drug and those with systemic fungal infections.

■ Use cautiously in breastfeeding patients and patients with active hepatitis, active or latent peptic ulcer, cirrhosis, diverticulitis, emotional instability, hypertension, hypothyroidism, myasthenia gravis, nonspecific ulcerative colitis,

ocular herpes simplex, osteoporosis, psychotic tendencies, recent intestinal anastomoses or MI, or renal insufficiency.

KEY POINTS

■ Drug is given with cortisone or hydrocortisone in adrenal insufficiency.

■ Glucose tolerance tests should be performed only if needed because addisonian patients tend to develop severe hypoglycemia within 3 hours after the test.

■ Drug may cause adverse effects similar to those of glucocorticoids.

hydrocortisone
CONTRAINDICATIONS AND CAUTIONS

■ Contraindicated in patients hypersensitive to drug or its ingredients, those with systemic fungal infections, and those receiving immunosuppressive doses with live-virus vaccines. Also contraindicated in premature infants (succinate).

■ Use with extreme caution if patient had a recent MI.

■ Use cautiously in breastfeeding patients and patients with active hepatitis, cirrhosis, diabetes mellitus, diverticulitis, emotional instability, GI ulcer, heart failure, hypertension, hypothyroidism, myasthenia gravis, nonspecific ulcerative colitis, ocular herpes simplex, osteoporosis, psychotic tendencies, recent intestinal anastomoses, renal disease, seizures, thromboembolic disorders, or tuberculosis.

KEY POINTS
■ Monitor patient for cushingoid effects, including moon face, buffalo hump, central obesity, thinning hair, hypertension, and infection.
■ Stress (fever, trauma, surgery, and emotional problems) may increase adrenal insufficiency, and the patient may need an increased dosage.
■ Periodic measurement of growth and development may be needed during high-dose or prolonged therapy in children.

triamcinolone
CONTRAINDICATIONS AND CAUTIONS
■ Contraindicated in patients hypersensitive to drug or its ingredients, those with systemic fungal infections, and those receiving immunosuppressive doses with live-virus vaccines.
■ Use cautiously in breastfeeding patients and patients with active hepatitis, cirrhosis, diabetes mellitus, diverticulitis, emotional instability, GI ulcer, heart failure, hypertension, hy-

pothyroidism, myasthenia gravis, nonspecific ulcerative colitis, ocular herpes simplex, osteoporosis, psychotic tendencies, recent intestinal anastomoses, recent MI, renal disease, seizures, thromboembolic disorders, or tuberculosis.

KEY POINTS
■ Monitor patient for cushingoid effects, including moon face, buffalo hump, central obesity, thinning hair, hypertension, and infection.
■ Check patient's weight, blood pressure, and electrolyte levels.
■ Explain signs and symptoms of early adrenal insufficiency, including fatigue, muscle weakness, joint pain, fever, anorexia, nausea, shortness of breath, dizziness, and fainting.

DIABETES MELLITUS

A chronic disturbance of carbohydrate, protein, and fat metabolism, diabetes mellitus is characterized by insulin resistance or deficiency. It occurs in two forms: type 1, which involves absolute insulin insufficiency, and type 2, which involves insulin resistance with varying degrees of insulin insufficiency. Diabetes mellitus affects nearly

16 million Americans, about one-third of whom are undiagnosed. The disease affects men and women equally and is more common with increasing age.

Type 1 diabetes usually starts before age 30. The patient typically is thin and needs exogenous insulin and diet management to maintain blood glucose levels.

Type 2 diabetes usually occurs in obese adults older than age 40, although it's becoming more common in North American youths. Besides obesity, which fosters insulin resistance, other conditions can raise the risk of type 2 diabetes as well:

■ Physiologic or emotional stress can raise levels of stress hormones, such as cortisol, epinephrine, glucagon, and growth hormone. Blood glucose levels rise as well, which places increased demands on the pancreas.

■ Pregnancy causes weight gain and increases levels of estrogen and placental hormones, which antagonize insulin.

■ Some drugs antagonize the effects of insulin, including thiazide diuretics, adrenal corticosteroids, and hormonal contraceptives.

Type 2 diabetes usually is treated with diet changes, exercise, antidiabetic drugs, and sometimes insulin therapy.

Nearly two-thirds of people with diabetes die of cardiovascular disease. It's also the leading cause of renal failure and new adult blindness. These effects result from the inability of insulin to accomplish its normal functions: transporting glucose into cells for use as energy and storage as glycogen, stimulating protein synthesis, and prompting storage of free fatty acids.

acarbose
CONTRAINDICATIONS AND CAUTIONS

■ Contraindicated in pregnant women, breast-feeding women, patients with a creatinine level above 2 mg/dl, patients hypersensitive to drug, patients with a condition that could deteriorate from increased intestinal gas, and patients with cirrhosis, colon ulceration, diabetic ketoacidosis, disordered digestion or absorption, inflammatory bowel disease, partial intestinal obstruction, predisposition to intestinal obstruction, or renal impairment.

■ Use cautiously in patients receiving a sulfonylurea or insulin. Acarbose may increase the risk of hypoglycemia.

KEY POINTS

■ Insulin therapy may be needed during times of increased stress (as from infection, fever, surgery, or trauma). Monitor patient closely for hyperglycemia.

■ Check patient's 1-hour postprandial glucose level to determine the effectiveness of acarbose and identify an appropriate dose. Report hyperglycemia to prescriber.

■ Assess glycosylated hemoglobin level every 3 months.

■ Assess transaminase level every 3 months during first year of therapy and periodically thereafter if patient receives more than 50 mg t.i.d. Report abnormalities; drug may need adjustment or withdrawal.

■ If patient takes acarbose with a sulfonylurea or insulin, take steps to prevent hypoglycemia. If it occurs, give oral glucose (dextrose) or, if needed, I.V. glucose or glucagons and notify prescriber. Dosage may need adjustment to prevent future episodes of hypoglycemia.

chlorpropamide
CONTRAINDICATIONS AND CAUTIONS

■ Contraindicated in pregnant women, breast-feeding women, patients hypersensitive to drug, and patients with type 2 diabetes complicated by acidosis, diabetic coma, ketosis, major surgery, severe infection, or trauma.

■ Also contraindicated for treating type 1 diabetes or diabetes that can be controlled by diet.

■ Use cautiously in patients allergic to sulfonamides; debilitated, malnourished, or elderly patients; and patients with porphyria or impaired hepatic or renal function.

KEY POINTS

■ Adverse effects of drug, especially hypoglycemia, may be more frequent, prolonged, or severe than with some other sulfonylureas because of this drug's long duration of action. If hypoglycemia occurs, monitor patient closely for 3 to 5 days or more.

■ Urge patient to avoid even small amounts of alcohol to prevent chlorpropamide-alcohol flush, which can cause facial flushing, headache, lightheadedness, and breathlessness.

■ Drug may accumulate if patient has renal insufficiency. Watch for and report evidence of impending renal insufficiency, such as dysuria, anuria, and hematuria.

glimepiride
CONTRAINDICATIONS AND CAUTIONS

■ Contraindicated in pregnant patients, patients hypersensitive to drug, and patients with diabetic ketoacidosis, which should be treated with insulin. Also contraindicated as sole therapy for type 1 diabetes.

■ Don't give to elderly patients.

■ Use cautiously in patients allergic to sulfonamides, debilitated or malnourished patients, and patients with adrenal, pituitary, hepatic, or renal insufficiency; these patients are more susceptible to the hypoglycemic action of glucose-lowering drugs.

KEY POINTS

■ Glimepiride and insulin may be used together in patients who lose glucose control after initially responding to therapy (secondary failure).

■ Check fasting glucose level periodically to determine patient's response to drug. Also assess glycosylated hemoglobin level, usually every 3 to 6 months, to determine long-term glycemic control.

■ Oral hypoglycemics may increase the risk of death from cardiovascular events compared with diet alone or with diet and insulin therapy.

glipizide
CONTRAINDICATIONS AND CAUTIONS

■ Contraindicated in pregnant women, breast-feeding women, patients hypersensitive to drug, and patients with diabetic ketoacidosis with or without coma. Also contraindicated as sole therapy in type 1 diabetes.

■ Use cautiously in patients with renal or hepatic disease; debilitated, malnourished, or elderly patients; and patients allergic to sulfonamides.

KEY POINTS

■ Some patients may attain effective control on a once-daily regimen; others respond better to divided doses.

■ Glipizide is a second-generation sulfonylurea and seems to cause fewer adverse effects than such first-generation drugs as chlorpropamide.

■ During periods of increased stress, patient may need insulin therapy and more frequent assessment for hyperglycemia.

glyburide
CONTRAINDICATIONS AND CAUTIONS

■ Contraindicated in pregnant women, breast-feeding women,

patients hypersensitive to drug, and patients with diabetic ketoacidosis with or without coma. Also contraindicated as sole therapy for type 1 diabetes.

■ Use cautiously in patients with hepatic or renal impairment; debilitated, malnourished, or elderly patients; and patients allergic to sulfonamides.

KEY POINTS

■ Drug is a second-generation sulfonylurea and seems to cause fewer adverse effects than such first-generation drugs as chlorpropamide.

■ During periods of increased stress, patient may need insulin therapy and more frequent assessment for hyperglycemia.

■ Instruct patient to report hypoglycemia to prescriber immediately; it may be severe or even fatal in patients taking as little as 2.5 to 5 mg glyburide daily.

insulin
CONTRAINDICATIONS AND CAUTIONS

■ Contraindicated in patients hypersensitive to any component of the preparation and in patients with hypoglycemia.

KEY POINTS

■ Dosage is always expressed in USP units. Remember to use only syringes calibrated for the particular form of insulin given, either U-100 or U-500.

■ Show patient and caregivers how to measure and give insulin. Stress the importance of measuring accurately, especially with concentrated regular insulin. If needed, suggest a magnifying sleeve, dose magnifier, or other aid to help improve accuracy.

■ Teach patient that glucose levels and urine ketone tests provide essential dosage guides. Explain the importance of knowing peak insulin times and detecting high and low glucose levels, and warn that hypoglycemia and may cause brain damage if prolonged.

metformin
CONTRAINDICATIONS AND CAUTIONS

■ Contraindicated in patients hypersensitive to drug; patients with renal disease, hepatic disease, or metabolic acidosis; patients with heart failure that needs drug therapy; patients having X-rays that involve iodinated contrast materials; and patients with an increased risk of renal dysfunction, cardiovascular collapse, myocardial infarction, hypoxia, and septicemia.

■ Use cautiously with elderly, debilitated, or malnourished patients and patients with adrenal or pituitary insufficiency because of the increased risk of hypoglycemia.

KEY POINTS

■ Before therapy starts and at least annually thereafter, assess patient's renal function. If it's impaired, expect prescriber to switch to a different antidiabetic, especially if patient is elderly.

■ If patient hasn't responded after 4 weeks of therapy at maximum dosage, prescriber may add an oral sulfonylurea while keeping metformin at maximum dosage. If patient still doesn't respond after several months of therapy with both drugs at maximum dosage, prescriber may discontinue both and start insulin therapy.

■ During periods of increased stress, patient may need insulin therapy and more frequent assessment for hyperglycemia.

pioglitazone
CONTRAINDICATIONS AND CAUTIONS

■ Contraindicated in patients hypersensitive to drug or its components, patients with diabetic ketoacidosis, patients who developed jaundice while taking troglitazone (now discontin-

ued), and patients with type 1 diabetes, active liver disease, an alanine transaminase (ALT) level more than 2½ times the upper limit of normal, or New York Heart Association (NYHA) Class III or IV heart failure.

■ Use cautiously in patients with edema or heart failure.

KEY POINTS

■ Measure liver enzyme levels when therapy starts, every 2 months for the first year, and periodically thereafter.

■ Obtain liver function tests if patient develops evidence of liver dysfunction, such as nausea, vomiting, abdominal pain, fatigue, anorexia, or dark urine.

■ Expect to discontinue drug if patient develops jaundice or if ALT levels are more than 3 times above normal.

ALERT Pioglitazone hydrochloride alone or with insulin can cause fluid retention that may trigger or worsen heart failure. Watch for evidence of heart failure, and stop the drug if the patient's cardiac status declines. This drug isn't recommended for patients with NYHA Class III or IV heart failure.

■ Hemoglobin level and hematocrit may decrease, especially in the first 4 to 12 weeks of therapy.

repaglinide

CONTRAINDICATIONS AND CAUTIONS

■ Contraindicated in patients hypersensitive to drug or its components and in those with type 1 diabetes or diabetic ketoacidosis.

■ Use cautiously in elderly, debilitated, or malnourished patients; patients with hepatic insufficiency (in whom reduced metabolism could cause hypoglycemia and increased repaglinide levels); and patients with adrenal or pituitary insufficiency (who have an increased risk of hypoglycemia from glucose-lowering drugs).

KEY POINTS

■ Metformin may be added if repaglinide alone is inadequate.

■ Oral antidiabetics, including repaglinide, may increase the risk of death from cardiovascular events over diet alone or diet plus insulin.

■ During periods of increased stress, patient may need insulin therapy and more frequent assessment for hyperglycemia.

rosiglitazone

CONTRAINDICATIONS AND CAUTIONS

■ Contraindicated in patients hypersensitive to drug or its components, patients who developed jaundice while taking troglitazone (now discontinued), and patients with active liver disease, an ALT level more than 2½ times the upper limit of normal, type 1 diabetes, or diabetic ketoacidosis. Also contraindicated in those with New York Heart Association Class III or IV heart failure unless expected benefits outweigh risks.

■ Rosiglitazone-metformin therapy is contraindicated in patients with renal impairment because metformin is contraindicated in these patients.

■ Use cautiously in patients with edema or heart failure.

KEY POINTS

■ Check liver enzyme levels before therapy starts, and don't give drug if liver enzyme levels are increased.

■ Check liver enzyme levels every 2 months for 12 months and periodically thereafter. If the ALT level rises during treatment, increase the frequency of blood testing. Drug should be discontinued if levels reach 3 times the upper limit of normal and remain elevated, or if jaundice develops.

ALERT *Rosiglitazone given alone or with insulin can cause fluid retention that may trigger or worsen heart failure. Watch for evidence of heart failure, and stop drug if patient's cardiac status declines. This drug isn't recommended for patients with NYHA Class III or IV heart failure.*

■ Hemoglobin level, hematocrit, and free fatty acid level may decrease during therapy, usually in the first 4 to 8 weeks. Total cholesterol, low-density lipoprotein, and high-density lipoprotein levels may increase.

14 / DRUGS FOR GASTROINTESTINAL DISORDERS

CHRONIC CONSTIPATION

Also known as *lazy colon, colonic stasis, colonic inertia,* and *atonic constipation,* chronic constipation may lead to fecal impaction if left untreated. Chronic constipation is common in elderly and disabled people because of their inactivity and can be relieved with diet changes and exercise. Untreated, it can result in hemorrhoids, fissures, and megacolon.

Chronic constipation usually results from some deficiency in the three elements needed for normal bowel activity: dietary bulk, fluid intake, and exercise. Other possible causes can include habitual disregard of the impulse to defecate, emotional conflicts, overuse of laxatives, or prolonged dependence on enemas, which dull rectal sensitivity to the presence of stool. Anal fissures can cause chronic constipation as well.

CLINICAL TIP *Certain drugs (such as tranquilizers, anticholinergics, opioids, and antacids) can cause chronic constipation, and patients with certain disorders (such as Parkinson's disease, multiple sclerosis, hypothyroidism, scleroderma, and lupus erythematosus) are more prone to develop it.*

bisacodyl
CONTRAINDICATIONS AND CAUTIONS
■ Contraindicated in patients hypersensitive to drug or its components and in those with gastroenteritis, intestinal obstruction, rectal bleeding, or evidence of appendicitis or acute surgical abdomen, such as abdominal pain, nausea, and vomiting.

KEY POINTS
■ Give suppository at times that don't interfere with scheduled activities or sleep. Soft, formed stools are usually produced 15 to 60 minutes after insertion.

■ Insert suppository as high as possible into the rectum, and try to position suppository against the rectal wall. Avoid embedding it in feces because doing so may delay onset of action.

■ Determine whether patient has adequate fluid intake, exercise, and diet.

calcium polycarbophil
CONTRAINDICATIONS AND CAUTIONS
■ Contraindicated in patients who have trouble swallowing or evidence of gastrointestinal (GI) obstruction.

KEY POINTS
■ Rectal bleeding or failure to respond to therapy may indicate need for surgery.

■ Full benefit of drug may take 1 to 3 days.

■ Determine whether patient has adequate fluid intake, exercise, and diet.

glycerin
CONTRAINDICATIONS AND CAUTIONS
■ Contraindicated in patients hypersensitive to drug and in those with abdominal pain, vomiting, or other evidence of intestinal obstruction, appendicitis, fecal impaction, or acute surgical abdomen.

KEY POINTS
■ Drug is used mainly to reestablish proper toilet habits in laxative-dependent patients.

■ Tell patient that drug must be retained for at least 15 minutes and that it usually acts within 1 hour. Entire suppository need not melt to be effective.

■ Warn patient about adverse GI reactions.

lactulose
CONTRAINDICATIONS AND CAUTIONS
■ Contraindicated in patients on a low-galactose diet.

■ Use cautiously in patients with diabetes mellitus.

KEY POINTS
■ Show patient how to mix and use the drug at home, if needed.

■ Review adverse reactions, and tell patient to notify prescriber if they become bothersome or if diarrhea develops.

■ Caution patient not to take other laxatives during lactulose therapy.

psyllium
CONTRAINDICATIONS AND CAUTIONS
■ Contraindicated in patients hypersensitive to drug and in those with intestinal obstruction, intestinal ulceration, dis-

abling adhesions, difficulty swallowing, or evidence of appendicitis, such as abdominal pain, nausea, or vomiting.

KEY POINTS

■ Mix with at least 8 ounces (240 ml) of cold, pleasant-tasting liquid—such as orange juice—to mask grittiness, and stir only a few seconds. Have patient drink mixture immediately so it doesn't congeal. Follow with another glass of liquid.

■ Determine whether patient has adequate fluid intake, exercise, and diet.

■ Drug isn't absorbed systemically and is nontoxic. It's especially useful in debilitated patients and those with postpartum constipation, irritable bowel syndrome, or diverticular disease. It's also used to treat chronic laxative abuse and, with other laxatives, to empty the colon before barium enema examinations.

CROHN'S DISEASE

Crohn's disease is an inflammation of the gastrointestinal tract characterized by flare-ups and remissions. It can affect any portion of the tract from the mouth to the anus. About half the time, it involves the colon and small intestine. About one-third of cases involve the terminal ileum, and 10% to 20% of cases involve only the colon.

As the disease progresses, lacteal blockage in the intestinal wall leads to edema, inflammation, ulcers, strictures, fistulas, and abscesses. The lesions create a characteristic cobblestone appearance. Absorption is impaired and small bowel obstruction may result. Eventually, deep ulcers and fissures may extend through all layers of the intestinal wall and may involve regional lymph nodes and the mesentery.

Crohn's disease is most common in adults ages 20 to 40. It's two to three times more common in people of Jewish ancestry and least common in blacks. Although the exact cause of Crohn's disease is unknown, possible causes include allergies and other immune disorders, and infection. However, no infecting organism has been isolated.

budesonide
CONTRAINDICATIONS AND CAUTIONS

■ Contraindicated in patients hypersensitive to budesonide.

■ Use cautiously in patients with cataracts, diabetes mellitus, glaucoma, hypertension, osteoporosis, peptic ulcer disease, or tuberculosis; those with a family history of diabetes or glaucoma; and those with any other condition in which glucocorticosteroids may have unwanted effects.

■ Because glucocorticoids appear in breast milk, the decision to breast-feed should be based on the mother's relative need for the drug.

KEY POINTS

■ During periods of increased stress, as during surgery, the patient may need systemic glucocorticoid therapy in addition to budesonide.

■ Watch carefully for evidence of corticosteroid withdrawal if patient is switching from systemic glucocorticoid therapy to budesonide. Stay alert for the effects of immunosuppression, especially in patients who haven't had such diseases as chickenpox or measles; these can be fatal in patients who are immunosuppressed or receiving glucocorticoids.

■ When used long-term, budesonide may cause hypercorticism and adrenal suppression.

infliximab

CONTRAINDICATIONS AND CAUTIONS

■ Contraindicated in patients with heart failure and those who are hypersensitive to the drug, its components, or murine proteins.

■ Use cautiously in elderly patients and those with active infection or a history of chronic or recurrent infection. If the patient has lived in a region where histoplasmosis is endemic, carefully consider the risks and benefits of infliximab before starting therapy.

KEY POINTS

ALERT Watch for infusion-related reactions (fever, chills, pruritus, urticaria, dyspnea, hypotension, hypertension, chest pain) during and for 2 hours after administration. If a reaction occurs, stop drug, notify prescriber, and be prepared to give acetaminophen, antihistamines, corticosteroids, and epinephrine.

■ Patients with chronic Crohn's disease and long-term exposure to immunosuppressants have an increased risk of developing lymphoma and infection.

■ Infliximab may affect immune responses, and the patient may develop autoimmune antibodies and lupus-like syndrome;

notify prescriber if this happens. Symptoms resolve when drug is stopped.

sulfasalazine

CONTRAINDICATIONS AND CAUTIONS

■ Contraindicated in patients hypersensitive to drug or its metabolites; those with porphyria, intestinal obstruction, or urinary obstruction; and children younger than age 2.

■ Use cautiously and in reduced amounts in patients with impaired hepatic or renal function, severe allergy, bronchial asthma, or G6PD deficiency.

KEY POINTS

■ Warn patient to avoid ultraviolet light.

■ Advise patient that drug may turn skin and urine orange-yellow and may turn contact lenses yellow. Instruct patient to notify prescriber immediately if this happens.

GASTROESOPHAGEAL REFLUX

The backflow or reflux of gastric and duodenal contents through the lower esophageal sphincter and into the esophagus is called gastroesophageal reflux. If this event becomes chronic, the disorder is known as gastroesophageal reflux disease, commonly known as GERD. Reflux occurs when the lower esophageal sphincter doesn't close tightly enough or when pressure in the stomach forces the sphincter open. Some of the causes of gastroesophageal reflux include the following:

■ delayed gastric emptying from partial gastric outlet obstruction or gastroparesis

■ abnormal esophageal clearance, in which acid isn't properly cleared and neutralized by esophageal peristalsis and salivary bicarbonates

■ pyloric surgery that allows reflux of bile or pancreatic juice

■ use of a nasogastric tube for more than 5 days

■ use of any substance that lowers pressure in the lower esophageal sphincter, such as certain foods, alcohol, cigarettes, anticholinergic drugs (such as atropine, belladonna, and propantheline), and certain other drugs (such as morphine, diazepam, and meperidine)

■ hiatal hernia, especially in children

■ any condition or body position that increases intraabdominal pressure.

Although reflux may cause no or only subtle symptoms, especially at first, it irritates the esophagus and may lead to reflux esophagitis (inflammation of the esophageal mucosa). The length of time the refluxed material stays in contact with the esophagus, as well as its potency, affects the amount of esophageal damage done. The prognosis varies with the underlying cause.

CLINICAL TIP Gastroesophageal reflux may cause unusual symptoms, such as a chronic cough, sore throat, asthma, laryngitis, and atypical chest pain.

cimetidine

CONTRAINDICATIONS AND CAUTIONS

■ Contraindicated in patients hypersensitive to drug.

■ Use cautiously in elderly or debilitated patients because they may be more susceptible to cimetidine-induced confusion.

KEY POINTS

■ Identify tablet strength when obtaining a drug history.

■ Assess patient for abdominal pain. Note blood in emesis, stool, or gastric aspirate.

■ Urge patient to avoid cigarette smoking because it may increase gastric acid secretion and worsen reflux.

esomeprazole

CONTRAINDICATIONS AND CAUTIONS

■ Contraindicated in patients hypersensitive to drug, its components, or omeprazole.

■ Use cautiously in pregnant women, breast-feeding women, and patients with hepatic insufficiency.

KEY POINTS

■ Give drug at least 1 hour before meals. If patient has trouble swallowing the capsule, empty its contents and mix with 1 tablespoon of applesauce. Have patient swallow the applesauce without chewing the enteric-coated pellets.

■ Watch patient for rash or other evidence of hypersensitivity. Monitor gastrointestinal (GI) symptoms for improvement or worsening. And assess liver function test results, especially if patient has hepatic disease.

■ Long-term therapy with omeprazole (of which esomeprazole is the s-isomer) may cause atrophic gastritis.

famotidine

CONTRAINDICATIONS AND CAUTIONS

■ Contraindicated in patients hypersensitive to drug.

KEY POINTS

■ Assess patient for abdominal pain. Note blood in emesis, stool, or gastric aspirate.

■ Advise patient to report abdominal pain or blood in stools or vomit.

■ Urge patient to avoid cigarette smoking because it may increase gastric acid secretion and worsen reflux.

lansoprazole

CONTRAINDICATIONS AND CAUTIONS

■ Contraindicated in patients hypersensitive to drug.

KEY POINTS

■ A symptomatic response to lansoprazole therapy doesn't preclude the presence of gastric cancer.

■ For best effect, instruct patient to take drug no more than 30 minutes before eating.

■ Caution patient not to crush or chew any form of lansoprazole.

metoclopramide

CONTRAINDICATIONS AND CAUTIONS

■ Contraindicated in patients hypersensitive to drug, patients for whom stimulation of GI motility might be dangerous (such as those with hemorrhage, obstruction, or perforation),

and patients with pheochromocytoma or seizure disorders.

■ Use cautiously in patients with a history of depression, Parkinson's disease, or hypertension.

KEY POINTS

■ Tell patient to avoid activities that require alertness for 2 hours after doses.

■ Urge patient to report persistent or serious adverse reactions promptly.

■ Tell patient to avoid alcohol consumption during therapy.

omeprazole

CONTRAINDICATIONS AND CAUTIONS

■ Contraindicated in patients hypersensitive to drug or its components.

KEY POINTS

■ Tell patient to swallow tablets or capsules whole and not to open, crush, or chew them.

■ Instruct patient to take drug 30 minutes before meals.

■ Caution patient to avoid hazardous activities if he gets dizzy.

pantoprazole

CONTRAINDICATIONS AND CAUTIONS

■ Contraindicated in patients hypersensitive to drug or its components.

KEY POINTS

■ Drug can be given without regard to meals.

■ A symptomatic response to pantoprazole doesn't preclude the presence of gastric cancer.

■ Instruct patient to take the drug exactly as prescribed and at about the same time every day.

rabeprazole

CONTRAINDICATIONS AND CAUTIONS

■ Contraindicated in patients hypersensitive to drug, to other benzimidazoles (lansoprazole, omeprazole), or to their components.

■ Use cautiously in patients with severe hepatic impairment.

KEY POINTS

■ Consider additional courses of therapy if duodenal ulcer or GERD isn't healed after the first course.

■ A symptomatic response to rabeprazole doesn't preclude the presence of gastric cancer.

■ Instruct patient that delayed-release tablets should be swallowed whole and not crushed, chewed, or split.

ranitidine

CONTRAINDICATIONS AND CAUTIONS

■ Contraindicated in patients hypersensitive to drug and those with acute porphyria.

■ Use cautiously in patients with hepatic dysfunction.

■ Adjust dosage in patients with impaired renal function.

KEY POINTS

■ Assess patient for abdominal pain. Note the presence of blood in emesis, stool, or gastric aspirate.

■ Urge patient to avoid cigarette smoking because it may increase gastric acid secretion and worsen reflux.

■ Instruct patient to take drug without regard to meals because absorption isn't affected by food.

IRRITABLE BOWEL SYNDROME

Once known as *spastic colon* or *spastic colitis*, irritable bowel syndrome (IBS) is marked by chronic abdominal pain, distention, and constipation, diarrhea, or an alternating pattern of both. IBS is common, but many patients don't seek medical attention for it. This disorder seems to be more common, and more severe, in women than in men.

The causes and mechanisms of this functional intestinal disorder remain poorly understood. What is clear is that the disorder involves altered intestinal motility and sensitivity, possibly in part through alterations in serotonin receptors in the intestinal wall. IBS also may be influenced by psychological stress, other intestinal disorders (such as diverticular disease), ingestion of irritants (such as coffee, chocolate, or raw fruits or vegetables), lactose intolerance, laxative abuse, food poisoning, or colon cancer.

alosetron

CONTRAINDICATIONS AND CAUTIONS

■ Contraindicated in patients hypersensitive to alosetron or its components; patients whose predominant symptom is constipation; patients unable to understand or comply with the required Patient-Physician Agreement; patients with current or previous Crohn's disease, ulcerative colitis, or diverticulitis; and patients with current or previous chronic or severe constipation, gastrointestinal (GI)

perforation or adhesion, hypercoagulation, impaired intestinal circulation, intestinal obstruction or stricture, ischemic colitis, sequelae from constipation, thrombophlebitis, or toxic megacolon.

■ Use cautiously in patients who are pregnant, planning to become pregnant, or breastfeeding.

■ Use in patients younger than age 18 hasn't been studied.

KEY POINTS

■ Drug is approved only for women with IBS whose predominant symptom is diarrhea. This drug isn't indicated for men or patients whose predominant symptom is constipation.

■ Diarrhea-predominant IBS is considered severe if the patient has one or more of the following: frequent, severe abdominal pain or discomfort; frequent bowel urgency or fecal incontinence; disability or restriction of daily activities.

■ Patients taking this drug may develop ischemic colitis and serious complications of constipation, resulting in death. If patient develops acute colitis, rectal bleeding, or sudden worsening of abdominal pain while taking drug, stop therapy immediately.

dicyclomine

CONTRAINDICATIONS AND CAUTIONS

■ Contraindicated in breast-feeding women, children younger than age 6 months, patients hypersensitive to anticholinergics, and patients with acute hemorrhage leading to an unstable cardiovascular status, glaucoma, myasthenia gravis, obstructive GI disease, obstructive uropathy, reflux esophagitis, severe ulcerative colitis, tachycardia from cardiac insufficiency or thyrotoxicosis, or toxic megacolon.

■ Use cautiously in patients in hot or humid environments (because of the risk of drug-induced heat stroke) and in patients with arrhythmias, autonomic neuropathy, coronary artery disease, GI infection (known or suspected), heart failure, hepatic or renal disease, hiatal hernia, hypertension, hyperthyroidism, prostatic hyperplasia, or ulcerative colitis.

KEY POINTS

■ Give drug 30 to 60 minutes before meals and at bedtime. Bedtime dose can be larger; give at least 2 hours after the last meal of the day.

■ Monitor patient's vital signs and urine output carefully.

■ Advise patient to avoid driving and other hazardous activities if drug causes drowsiness, dizziness, or blurred vision; to drink plenty of fluids to help prevent constipation; and to report rash or other skin problems.

tegaserod

CONTRAINDICATIONS AND CAUTIONS

■ Contraindicated in patients hypersensitive to drug or its components and in patients with abdominal adhesions, bowel obstruction (current or previous), frequent diarrhea, moderate or severe hepatic impairment, severe renal impairment, suspected sphincter of Oddi dysfunction, or symptomatic gallbladder disease.

■ Use cautiously in patient who now has or often has diarrhea.

KEY POINTS

■ Drug is indicated for use in women.

■ Stop drug if patient has new or sudden worsening of abdominal pain.

■ Patient may develop diarrhea during therapy. Usually, it occurs in the first week of treatment and resolves as therapy continues.

PEPTIC ULCER

A peptic ulcer—which may be gastric or duodenal—is a circumscribed lesion in the gastric or duodenal mucosa that extends through the muscularis mucosa. Typically, an ulcer results when mucosal defense mechanisms are overwhelmed or impaired by acid or pepsin. Peptic ulcers are five times more common in the duodenum and are most common among people ages 30 to 55. Gastric ulcers are most common among people ages 55 to 70.

Infection with the bacterium *Helicobacter pylori* is the most common cause of duodenal and gastric ulcers and is somewhat difficult to eradicate permanently. In fact, 70% to 85% of patients have a recurrence of the ulcer (confirmed by endoscopy) within 1 year of treatment. Nonsteroidal antiinflammatory drugs are another common cause of peptic ulcer because they inhibit prostaglandin secretion. Certain illnesses—such as pancreatitis, hepatic disease, Crohn's disease, Zollinger-Ellison syndrome, and gastritis—are also known causes. Also, psychological states that affect the autonomic nervous system (stress, anger, a "type A" personality) may affect the gastric mucosa as well.

cimetidine

CONTRAINDICATIONS AND CAUTIONS
■ Contraindicated in patients hypersensitive to drug.
■ Use cautiously in elderly or debilitated patients because they may be more susceptible to cimetidine-induced confusion.

KEY POINTS
■ Identify tablet strength when obtaining a drug history.
■ Assess patient for abdominal pain. Note blood in emesis, stool, or gastric aspirate.
■ Advise patient to report abdominal pain or blood in stools or vomit.
■ Urge patient to avoid cigarette smoking because it may increase gastric acid secretion and worsen disease.

famotidine

CONTRAINDICATIONS AND CAUTIONS
■ Contraindicated in patients hypersensitive to drug.

KEY POINTS
■ Assess patient for abdominal pain. Note blood in emesis, stool, or gastric aspirate.

balsalazide
CONTRAINDICATIONS AND CAUTIONS

■ Contraindicated in patients hypersensitive to salicylates or to any component of balsalazide disodium or balsalazide metabolites.

■ Use cautiously in breast-feeding patients and patients with a history of renal disease or dysfunction.

■ The safety and effectiveness of therapy lasting longer than 12 weeks aren't known.

KEY POINTS

■ Watch closely for evidence of hepatic dysfunction. Although no signs of hepatotoxicity have been reported with balsalazide disodium, hepatotoxicity (elevated liver function test values, jaundice, cirrhosis, liver necrosis, and liver failure) has occurred with other products containing mesalamine or metabolized to it.

■ Advise patient not to take drug if he's allergic to aspirin.

■ Instruct patient to swallow capsules whole.

hydrocortisone
CONTRAINDICATIONS AND CAUTIONS

■ Contraindicated in premature infants (succinate), patients hypersensitive to the drug or its ingredients, patients with systemic fungal infections, and patients receiving immunosuppressive doses with live-virus vaccines.

■ Use with extreme caution if patient has had a recent myocardial infarction.

■ Use cautiously in breast-feeding patients and patients with active hepatitis, cirrhosis, diabetes mellitus, diverticulitis, emotional instability, gastrointestinal (GI) ulcer, heart failure, hypertension, hypothyroidism, myasthenia gravis, ocular herpes simplex, osteoporosis, psychotic tendencies, recent intestinal anastomoses, renal disease, seizures, thromboembolic disorders, ulcerative colitis, or tuberculosis.

KEY POINTS

■ Administration by enema may produce the same systemic effects as other forms of hydrocortisone. If enema therapy must exceed 21 days, stop gradually by reducing use to every other night for 2 to 3 weeks.

■ Most adverse reactions to corticosteroids are dose- or duration-dependent.

■ Always adjust to lowest effective dose.

mesalamine

CONTRAINDICATIONS AND CAUTIONS

■ Contraindicated in children and in patients allergic to mesalamine, salicylates, or their components.

■ Use cautiously in elderly, pregnant, and breast-feeding patients and in those with renal impairment.

KEY POINTS

■ Intact or partially intact tablets may be seen in the stool. Notify prescriber if this occurs repeatedly.

■ Monitor renal function studies periodically in patients on long-term therapy.

■ Advise patient to stop drug if fever or rash occurs.

■ A patient intolerant of sulfasalazine may also be hypersensitive to mesalamine.

olsalazine

CONTRAINDICATIONS AND CAUTIONS

■ Contraindicated in patients hypersensitive to salicylates.

■ Use cautiously in patients with renal disease. Although problems haven't been reported, the possibility of renal tubular damage from absorbed drug or its metabolites must be considered.

KEY POINTS

■ Some patients develop diarrhea during therapy. Although it appears to be dose-related, it's difficult to distinguish from worsening of disease symptoms.

■ Similar drugs have caused worsening of disease.

■ Teach patient to take drug in evenly divided doses and with food to minimize adverse GI reactions.

sulfasalazine

CONTRAINDICATIONS AND CAUTIONS

■ Contraindicated in children younger than age 2, patients hypersensitive to drug or its metabolites, and patients with porphyria, intestinal obstruction, or urinary obstruction.

■ Use cautiously and in reduced amounts in patients with impaired hepatic or renal function, severe allergy, bronchial asthma, or G6PD deficiency.

KEY POINTS

■ Stop drug immediately and notify prescriber if patient shows evidence of hypersensitivity.

■ Give drug with food to decrease GI irritation.

■ Drug may cause urine discoloration.

15 / DRUGS FOR GENITOURINARY DISORDERS

BENIGN PROSTATIC HYPERPLASIA .

Although most men older than age 50 have some enlargement of the prostate gland, benign prostatic hyperplasia (BPH) refers to a condition in which the gland is enlarged enough to compress the urethra and cause some amount of urinary obstruction. BPH also may cause a pouch to form in the bladder that retains urine and increases the risk of calculus formation or cystitis.

Recent evidence suggests that BPH may be related to hormonal activity. As men age, production of androgenic hormones decreases, causing an imbalance in androgen and estrogen levels and high levels of dihydrotestosterone, the main prostatic intracellular androgen. Other causes include neoplasm, arteriosclerosis, inflammation, and metabolic or nutritional disturbances.

Depending on the cause and degree of enlargement, the age and health of the patient, and the extent of obstruction, BPH is treated symptomatically or surgically.

doxazosin
CONTRAINDICATIONS AND CAUTIONS
■ Contraindicated in patients hypersensitive to drug or to quinazoline derivatives (including prazosin and terazosin).
■ Use cautiously in patients with impaired hepatic function.

KEY POINTS
■ Monitor blood pressure closely.
■ If syncope occurs, place patient in a recumbent position and treat supportively.
■ Advise patient about a possible first-dose effect (marked low blood pressure, dizziness, or fainting when he stands up) similar to that produced by other alpha blockers. Explain that it's most common after the first

dose but can also occur when the dosage is changed or therapy interrupted.

dutasteride

CONTRAINDICATIONS AND CAUTIONS

■ Contraindicated in women and children and in patients hypersensitive to dutasteride, its ingredients, or other 5-alpha-reductase inhibitors.

■ Use cautiously in patients with hepatic disease and in those taking long-term potent CYP 3A4 inhibitors.

KEY POINTS

■ Other urological diseases should be ruled out before therapy starts.

■ Patients with a large residual urine volume, severely diminished urine flow, or both, should be monitored carefully for obstructive uropathy.

■ Patient should wait at least 6 months after the last dose before donating blood.

finasteride

CONTRAINDICATIONS AND CAUTIONS

■ Contraindicated in patients hypersensitive to drug or to other 5-alpha-reductase inhibitors, such as dutasteride. Although drug isn't used in women or children, manufac-

turer indicates pregnancy as a contraindication.

■ Use cautiously in patients with liver dysfunction.

KEY POINTS

■ Before therapy, patient should be evaluated for conditions that mimic BPH, including hypotonic bladder; prostate cancer, infection, or stricture; and relevant neurologic conditions.

■ Carefully monitor patients who have a large residual urine volume or severely diminished urine flow; these patients may not be candidates for therapy.

■ Carefully assess sustained increases in prostate-specific antigen levels, which could indicate noncompliance with therapy.

prazosin

CONTRAINDICATIONS AND CAUTIONS

■ Contraindicated in patients hypersensitive to drug or other alpha blockers.

■ Use cautiously in patients receiving other antihypertensives.

KEY POINTS

■ Monitor patient's blood pressure and pulse frequently.

■ If initial dose is more than 1 mg, first-dose syncope may occur.

■ Tell patient not to stop taking drug suddenly, but to notify prescriber if unpleasant adverse reactions occur.

tamsulosin

CONTRAINDICATIONS AND CAUTIONS

■ Contraindicated in patients hypersensitive to drug or its components.

KEY POINTS

■ Monitor patient for decreases in blood pressure.

■ Symptoms of BPH and prostate cancer are similar; cancer should be ruled out before therapy starts.

■ Tell patient to rise slowly at the start of therapy and to avoid situations in which fainting could cause injury. Explain that the drug may cause sudden drops in blood pressure, especially after the first dose or when changing doses.

terazosin

CONTRAINDICATIONS AND CAUTIONS

■ Contraindicated in patients hypersensitive to drug.

KEY POINTS

■ Monitor blood pressure frequently.

■ Tell patient not to stop taking drug suddenly, but to notify prescriber if unpleasant adverse reactions occur.

■ Advise patient that light-headedness may occur, especially during the first few days of therapy. Advise him to rise slowly to minimize this effect and to report signs and symptoms to the prescriber.

CHLAMYDIAL INFECTION

Infection with the bacterium *Chlamydia trachomatis* is the most common sexually transmitted disease in the United States, affecting an estimated 4 million Americans each year. It causes urethritis in men and urethritis and cervicitis in women. This bacterium also causes two diseases that are rare in the United States but common elsewhere in the world: trachoma inclusion conjunctivitis, a leading cause of blindness in third-world countries, and lymphogranuloma venereum.

Untreated, chlamydial infection can lead to such complications as acute epididymitis, salpingitis, pelvic inflammatory disease and, eventually, sterility. Some evidence exists that it may cause spontaneous abortion and premature delivery as well. Children born to mothers with chlamydial infections may develop conjunctivitis, otitis media, and pneumonia in the birth canal.

Transmission of *C. trachomatis* occurs mainly through vaginal or rectal intercourse or oral contact with an infected person's genitals. Because signs and symptoms typically appear late in the course of the disease, transmission may occur without any awareness of it.

doxycycline

CONTRAINDICATIONS AND CAUTIONS

■ Contraindicated in patients hypersensitive to drug or other tetracyclines.

■ Use cautiously in patients with impaired renal or hepatic function.

■ Use of this drug during the last half of pregnancy and in children younger than age 8 may retard bone growth and cause permanent tooth discoloration and enamel defects.

KEY POINTS

■ Check the expiration date. Outdated or deteriorated tetracyclines may cause reversible nephrotoxicity (Fanconi's syndrome).

■ Check patient's tongue for signs of fungal infection, and stress the importance of oral hygiene.

■ Photosensitivity reactions may occur within a few minutes to several hours after exposure. Explain that susceptibility may last for some time after therapy ends.

erythromycin

CONTRAINDICATIONS AND CAUTIONS

■ Contraindicated in pregnant patients and in those hypersensitive to drug or other macrolides.

■ Use cautiously in breast-feeding patients and patients with impaired hepatic function. Monitor liver function test results.

KEY POINTS

■ Assess patient for superinfection because drug may cause overgrowth of nonsusceptible bacteria or fungi.

■ Monitor hepatic function to detect increased levels of alkaline phosphatase, alanine transaminase, aspartate transaminase, and bilirubin.

■ Watch for ototoxicity, especially in patients with renal or hepatic insufficiency and in those receiving high doses of drug.

minocycline
CONTRAINDICATIONS AND CAUTIONS

■ Contraindicated in patients hypersensitive to drug or other tetracyclines.

■ Use cautiously in patients with impaired renal or hepatic function.

■ Use of this drug during the last half of pregnancy and in children younger than age 8 may retard bone growth and cause permanent tooth discoloration and enamel defects.

KEY POINTS

■ Check the expiration date. Outdated or deteriorated tetracyclines may cause reversible nephrotoxicity (Fanconi's syndrome).

■ Monitor renal and liver function test results.

■ Photosensitivity reactions may occur within a few minutes to several hours after exposure. Explain that susceptibility may last for some time after therapy ends.

tetracycline
CONTRAINDICATIONS AND CAUTIONS

■ Contraindicated in patients hypersensitive to drug or other tetracyclines.

■ Use with extreme caution in patients with renal or hepatic impairment, and monitor renal and liver function test results.

■ Use of this drug during the last half of pregnancy and in children younger than age 8 may retard bone growth and cause permanent tooth discoloration and enamel defects.

KEY POINTS

■ Check the expiration date. Outdated or deteriorated tetracyclines may cause reversible nephrotoxicity (Fanconi's syndrome).

■ Check the patient's tongue for evidence of candidal infection. Stress the importance of oral hygiene.

■ Photosensitivity reactions may occur within a few minutes to several hours after sun exposure. Explain that susceptibility may last for some time after therapy ends.

FORMS OF PELVIC INFLAMMATORY DISEASE

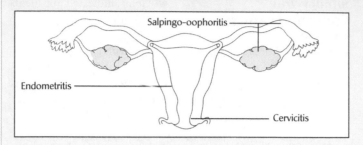

CAUSE AND CLINICAL FEATURES

Salpingo–oophoritis
■ Acute: sudden onset of lower abdominal and pelvic pain, usually following menses; increased vaginal discharge; fever; malaise; lower abdominal pressure and tenderness; tachycardia; pelvic peritonitis
■ Chronic: recurring acute episodes

Cervicitis
■ Acute: purulent, foul-smelling vaginal discharge; vulvovaginitis, with itching or burning; red, edematous cervix; pelvic discomfort; sexual dysfunction; metrorrhagia; infertility; spontaneous abortion
■ Chronic: cervical dystocia, laceration or eversion of the cervix, ulcerative vesicular lesion (when cervicitis results from herpes simplex virus II)

Endometritis
(usually postpartum or postabortion)
■ Acute: mucopurulent or purulent vaginal discharge oozing from the cervix; edematous, hyperemic endometrium, possibly leading to ulceration and necrosis (with virulent organisms); lower abdominal pain and tenderness; fever; rebound pain; abdominal muscle spasm; thrombophlebitis of uterine and pelvic vessels (in severe forms)
■ Chronic: recurring acute episodes (increasingly common because of widespread use of intrauterine devices)

PELVIC INFLAMMATORY DISEASE

Pelvic inflammatory disease (PID) is any acute, subacute, recurrent, or chronic infection of the oviducts, ovaries, and adjacent tissue. It may involve the cervix (cervicitis), uterus (endometritis), fallopian tubes (salpingitis), and ovaries (oophoritis) and may extend to the connective tissue between the broad ligaments (parametritis). (See *Forms of pelvic inflammatory disease*.)

PID can result from infection with aerobic or anaerobic organisms. *Neisseria gonorrhoeae* is a common culprit because it readily penetrates the barrier of cervical mucus that normally protects the cervix. Other bacteria found in cervical mucus include staphylococci, streptococci, diphtheroids, chlamydiae, and coliforms, including *Pseudomonas* and *Escherichia coli*. Infection can result from one or more of these organisms or from normally nonpathogenic bacteria that overgrow in an altered endometrial environment. Bacterial multiplication is most common during parturition, because the endometrium is at-

DIAGNOSTIC FINDINGS

- Blood studies show leukocytosis or normal white blood cell (WBC) count.
- X-ray may show ileus.
- Pelvic examination reveals extreme tenderness.
- Smear of cervical or periurethral gland exudate shows gram-negative intracellular diplococci.

- Cultures for *Neisseria gonorrhoeae* are positive in more than 90% of patients.
- Cytologic smears may reveal severe inflammation.
- If cervicitis isn't complicated by salpingitis, WBC count is normal or slightly elevated; erythrocyte sedimentation rate (ESR) is elevated.
- With acute cervicitis, cervical palpation reveals tenderness.
- With chronic cervicitis, causative organisms are usually staphylococci or streptococci.

- With severe infection, palpation may reveal a boggy uterus.
- Uterine and blood samples are positive for the causative organism, usually staphylococcus.
- WBC count and ESR are elevated.

■ Safety and efficacy haven't been established in children younger than age 18.

KEY POINTS
■ Give drug I.V. for no longer than 10 days; after 10 days, change I.V. to P.O.

■ Warn patient that hypersensitivity reactions may follow the first dose. Tell patient to stop drug and call prescriber immediately at the first sign of rash or other allergic reaction.

■ Urge patient to avoid prolonged exposure to direct sunlight and to use a sunscreen when outdoors.

piperacillin and tazobactam
CONTRAINDICATIONS AND CAUTIONS
■ Contraindicated in patients hypersensitive to drug or other penicillins.

■ Use cautiously in patients with bleeding tendencies, drug allergies (especially to cephalosporins) because of possible cross-sensitivity, hypokalemia, or uremia.

KEY POINTS
■ Obtain specimen for culture and sensitivity tests before giving first dose. Therapy may begin pending results.

■ If large doses are given or therapy is prolonged, bacterial or fungal superinfection may occur, especially in elderly, debilitated, or immunosuppressed patients.

16 / DRUGS FOR IMMUNE DISORDERS

ALLERGIC RHINITIS

An immune reaction to inhaled allergens, allergic rhinitis affects more than 20 million Americans, making it the most common atopic allergic reaction. Depending on the allergen, the resulting rhinitis and conjunctivitis may be seasonal (hay fever) or year-round (perennial allergic rhinitis).

Hay fever reflects an immunoglobulin E–mediated, type I hypersensitivity response. Usually, it's induced by windborne pollens: in spring, by tree pollens (oak, elm, maple, alder, birch, cottonwood); in summer, by grass pollens (crabgrass, bluegrass, fescue, and ryegrass); and in fall, by weed pollens (ragweed). Occasionally, hay fever is induced by allergy to fungal spores.

With perennial allergic rhinitis, the major allergens and irritants include dust mites, feather pillows, mold, cigarette smoke, upholstery, and animal dander. Seasonal pollen allergy may worsen symptoms of perennial rhinitis.

beclomethasone
CONTRAINDICATIONS AND CAUTIONS
■ Contraindicated in patients hypersensitive to drug and in those with untreated infection of the nasal mucosa.
■ Use with extreme caution, if at all, in patients with tuberculosis of the respiratory tract, ocular herpes simplex, or untreated fungal, bacterial, or systemic viral infections. Also use cautiously in patients with recent nasal septal ulcers, nasal surgery, or trauma.

KEY POINTS
■ Assess patient for fungal infections.
■ Drug isn't effective for acute exacerbations of rhinitis. Decongestants or antihistamines may be needed.

■ Explain that, unlike decongestants, this drug doesn't work right away. Most patients notice improvement in a few days, but some may need 2 to 3 weeks.

budesonide

CONTRAINDICATIONS AND CAUTIONS

■ Contraindicated in patients hypersensitive to drug or its components and in those with recent septal ulcers, nasal surgery, or nasal trauma that may not be completely healed.

■ Use with extreme caution in patients with tuberculosis of the respiratory tract, ocular herpes simplex, or untreated fungal, bacterial, or systemic viral infections.

KEY POINTS

■ Systemic corticosteroid effects may occur if patient exceeds recommended inhaled dose.

■ Tell patient to contact prescriber if signs or symptoms don't improve in 3 weeks or if condition worsens.

■ Teach patient good nasal and oral hygiene.

cetirizine

CONTRAINDICATIONS AND CAUTIONS

■ Contraindicated in patients hypersensitive to drug or to hydroxyzine.

■ Drug isn't recommended for breast-feeding women.

■ Use cautiously in patients with renal or liver impairment.

KEY POINTS

■ Stop drug 4 days before patient undergoes diagnostic skin tests for allergies. Drug can prevent, reduce, or mask positive skin test response.

■ Warn patient not to perform hazardous activities until central nervous system (CNS) effects of drug are known. Somnolence is a common adverse reaction.

■ Inform patient that sugarless gum, hard candy, or ice chips may relieve dry mouth.

desloratadine

CONTRAINDICATIONS AND CAUTIONS

■ Contraindicated in patients hypersensitive to drug, to loratadine, or to their components.

■ Use cautiously in geriatric patients because of the greater likelihood of other diseases, other drug therapy, and decreased hepatic, renal, or cardiac function.

■ Drug appears in breast milk. Depending on the patient's need for drug, she should either stop breast-feeding or stop taking the drug.

KEY POINTS

■ Advise patient not to exceed recommended dosage. Higher doses don't increase effectiveness and may cause somnolence.
■ Tell patient that drug can be taken without regard to meals.

fexofenadine

CONTRAINDICATIONS AND CAUTIONS

■ Contraindicated in patients hypersensitive to drug or its components.
■ Use cautiously in patients with impaired renal function.

KEY POINTS

■ Stop drug 4 days before patient undergoes diagnostic skin tests for allergies because drug can prevent, reduce, or mask positive skin test response.
■ Warn patient to avoid alcohol and hazardous activities until CNS effects of drug are known. Explain that drug may cause drowsiness.
■ Inform patient that sugarless gum, hard candy, or ice chips may relieve dry mouth.

loratadine

CONTRAINDICATIONS AND CAUTIONS

■ Contraindicated in patients hypersensitive to drug.
■ Use cautiously in breast-feeding patients and patients with liver or renal impairment.

KEY POINTS

■ Stop drug 4 days before patient undergoes diagnostic skin tests for allergies because drug can prevent, reduce, or mask positive skin test response.
■ Warn patient to avoid alcohol and hazardous activities until CNS effects of drug are known.
■ Tell patient that dry mouth can be relieved with sugarless gum, hard candy, or ice chips.

triamcinolone

CONTRAINDICATIONS AND CAUTIONS

■ Contraindicated in patients hypersensitive to drug or its ingredients and in those with status asthmaticus.
■ Use with extreme caution, if at all, in patients with tuberculosis of the respiratory tract, ocular herpes simplex, or untreated fungal, bacterial, or systemic viral infections.
■ Use cautiously in patients receiving systemic corticosteroids.

■ It's unknown whether drug appears in breast milk. Because of risk of severe adverse effects, breast-feeding isn't recommended during therapy.

KEY POINTS
■ For nasal spray, if improvement isn't evident after 2 to 3 weeks, the patient should be reevaluated.

■ Patient should use drug at regular intervals to obtain full therapeutic effect.

■ For best results, patient should clear nasal passages before using drug.

ANKYLOSING SPONDYLITIS

A chronic inflammatory disease, ankylosing spondylitis affects mainly the sacroiliac, apophyseal, and costovertebral joints and adjacent soft tissue. It usually starts in the sacroiliac joints and gradually progresses to the lumbar, thoracic, and cervical regions of the spine. Deterioration of bone and cartilage can lead to fibrous tissue formation and eventual fusion of the spine or peripheral joints.

Ankylosing spondylitis affects five times as many men as women and, among whites, may affect up to 1% of the population. Recent evidence strongly suggests a family tendency. And because more than 90% of patients with this disease have circulating immune complexes and test positive for histocompatibility antigen HLA-B27, it probably has an immunologic component. A possible link to underlying infection is being investigated as well.

diclofenac
CONTRAINDICATIONS AND CAUTIONS
■ Contraindicated in patients hypersensitive to drug and in those with hepatic porphyria or a history of asthma, urticaria, or other allergic reaction after taking aspirin or a nonsteroidal anti-inflammatory drug (NSAID).

■ Drug isn't recommended for use during late pregnancy or breast-feeding.

■ Use drug cautiously in patients with a history of cardiac disease, fluid retention, hepatic dysfunction, hypertension, impaired renal function, or peptic ulcer disease.

KEY POINTS
■ Monitor transaminase, especially alanine transaminase, levels in patients undergoing long-term therapy. The first transaminase measurement should be

no more than 8 weeks after therapy starts.

🌀 **ALERT** *Serious gastrointestinal (GI) toxicity, including peptic ulcers and bleeding, can occur in patients taking NSAIDs, without causing symptoms.*

■ Because of their antipyretic and anti-inflammatory actions, NSAIDs may mask the signs and symptoms of infection.

indomethacin
CONTRAINDICATIONS AND CAUTIONS

■ Contraindicated in pregnant women; breast-feeding women; patients hypersensitive to drug; patients with a history of aspirin- or NSAID-induced asthma, rhinitis, or urticaria; and neonates with active bleeding, coagulation defects, congenital heart disease for whom patency of the ductus arteriosus is needed, necrotizing enterocolitis, significant renal impairment, thrombocytopenia, or untreated infection.

■ Suppositories are contraindicated in patients with a history of proctitis or recent rectal bleeding.

■ Use cautiously in elderly patients, patients with a history of GI disease, and patients with cardiovascular (CV) disease, depression, epilepsy, hepatic dis-

ease, infection, mental illness, parkinsonism, or renal disease.

KEY POINTS

■ Drug causes sodium retention; watch for weight gain (especially in elderly patients) and increased pressure in patients with hypertension.

■ Because of their antipyretic and anti-inflammatory actions, NSAIDs may mask the signs and symptoms of infection.

🌀 **ALERT** *Serious GI toxicity, including peptic ulcers and bleeding, can occur in patients taking NSAIDs, without causing symptoms.*

naproxen
CONTRAINDICATIONS AND CAUTIONS

■ Contraindicated in patients hypersensitive to drug and in those with asthma, rhinitis, and nasal polyps.

■ Use cautiously in elderly patients, patients with a history of peptic ulcer disease, and patients with CV disease, GI disorders, hepatic disease, or renal disease.

■ Drug should be avoided during last trimester of pregnancy.

KEY POINTS

■ Monitor complete blood count (CBC) and renal and hepatic function every 4 to 6 months in long-term therapy.

🌀 ALERT   *Serious GI toxicity, including peptic ulcers and bleeding, can occur in patients taking NSAIDs, without causing symptoms.*

■ Because of their antipyretic and anti-inflammatory actions, NSAIDs may mask the signs and symptoms of infection.

sulindac

CONTRAINDICATIONS AND CAUTIONS

■ Contraindicated in patients hypersensitive to drug and in those for whom aspirin or NSAIDs cause acute asthmatic attacks, urticaria, or rhinitis.

■ Don't give drug to pregnant women.

■ Use cautiously in patients with a history of ulcers and GI bleeding, patients with conditions predisposing them to fluid retention, and patients with compromised cardiac function, hypertension, or renal dysfunction.

KEY POINTS

■ Periodically monitor hepatic function, renal function, and CBC in a patient receiving long-term therapy.

🌀 ALERT   *Serious GI toxicity, including peptic ulcers and bleeding, can occur in patients taking NSAIDs, without causing symptoms.*

■ Because of their antipyretic and anti-inflammatory actions, NSAIDs may mask the signs and symptoms of infection.

HUMAN IMMUNODEFICIENCY VIRUS INFECTION

Human immunodeficiency virus (HIV) infection and its terminal condition, acquired immunodeficiency syndrome (AIDS), involve progressive failure of the immune system after infection with the HIV retrovirus. Immunodeficiency makes the patient susceptible to opportunistic infections, unusual cancers, and other abnormalities that define AIDS.

HIV is transmitted by contact with infected blood or body fluids and not by casual household or social contact. For example, it can be transmitted during intimate sexual contact, especially receptive rectal intercourse; transfusion of contaminated blood or blood products; sharing of contaminated needles; or transplacental or postpartum transmission from an infected mother to the fetus (by cervical or blood contact at delivery and in breast milk).

The virus gains access by binding to the CD4+ molecule on the surface of lymphocytes, macrophages, or other cells bearing CD4+ antigens. After invading a cell, HIV either replicates, which leads to cell death, or becomes latent. HIV infection leads to profound pathology, either directly, through destruction of CD4+ T cells, other immune cells, and neuroglial cells, or indirectly, through the secondary effects of CD4+ T-cell dysfunction and immunosuppression. The infection may involve immunodeficiency (opportunistic infections and unusual cancers), autoimmunity (lymphoid interstitial pneumonia, arthritis, hypergammaglobulinemia), and neurologic dysfunction (AIDS dementia complex, HIV encephalopathy, peripheral neuropathy).

Most people develop antibodies within 6 to 8 weeks of contracting the virus, but evidence of immunodeficiency may not surface for 8 to 10 years, perhaps longer. Indeed, with current combination antiretroviral therapies, many authorities are beginning to consider HIV/AIDS a chronic disease rather than an inevitable death sentence.

abacavir

CONTRAINDICATIONS AND CAUTIONS

■ Contraindicated in patients hypersensitive to drug or its components.

■ Use cautiously in patients at risk for liver disease because nucleoside analogues have been linked to lactic acidosis and life-threatening hepatomegaly with steatosis.

■ Use cautiously in pregnant women and only if potential benefits outweigh risks.

KEY POINTS

■ Women are more likely than men to experience lactic acidosis and severe hepatomegaly with steatosis. Obesity and prolonged nucleoside exposure may be risk factors. Stop the drug if these problems occur.

ALERT Abacavir can cause fatal hypersensitivity reactions; if patient develops evidence of hypersensitivity (fever, rash, fatigue, nausea, vomiting, diarrhea, abdominal pain), patient should stop drug and seek medical attention immediately.

■ Don't restart drug after a hypersensitivity reaction because severe signs and symptoms will recur within hours and may include severe hypotension and death.

amprenavir

CONTRAINDICATIONS AND CAUTIONS

■ Contraindicated in infants, children younger than age 4, pregnant women, patients hypersensitive to drug or its components, patients with liver or kidney failure, and patients treated with disulfiram or metronidazole.

■ Use cautiously in patients with moderate or severe hepatic impairment, diabetes mellitus, sulfonamide allergy, or hemophilia A or B.

■ Use cautiously in pregnant women and only when potential benefits outweigh the risks.

KEY POINTS

◎ *ALERT Drug can cause severe or life-threatening rash, including Stevens-Johnson syndrome. Stop therapy if patient develops a severe or life-threatening rash or a moderate rash accompanied by systemic signs and symptoms.*

■ Because amprenavir may interact with many drugs, obtain patient's complete drug history. Ask to see which drugs the patient takes.

■ Protease inhibitors may cause redistribution of body fat, including central obesity, dorsocervical fat enlargement (buffalo hump), peripheral wasting, breast enlargement, and cushingoid appearance. The mechanism and long-term consequences of these effects are unknown.

efavirenz

CONTRAINDICATIONS AND CAUTIONS

■ Contraindicated in patients hypersensitive to drug or its components.

■ Use cautiously in patients with hepatic impairment and in those receiving hepatotoxic drugs.

KEY POINTS

■ Drug shouldn't be used as monotherapy or added on as a single drug when a regimen is failing because of viral resistance.

■ Monitor liver function test results in patients with history of hepatitis B or C and in those taking ritonavir.

■ Pregnancy must be ruled out before therapy starts.

■ Children may be more prone to adverse reactions, especially diarrhea, nausea, vomiting, and rash.

lamivudine and zidovudine

CONTRAINDICATIONS AND CAUTIONS

■ Contraindicated in patients hypersensitive to drug or its

components, patients younger than age 12, patients who weigh less than 50 kg (110 lb), patients with a creatinine clearance below 50 ml/minute, and patients with dose-limiting adverse effects.

■ Use combination cautiously in patients with bone marrow suppression (granulocyte count below 1,000 cells/mm³ or hemoglobin level below 9.5 g/dl).

KEY POINTS
■ Lactic acidosis and severe hepatomegaly with steatosis may occur in patients receiving lamivudine and zidovudine alone and as adjunctive therapy. Notify prescriber if evidence of lactic acidosis or hepatotoxicity (abdominal pain, jaundice) develops.

ALERT Monitor patient for bone marrow toxicity with frequent blood counts, particularly during advanced HIV infection. Watch for evidence of lactic acidosis and hepatotoxicity.

■ Assess patient's fine motor skills and peripheral sensation for evidence of peripheral neuropathies. Assess patient for myopathy and myositis.

lopinavir and ritonavir
CONTRAINDICATIONS AND CAUTIONS
■ Contraindicated in patients hypersensitive to drug or its components.

■ Use cautiously in patients with a history of pancreatitis and patients with hepatic impairment, hepatitis B or C, hemophilia, or marked elevations in liver enzyme levels.

■ Use cautiously in elderly patients.

KEY POINTS
■ Watch for signs of fat redistribution, including central obesity, buffalo hump, peripheral wasting, breast enlargement, and cushingoid appearance.

ALERT Assess patient for signs and symptoms of pancreatitis (nausea, vomiting, abdominal pain, or increased lipase and amylase values).

■ Watch for evidence of bleeding (hypotension, rapid heart rate).

saquinavir
CONTRAINDICATIONS AND CAUTIONS
■ Contraindicated in patients hypersensitive to drug or its components.

■ Safety hasn't been established in pregnant or breast-feeding women or in children younger than age 16.

KEY POINTS

- Evaluate complete blood count (CBC), platelets, electrolytes, uric acid, liver enzymes, and bilirubin before therapy begins and at appropriate intervals during therapy.

- If serious toxicity occurs during treatment, stop drug until cause is identified or toxicity resolves. Drug may be resumed without dosage modification.

- Monitor patient's hydration if adverse gastrointestinal (GI) reactions occur.

stavudine
CONTRAINDICATIONS AND CAUTIONS

- Contraindicated in patients hypersensitive to drug.

- Use cautiously in patients with renal impairment, patients with a history of peripheral neuropathy, and pregnant women, who may have an increased risk of fatal lactic acidosis if they receive stavudine and didanosine with other antiretrovirals.

- Adjust dosage if creatinine clearance is below 50 ml/minute. Adjust dosage or stop drug if peripheral neuropathy occurs.

KEY POINTS

- Watch for evidence of pancreatitis, especially if patient takes stavudine with didanosine or hydroxyurea. If patient has pancreatitis, reinstate drug cautiously.

🌀 *ALERT Motor weakness that mimics Guillain-Barré syndrome (including respiratory failure) may occur in HIV patients who take stavudine with other antiretrovirals, usually when the patient also has lactic acidosis. Watch for evidence of lactic acidosis, including generalized fatigue, GI problems, tachypnea, or dyspnea. Interrupt antiretroviral therapy and obtain a full medical work-up. Stavudine may be discontinued permanently.*

- Peripheral neuropathy appears to be the major dose-limiting adverse effect of stavudine. It may or may not resolve after drug is stopped.

tenofovir
CONTRAINDICATIONS AND CAUTIONS

- Contraindicated in patients hypersensitive to the drug or its components and in patients with a creatinine clearance less than 60 ml/minute.

- Use very cautiously in patients with risk factors for liver disease or with hepatic impairment.

■ Because the effects of tenofovir on pregnant women and breast-feeding infants aren't known, give this drug to pregnant women only if its benefits clearly outweigh the risks. Mothers receiving tenofovir for HIV infection shouldn't breast-feed.

■ Safety and efficacy haven't been studied in children.

KEY POINTS

🌀 *ALERT Antiretrovirals have been linked to lactic acidosis and life-threatening hepatomegaly with steatosis. These effects may occur without elevated transaminase levels. Risk factors may include long-term antiretroviral use, obesity, and being female. Monitor all patients for hepatotoxicity.*

■ Antiretrovirals may cause redistribution of body fat, resulting in central obesity, peripheral wasting, and a buffalo hump. The long-term effects of these changes are unknown. Monitor patients for changes in body fat.

■ Tenofovir may be linked to bone abnormalities (osteomalacia and decreased bone mineral density) and renal toxicity (increased creatinine and phosphaturia levels). Monitor patient carefully during long-term treatment.

zalcitabine

CONTRAINDICATIONS AND CAUTIONS

■ Contraindicated in patients hypersensitive to drug or its components.

■ Use with extreme caution in patients with peripheral neuropathy.

■ Use cautiously in patients with cardiomyopathy, hepatic failure, or a history of pancreatitis or heart failure. Monitor liver function test results and pancreatic enzymes.

KEY POINTS

🌀 *ALERT Life-threatening lactic acidosis, severe hepatomegaly with steatosis, and hepatic failure may occur. Monitor patient closely.*

■ Toxic drug effects may cause abnormalities in CBC; hemoglobin; leukocyte, reticulocyte, granulocyte, and platelet counts; and alanine transaminase, aspartate transaminase, and alkaline phosphatase levels.

■ Assess patient for peripheral neuropathy, characterized by numbness and burning in the limbs, the drug's major toxic effects. If drug isn't withdrawn, peripheral neuropathy can progress to sharp shooting pain or severe continuous burning pain requiring opioid analgesics.

The pain may or may not be reversible.

zidovudine

CONTRAINDICATIONS AND CAUTIONS

■ Contraindicated in patients hypersensitive to drug.

■ Use cautiously and with close monitoring in patients with advanced symptomatic HIV infection and patients with severe bone marrow depression.

■ Use cautiously in patients with hepatomegaly, hepatitis, or other risk factors for liver disease and in those with renal insufficiency. Monitor renal and liver function test results.

KEY POINTS

ALERT Although rare, lactic acidosis without hypoxemia may occur with the use of antiretroviral nucleoside analogues, including zidovudine. Notify prescriber if patient develops unexplained tachypnea, dyspnea, or decreased bicarbonate level. Drug may need to be suspended until lactic acidosis is ruled out.

■ Monitor blood studies every 2 weeks to detect anemia or agranulocytosis. Patient may need dosage reduction or temporary discontinuation of drug.

■ Advise patient that blood transfusions may be needed during treatment. Zidovudine often causes a low red blood cell count.

RHEUMATOID ARTHRITIS

A chronic, systemic inflammatory disease, rheumatoid arthritis (RA) primarily attacks peripheral joints and surrounding muscles, tendons, ligaments, and blood vessels. Partial remissions and unpredictable exacerbations mark the course of this potentially crippling disease.

RA occurs worldwide, striking nearly three times more women than men. It can occur at any age but is most common among 25- to 55-year-olds. RA affects 1% to 2% of the total population.

This disease usually requires lifelong treatment and sometimes surgery. In most patients, it follows an intermittent course and allows normal activity, although 10% suffer total disability from severe articular deformity, extra-articular symptoms, or both. The prognosis worsens with the development of nodules, vasculitis, and high titers of rheumatoid factor (RF), which reflects development of an immunoglobulin (Ig) M antibody against the patient's own IgG.

Much more is known about the course of RA than its causes. If unarrested, the inflammatory process in the joints occurs in four stages. In the first stage, synovitis develops from congestion and edema of the synovial membrane and joint capsule. Infiltration by lymphocytes, macrophages, and neutrophils perpetuates the local inflammatory response. These cells, as well as fibroblast-like synovial cells, produce enzymes that help to degrade bone and cartilage.

Formation of pannus—thickened layers of granulation tissue—marks the onset of the second stage. Pannus covers and invades cartilage and eventually destroys the joint capsule and bone.

The third stage is characterized by fibrous ankylosis—fibrous invasion of the pannus and scar formation that occludes the joint space. Bone atrophy and malalignment cause visible deformities and disrupt the articulation of opposing bones, causing muscle atrophy and imbalance and, possibly, partial dislocations or subluxations.

In the fourth stage, fibrous tissue calcifies, resulting in bony ankylosis and total immobility.

anakinra

CONTRAINDICATIONS AND CAUTIONS

■ Contraindicated in immunosuppressed patients, patients with chronic infections, and patients hypersensitive to *Escherichia coli*–derived proteins or any component of the product.

■ Use cautiously in elderly patients because they have a greater risk of infection and are more likely to have renal impairment.

■ Use cautiously in breastfeeding women because it isn't known whether drug appears in breast milk.

■ Use drug cautiously with other tumor necrosis factor–blocking drugs because of the increased risk of neutropenia.

KEY POINTS

■ Don't start drug if patient has an active infection.

■ Obtain neutrophil count before treatment, monthly for the first 3 months of treatment, and then quarterly for up to 1 year.

■ Stop drug if patient develops a serious infection.

auranofin

CONTRAINDICATIONS AND CAUTIONS

■ Contraindicated in pregnant women; patients with a history of severe gold toxicity or toxicity from previous exposure to other heavy metals; patients who have recently undergone radiation therapy; patients with bone marrow aplasia, exfoliative dermatitis, necrotizing enterocolitis, pulmonary fibrosis, or severe hematologic disorders; and patients with colitis, eczema, hemorrhagic conditions, severe debilitation, systemic lupus erythematosus, or urticaria.

■ Use cautiously in patients taking other drugs that cause blood dyscrasias and in patients with a history of bone marrow depression, rash, or renal, hepatic, or inflammatory bowel disease.

KEY POINTS

■ Monitor patient's platelet count monthly. Stop drug if platelet count falls below 100,000/mm³, hemoglobin drops suddenly, granulocytes are less than 1,500/mm³, or leukopenia (WBC count less than 4,000/mm³) or eosinophilia develops.

■ Monitor patient's urinalysis results monthly. If proteinuria or hematuria develops, stop drug (because it can cause nephrotic syndrome or glomerulonephritis) and notify prescriber.

■ Monitor renal and liver function test results.

aurothioglucose
CONTRAINDICATIONS AND CAUTIONS

■ Contraindicated in patients hypersensitive to drug, patients with a history of severe toxicity from previous exposure to gold or other heavy metals, patients who have recently undergone radiation therapy, and patients with colitis, eczema, exfoliative dermatitis, hemorrhagic conditions, hepatic dysfunction, hepatitis, renal disease, severe hematologic disorders, severe uncontrollable diabetes, Sjögren's syndrome, systemic lupus erythematosus, uncontrolled heart failure, or urticaria.

■ Use with extreme caution, if at all, in patients with rash, marked hypertension, compromised cerebral or cardiovascular circulation, or a history of renal or hepatic disease, drug allergies, or blood dyscrasias.

KEY POINTS

■ Analyze urine for protein and sediment changes before each injection.

■ Monitor complete blood count (CBC), including platelet count, before every second injection.

■ Warn women of childbearing potential about the risks of gold therapy during pregnancy.

azathioprine

CONTRAINDICATIONS AND CAUTIONS

■ Contraindicated in patients hypersensitive to drug or its components.

■ Use cautiously in patients with hepatic or renal dysfunction.

KEY POINTS

■ Monitor CBC and platelet counts weekly for 1 month, and then twice monthly. Notify prescriber if counts drop suddenly or become dangerously low. Drug may need to be withheld temporarily.

■ Watch for early evidence of hepatotoxicity, such as clay-colored stools, dark urine, pruritus, and yellow skin and sclera; also watch for increased alkaline phosphatase, bilirubin, aspartate transaminase (AST), and alanine transaminase (ALT) levels.

■ Therapeutic response usually occurs within 8 weeks.

etanercept

CONTRAINDICATIONS AND CAUTIONS

■ Contraindicated in patients hypersensitive to drug or its components and in those with sepsis.

■ Use cautiously if patient has RA and a demyclinating disorder, such as multiple sclerosis, myelitis, or optic neuritis.

KEY POINTS

■ Drug may alter the ability to fight against infection. Notify prescriber and stop therapy if serious infection occurs.

■ Don't give live-virus vaccines during therapy.

■ Patients with juvenile RA should, if possible, be brought up-to-date with all immunizations before starting treatment.

infliximab

CONTRAINDICATIONS AND CAUTIONS

■ Contraindicated in patients hypersensitive to murine proteins or other components of drug and in those with congestive heart failure.

■ Use cautiously in elderly patients, patients with a history of chronic or recurrent infection, and patients who have lived in regions where histoplasmosis is endemic.

KEY POINTS

 ALERT *Watch for infusion-related reactions, including fever, chills, pruritus, urticaria, dyspnea, hypotension, hypertension, and* chest pain, during and for 2 hours after administration. If a reaction occurs, stop drug, notify prescriber, and be prepared to give acetaminophen, antihistamines, corticosteroids, and epinephrine.

■ Watch for development of lymphoma and infection.

■ Patient should be evaluated for latent tuberculosis infection with a tuberculosis skin test. Treatment of latent tuberculosis infection should be started before infliximab.

leflunomide
CONTRAINDICATIONS AND CAUTIONS

■ Contraindicated in patients hypersensitive to drug or its components and in women who are or may become pregnant or who are breast-feeding.

■ Drug isn't recommended for patients younger than age 18, men attempting to father a child, and patients with bone marrow dysplasia, hepatic insufficiency, hepatitis B or C, severe immunodeficiency, or severe uncontrolled infection.

■ Use cautiously in patients with renal insufficiency.

KEY POINTS

ALERT Men trying to father a child should stop drug therapy and follow recommended leflunomide removal protocol

(cholestyramine 8 g P.O. t.i.d. for 11 days). In addition to following cholestyramine protocol, verify that drug levels are less than 0.02 mg/L by two separate tests at least 14 days apart. If level exceeds 0.02 mg/L, consider additional cholestyramine treatment.

■ Monitor liver enzyme (ALT and AST) levels before starting therapy and monthly thereafter until stable.

methotrexate
CONTRAINDICATIONS AND CAUTIONS

■ Contraindicated in pregnant women, breast-feeding women, patients hypersensitive to drug, and patients with psoriasis or RA who also have alcoholic liver, alcoholism, blood dyscrasias, chronic liver disease, or immunodeficiency syndromes.

■ Use cautiously and possibly at modified dosage in very young, elderly, or debilitated patients; patients with infection, peptic ulceration, or ulcerative colitis; and patients with anemia, aplasia, bone marrow suppression, impaired hepatic or renal function, leukopenia, or thrombocytopenia.

KEY POINTS

■ Monitor pulmonary function tests periodically and fluid intake and output daily. Encourage fluid intake of 2 to 3 L daily.

■ Watch for increases in AST, ALT, and alkaline phosphatase levels, which may signal hepatic dysfunction.

■ To prevent precipitation of drug, especially at high doses, keep urine pH above 7 by giving sodium bicarbonate tablets or I.V. fluids containing sodium bicarbonate. Reduce dosage if blood urea nitrogen (BUN) level is 20 to 30 mg/dl or creatinine level is 1.2 to 2 mg/dl. Stop drug and notify prescriber if BUN level exceeds 30 mg/dl or creatinine level exceeds 2 mg/dl.

rofecoxib

CONTRAINDICATIONS AND CAUTIONS

■ Contraindicated in pregnant women (because drug may cause ductus arteriosus to close prematurely), patients hypersensitive to drug or its components, patients with advanced kidney disease, patients with moderate or severe hepatic insufficiency, and patients in whom aspirin or nonsteroidal anti-inflammatory drugs (NSAIDs) have caused asthma, urticaria, or allergic reactions.

■ Use cautiously in dehydrated patients (rehydrate before therapy), patients with a history of ulcer disease or gastrointestinal (GI) bleeding, patients taking such drugs as oral corticosteroids and anticoagulants, and patients with an increased risk of GI bleeding, such as elderly patients, alcoholic patients, smokers, and those in poor general health.

■ Use cautiously in patients with a history of ischemic heart disease. Because rofecoxib has no platelet effects, it doesn't substitute for aspirin in preventing cardiovascular events. Antiplatelet therapy may continue.

■ Use cautiously in patients with fluid retention, hypertension, or heart failure, and start therapy at the lowest recommended dosage.

KEY POINTS

■ Monitor blood pressure and check patient for fluid retention or worsening heart failure.

■ NSAIDs may cause serious GI toxicity, including bleeding, ulceration, and perforation of the stomach, small intestine, and large intestine.

■ Drug may be hepatotoxic. Monitor patient for evidence of liver toxicity. Stop drug if evidence of liver disease develops.

sulfasalazine
CONTRAINDICATIONS AND CAUTIONS

■ Contraindicated in children younger than age 2, patients hypersensitive to drug or its metabolites, and patients with porphyria, intestinal obstruction, or urinary obstruction.

■ Use cautiously and in reduced amounts in patients with impaired hepatic or renal function, severe allergy, bronchial asthma, or G6PD deficiency.

KEY POINTS

■ Although therapeutic response has been noted as soon as 4 weeks after starting therapy, it may take 12 weeks of therapy before some RA patients show benefit.

■ Drug may discolor urine.

■ Stop drug immediately and notify prescriber if patient shows evidence of hypersensitivity.

17 / DRUGS FOR INFECTIOUS DISORDERS

ANTHRAX

Anthrax is an acute infection caused by the bacterium *Bacillus anthracis*, which exists in the soil as spores that may be viable for years. The infection is most common in grazing animals, such as cattle, sheep, goats, and horses. It can also affect people who contact contaminated animals or their hides, bones, fur, hair, or wool. It also can be transmitted intentionally, as an agent of bioterrorism or biological warfare.

Anthrax occurs worldwide but is most common in developing countries. In humans, it occurs in three forms, depending on the mode of transmission. The spores can enter the body through abraded or broken skin (cutaneous anthrax), by inhalation (inhalational anthrax), or through ingestion of undercooked meat from an infected animal (gastrointestinal anthrax). Anthrax isn't known to spread from person to person.

amoxicillin

CONTRAINDICATIONS AND CAUTIONS

■ Contraindicated in patients hypersensitive to drug or other penicillins.

■ Use cautiously in patients with allergies to other drugs (especially cephalosporins) because of possible cross-sensitivity and in those with mononucleosis because of the high risk of maculopapular rash.

KEY POINTS

■ Before giving drug, ask patient about allergic reactions to penicillin; however, a negative history doesn't rule out future reactions.

■ If large doses are given or therapy is prolonged, bacterial or fungal superinfection may occur, especially in elderly, debilitated, or immunosuppressed patients.

■ Tell patient to take full quantity of drug exactly as prescribed, even if he feels better before the prescription is finished.

ciprofloxacin
CONTRAINDICATIONS AND CAUTIONS
■ Contraindicated in patients sensitive to fluoroquinolones.

■ Use cautiously in patients with central nervous system (CNS) disorders, such as severe cerebral arteriosclerosis or seizure disorders, and in those at risk for seizures. Drug may cause CNS stimulation.

■ Safety in children younger than age 18 hasn't been established; however, drug may be used as recommended by the Centers for Disease Control and Prevention (CDC) for inhalational or cutaneous anthrax as indicated. Drug may cause cartilage erosion.

KEY POINTS
■ Follow current CDC recommendations for anthrax.

■ Cutaneous anthrax with systemic involvement, extensive edema, or lesions on the head or neck needs I.V. therapy and a multidrug approach.

■ Multidrug regimens may include rifampin, vancomycin, penicillin, ampicillin, chloram-

phenicol, imipenem, clindamycin, and clarithromycin.

■ Corticosteroids may be considered as adjunctive therapy for anthrax patients with severe edema and for meningitis, based on experience with bacterial meningitis of other etiologies.

doxycycline
CONTRAINDICATIONS AND CAUTIONS
■ Contraindicated in patients hypersensitive to drug or other tetracyclines.

■ Use cautiously in patients with impaired renal or hepatic function.

■ Use of this drug during the last half of pregnancy and in children younger than age 8 may retard bone growth and cause permanent tooth discoloration and enamel defects.

KEY POINTS
■ Cutaneous anthrax with systemic involvement, extensive edema, or lesions on the head or neck needs I.V. therapy and a multidrug approach.

■ Multidrug regimen may include rifampin, vancomycin, penicillin, ampicillin, chloramphenicol, imipenem, clindamycin, and clarithromycin.

■ Corticosteroids may be considered as adjunctive therapy for anthrax patients with severe edema and for meningitis, based on experience with bacterial meningitis of other etiologies.

penicillin G potassium

CONTRAINDICATIONS AND CAUTIONS

- Contraindicated in patients hypersensitive to drug or other penicillins.
- Use cautiously in patients with allergies to other drugs, especially cephalosporins, because of possible cross-sensitivity.

KEY POINTS

- Monitor renal function closely. Patients with poor renal function are predisposed to high blood levels of drug.
- Monitor potassium and sodium levels closely in patients receiving more than 10 million units I.V. daily.
- Observe patient closely. With large doses and prolonged therapy, bacterial or fungal superinfection may occur, especially in elderly, debilitated, or immunosuppressed patients.

penicillin G procaine

CONTRAINDICATIONS AND CAUTIONS

- Contraindicated in patients hypersensitive to drug or other penicillins.
- Use cautiously in patients with allergies to other drugs, especially cephalosporins, because of possible cross-sensitivity. Some forms contain sulfites, which may cause allergic reactions in sensitive persons.

KEY POINTS

- *ALERT Treatment for inhalational anthrax (postexposure) must last 60 days. Prescriber should consider the risk-benefit ratio of continuing penicillin longer than 2 weeks, compared with switching to an effective alternate drug.*
- Allergic reactions are hard to treat because of drug's slow absorption rate.
- Monitor renal and hematopoietic function periodically.

CANDIDIASIS

Candidiasis is usually a mild, superficial fungal infection caused by a yeast-like fungus of the genus *Candida*. The infection usually affects the nails (onychomycosis), skin (diaper rash), or mucous membranes, especially the oropharynx (thrush), vagina (candidiasis), esophagus, and gastrointestinal (GI) tract. Rarely, fungi enter the bloodstream and invade the kidneys, lungs, endocardium, brain, or other structures, causing serious infection. Systemic infection occurs mainly in drug abusers and patients already hospitalized, particularly diabetics and immunosuppressed patients.

Although various strains of *Candida* are part of the normal flora of the GI tract, mouth, vagina, and skin, they can cause infection when a change in the body permits their sudden proliferation. The usual trigger is the use of broad-spectrum antibiotics, which decreases the number of normal flora and allows candidal organisms to proliferate. Other triggers include rising blood glucose levels from diabetes mellitus; lowered resistance from a disease (such as cancer), an immunosuppressant, radiation, aging, or human immunodeficiency virus (HIV) infection; or systemic introduction through I.V. or urinary catheter use, drug abuse, hyperalimentation, or surgery. The occurrence of candidiasis is rising because I.V. therapy is more widely used and because there are more immunocompromised patients, especially those with HIV infection.

amphotericin B desoxycholate
CONTRAINDICATIONS AND CAUTIONS
■ Contraindicated in patients hypersensitive to drug.

■ Use cautiously in patients with impaired renal function.

KEY POINTS
■ Because of drug's dangerous adverse effects, it's used mainly for patients with progressive, potentially fatal fungal infections.

■ Infusion-related reactions, including fever, shaking chills, hypotension, anorexia, nausea, vomiting, headache, dyspnea, and tachypnea, may occur 1 to 3 hours after starting infusion.

ALERT *Amphotericin B preparations and dosages aren't interchangeable. Confusing them may cause permanent damage or death.*

clotrimazole
CONTRAINDICATIONS AND CAUTIONS
■ Contraindicated in patients hypersensitive to drug. Also contraindicated for ophthalmic use.

■ Watch for and report irritation or sensitivity; stop drug if irritation occurs, and notify prescriber.

■ Improvement usually occurs within 1 week; if no improvement occurs after 4 weeks, diagnosis should be reviewed.

■ Warn patient not to use occlusive wraps or dressings.

econazole

CONTRAINDICATIONS AND CAUTIONS

■ Contraindicated in patients hypersensitive to drug or its components.

■ Clean and dry affected area before applying.

■ Don't use occlusive dressings.

■ Tell patient to stop drug and call prescriber if condition persists or worsens or if irritation occurs.

fluconazole

CONTRAINDICATIONS AND CAUTIONS

■ Contraindicated in patients hypersensitive to drug and in breast-feeding patients.

■ Use cautiously in patients hypersensitive to other antifungal azole compounds.

KEY POINTS

■ Serious hepatotoxicity has occurred in patients with underlying medical conditions.

■ Periodically monitor liver function during prolonged therapy.

■ If mild rash develops, monitor patient closely. Stop drug if lesions progress, and notify prescriber.

ketoconazole

CONTRAINDICATIONS AND CAUTIONS

■ Contraindicated in patients hypersensitive to drug.

■ Use oral form cautiously in patients with hepatic disease and in those taking other hepatotoxic drugs.

■ Use topical form cautiously in breast-feeding women.

KEY POINTS

■ Oral doses up to 800 mg/day can be used to treat fungal meningitis and intracerebral fungal lesions.

■ Because of potential for hepatotoxicity, oral ketoconazole shouldn't be used for minor conditions, such as fungal infections of skin or nails.

■ Monitor patient taking oral form for evidence of hepatotoxicity, including elevated liver enzyme levels, nausea that won't subside, and unusual fatigue, jaundice, dark urine, or pale stool.

nystatin

CONTRAINDICATIONS AND CAUTIONS

■ Contraindicated in patients hypersensitive to drug.

KEY POINTS

■ Nystatin isn't effective against systemic infections.

- Don't use occlusive dressings.
- Cream is recommended for skinfolds; powder for moist areas; ointment for dry areas.

CONJUNCTIVITIS

In conjunctivitis, hyperemia of the conjunctiva stems from infection, allergy, or a chemical reaction. Infectious conjunctivitis typically results from bacteria (most commonly *Staphylococcus aureus*, *Streptococcus pneumoniae*, *Neisseria gonorrhoeae*, or *Neisseria meningitides*) or one of a number of viruses, including herpes simplex type 1. Bacterial and viral conjunctivitis are highly contagious but typically resolve after about 2 weeks. The infection may start in one eye but typically spreads to both.

Allergic conjunctivitis typically stems from a reaction to pollen, grass, a topical drug, an air pollutant, or smoke. It's bilateral, may be seasonal, and typically starts before puberty and lasts about 10 years. Some patients have other evidence of allergy to grass or pollen.

Chemical conjunctivitis may follow exposure to an occupational irritant, such as an acid or alkali and may affect only one eye. Conjunctivitis also may result from rickettsial disease (Rocky Mountain spotted fever) or parasitic disease caused by *Phthirus pubis* or *Schistosoma haematobium*. And an idiopathic form of conjunctivitis may result from certain systemic diseases, such as erythema multiforme, chronic follicular (orphan's) conjunctivitis, thyroid disease, and Stevens-Johnson syndrome.

azelastine
CONTRAINDICATIONS AND CAUTIONS
- Contraindicated in patients hypersensitive to any component of the drug.

KEY POINTS
- Drug is indicated only for ocular use.
- Don't use to treat contact lens–related irritation.
- The preservative benzalkonium may be absorbed by soft contact lenses.

ciprofloxacin
CONTRAINDICATIONS AND CAUTIONS
- Contraindicated in patients hypersensitive to ciprofloxacin or other fluoroquinolone antibiotics.
- Use cautiously in breast-feeding women.

KEY POINTS

■ A topical overdose may be flushed from eyes with warm tap water.

■ If the corneal epithelium is still compromised after 14 days of treatment, continue therapy.

■ Prolonged use may result in overgrowth of nonsusceptible organisms, including fungi. Start appropriate treatment if superinfection occurs.

erythromycin

CONTRAINDICATIONS AND CAUTIONS

■ Contraindicated in patients hypersensitive to drug.

■ Use cautiously in breast-feeding women.

KEY POINTS

■ Drug should be used only when sensitivity studies show it's effective against infecting organisms; it shouldn't be used in infections of unknown cause.

■ Advise patient to watch for and report evidence of sensitivity (itching, red lids, swelling or constant burning).

■ Tell patient that vision may be blurred for a few minutes after applying ointment.

gentamicin

CONTRAINDICATIONS AND CAUTIONS

■ Contraindicated in patients hypersensitive to drug.

■ Use cautiously in patients with history of sensitivity to aminoglycosides because cross-sensitivity may occur.

KEY POINTS

■ Obtain specimen for culture before giving drug. Therapy may begin before culture results are known.

■ Systemic absorption from overuse may cause toxicities.

■ If ophthalmic gentamicin is given with systemic gentamicin, monitor gentamicin levels.

ofloxacin

CONTRAINDICATIONS AND CAUTIONS

■ Contraindicated in patients hypersensitive to ofloxacin, other fluoroquinolones, or other components of drug; also contraindicated in breast-feeding women.

KEY POINTS

■ Stop drug if improvement doesn't occur within 7 days. Prolonged use may result in overgrowth of nonsusceptible organisms, including fungi.

■ If an allergic reaction occurs, tell patient to stop drug and notify prescriber. Serious acute hypersensitivity reactions may need emergency treatment.

■ Warn patient not to use leftover drug for new eye infection.

CYTOMEGALOVIRUS INFECTION

Also called *cytomegalic inclusion disease*, cytomegalovirus (CMV) infection is caused by a DNA, ether-sensitive virus of the herpes family. About four out of five persons older than age 35 have been infected with CMV, usually during childhood or early adulthood. Usually, the disease is so mild that it's overlooked. The disease occurs worldwide and is transmitted by human contact.

CMV has been found in the saliva, urine, semen, breast milk, stool, blood, and vaginal and cervical secretions of infected persons. Transmission usually happens through contact with these infected secretions, which harbor the virus for months or even years.

ALERT *CMV infection during pregnancy can be hazardous to the fetus, possibly leading to birth defects, brain damage, severe neonatal illness, or stillbirth.*

The virus may be transmitted by sexual contact and can cross the placenta to cause a congenital infection. Immunosuppressed patients, especially those who have received organ transplants, run a 90% chance of contracting CMV infection. Recipients of blood transfusions from donors with positive CMV antibodies are at some risk. And pregnant women who develop mononucleosis should also be evaluated for CMV infection.

cidofovir

CONTRAINDICATIONS AND CAUTIONS

■ Contraindicated in patients hypersensitive to drug, patients with a history of severe hypersensitivity to probenecid or other sulfur-containing drugs, patients receiving drugs with nephrotoxic potential, and patients with a creatinine level above 1.5 mg/dl, a calculated creatinine clearance of 55 ml/minute or less, or a urine protein level of 100 mg/dl or more (equivalent to 2+ proteinuria or more).

■ Use cautiously in patients with impaired renal function. Monitor renal function tests and patient's fluid balance.

■ Safety and effectiveness in children haven't been established.

■ It's unknown if cidofovir appears in breast milk. Don't give drug to breast-feeding women.

KEY POINTS

■ Cidofovir is indicated only for CMV retinitis in patients with acquired immunodeficiency syndrome. Safety and efficacy haven't been established for other CMV infections, congenital or neonatal CMV disease, or CMV disease in patients not infected with human immunodeficiency virus.

■ Drug shouldn't be given as a direct intraocular injection because it may cause vision impairment and significant decreases in intraocular pressure.

■ Monitor renal function (serum creatinine and urine protein levels) before each dose. Dosage may be modified by a prescriber if renal function changes.

■ Fanconi's syndrome and decreased bicarbonate levels with renal tubular damage have been reported in patients receiving cidofovir. Monitor patient closely.

fomivirsen
CONTRAINDICATIONS AND CAUTIONS

■ Contraindicated in patients hypersensitive to drug or its components and in those treated with I.V. or intravitreal cidofovir during previous 2 to 4 weeks because of the risk of exaggerated ocular inflammation.

KEY POINTS

■ Drug is for ophthalmic use only by intravitreal injection.

■ Drug provides localized therapy for the treated eye and not for the other eye or for systemic CMV disease. Monitor patient for extraocular CMV disease or disease in the other eye.

■ Monitor light perception and optic nerve head perfusion after injection.

foscarnet
CONTRAINDICATIONS AND CAUTIONS

■ Contraindicated in patients hypersensitive to drug.

■ Because drug is nephrotoxic, use it cautiously and at reduced amounts in patients with abnormal renal function. Some degree of nephrotoxicity occurs in most patients who receive this drug.

KEY POINTS

■ Because drug is highly toxic and toxicity is probably dose-related, always use the lowest effective dosage.

■ Monitor creatinine clearance often during therapy because of drug's adverse effects on renal function. A baseline 24-hour creatinine clearance is recommended, and then regular determinations two to three times weekly during induction and at least once every 1 to 2 weeks during maintenance.

■ Because drug can alter electrolytes, monitor levels using a schedule similar to that for creatinine clearance. Assess patient for tetany and seizures caused by abnormal electrolyte levels.

ALERT Monitor patient's hemoglobin level and hematocrit. Anemia occurs in up to 33% of patients treated with drug. It may be severe enough to need transfusions.

ganciclovir

CONTRAINDICATIONS AND CAUTIONS

■ Contraindicated in patients hypersensitive to drug or to acyclovir, patients with an absolute neutrophil count below 500/mm³, and patients with a platelet count below 25,000/mm³.

■ Use cautiously and at a reduced dosage in patients with renal dysfunction. Monitor renal function tests.

KEY POINTS

■ Because of the risk of agranulocytosis and thrombocytopenia, obtain neutrophil and platelet counts every 2 days during twice-daily ganciclovir dosing and at least weekly thereafter.

■ Explain the importance of drinking plenty of fluids during therapy.

■ Advise patient that drug causes birth defects. Instruct women to use effective birth control during treatment; instruct men to use barrier contraception during and for at least 90 days after taking ganciclovir.

valganciclovir

CONTRAINDICATIONS AND CAUTIONS

■ Contraindicated in patients hypersensitive to valganciclovir or ganciclovir.

■ Don't use in patients receiving hemodialysis.

■ Use cautiously in patients with cytopenias and in those who have received immunosuppressants or radiation.

KEY POINTS

■ Follow the dosing guidelines for valganciclovir because ganciclovir and valganciclovir aren't interchangeable and overdose may occur.

ALERT Toxicities include severe leukopenia, neutropenia, anemia, pancytopenia, bone marrow depression, aplastic anemia, and thrombocytopenia. Don't give drug if patient's absolute neutrophil count is less than 500 cells/mm³, platelet count is less than 25,000/mm³, or hemoglobin is less than 8 g/dl.

■ Monitor complete blood count, platelet counts, and creatinine levels or clearance often during treatment.

GONORRHEA

A common sexually transmitted disease, gonorrhea is an infection of the genitourinary tract, especially the urethra and cervix and occasionally the rectum, pharynx, and eyes. Untreated gonorrhea can spread through the blood to the joints, tendons, meninges, and endocardium; in women, it can lead to chronic pelvic inflammatory disease and sterility.

Transmission of *Neisseria gonorrhoeae* almost always follows sexual contact with an infected person. Children born to infected mothers can contract gonococcal ophthalmia neonatorum during passage through the birth canal. Children and adults with gonorrhea can contract gonococcal conjunctivitis by touching their eyes with contaminated hands.

After adequate treatment, the prognosis is excellent, although reinfection is common. Gonorrhea is most common among people with multiple sex partners and among young people, particularly those ages 19 to 25.

amoxicillin
CONTRAINDICATIONS AND CAUTIONS
■ Contraindicated in patients hypersensitive to drug or other penicillins.
■ Use cautiously in patients with other drug allergies (especially to cephalosporins) because of possible cross-sensitivity and in those with mononucleosis because of a high risk of maculopapular rash.

KEY POINTS
■ Before giving drug, ask patient about allergic reactions to penicillin, although a negative history doesn't guarantee freedom from future reactions.
■ If large doses are given or therapy is prolonged, bacterial or fungal superinfection may occur, especially in elderly, debilitated, or immunosuppressed patients.
■ Tell patient to take entire quantity of drug exactly as prescribed, even if he feels better before prescription is finished.

azithromycin

CONTRAINDICATIONS AND CAUTIONS

■ Contraindicated in patients hypersensitive to erythromycin or other macrolides.

■ Use cautiously in patients with impaired hepatic function.

KEY POINTS

■ Obtain specimen for culture and sensitivity tests before giving first dose. Therapy may begin pending results.

■ Monitor patient for superinfection. Drug may cause overgrowth of nonsusceptible bacteria or fungi.

■ May cause photosensitivity. Advise patient to avoid excessive sunlight exposure.

cefotaxime

CONTRAINDICATIONS AND CAUTIONS

■ Contraindicated in patients hypersensitive to drug or other cephalosporins.

■ Use cautiously in patients hypersensitive to penicillin because of the possibility of cross-sensitivity with other beta-lactam antibiotics. Also use cautiously in breast-feeding women and patients with a history of colitis or renal insufficiency.

KEY POINTS

■ Obtain specimen for culture and sensitivity tests before giving first dose. Therapy may begin pending results.

■ If large doses are given, therapy is prolonged, or patient is at high risk, watch for superinfection.

■ Instruct patient to report discomfort at I.V. insertion site.

ceftizoxime

CONTRAINDICATIONS AND CAUTIONS

■ Contraindicated in patients hypersensitive to drug or other cephalosporins.

■ Use cautiously in patients hypersensitive to penicillin because of possible cross-sensitivity with other beta-lactam antibiotics. Also use cautiously in breast-feeding women and patients with a history of colitis or renal insufficiency.

KEY POINTS

■ Obtain specimen for culture and sensitivity tests before giving first dose. Therapy may begin pending results.

■ If large doses are given, therapy is prolonged, or patient is at high risk, watch for superinfection.

■ Instruct patient to report discomfort at I.V. insertion site.

ceftriaxone

CONTRAINDICATIONS AND CAUTIONS

■ Contraindicated in patients hypersensitive to drug or other cephalosporins.

■ Use cautiously in patients hypersensitive to penicillin because of possible cross-sensitivity with other beta-lactam antibiotics. Also use cautiously in breast-feeding women and patients with a history of colitis or renal insufficiency.

KEY POINTS

■ Obtain specimen for culture and sensitivity tests before giving first dose. Therapy may begin pending results.

■ If large doses are given, therapy is prolonged, or patient is at high risk, watch for superinfection.

■ Monitor prothrombin time and international normalized ratio in patients with impaired vitamin K synthesis or low vitamin K stores. Vitamin K therapy may be needed.

doxycycline

CONTRAINDICATIONS AND CAUTIONS

■ Contraindicated in patients hypersensitive to drug or other tetracyclines.

■ Use cautiously in patients with impaired renal or hepatic function. Use of these drugs during the last half of pregnancy and in children younger than age 8 may retard bone growth and cause permanent tooth discoloration and enamel defects.

KEY POINTS

■ Check expiration date. Outdated or deteriorated tetracyclines may cause reversible nephrotoxicity (Fanconi's syndrome).

■ Check patient's tongue for signs of fungal infection. Stress good oral hygiene.

■ Photosensitivity reactions may occur within a few minutes to several hours after exposure. Explain that susceptibility may last some time after therapy ends.

erythromycin

CONTRAINDICATIONS AND CAUTIONS

■ Contraindicated in pregnant patients and in patients hypersensitive to drug or to other macrolides.

■ Use erythromycin cautiously in patients with impaired hepatic function, and monitor liver function test results.

■ Drug appears in breast milk. Use cautiously in breast-feeding women.

KEY POINTS

■ Obtain urine specimen for culture and sensitivity tests before giving first dose. Therapy may begin pending results.

■ Monitor hepatic function (increased levels of alkaline phosphatase, alanine transaminase, aspartate transaminase, and bilirubin may occur).

■ Ototoxicity may occur, especially in patients with renal or hepatic insufficiency and in those receiving high doses of drug.

gatifloxacin
CONTRAINDICATIONS AND CAUTIONS

■ Contraindicated in patients hypersensitive to fluoroquinolones. Don't use in patients with prolonged QTc interval or uncorrected hypokalemia.

■ Use cautiously in patients with clinically significant bradycardia, acute myocardial ischemia, known or suspected central nervous system (CNS) disorders, or renal insufficiency.

KEY POINTS

■ In patients being treated for gonorrhea, test for syphilis at time of diagnosis.

■ Stop drug if patient has CNS stimulation with tremors, confusion, depression, hallucinations, increased intracranial pressure, insomnia, lightheadedness, nightmares, paranoia, psychosis, restlessness, or seizures. Also stop drug if patient has pain, inflammation, or tendon rupture.

■ Advise patient to use sunblock and protective clothing to reduce excessive exposure to sunlight.

ofloxacin
CONTRAINDICATIONS AND CAUTIONS

■ Contraindicated in patients hypersensitive to drug or other fluoroquinolones.

■ Use cautiously in pregnant women and in patients with seizure disorders, CNS diseases (such as cerebral arteriosclerosis), hepatic disorders, or renal impairment.

■ Ofloxacin appears in breast milk in levels similar to those found in plasma. Safety hasn't been established in breast-feeding women.

■ Safety and efficacy in children younger than age 18 haven't been established.

KEY POINTS

■ Patients treated for gonorrhea should have a serologic test for syphilis. Drug isn't effective against syphilis, and treatment of gonorrhea may mask or delay symptoms of syphilis.

■ Monitor renal and hepatic studies and complete blood count in prolonged therapy.

■ Advise patient to avoid prolonged exposure to direct sunlight and to use a sunscreen when outdoors.

penicillin G procaine
CONTRAINDICATIONS AND CAUTIONS

■ Contraindicated in patients hypersensitive to drug or other penicillins.

■ Use cautiously in patients allergic to other drugs, especially cephalosporins, because of possible cross-sensitivity. Some forms contain sulfites, which may cause allergic reactions in sensitive persons.

KEY POINTS

🌀 *ALERT Never give by I.V. route. Inadvertent I.V. administration may cause death from CNS toxicity.*

■ Allergic reactions are hard to treat because of drug's slow absorption rate.

■ Monitor renal and hematopoietic function periodically.

HERPES SIMPLEX

A recurrent viral infection, herpes simplex is subclinical in about 85% of cases. The others produce localized lesions and systemic reactions. After the first infection, a patient is a carrier susceptible to recurrent infections, which may be provoked by fever, menses, stress, heat, and cold. In recurrent infections, the patient usually has no systemic signs and symptoms.

Herpes simplex is caused by *Herpes-virus hominis* (HVH), a widespread infectious agent. Type 1 herpes, which is transmitted by oral and respiratory secretions, affects the skin and mucous membranes and commonly produces cold sores and fever blisters. Type 2 herpes primarily affects the genital area and is transmitted by sexual contact. Cross-infection may result from orogenital sex.

Primary HVH is the leading cause of gingivostomatitis in children ages 1 to 3. It causes the most common nonepidemic encephalitis and is the second most common viral infection in pregnant women. It can pass to the fetus across the placenta and, in early pregnancy, may cause spontaneous abortion or premature birth.

Herpes is equally common in men and women. It occurs worldwide and is most prevalent among children in lower socioeconomic groups who live in

Safety and efficacy in children haven't been established.

Use of drug during pregnancy should be considered only if the benefits outweigh the risks.

If patient is breast-feeding, drug may need to be stopped.

KEY POINTS

Teach patient the signs and symptoms of herpes infection (rash, tingling, itching, and pain), and advise him to notify prescriber immediately if they occur. Treatment should begin as soon as possible after symptoms appear, preferably within 48 hours of the onset of zoster rash.

Tell patient that valacyclovir doesn't cure herpes but may decrease the length and severity of symptoms.

Don't confuse valacyclovir (Valtrex) with valganciclovir (Valcyte).

vidarabine
CONTRAINDICATIONS AND CAUTIONS

Contraindicated in patients hypersensitive to drug.

KEY POINTS

Explain to patient that ointment may cause a temporary visual haze.

Advise patient to watch for signs of sensitivity, such as itch-ing lids, swelling, or constant burning.

Tell patient to minimize sensitivity to sunlight by wearing sunglasses and avoiding prolonged exposure to sunlight.

MENINGITIS

With meningitis, the brain and the spinal cord meninges become inflamed, usually as a result of bacterial infection. Such inflammation may involve all three meningeal membranes — the dura mater, arachnoid, and pia mater — along with adjacent tissues and nerve cells. About 70% of cases occur in children younger than age 5, and meningitis is increasing among college students who live in dormitories.

Meningitis is almost always a complication of another bacterial infection caused by *Neisseria meningitidis, Haemophilus influenzae, Streptococcus pneumoniae,* or *Escherichia coli.* Examples of such infections include bacteremia (especially from pneumonia, empyema, osteomyelitis, and endocarditis), sinusitis, otitis media, tooth abscess, encephalitis, myelitis, or brain abscess. Viral meningitis usually is less severe and usually is a com-

TELLTALE SIGNS OF MENINGITIS

Brudzinski's sign

To test for *Brudzinski's sign*, place the patient in a dorsal recumbent position, and then put your hands behind his neck and bend it forward. Pain and resistance may indicate meningeal inflammation, neck injury, or arthritis. However, if the patient also flexes the hips and knees in response to this manipulation, chances are he has meningitis.

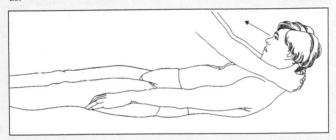

Kernig's sign

To test for *Kernig's sign*, place the patient in a supine position. Flex his leg at the hip and knee, and then straighten the knee. Pain or resistance points to meningitis.

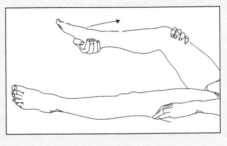

plication of an existing viral infection.

Meningitis also may follow a skull fracture, penetrating head wound, lumbar puncture, or ventricular shunting procedure. Aseptic meningitis may result from a virus or other organism. Sometimes no causative organism can be found.

The diagnosis usually relies on the results of a lumbar puncture and positive Brudzinski's and Kernig's signs. (See *Telltale signs of meningitis*.) The prognosis is good and complications are rare, especially if the disease is recognized early and the infecting organism responds to an antibiotic. However, mortality in patients with untreated meningitis is 70% to 100%. The prognosis is poorer for infants, elderly people, and those who are immunocompromised.

amphotericin B desoxycholate

CONTRAINDICATIONS AND CAUTIONS

■ Contraindicated in patients hypersensitive to drug.

■ Use cautiously in patients with impaired renal function.

KEY POINTS

■ Because of drug's dangerous adverse effects, it's used mainly for patients with progressive and potentially fatal fungal infections.

■ Infusion-related reactions, including fever, shaking chills, hypotension, anorexia, nausea, vomiting, headache, dyspnea, and tachypnea, may occur 1 to 3 hours after starting infusion.

ALERT Amphotericin B preparations and dosages aren't interchangeable. Confusing them may cause permanent damage or death.

ampicillin

CONTRAINDICATIONS AND CAUTIONS

■ Contraindicated in patients hypersensitive to drug or other penicillins.

■ Use cautiously in patients with allergies to other drugs (especially cephalosporins) because of possible cross-sensitivity and in those with mononucleosis because of a high risk of maculopapular rash.

KEY POINTS

■ In pediatric meningitis, ampicillin may be given with parenteral chloramphenicol for 24 hours pending cultures.

■ If large doses are given or therapy is prolonged, bacterial or fungal superinfection may occur, especially in elderly, debilitated, or immunosuppressed patients.

■ Watch for evidence of hypersensitivity, such as erythematous maculopapular rash, urticaria, and anaphylaxis.

ceftizoxime

CONTRAINDICATIONS AND CAUTIONS

■ Contraindicated in patients hypersensitive to drug or other cephalosporins.

■ Use cautiously in patients hypersensitive to penicillin because of possibility of cross-sensitivity with other beta-lactam antibiotics. Also use cautiously in breast-feeding women and patients with a history of colitis or renal insufficiency.

KEY POINTS

■ Obtain specimen for culture and sensitivity tests before giving first dose. Therapy may begin pending results.

■ If large doses are given, therapy is prolonged, or patient is at high risk, monitor patient for superinfection.

■ Instruct patient to report discomfort at I.V. insertion site.

ceftriaxone

CONTRAINDICATIONS AND CAUTIONS

■ Contraindicated in patients hypersensitive to drug or other cephalosporins.

■ Use cautiously in patients hypersensitive to penicillin because of possibility of cross-sensitivity with other beta-lactam antibiotics. Also use cautiously in breast-feeding women and in patients with a history of colitis or renal insufficiency.

KEY POINTS

■ Obtain specimen for culture and sensitivity tests before giving first dose. Therapy may begin pending results.

■ If large doses are given, therapy is prolonged, or patient is at high risk, monitor patient for signs and symptoms of superinfection.

■ Monitor prothrombin time and international normalized ratio in patients with impaired vitamin K synthesis or low vitamin K stores. Vitamin K therapy may be needed.

cefuroxime

CONTRAINDICATIONS AND CAUTIONS

■ Contraindicated in patients hypersensitive to drug or other cephalosporins.

■ Use cautiously in patients hypersensitive to penicillin because of possibility of cross-sensitivity with other beta-lactam antibiotics. Also use cautiously in breast-feeding women and in patients with a history of colitis or renal insufficiency.

KEY POINTS

■ Obtain specimen for culture and sensitivity tests before giving first dose. Therapy may begin pending results.

■ If large doses are given, therapy is prolonged, or patient is at high risk, monitor patient for signs and symptoms of superinfection.

■ Advise patient receiving drug I.V. to report discomfort at I.V. insertion site.

chloramphenicol

CONTRAINDICATIONS AND CAUTIONS

■ Contraindicated in patients hypersensitive to drug.

■ Use cautiously in patients with impaired hepatic or renal function, acute intermittent porphyria, or G6PD deficiency; also use cautiously with other drugs that cause bone marrow suppression or blood disorders.

■ Use cautiously in premature infants and newborns because potentially fatal gray syndrome may occur. Symptoms include abdominal distention, gray cyanosis, vasomotor collapse, respiratory distress, and death within a few hours of symptom onset.

KEY POINTS

■ Obtain plasma levels. Maintain levels at 5 to 20 mcg/ml.

ALERT *Monitor complete blood count and levels of platelets, iron, and reticulocytes before and every 2 days during therapy. Stop drug immediately if anemia, reticulocytopenia, leukopenia, or thrombocytopenia develops, and notify prescriber.*

■ Monitor patient for evidence of superinfection.

fluconazole
CONTRAINDICATIONS AND CAUTIONS

■ Contraindicated in breast-feeding women and patients hypersensitive to drug.

■ Use cautiously in patients hypersensitive to other antifungal azole compounds.

KEY POINTS

■ Serious hepatotoxicity has occurred in patients with underlying medical conditions.

■ Periodically monitor liver function in prolonged therapy.

■ If patient develops mild rash, monitor him closely. Stop drug if lesions progress, and notify prescriber.

flucytosine
CONTRAINDICATIONS AND CAUTIONS

■ Contraindicated in patients hypersensitive to drug.

■ Use with extreme caution in patients with impaired hepatic or renal function or bone marrow suppression.

KEY POINTS

■ Monitor blood, liver, and renal function studies often during therapy; obtain susceptibility tests weekly to monitor drug resistance.

■ If possible, obtain blood level assays of drug regularly to maintain flucytosine at therapeutic level of 40 to 60 mcg/ml. Blood levels above 100 mcg/ml may be toxic.

■ Monitor fluid intake and output; report marked changes.

meropenem

CONTRAINDICATIONS AND CAUTIONS

■ Contraindicated in patients hypersensitive to components of drug or other drugs in same class and in patients who have had anaphylactic reactions to beta-lactams.

■ For bacterial meningitis, drug is approved only for children age 3 months and older.

KEY POINTS

■ Serious and occasionally fatal hypersensitivity reactions may occur in patients receiving therapy with beta-lactams. Before therapy begins, determine whether patient has had hypersensitivity reactions to penicillins, cephalosporins, other beta-lactams, or other allergens.

■ Seizures and other adverse central nervous system (CNS) reactions may be caused by meropenem therapy in patients with CNS disorders, bacterial meningitis, or compromised renal function.

■ Periodic assessment of organ system functions, including renal, hepatic, and hematopoietic function, is recommended during prolonged therapy.

nafcillin

CONTRAINDICATIONS AND CAUTIONS

■ Contraindicated in patients hypersensitive to drug or other penicillins.

■ Use cautiously in patients with gastrointestinal distress and in those with other drug allergies (especially to cephalosporins) because of possible cross-sensitivity.

KEY POINTS

■ If large doses are given or therapy is prolonged, bacterial or fungal superinfection may occur, especially in elderly, debilitated, or immunosuppressed patients.

■ Monitor white blood cell counts twice weekly in patients receiving nafcillin for longer than 2 weeks. Neutropenia commonly occurs in the third week.

■ An abnormal urinalysis result may indicate drug-induced interstitial nephritis.

OTITIS MEDIA

Inflammation of the middle ear, otitis media may be acute or chronic, suppurative or secretory. Acute otitis media is common in children, particularly during the winter months, paralleling the seasonal rise in non-bacterial respiratory tract infections. With prompt treatment, it typically clears up completely; however, prolonged accumulation of fluid in the middle ear cavity can lead to chronic otitis media with possible scarring, adhesions, and hearing loss.

In the suppurative form of otitis media, nasopharyngeal flora reflux through the eustachian tube and colonize the middle ear, usually aided by a respiratory tract infection, allergic reaction, nasotracheal intubation, or positional change. The most common causative organisms are pneumococci, *Haemophilus influenzae* (the most common in children younger than age 6), *Moraxella catarrhalis*, beta-hemolytic streptococci, staphylococci (the most common in children age 6 or older), and gram-negative bacteria.

In the secretory form of otitis media, obstruction of the eustachian tube creates negative pressure in the middle ear that promotes transudation of sterile serous fluid from blood vessels in the membrane of the middle ear. The effusion may stem from eustachian tube dysfunction from viral infection or allergy. It also may follow barotrauma (pressure injury caused by inability to equalize pressures between the environment and the middle ear), as during rapid aircraft descent in a person with an upper respiratory tract infection or during rapid underwater ascent in scuba diving (barotitis media).

amoxicillin and clavulanate potassium
CONTRAINDICATIONS AND CAUTIONS

■ Contraindicated in patients hypersensitive to drug or other penicillins, patients on hemodialysis, patients with creatinine clearance less than 30 ml/minute, and patients with a history of amoxicillin-related cholestatic jaundice or hepatic dysfunction.

■ Use cautiously in patients with allergies to other drugs (especially to cephalosporins) because of possibility of cross-sensitivity, patients with mononucleosis because of the high risk of maculopapular rash, and patients with hepatic impairment. Monitor hepatic function.

■ Use cautiously in breast-feeding women; drug appears in breast milk.

KEY POINTS

- Don't interchange the oral suspensions because of varying clavulanic acid contents.
- Augmentin ES-600 is intended only for persistent or recurrent acute otitis media in children age 3 months to 12 years.
- Avoid use of 250-mg tablet in children who weigh less than 40 kg (88 lb). Use chewable form instead.

CLINICAL TIP The 250- and 500-mg film-coated tablets contain the same amount of clavulanic acid (125 mg). Therefore, two 250-mg tablets aren't equivalent to one 500-mg tablet. And regular tablets aren't equivalent to Augmentin XR.

azithromycin

CONTRAINDICATIONS AND CAUTIONS

- Contraindicated in patients hypersensitive to erythromycin or other macrolides.
- Use cautiously in patients with impaired hepatic function.

KEY POINTS

- May cause photosensitivity. Advise patient to avoid excessive sunlight exposure.
- Monitor patient for superinfection. Drug may cause overgrowth of nonsusceptible bacteria or fungi.

- Tell patient to take all of the drug as prescribed, even if he feels better before the prescription is finished.

cefaclor

CONTRAINDICATIONS AND CAUTIONS

- Contraindicated in patients hypersensitive to drug or other cephalosporins.
- Use cautiously in patients hypersensitive to penicillin because of the possibility of cross-sensitivity with other beta-lactam antibiotics. Also use cautiously in breast-feeding women and in patients with a history of colitis or renal insufficiency.

KEY POINTS

- If large doses are given, therapy is prolonged, or patient is at high risk, watch for signs and symptoms of superinfection.
- Tell patient to take entire amount of drug exactly as prescribed, even if he feels better before the prescription is finished.
- Drug may cause photosensitivity. Advise patient to avoid excessive exposure to sunlight.

cefpodoxime

CONTRAINDICATIONS AND CAUTIONS

■ Contraindicated in patients hypersensitive to drug or other cephalosporins.

■ Use cautiously in breast-feeding women, patients with a history of penicillin hypersensitivity because of the risk of cross-sensitivity, and patients receiving nephrotoxic drugs because other cephalosporins have nephrotoxic potential.

KEY POINTS

■ Monitor renal function and compare with baseline.

■ Give drug with food to enhance absorption.

■ Monitor patient for superinfection because drug may cause overgrowth of nonsusceptible bacteria or fungi.

cefprozil

CONTRAINDICATIONS AND CAUTIONS

■ Contraindicated in patients hypersensitive to drug or other cephalosporins.

■ Use cautiously in breast-feeding women, patients hypersensitive to penicillin because of possible cross-sensitivity with other beta-lactam antibiotics, and patients with history of colitis or renal insufficiency.

KEY POINTS

■ Monitor renal and liver function test results.

■ Monitor patient for superinfection because drug may cause overgrowth of nonsusceptible bacteria or fungi.

■ Advise patient to take drug as prescribed, even after he feels better.

cefuroxime

CONTRAINDICATIONS AND CAUTIONS

■ Contraindicated in patients hypersensitive to drug or other cephalosporins.

■ Use cautiously in breast-feeding women, patients hypersensitive to penicillin because of possible cross-sensitivity with other beta-lactam antibiotics, and patients with a history of colitis or renal insufficiency.

KEY POINTS

■ Cefuroxime axetil absorption is enhanced by food.

🌀 *ALERT Cefuroxime axetil film-coated tablet and oral suspension aren't bioequivalent. Don't substitute on a mg/mg basis.*

■ Tell patient to take all of the drug prescribed, even if he feels better before the prescription is finished.

cephalexin

CONTRAINDICATIONS AND CAUTIONS

■ Contraindicated in patients hypersensitive to cephalosporins.

■ Use cautiously in breast-feeding women, patients hypersensitive to penicillin because of possible cross-sensitivity with other beta-lactam antibiotics, and patients with a history of colitis or renal insufficiency.

KEY POINTS

■ If large doses are given, therapy is prolonged, or patient is at high risk, watch for superinfection.

■ Tell patient to take all the drug prescribed, even if he feels better before the prescription is finished.

■ Instruct patient to take drug with food or milk to lessen gastrointestinal (GI) discomfort.

clarithromycin

CONTRAINDICATIONS AND CAUTIONS

■ Contraindicated in patients hypersensitive to clarithromycin, erythromycin, or other macrolides and in those receiving pimozide or other drugs that cause prolonged QT interval or cardiac arrhythmias.

■ Use cautiously in patients with hepatic or renal impairment.

KEY POINTS

■ Drug may cause allergic reactions (including anaphylaxis, Stevens-Johnson syndrome, and toxic epidermal necrolysis), central nervous system (CNS) effects, GI effects, hepatic dysfunction, neutropenia, QT interval prolongation, thrombocytopenia, and ventricular arrhythmias.

■ Monitor patient for superinfection because drug may cause overgrowth of nonsusceptible bacteria or fungi.

co-trimoxazole

CONTRAINDICATIONS AND CAUTIONS

■ Contraindicated in pregnant women at term, breast-feeding women, infants younger than age 2 months, patients hypersensitive to trimethoprim or sulfonamides, patients with a creatinine clearance less than 15 ml/minute, and patients with porphyria or megaloblastic anemia from folate deficiency.

■ Use cautiously and in reduced dosages in patients with impaired hepatic function, a creatinine clearance of 15 to 30 ml/minute, severe allergy,

bronchial asthma, G6PD deficiency, or blood dyscrasia.

KEY POINTS

■ Double-check dosage, which
may be written as trimethoprim
component.
■ "DS" product means "double strength."
■ Monitor renal and liver
function test results.

  ALERT *Promptly report
rash, sore throat, fever, cough,
mouth sores, or iris lesions—early
signs and symptoms of erythema
multiforme, which may progress to
the sometimes fatal Stevens-Johnson
syndrome. These symptoms also
may be early evidence of blood
dyscrasias.*

loracarbef
**CONTRAINDICATIONS AND
CAUTIONS**

■ Contraindicated in patients
hypersensitive to drug or other
cephalosporins.
■ Use cautiously in patients
hypersensitive to penicillin
because of possible cross-
sensitivity with other beta-
lactam antibiotics. Also use cautiously in breast-feeding women
and patients with a history of
colitis and renal insufficiency.
■ Safety and efficacy of drug
haven't been established in infants younger than age 6
months.

KEY POINTS

■ Monitor renal function.
■ For otitis media, the more
rapidly absorbed oral suspension produces higher peak drug
levels than capsules do.
■ Food decreases absorption.
Have patient take drug on empty stomach at least 1 hour before or 2 hours after a meal.

PHARYNGITIS

The most common throat disorder, pharyngitis is an acute or
chronic inflammation of the
pharynx. It's widespread among
adults who live or work in dusty
or dry environments, use their
voices excessively, habitually use
tobacco or alcohol, or have
chronic sinusitis, persistent
coughs, or allergies.

Pharyngitis is usually caused
by a virus. The most common
viral agents are rhinovirus,
coronavirus, adenovirus, influenza, and parainfluenza. The
most common bacterial cause is
group A beta-hemolytic streptococci. Other common causes
are *Mycoplasma* and *Chlamydia*.

azithromycin

CONTRAINDICATIONS AND CAUTIONS

■ Contraindicated in patients hypersensitive to erythromycin or other macrolides.

■ Use cautiously in patients with impaired hepatic function.

KEY POINTS

■ May cause photosensitivity. Advise patient to avoid excessive exposure to sunlight.

■ Monitor patient for superinfection because drug may cause overgrowth of nonsusceptible bacteria or fungi.

■ Tell patient to take entire amount of drug exactly as prescribed, even if he feels better before the prescription is finished.

cefadroxil

CONTRAINDICATIONS AND CAUTIONS

■ Contraindicated in patients hypersensitive to drug or other cephalosporins.

■ Use cautiously in patients with a history of sensitivity to penicillin and in breast-feeding women. Also use cautiously in patients with impaired renal function; dosage adjustments may be necessary.

KEY POINTS

■ If creatinine clearance is less than 50 ml/minute, dosage interval should be lengthened so drug doesn't accumulate. Monitor renal function in patients with renal dysfunction.

■ Instruct patient to take drug with food or milk to lessen gastrointestinal (GI) discomfort.

■ Tell patient to take entire amount of drug exactly as prescribed, even if he feels better before the prescription is finished.

■ Advise patient to notify prescriber if rash develops or signs and symptoms of superinfection appear, such as recurring fever, chills, and malaise.

cefdinir

CONTRAINDICATIONS AND CAUTIONS

■ Contraindicated in patients hypersensitive to drug or other cephalosporins.

■ Use cautiously in patients hypersensitive to penicillin because of possibility of cross-sensitivity with other beta-lactam antibiotics. Also use cautiously in patients with a history of colitis or renal insufficiency.

KEY POINTS

■ Pseudomembranous colitis may occur with cefdinir and

should be considered in patients with diarrhea after antibiotic therapy and in those with a history of colitis.

■ Advise patient to report severe diarrhea or diarrhea with abdominal pain.

■ Tell patient to report adverse reactions or evidence of superinfection promptly.

cefditoren

CONTRAINDICATIONS AND CAUTIONS

■ Contraindicated in patients hypersensitive to drug or other cephalosporins, patients with carnitine deficiency or an inborn error of metabolism that could lead to carnitine deficiency, and patients hypersensitive to milk protein (as distinct from those with lactose intolerance) because cefditoren tablets contain sodium caseinate, a milk protein.

■ Cephalosporins appear in breast milk and should be used cautiously in breast-feeding women. Safe use hasn't been established.

■ Use cautiously in patients with impaired renal function or penicillin allergy.

KEY POINTS

■ If patient develops diarrhea after receiving cefditoren, keep in mind that drug may cause pseudomembranous colitis.

■ Monitor patient for overgrowth of resistant organisms.

■ Patients who have renal impairment, hepatic impairment, or a poor nutritional state, and patients receiving a protracted course of antibiotics or who have been stabilized on anticoagulants may be at risk for decreased prothrombin activity. Monitor prothrombin time in these patients.

cefpodoxime

CONTRAINDICATIONS AND CAUTIONS

■ Contraindicated in patients hypersensitive to drug or other cephalosporins.

■ Use cautiously in patients with a history of penicillin hypersensitivity because of possible cross-sensitivity and in patients receiving nephrotoxic drugs because other cephalosporins have nephrotoxic potential. Because drug appears in breast milk, use cautiously in breast-feeding women.

KEY POINTS

■ Monitor renal function and compare with baseline.

■ Give drug with food to enhance absorption.

■ Monitor patient for superinfection because drug may cause

overgrowth of nonsusceptible bacteria or fungi.

cefprozil

CONTRAINDICATIONS AND CAUTIONS

■ Contraindicated in patients hypersensitive to drug or other cephalosporins.

■ Use cautiously in patients hypersensitive to penicillin because of possible cross-sensitivity with other beta-lactam antibiotics. Also use cautiously in breast-feeding women and in patients with a history of colitis or renal insufficiency.

KEY POINTS

■ Monitor renal function and liver function test results.

■ Monitor patient for superinfection because drug may cause overgrowth of nonsusceptible bacteria or fungi.

■ Advise patient to take entire amount of drug exactly as prescribed, even if he feels better before the prescription is finished.

cefuroxime

CONTRAINDICATIONS AND CAUTIONS

■ Contraindicated in patients hypersensitive to drug or other cephalosporins.

■ Use cautiously in patients hypersensitive to penicillin because of possible cross-sensitivity with other beta-lactam antibiotics. Also use cautiously in breast-feeding women and patients with a history of colitis or renal insufficiency.

KEY POINTS

■ Absorption of cefuroxime axetil is enhanced by food.

■ Cefuroxime axetil film-coated tablet and oral suspension aren't bioequivalent. Don't substitute on a mg/mg basis.

■ Tell patient to take entire amount of drug exactly as prescribed, even if he feels better before the prescription is finished.

clarithromycin

CONTRAINDICATIONS AND CAUTIONS

■ Contraindicated in patients hypersensitive to clarithromycin, erythromycin, or other macrolides and in those receiving pimozide or other drugs that cause prolonged QT interval or cardiac arrhythmias.

■ Use cautiously in patients with hepatic or renal impairment.

KEY POINTS

■ Drug may cause allergic reactions (including anaphylaxis, Stevens-Johnson syndrome, and toxic epidermal necrolysis), central nervous system effects, GI effects, hepatic dysfunction, neutropenia, QT interval prolongation, thrombocytopenia, and ventricular arrhythmias.

■ Monitor patient for superinfection because drug may cause overgrowth of nonsusceptible bacteria or fungi.

loracarbef

CONTRAINDICATIONS AND CAUTIONS

■ Contraindicated in patients hypersensitive to drug or other cephalosporins.

■ Use cautiously in patients hypersensitive to penicillin because of possibility of cross-sensitivity with other beta-lactam antibiotics. Also use cautiously in breast-feeding women and patients with a history of colitis or renal insufficiency.

■ Safety and efficacy of drug haven't been established in infants younger than age 6 months.

KEY POINTS

■ Monitor renal function.

■ Food decreases absorption. Have patient take drug on empty stomach at least 1 hour before or 2 hours after a meal.

■ Instruct patient to take entire amount of drug prescribed, even if he feels better before the prescription is finished.

18 / DRUGS FOR MUSCULOSKELETAL DISORDERS

GOUT

Also known as *gouty arthritis*, gout is a metabolic disease in which urate deposits lead to painfully arthritic joints. Although gout can occur in any joint, it usually affects the feet and legs. It may be primary or secondary.

Primary gout usually occurs in men older than age 30 and postmenopausal women. The exact cause remains unknown but may involve a genetic defect in purine metabolism that leads to overproduction of uric acid (hyperuricemia), retention of uric acid, or both.

Secondary gout occurs in older people. It may develop during the course of another disease (such as obesity, diabetes mellitus, hypertension, sickle cell anemia, or renal disease); hyperuricemia results from the breakdown of nucleic acid. It also may follow drug therapy, especially with hydrochlorothi-azide or pyrazinamide, which interferes with urate excretion. An increased uric acid level leads to urate deposits, called tophi, in joints or tissues, causing local necrosis or fibrosis.

Gout follows an intermittent course and commonly leaves patients symptom-free for years between attacks. Over time, however, gout can lead to chronic disability or incapacitation and, rarely, to severe hypertension and progressive renal disease. The prognosis is good with treatment.

allopurinol
CONTRAINDICATIONS AND CAUTIONS
■ Contraindicated in patients hypersensitive to drug and in those with idiopathic hemochromatosis.

KEY POINTS
■ Assess uric acid levels to evaluate drug's effectiveness.
■ Monitor fluid intake and output, and maintain daily urine

output of at least 2 L and neutral or slightly alkaline urine.

■ Periodically check complete blood count (CBC) and hepatic and renal function, especially at start of therapy.

colchicine
CONTRAINDICATIONS AND CAUTIONS

■ Contraindicated in patients hypersensitive to drug and in those with blood dyscrasias, serious cardiovascular (CV) disease, gastrointestinal (GI) disorders, or renal disease.

■ Use cautiously in elderly or debilitated patients and in those with early signs of CV, GI, or renal disease.

KEY POINTS

■ Obtain baseline laboratory test results, including CBC, before and periodically during therapy.

ALERT After full course of I.V. colchicine (4 mg), don't give colchicine by any route for at least 7 days. Colchicine is a toxic drug and may be lethal if given in overdose.

■ The first evidence of acute overdose may be GI symptoms, followed by vascular damage, muscle weakness, and ascending paralysis. Delirium and seizures may occur without the patient losing consciousness.

indomethacin
CONTRAINDICATIONS AND CAUTIONS

■ Contraindicated in pregnant women; breast-feeding women; patients hypersensitive to drug; patients with a history of asthma, rhinitis, or urticaria from aspirin or nonsteroidal anti-inflammatory drugs (NSAIDs); and neonates with active bleeding, coagulation defects, congenital heart disease (for whom patency of the ductus arteriosus is needed), necrotizing enterocolitis, significant renal impairment, thrombocytopenia, or untreated infection.

■ Suppositories are contraindicated in patients with a history of proctitis or recent rectal bleeding.

■ Because of its high risk of adverse effects with long-term use, indomethacin shouldn't be used routinely as an analgesic or antipyretic.

■ Use cautiously in elderly patients, patients with a history of GI disease, and patients with CV disease, depression, epilepsy, hepatic disease, infection, mental illness, parkinsonism, or renal disease.

KEY POINTS

■ Don't give sustained-release capsules to treat acute gouty arthritis.

■ Drug causes sodium retention; watch for weight gain (especially in elderly patients) and increased blood pressure in patients with hypertension.

■ NSAIDs may cause serious GI toxicity, including peptic ulcers and bleeding, without causing symptoms.

naproxen
CONTRAINDICATIONS AND CAUTIONS

■ Contraindicated in patients hypersensitive to drug and in those with the syndrome of asthma, rhinitis, and nasal polyps.

■ Drug should be avoided during last trimester of pregnancy.

■ Use cautiously in elderly patients and patients with CV disease, GI disorders, hepatic disease, a history of peptic ulcer disease, or renal disease.

KEY POINTS

■ Because NSAIDs impair synthesis of renal prostaglandins, they can decrease renal blood flow and lead to reversible renal impairment, especially in elderly patients, patients taking diuretics, and patients with renal failure, heart failure, or liver dysfunction. Monitor these patients closely.

■ NSAIDs may cause serious GI toxicity, including peptic ulcers and bleeding, without causing symptoms.

■ Because of their antipyretic and anti-inflammatory actions, NSAIDs may mask evidence of infection.

sulindac
CONTRAINDICATIONS AND CAUTIONS

■ Contraindicated in patients hypersensitive to drug, pregnant women, and patients for whom aspirin or NSAIDs precipitate acute asthma attacks, urticaria, or rhinitis.

■ Use cautiously in patients with a history of ulcers and GI bleeding and patients with compromised cardiac function or conditions predisposing them to fluid retention, hypertension, or renal dysfunction.

KEY POINTS

■ NSAIDs may cause serious GI toxicity, including peptic ulcers and bleeding, without causing symptoms.

■ Drug causes sodium retention but probably has less effect on the kidneys than other NSAIDs.

■ NSAIDs may mask evidence of infection.

OSTEOARTHRITIS

Osteoarthritis, also known as *hypertrophic osteoarthritis, osteoarthrosis,* and *degenerative joint disease,* is the most common form of arthritis. A chronic disease, it causes deterioration of the joint cartilage and formation of reactive new bone at the margins and subchondral areas of the joints. This degeneration results from a breakdown of chondrocytes, usually in the hips and knees.

Osteoarthritis is widespread, occurring equally in both sexes until age 55. After age 55, women are more likely to have it. Primary osteoarthritis is a normal part of aging and may result from metabolic, genetic, chemical, and mechanical factors. Secondary osteoarthritis usually follows an identifiable predisposing event—usually traumatic injury, congenital deformity, or obesity—and leads to degenerative changes.

The earliest symptoms typically begin in middle age and may progress as the person ages. The eventual degree of disability depends on the site and severity of involvement; it can range from minor limitation of the fingers to severe disability if the hips or knees are involved. The rate of progression varies, and joints may remain stable for years in an early stage of deterioration.

celecoxib

CONTRAINDICATIONS AND CAUTIONS

■ Contraindicated in pregnant women in the third trimester, patients with severe hepatic impairment, and patients hypersensitive to celecoxib, sulfonamides, aspirin, or other nonsteroidal anti-inflammatory drugs (NSAIDs).

■ Use cautiously in elderly or debilitated patients, patients with a history of ulcers or gastrointestinal (GI) bleeding, patients known or suspected to be poor metabolizers via P-450 2C9 enzymes, and patients with advanced renal disease, anemia, asthma, dehydration, edema, heart failure, hypertension, or symptomatic liver disease.

KEY POINTS

■ A patient with a history of ulcers or GI bleeding has an increased risk of GI bleeding while taking NSAIDs such as celecoxib. Other risk factors for GI bleeding include alcoholism, older age, poor overall health, smoking, corticosteroid or anticoagulant therapy, and longer duration of NSAID therapy.

- NSAIDs such as celecoxib can cause fluid retention; monitor a patient who has hypertension, edema, or heart failure.
- Drug may be hepatotoxic; watch for evidence of liver toxicity.

diclofenac

CONTRAINDICATIONS AND CAUTIONS

- Contraindicated in patients hypersensitive to drug and in those with hepatic porphyria or a history of asthma, urticaria, or other allergic reactions after taking aspirin or other NSAIDs.
- Drug isn't recommended during late pregnancy or breast-feeding.
- Use cautiously in patients with a history of peptic ulcer disease and patients with cardiac disease, fluid retention, hepatic dysfunction, hypertension, or impaired renal function.

KEY POINTS

- Because NSAIDs impair synthesis of renal prostaglandins, they can decrease renal blood flow and lead to reversible renal impairment, especially in elderly patients, patients who take diuretics, and patients with renal failure, heart failure, or liver dysfunction. Monitor these patients closely.

- Liver function test values may increase during therapy. Monitor transaminase, especially alanine transaminase (ALT), levels periodically in patients receiving long-term therapy. The first transaminase measurement should take place no more than 8 weeks after therapy begins.
- NSAIDs may cause serious GI toxicity, including peptic ulcers and bleeding, without causing symptoms.

diflunisal

CONTRAINDICATIONS AND CAUTIONS

- Contraindicated in patients hypersensitive to drug and in those for whom aspirin or other NSAIDs cause acute asthma attacks, urticaria, or rhinitis.
- Use cautiously in patients with a history of peptic ulcer disease and patients with compromised cardiac function, GI bleeding, hypertension, renal impairment, or other conditions predisposing them to fluid retention.

KEY POINTS

- Give drug with water, milk, or meals to reduce GI upset.
- Tablets must be swallowed whole.

  ALERT Because of the risk of Reye's syndrome, the Cen-

ters for Disease Control and Prevention warns against giving salicylates to children and teenagers with chickenpox or flu-like illness.

indomethacin

CONTRAINDICATIONS AND CAUTIONS

■ Contraindicated in pregnant women; breast-feeding women; patients hypersensitive to drug; patients with a history of aspirin- or NSAID-induced asthma, rhinitis, or urticaria; and neonates with active bleeding, coagulation defects, congenital heart disease (for whom patency of the ductus arteriosus is needed), necrotizing enterocolitis, significant renal impairment, thrombocytopenia, or untreated infection.

■ Suppositories are contraindicated in patients with a history of proctitis or recent rectal bleeding.

■ Use cautiously in elderly patients, patients with a history of GI disease, and patients with cardiovascular (CV) disease, depression, epilepsy, hepatic disease, infection, mental illness, parkinsonism, or renal disease.

■ Because of the high risk of adverse effects during long-term therapy, indomethacin shouldn't be used routinely as an analgesic or antipyretic.

KEY POINTS

■ Many drug interactions are possible. Check patient's medication orders to avoid potential dangers.

■ Drug causes sodium retention; watch for weight gain (especially in elderly patients) and increased blood pressure in patients with hypertension.

■ NSAIDs may cause serious GI toxicity, including peptic ulcers and bleeding, without causing symptoms.

ketoprofen

CONTRAINDICATIONS AND CAUTIONS

■ Contraindicated in patients hypersensitive to drug and in those with history of aspirin- or NSAID-induced asthma, urticaria, or other allergic reactions.

■ Avoid use during last trimester of pregnancy.

■ Drug isn't recommended for children or breast-feeding women.

■ Use cautiously in patients with a history of peptic ulcer disease and patients with fluid retention, heart failure, hypertension, or renal dysfunction.

KEY POINTS

■ Because NSAIDs impair synthesis of renal prostaglandins, they can decrease renal blood flow and lead to reversible renal impairment, especially in elderly patients, patients who take diuretics, and patients with renal failure, heart failure, or liver dysfunction. Monitor these patients closely.

■ Drug decreases platelet adhesion and aggregation and can prolong bleeding time by about 3 to 4 minutes from baseline.

■ NSAIDs may cause serious GI toxicity, including peptic ulcers and bleeding, without causing symptoms.

meloxicam
CONTRAINDICATIONS AND CAUTIONS

■ Contraindicated in patients late in pregnancy, patients hypersensitive to drug, and patients who have developed asthma, urticaria, or allergic-type reactions after taking aspirin or other NSAIDs.

■ Use with extreme caution in patients with a history of ulcers, GI bleeding, or asthma.

■ Use cautiously in elderly and debilitated patients (because of increased risk of fatal GI bleeding) and in patients with anemia, asthma, dehydration, fluid retention, heart failure, hepatic disease, hypertension, or renal disease.

KEY POINTS

■ NSAIDs can cause fluid retention; closely monitor patients who have hypertension, edema, or heart failure.

■ Drug may be hepatotoxic. Watch for elevated ALT and aspartate transaminase levels. If evidence of liver disease develops or systemic signs and symptoms occur (such as eosinophilia rash), stop drug and call prescriber.

■ Rehydrate dehydrated patients before starting drug.

nabumetone
CONTRAINDICATIONS AND CAUTIONS

■ Contraindicated in patients hypersensitive to drug and patients with a history of aspirin- or NSAID-induced asthma, urticaria, or other allergic-type reactions.

■ Drug isn't recommended for children or patients in the third trimester of pregnancy.

■ Use cautiously in patients with a history of peptic ulcer disease, patients with renal or hepatic impairment, and patients with heart failure, hypertension, or other conditions that may predispose them to fluid retention.

KEY POINTS

■ Because NSAIDs impair synthesis of renal prostaglandins, they can decrease renal blood flow and lead to reversible renal impairment, especially in elderly patients, patients taking diuretics, and patients with renal failure, heart failure, or liver dysfunction. Monitor these patients closely.

CLINICAL TIP Give drug with food, milk, or antacids. Drug is absorbed more rapidly when taken with food or milk.

■ During long-term therapy, periodically monitor renal and liver function, complete blood count, and hematocrit; assess patient for evidence of GI bleeding. NSAIDs can cause serious GI toxicity, including peptic ulcers and bleeding, without causing symptoms.

naproxen

CONTRAINDICATIONS AND CAUTIONS

■ Contraindicated in patients hypersensitive to drug and in those with the syndrome of asthma, rhinitis, and nasal polyps.

■ Drug should be avoided during last trimester of pregnancy.

■ Use cautiously in elderly patients, patients with a history of peptic ulcer disease, and patients with CV disease, GI disorders, hepatic disease, or renal disease.

KEY POINTS

■ Because NSAIDs impair synthesis of renal prostaglandins, they can decrease renal blood flow and lead to reversible renal impairment, especially in elderly patients, patients taking diuretics, and patients with renal failure, heart failure, or liver dysfunction. Monitor these patients closely.

■ NSAIDs may cause serious GI toxicity, including peptic ulcers and bleeding, without causing symptoms.

■ Because of their antipyretic and anti-inflammatory actions, NSAIDs may mask evidence of infection.

rofecoxib

CONTRAINDICATIONS AND CAUTIONS

■ Contraindicated in patients hypersensitive to drug or its components, pregnant women (because drug may cause ductus arteriosus to close prematurely), patients with advanced kidney disease or moderate to severe hepatic insufficiency, and patients who have had asthma, urticaria, or allergic reactions after taking aspirin or other NSAIDs.

■ Drug isn't recommended for breast-feeding women.

■ Use cautiously in patients with a history of ulcer disease, GI bleeding, or ischemic heart disease; patients taking such drugs as oral corticosteroids or anticoagulants; patients who are considerably dehydrated; patients with fluid retention, hypertension, or heart failure; and patients with risk factors that may increase the risk of GI bleeding, such as older age, alcoholism, poor general health, and smoking.

KEY POINTS

■ Rehydrate dehydrated patient before therapy starts.

■ If patient has fluid retention, hypertension, or heart failure, start therapy at lowest recommended dosage. Monitor blood pressure, and check patient for fluid retention or worsening heart failure.

■ Drug may be hepatotoxic. Watch for evidence of liver toxicity, and stop drug if it occurs.

■ The risk of GI toxicity with rofecoxib 50 mg once daily is significantly less than with naproxen 500 mg twice daily, but rofecoxib may cause more than twice as many adverse cardiac events as naproxen.

ALERT Because it has no effect on platelets, rofecoxib isn't a substitute for aspirin in preventing CV events.

valdecoxib

CONTRAINDICATIONS AND CAUTIONS

■ Contraindicated in patients hypersensitive to drug, patients with advanced renal or hepatic disease, and patients who have experienced asthma, urticaria, or allergic reactions to aspirin, sulfonamides, or NSAIDs.

■ Use with extreme caution in patients with a history of GI bleeding or peptic ulcer disease.

■ Use cautiously in elderly patients; debilitated patients; dehydrated patients; patients with fluid retention; patients with asthma, renal impairment, heart failure, hepatic dysfunction, or hypertension; patients taking angiotensin-converting enzyme inhibitors, anticoagulants, corticosteroids, diuretics, or long-term NSAIDs; and patients with risk factors that increase the risk of GI bleeding, such as smoking, alcoholism, and poor general health.

KEY POINTS

■ Monitor hemoglobin and hematocrit in patients on long-term therapy; watch for evidence of anemia.

■ Liver function test values may be elevated, progressing to more serious hepatic abnormalities. Notify prescriber about evidence of hepatic dysfunction.

■ Fluid retention and edema may occur.

OSTEOPOROSIS

In this metabolic bone disorder, the rate of bone resorption increases while the rate of bone formation decreases, causing bone mass to decline. Bones affected by this disease lose calcium and phosphate salts and thus become porous, brittle, and abnormally vulnerable to fracture. Osteoporosis may be primary or secondary to an underlying disease.

Primary osteoporosis is commonly called *senile* or *postmenopausal osteoporosis* because it's most common in elderly, postmenopausal women. Its cause is unknown; however, a mild but prolonged negative calcium balance from inadequate dietary calcium intake may be an important contributing factor—as may declining gonadal adrenal function, faulty protein metabolism from estrogen deficiency, and a sedentary lifestyle.

Causes of secondary osteoporosis include prolonged therapy with corticosteroids or heparin, total immobilization or disuse of a bone (as with hemiplegia, for example), alcoholism, malnutrition, malabsorption, scurvy, lactose intolerance, hyperthyroidism, osteogenesis imperfecta, and Sudeck's atrophy (localized to hands and feet, with recurring attacks).

alendronate

CONTRAINDICATIONS AND CAUTIONS

■ Contraindicated in patients hypersensitive to drug and in those with hypocalcemia, severe renal insufficiency, or abnormalities of the esophagus that delay esophageal emptying.

■ Use cautiously in patients with active upper gastrointestinal (GI) problems (dysphagia, symptomatic esophageal diseases, gastritis, duodenitis, ulcers) or mild to moderate renal insufficiency.

KEY POINTS

■ Osteoporosis may be confirmed by diagnostic tests that show low bone mass or by a history of osteoporotic fracture.

■ Correct hypocalcemia and other disturbances of mineral metabolism (such as vitamin D deficiency) before therapy begins.

■ Give drug with 6 to 8 ounces of water at least 30 minutes before patient's first food or drink of the day to facilitate delivery to the stomach. Don't let patient lie down for 30 minutes after taking drug.

calcitonin

CONTRAINDICATIONS AND CAUTIONS

■ Contraindicated in patients hypersensitive to drug.

KEY POINTS

■ Skin test is usually done before therapy starts. Systemic allergic reactions are possible because hormone is protein. Keep epinephrine nearby.

■ Give at bedtime, when possible, to minimize nausea and vomiting.

■ Patient should receive adequate vitamin D and calcium supplements daily.

estrogens, conjugated

CONTRAINDICATIONS AND CAUTIONS

■ Contraindicated in pregnant patients and patients with breast or reproductive cancer (except palliative treatment), estrogen-dependent neoplasia, thromboembolic disorders, thrombophlebitis, or undiagnosed abnormal genital bleeding.

■ Use cautiously in patients with asthma, bone disease, cardiac dysfunction, cerebrovascular or coronary artery disease, hepatic dysfunction, migraine, renal dysfunction, or seizures. Also use cautiously in women with a strong family history (mother, grandmother, sister) of breast or genital tract cancer or who have breast nodules, fibrocystic breasts, or abnormal mammogram findings.

KEY POINTS

■ Make sure patient has a thorough physical examination before starting estrogen therapy. Patients receiving long-term therapy should have annual examinations. Periodically monitor lipid levels, blood pressure, body weight, and hepatic function.

CLINICAL TIP Notify pathologist about estrogen therapy when sending specimens to laboratory for evaluation.

■ Because of thromboembolism risk, stop therapy at least 1 month before procedures that require prolonged immobilization or raise the risk of thromboembolism, such as knee or hip surgery.

raloxifene

CONTRAINDICATIONS AND CAUTIONS

■ Contraindicated in women hypersensitive to drug or its components, women who are pregnant or planning to get pregnant, women who are breast-feeding, children, and patients with previous or current venous thromboembolic events, including deep vein thrombosis, pulmonary embolism, and retinal vein thrombosis.

■ Use cautiously in patients with severe hepatic impairment.

■ Safety and efficacy of drug haven't been evaluated in men.

KEY POINTS

■ Watch for evidence of blood clots. The risk of thromboembolic events is greatest during the first 4 months of treatment.

■ Stop drug at least 72 hours before prolonged immobilization and resume only after patient is fully mobile.

■ Report unexplained uterine bleeding; drug isn't known to cause endometrial proliferation.

■ Watch for breast abnormalities; drug isn't known to cause breast enlargement, breast pain, or an increased risk of breast cancer.

risedronate
CONTRAINDICATIONS AND CAUTIONS

■ Contraindicated in patients hypersensitive to any component of the product, hypocalcemic patients, patients with creatinine clearance less than 30 ml/minute, and patients who can't stand or sit upright for 30 minutes after administration.

■ Use cautiously in patients with upper GI disorders such as dysphagia, esophagitis, and esophageal or gastric ulcers.

KEY POINTS

■ Give drug with 6 to 8 ounces of water at least 30 minutes before patient's first food or drink of the day to facilitate delivery to the stomach. Don't let patient lie down for 30 minutes after taking drug.

■ Bisphosphonates have been linked to such GI disorders as dysphagia, esophagitis, and esophageal or gastric ulcers. Assess patient for evidence of esophageal disease (such as dysphagia, retrosternal pain, or severe persistent or worsening heartburn).

■ Patients should receive supplemental calcium and vitamin D if dietary intake is inadequate. Because calcium supplements and drugs containing calcium, aluminum, or magnesium may interfere with risedronate absorption, separate dosing times.

PAGET'S DISEASE

Also known as *osteitis deformans*, Paget's disease is a slowly progressive metabolic bone disease characterized by an initial phase of excessive bone resorption (osteoclastic phase), followed by a reactive phase of excessive abnormal bone formation (osteoblastic phase). The new bone structure, which is chaotic, fragile, and weak, causes painful deformities of both external contour and internal structure.

Paget's disease occurs worldwide but is more common in Europe, Australia, and New Zealand, where it occurs in up to 5% of elderly people. Although its cause is unknown, one theory holds that early viral infection (possibly with mumps virus) causes a dormant skeletal infection that erupts many years later as Paget's disease. In 5% of patients, the involved bone becomes malignant.

Paget's disease usually localizes in one or more areas of the skeleton, usually the lower torso; however, occasionally, skeletal deformity is widely distributed. The disease can be fatal, especially when accompanied by heart failure (widespread disease creates a continuous need for high cardiac output), bone sarcoma, or giant cell tumors.

alendronate

CONTRAINDICATIONS AND CAUTIONS

■ Contraindicated in patients hypersensitive to drug and those with hypocalcemia, severe renal insufficiency, or abnormalities of the esophagus that delay esophageal emptying.

■ Use cautiously in patients with active upper gastrointestinal (GI) problems (dysphagia, symptomatic esophageal diseases, gastritis, duodenitis, ulcers) or mild to moderate renal insufficiency.

KEY POINTS

■ Use drug for patients with alkaline phosphatase level at least twice the upper limit of normal, patients who are symptomatic, and patients at risk for future complications from the disease.

■ Give drug with 6 to 8 ounces of water at least 30 minutes before patient's first food or drink of the day to facilitate delivery to the stomach. Don't let patient lie down for 30 minutes after taking drug.

■ Monitor patient's calcium and phosphate levels throughout therapy.

calcitonin

CONTRAINDICATIONS AND CAUTIONS

■ Contraindicated in patients hypersensitive to salmon calcitonin.

KEY POINTS

■ Skin test is usually done before starting therapy. Systemic allergic reactions are possible because hormone is protein. Keep epinephrine nearby.

■ Give at bedtime, when possible, to minimize nausea and vomiting.

■ Maximum reductions of alkaline phosphatase levels and urinary hydroxyproline excretion may take 6 to 24 months of continuous treatment.

pamidronate

CONTRAINDICATIONS AND CAUTIONS

■ Contraindicated in patients hypersensitive to drug or other bisphosphonates, such as etidronate.

■ Use with extreme caution, and only after considering risks and benefits, in patients with renal impairment.

■ Use cautiously in breast-feeding women.

KEY POINTS

■ Because drug can cause electrolyte disturbances, carefully monitor electrolyte levels, especially calcium, phosphate, and magnesium. Short-term administration of calcium may be needed in patients with severe hypocalcemia. Also monitor creatinine level, complete blood count and differential, hemoglobin, and hematocrit.

ALERT Give drug only by slow I.V. infusion. Injecting a bolus may cause nephropathy.

■ Assess patient's temperature. Some patients develop a slight elevation for 24 to 48 hours after taking drug.

risedronate

CONTRAINDICATIONS AND CAUTIONS

■ Contraindicated in patients hypersensitive to any component of the product, hypocalcemic patients, patients with creatinine clearance less than 30 ml/minute, and patients who can't stand or sit upright for 30 minutes after administration.

■ Use cautiously in patients with upper GI disorders such as dysphagia, esophagitis, and esophageal or gastric ulcers.

KEY POINTS

■ Give drug with 6 to 8 ounces of water at least 30 minutes before patient's first food or drink of the day to facilitate delivery to the stomach. Don't let patient lie down for 30 minutes after taking drug.

■ Bisphosphonates have been linked to such GI disorders as dysphagia, esophagitis, and esophageal or gastric ulcers. Monitor patient for evidence of esophageal disease (such as dysphagia, retrosternal pain, or severe persistent or worsening heartburn).

■ Patients should receive supplemental calcium and vitamin D if dietary intake is inadequate. Because calcium supplements and drugs containing calcium, aluminum, or magnesium may interfere with risedronate absorption, separate dosing times.

DRUGS FOR RESPIRATORY DISORDERS

ASTHMA

A reversible lung disease, asthma is characterized by obstruction or narrowing of inflamed, hyperresponsive airways. Although asthma can arise at any age, half of all cases arise in children under age 10. In this age group, asthma affects twice as many boys as girls; however, the sex ratio equalizes by age 30.

Asthma that results from sensitivity to identified external allergens is called extrinsic (atopic) asthma. Asthma that results from an unknown allergen is called intrinsic (nonatopic) asthma. Many people with asthma have qualities of both the intrinsic and extrinsic types.

Allergens that cause extrinsic asthma include pollen, animal dander, house dust, mold, kapok or feather pillows, sulfite-containing food additives, and other sensitizing substances. This type of asthma typically begins in childhood, and the child typically has other evidence of atopy (type I, immunoglobulin [Ig] E–mediated allergy), such as eczema and allergic rhinitis. When the person inhales an allergen, sensitized IgE antibodies trigger mast cell degranulation in the lung interstitium, releasing histamine, cytokines, prostaglandins, thromboxanes, leukotrienes, and eosinophil chemotaxic factors. Histamine then attaches to receptor sites in larger bronchi, causing irritation, inflammation, and edema. In the late phase, inflammatory cells flow in. The influx of eosinophils brings more inflammatory mediators and contributes to local injury.

With intrinsic asthma, no extrinsic allergen can be identified. Usually, it starts with a severe respiratory tract infection, and many different forces can cause an asthma attack. Irritants, emotional stress, fatigue, exposure to noxious fumes, and changes in endocrine components, temperature, and humidity may aggravate attacks. Other substances may trigger an attack by inhibiting prostaglandins and releasing mast cell mediators; examples include aspirin, nonsteroidal anti-inflammatory drugs, and tartrazine. Exercise may also provoke an attack. In exercise-induced asthma, bronchospasm may occur after heat and moisture loss in the upper airways. An asthma attack may resolve spontaneously or with drug treatment.

albuterol

CONTRAINDICATIONS AND CAUTIONS
■ Contraindicated in patients hypersensitive to drug or its ingredients.
■ Use cautiously in patients overly responsive to adrenergics and those with cardiovascular (CV) disorders (including coronary insufficiency and hypertension), hyperthyroidism, or diabetes mellitus.
■ Give extended-release tablets cautiously to patients with GI narrowing.

KEY POINTS
■ Warn patient about possible paradoxical bronchospasm, and tell him to stop drug immediately if it occurs.
■ If prescriber orders more than one inhalation, tell patient

to wait at least 2 minutes between inhalations.
■ If patient also uses a corticosteroid inhaler, instruct him to use the bronchodilator first and then wait about 5 minutes before using the corticosteroid.

budesonide

CONTRAINDICATIONS AND CAUTIONS
■ Contraindicated in patients hypersensitive to drug and in those with status asthmaticus or other acute asthma episodes.
■ Use cautiously in patients with active or quiescent tuberculosis of the respiratory tract, ocular herpes simplex, or untreated systemic fungal, bacterial, viral, or parasitic infections.

KEY POINTS
■ When changing from systemic corticosteroid to budesonide, use caution and gradually decrease corticosteroid dose to prevent adrenal insufficiency.
■ Drug doesn't remove the need for systemic corticosteroid therapy in some patients.
■ If bronchospasm occurs after using budesonide, stop therapy and give a bronchodilator.
■ Lung function may improve within 24 hours, but maximum benefit may not occur for 1 to 2 weeks or longer.

flunisolide

CONTRAINDICATIONS AND CAUTIONS

■ Contraindicated in patients hypersensitive to drug and in those with status asthmaticus or respiratory tract infections.

■ Drug isn't recommended for patients with nonasthmatic bronchial diseases or asthma controlled by bronchodilators or noncorticosteroids alone.

KEY POINTS

■ Flunisolide doesn't relieve acute asthma attacks.

🍀 *CLINICAL TIP A spacer device helps ensure proper dosage and decreases adverse effects.*

■ Withdraw drug slowly in patients who have received long-term oral corticosteroid therapy. After withdrawing systemic corticosteroids, patient may need supplemental systemic corticosteroids if stress causes adrenal insufficiency.

fluticasone

CONTRAINDICATIONS AND CAUTIONS

■ Contraindicated in patients hypersensitive to drug or its components.

■ Contraindicated as primary treatment of patients with status asthmaticus or other acute episodes of asthma requiring more intensive measures.

■ Use cautiously in breast-feeding patients.

KEY POINTS

■ During withdrawal from oral corticosteroids, some patients may have signs and symptoms of systemically active corticosteroid withdrawal, such as joint or muscle pain, lassitude, and depression, despite maintenance or even improvement of respiratory function.

■ For patients starting therapy who are already taking an oral corticosteroid, expect to reduce prednisone dosage weekly, beginning 1 week or more after fluticasone therapy starts, until prednisone dosage is no more than 2.5 mg/day.

■ As with other inhaled asthma drugs, bronchospasm may occur with an immediate increase in wheezing after dosing. If bronchospasm occurs after patient uses fluticasone inhalation aerosol, immediately give a fast-acting inhaled bronchodilator.

fluticasone and salmeterol inhalation powder

CONTRAINDICATIONS AND CAUTIONS

■ Contraindicated in patients hypersensitive to drug or its components.

■ Contraindicated as primary treatment of status asthmaticus or acute asthmatic episodes.

■ Use very cautiously in patients with active or quiescent respiratory tuberculosis, ocular herpes simplex, or untreated systemic fungal, bacterial, viral, or parasitic infection.

■ Use cautiously in patients with CV disorders, seizures, or thyrotoxicosis; patients unusually responsive to sympathomimetic amines; and patients with hepatic impairment.

KEY POINTS

■ Don't use Advair Diskus to stop an asthma attack. Patient should carry an inhaled, short-acting beta$_2$ agonist (such as albuterol) for acute symptoms.

■ If drug causes paradoxical bronchospasm, immediately give a short-acting inhaled bronchodilator (such as albuterol) and notify prescriber.

■ Monitor patient for increased use of an inhaled short-acting beta$_2$ agonist. The dose of Advair Diskus may need to be increased.

metaproterenol

CONTRAINDICATIONS AND CAUTIONS

■ Contraindicated in patients hypersensitive to drug or its components, patients receiving general anesthesia with cyclopropane or halogenated hydrocarbon anesthetics, and patients with tachycardia, arrhythmias linked to tachycardia, peripheral or mesenteric vascular thrombosis, profound hypoxia, or hypercapnia.

■ Use cautiously in patients receiving cardiac glycosides and in patients with cirrhosis, diabetes, heart disease, hypertension, or hyperthyroidism.

KEY POINTS

■ Patients may use tablets and aerosol together. Watch closely for toxicity.

■ Teach patient to perform oral inhalation correctly with a metered-dose inhaler by giving these instructions:

– Shake the canister.

– Clear your nasal passages and throat.

– Breathe out, expelling as much air as possible from your lungs.

– Place the mouthpiece well into your mouth, and inhale deeply as you release a dose from the inhaler. Or, hold the inhaler about 1 inch (two finger widths) from your open mouth; inhale through your mouth as you release a dose.

– Hold your breath for several seconds, remove the mouthpiece from your mouth, and exhale slowly. Allow 2 minutes between inhalations.

■ Inhalant solution can be given by intermittent positive-pressure breathing device with the drug diluted in normal saline solution or with a hand nebulizer at full strength.

montelukast
CONTRAINDICATIONS AND CAUTIONS

■ Contraindicated in patients hypersensitive to drug or its components.

■ Use cautiously and with appropriate monitoring in patients whose dosages of systemic corticosteroids are reduced.

KEY POINTS

■ Drug isn't indicated for patients with acute asthma attacks, status asthmaticus, or as monotherapy for managing exercise-induced bronchospasm. Continue appropriate rescue drug for acute worsening.

■ Give oral granules either directly in the mouth or mixed with a teaspoonful of cold or room-temperature applesauce, carrots, rice, or ice cream. Don't open the packet until ready to use. After opening the packet, give full dose within 15 minutes. If mixed with food, don't store excess for future use; discard any unused portion.

■ Don't dissolve oral granules in liquid; let the patient take a drink after receiving the granules. Oral granules may be given without regard to meals.

salmeterol
CONTRAINDICATIONS AND CAUTIONS

■ Contraindicated in patients hypersensitive to drug or its components.

■ Use cautiously in patients unusually responsive to sympathomimetics and in patients with arrhythmias, coronary insufficiency, hypertension, other CV disorders, seizure disorders, or thyrotoxicosis.

KEY POINTS

■ Although drug is a beta agonist, it shouldn't be used to treat acute bronchospasm; a short-acting beta agonist, such as albuterol, should be given for worsening symptoms.

CLINICAL TIP *Remind patient to take drug at about 12-hour intervals for optimal effect and to take drug even when feeling better.*

■ Monitor patient for rash and urticaria, which may signal a hypersensitivity reaction. Rare serious asthma episodes or asthma-related deaths have occurred in patients using salmeterol, with African Americans at greatest risk.

zafirlukast
CONTRAINDICATIONS AND CAUTIONS
■ Contraindicated in patients hypersensitive to drug.

■ Drug isn't indicated for reversing bronchospasm in acute asthma attacks.

■ Give cautiously to geriatric patients and those with hepatic impairment.

KEY POINTS
■ Give drug 1 hour before or 2 hours after meals.

■ Reducing oral corticosteroid dose has been followed in rare cases by eosinophilia, vasculitic rash, worsening pulmonary symptoms, cardiac complications, or neuropathy, sometimes presenting as Churg-Strauss syndrome.

PNEUMOCYSTIS CARINII *PNEUMONIA*

Because of its link with human immunodeficiency virus (HIV) infection, *Pneumocystis carinii* pneumonia (PCP), an opportunistic infection, has become more widespread since the 1980s. Before the advent of PCP prophylaxis, PCP was the first evidence of HIV infection in about 60% of patients.

PCP occurs in up to 90% of HIV-infected patients in the United States at some point during their lifetime and is the leading cause of death in these patients. Disseminated infection doesn't occur. PCP also occurs with other immunocompromised conditions, including organ transplantation, leukemia, and lymphoma.

P. carinii usually is classified as a protozoan, although some experts consider it more closely related to fungi. It exists as a saprophyte in the lungs of humans and some animals.

Part of the normal flora in most healthy people, *P. carinii* becomes an aggressive pathogen in an immunocompromised person. Impaired cell-mediated (T-cell) immunity probably is more important than impaired humoral (B-cell) immunity in predisposing a person to PCP; however, the immune defects involved are poorly understood.

The organism invades the lungs bilaterally and multiplies extracellularly. As the infestation grows, alveoli fill with organisms and exudate, impairing gas exchange. The alveoli hypertrophy and thicken progressively, eventually leading to extensive consolidation.

The main transmission route seems to be air, although the organism already lives in most people. The incubation period probably lasts 4 to 8 weeks.

atovaquone

CONTRAINDICATIONS AND CAUTIONS

■ Contraindicated in patients hypersensitive to drug.

■ Use cautiously in breast-feeding women because drug appears in breast milk. Also use cautiously with other highly protein-bound drugs, and assess the patient for toxicity when used together.

KEY POINTS

■ Give drug with meals because food significantly enhances absorption.

■ Monitor patient closely during therapy because of risk of concurrent pulmonary infections.

co-trimoxazole

CONTRAINDICATIONS AND CAUTIONS

■ Contraindicated in patients hypersensitive to trimethoprim or sulfonamides, pregnant women at term, breast-feeding women, infants younger than age 2 months, and patients with creatinine clearance less than 15 ml/minute, porphyria, or megaloblastic anemia from folate deficiency.

■ Use cautiously and in reduced dosages in patients with impaired hepatic function, a creatinine clearance of 15 to 30 ml/minute, severe allergy or bronchial asthma, G6PD deficiency, or blood dyscrasia.

KEY POINTS

■ Double-check dosage, which may be written as trimethoprim component.

■ "DS" product means "double strength."

■ Promptly report rash, sore throat, fever, cough, mouth sores, or iris lesions—early evidence of erythema multiforme, which may progress to the life-threatening Stevens-Johnson syndrome. These changes also may represent early signs of blood dyscrasias.

■ Adverse reactions, especially hypersensitivity reactions, rash, and fever, occur much more often in patients with acquired immunodeficiency syndrome (AIDS).

pentamidine

CONTRAINDICATIONS AND CAUTIONS

■ Contraindicated in patients with history of anaphylactic reaction to drug.

■ Use cautiously in patients with anemia, diabetes, hepatic dysfunction, hypertension, hypocalcemia, hypoglycemia, hypotension, leukopenia, pancreatitis, renal dysfunction, Stevens-Johnson syndrome, or thrombocytopenia.

■ It's unknown if drug appears in breast milk. Use cautiously in breast-feeding women.

KEY POINTS

■ Give aerosol form only by Respirgard II nebulizer because dosage recommendations are based on particle size and delivery rate of this device. To give aerosol, mix contents of one vial in 6 ml sterile water for injection. Don't use normal saline solution. Don't mix with other drugs. Don't use low-pressure (less than 20 pounds per square inch [psi]) compressors. The flow rate should be 5 to 7 L/minute from a 40- to 50-psi air or oxygen source.

■ For I.V. use, infuse drug slowly with patient lying down to minimize the risk of hypotension. Closely monitor blood pressure.

■ For I.M. injection, reconstitute drug with 3 ml sterile water for a solution containing 100 mg/ml; give deep into muscle. Expect patient to report pain and induration at injection site. Rotate injection sites.

■ In patients with AIDS, pentamidine may produce less severe adverse reactions than cotrimoxazole.

PNEUMONIA

Pneumonia is an acute infection of the lung parenchyma that typically impairs gas exchange.

It can be viral, bacterial, fungal, protozoal, mycobacterial, mycoplasmal, or rickettsial in origin. Predisposing factors for bacterial and viral pneumonia include chronic illness and debilitation, cancer (particularly lung cancer), abdominal or thoracic surgery, atelectasis, common colds or other viral respiratory tract infections, chronic respiratory disease (asthma, bronchiectasis, chronic obstructive pulmonary disease, cystic fibrosis), influenza, smoking, malnutrition, alcoholism, sickle cell disease, tracheostomy, exposure to noxious gases, aspiration, and immunosuppressant therapy.

Pneumonia also may be classified by location or by type. For instance, bronchopneumonia involves the distal airways and alveoli; lobular pneumonia, part of a lobe; and lobar pneumonia, an entire lobe. The type may be primary or secondary. Primary pneumonia results from inhalation or aspiration of a pathogen; it includes pneumococcal and viral pneumonia. Secondary pneumonia may follow initial lung damage from a noxious chemical or other insult (superinfection), or may result from hematogenous spread of bacteria from a distant focus. (See *Types of pneumonia*, pages 494 to 497.) Predisposing factors for aspiration pneumonia include old age, debilitation, nasogastric tube feedings, impaired gag reflex, poor oral hygiene, and decreased level of consciousness.

The prognosis is generally good for people with normal lungs and adequate host defenses before pneumonia begins. However, pneumonia is the seventh leading cause of death in the United States and, in 2003, a new and deadly type of pneumonia emerged known as severe acute respiratory syndrome.

azithromycin
CONTRAINDICATIONS AND CAUTIONS
■ Contraindicated in patients hypersensitive to erythromycin or other macrolides.
■ Use cautiously in patients with impaired hepatic function.

KEY POINTS
■ Give multidose oral suspension 1 hour before or 2 hours after meals, not with antacids. Tablets and single-dose packets for oral suspension can be taken with or without food.
■ Reconstitute single-dose, 1 g packets for suspension with 2 ounces (60 ml) of water. Patient should rinse glass with another 2 ounces of water and drink it to make sure he has consumed entire dose. Packets aren't for pediatric use.

cefpodoxime
CONTRAINDICATIONS AND CAUTIONS
■ Contraindicated in patients hypersensitive to drug or other cephalosporins.
■ Use cautiously in breastfeeding women, patients with a history of penicillin hypersensitivity because of the risk of cross-sensitivity, and patients receiving nephrotoxic drugs because other cephalosporins have nephrotoxic potential.

KEY POINTS
■ Monitor renal function and compare with baseline.
■ Give drug with food to enhance absorption.
■ Refrigerate suspension at 36° to 46° F (2° to 8° C). Shake it
(Text continues on page 496.)

TYPES OF PNEUMONIA

TYPE	SIGNS AND SYMPTOMS
Viral	
Influenza (prognosis poor even with treatment; 50% mortality)	■ Cough (initially nonproductive; later, purulent sputum), marked cyanosis, dyspnea, high fever, chills, substernal pain and discomfort, moist crackles, frontal headache, myalgia ■ Death from cardiopulmonary collapse
Adenovirus (insidious onset; typically affects young adults)	■ Sore throat, fever, cough, chills, malaise, small amounts of mucoid sputum, retrosternal chest pain, anorexia, rhinitis, adenopathy, scattered crackles, and rhonchi
Respiratory syncytial virus (most common in infants and children)	■ Listlessness, irritability, tachypnea with retraction of intercostal muscles, slight sputum production, fine moist crackles, fever, severe malaise and, possibly, cough or croup
Measles (rubeola)	■ Fever, dyspnea, cough, small amounts of sputum, coryza, rash, and cervical adenopathy
Chickenpox (varicella) (uncommon in children, but present in 30% of adults with varicella)	■ Cough, dyspnea, cyanosis, tachypnea, pleuritic chest pain, hemoptysis, and rhonchi 1 to 6 days after onset of rash
Cytomegalovirus	■ Difficult to distinguish from other nonbacterial pneumonias ■ Fever, cough, shaking chills, dyspnea, cyanosis, weakness, and diffuse crackles ■ Occurs in neonates as devastating multisystemic infection; in normal adults, resembles mononucleosis; in immunocompromised hosts, varies from clinically inapparent to devastating

DIAGNOSIS	TREATMENT
■ Chest X-ray: diffuse bilateral broncho-pneumonia from hilus ■ White blood cell (WBC) count: normal to slightly elevated ■ Sputum smears: no specific organisms	■ Supportive: for respiratory failure, endotracheal intubation and ventilator assistance; for fever, hypothermia blanket or antipyretics; for influenza A, amantadine or rimantadine
■ Chest X-ray: patchy distribution of pneumonia, more severe than indicated by physical examination ■ WBC count: normal to slightly elevated	■ Treat only symptoms ■ Mortality low, usually clears with no residual effects
■ Chest X-ray: patchy bilateral consolidation ■ WBC count: normal to slightly elevated	■ Supportive: humidified air, oxygen, antimicrobials commonly given until viral cause confirmed, aerosolized ribavirin ■ Complete recovery in 1 to 3 weeks
■ Chest X-ray: reticular infiltrates, sometimes with hilar lymph node enlargement ■ Lung tissue specimen: characteristic giant cells	■ Supportive: bed rest, adequate hydration, antimicrobials, assisted ventilation, if necessary
■ Chest X-ray: shows more extensive pneumonia than indicated by physical examination, and bilateral, patchy, diffuse, nodular infiltrates ■ Sputum analysis: predominant mononuclear cells and characteristic intranuclear inclusion bodies with skin rash confirm diagnosis	■ Supportive: adequate hydration, oxygen therapy in critically ill patients ■ Therapy with I.V. acyclovir
■ Chest X-ray: in early stages, variable patchy infiltrates; later, bilateral, nodular, and more predominant in lower lobes ■ Percutaneous aspiration of lung tissue, transbronchial biopsy or open-lung biopsy: microscopic examination shows intranuclear and cytoplasmic inclusions; virus can be cultured from lung tissue	■ Supportive: adequate hydration and nutrition, oxygen therapy, bed rest ■ Generally, benign and self-limiting in mononucleosis-like form ■ Immunosuppressed patients: more severe, possibly fatal disease; ganciclovir or foscarnet treatment warranted

(continued)

TYPES OF PNEUMONIA (continued)

TYPE	SIGNS AND SYMPTOMS
Bacterial	
Streptococcus (*Streptococcus pneumoniae*)	■ Sudden onset of a single, shaking chill and sustained temperature of 102° to 104° F (38.9° to 40° C), commonly preceded by upper respiratory tract infection
Klebsiella	■ Fever and recurrent chills; cough producing rusty, bloody, viscous sputum (currant jelly); cyanosis of lips and nail beds from hypoxemia; shallow, grunting respirations ■ Likely in patients with chronic alcoholism, pulmonary disease, and diabetes
Staphylococcus	■ Temperature of 102° to 104° F (38.9° to 40° C), recurrent shaking chills, bloody sputum, dyspnea, tachypnea, and hypoxemia ■ Should be suspected with viral illness, such as influenza or measles, and in patients with cystic fibrosis
Aspiration	
Results from vomiting and aspiration of gastric or oropharyngeal contents into trachea and lungs	■ Noncardiogenic pulmonary edema may follow damage to respiratory epithelium from contact with stomach acid ■ Crackles, dyspnea, cyanosis, hypotension, and tachycardia ■ May be subacute pneumonia with cavity formation, or lung abscess may occur if foreign body is present

well before using, and discard unused portion after 14 days.

clarithromycin
CONTRAINDICATIONS AND CAUTIONS

■ Contraindicated in patients hypersensitive to clarithromycin, erythromycin, or other macrolides and in those receiving pimozide or other drugs that cause a prolonged QT interval or cardiac arrhythmias.

■ Use cautiously in patients with hepatic or renal impairment.

Diagnosis	Treatment
■ Chest X-ray: areas of consolidation, often lobar ■ WBC count: elevated ■ Sputum culture: may show gram-positive *S. pneumoniae;* this organism isn't always recovered	■ Antimicrobial therapy: macrolide for 7 to 10 days (starting after culture specimen obtained but before results available)
■ Chest X-ray: typically, but not always, consolidation in the upper lobe that causes bulging of fissures ■ WBC count: elevated ■ Sputum culture and Gram's stain: may show gram-negative cocci *(Klebsiella)*	■ Antimicrobial therapy: an aminoglycoside and a cephalosporin
■ Chest X-ray: multiple abscesses and infiltrates; high likelihood of empyema ■ WBC count: elevated ■ Sputum culture and Gram's stain: may show gram-positive staphylococci	■ Antimicrobial therapy: nafcillin or oxacillin for 14 days if staphylococci are penicillinase producing ■ Chest tube drainage of empyema
■ Chest X-ray: locates areas of infiltrates, which suggest diagnosis	■ Antimicrobial therapy: penicillin G or clindamycin ■ Supportive: oxygen therapy, suctioning, coughing, deep-breathing, adequate hydration

Key points

■ Drug may be taken with or without food. Don't refrigerate the suspension form.

■ Hexobarbital, phenytoin, valproate, and drugs metabolized by CYP3A may interact with clarithromycin.

■ Monitor patient for superinfection.

ertapenem

Contraindications and cautions

■ Contraindicated in patients who have had anaphylactic reactions to beta-lactams and patients hypersensitive to drug or its components, drugs in the same class, or local anesthetics of the amide type (intramuscular [I.M.] use).

■ Use cautiously in patients with central nervous system (CNS) disorders, compromised renal function, or both, because seizures may occur.

KEY POINTS

■ Anticonvulsant therapy may continue in patients with seizure disorders. If focal tremors, myoclonus, or seizures occur, notify prescriber. Ertapenem dosage may need to be decreased or stopped.

■ Methicillin-resistant staphylococci and *Enterococcus* species are resistant to ertapenem.

■ Monitor renal, hepatic, and hematopoietic function during prolonged therapy.

gatifloxacin
CONTRAINDICATIONS AND CAUTIONS

■ Contraindicated in patients hypersensitive to fluoroquinolones, patients with a prolonged QTc interval, and patients with uncorrected hypokalemia.

■ Use cautiously in patients with acute myocardial ischemia, clinically significant bradycar-

dia, known or suspected CNS disorders, or renal insufficiency.

KEY POINTS

■ Monitor patients also taking digoxin for signs and symptoms of digoxin toxicity.

■ Stop drug if patient has seizures, increased intracranial pressure, psychosis, or CNS stimulation leading to confusion, depression, hallucinations, insomnia, light-headedness, nightmares, paranoia, restlessness, or tremors.

■ Stop drug if patient develops pain, inflammation, or rupture of a tendon.

levofloxacin
CONTRAINDICATIONS AND CAUTIONS

■ Contraindicated in patients hypersensitive to drug, its components, or other fluoroquinolones.

■ Safety and efficacy of drug in children younger than age 18 and in pregnant and breast-feeding women haven't been established.

■ Use cautiously in patients with history of seizure disorders or other CNS diseases, such as cerebral arteriosclerosis.

■ Use cautiously and at adjusted dosage in patients with renal impairment.

KEY POINTS

■ If patient has evidence of excessive CNS stimulation (restlessness, tremor, confusion, hallucinations), stop drug and notify prescriber. Begin seizure precautions.

■ Drug may cause an abnormal electrocardiogram.

■ If *Pseudomonas aeruginosa* is a confirmed or suspected pathogen, use combination therapy with a beta-lactam.

linezolid
CONTRAINDICATIONS AND CAUTIONS

■ Contraindicated in patients hypersensitive to drug or its components.

KEY POINTS

■ No dosage adjustment is needed when switching from I.V. to P.O. forms.

■ Drug may cause thrombocytopenia. Monitor platelet count in patients at increased risk for bleeding, patients with thrombocytopenia, patients taking other drugs that may cause thrombocytopenia, and patients taking linezolid for more than 14 days.

■ Drug may lead to myelosuppression. Monitor complete blood count weekly in patients taking linezolid.

PULMONARY EMBOLISM AND INFARCTION

Pulmonary embolism is an obstruction of the pulmonary arterial bed by a dislodged thrombus or foreign substance. More than half the time, pulmonary embolism results from thrombi in the deep leg veins that embolize and float to the lungs. Less common sources of emboli are the pelvic veins, renal veins, hepatic vein, right side of the heart, and arms. Rarely, emboli contain air, fat, amniotic fluid, talc (from drugs intended for oral administration that are injected I.V. by addicts), or tumor cells.

Thrombi typically form as a result of vascular wall damage, venostasis, or hypercoagulability of the blood. They may embolize spontaneously during clot dissolution or may be dislodged during trauma, sudden muscular action, or a change in peripheral blood flow. Risk factors for pulmonary embolism include the following:

– atrial fibrillation
– autoimmune hemolytic anemia
– burns
– chronic pulmonary disease
– heart failure

- hormonal contraceptives
- leg fractures or surgery
- long-term immobility
- malignancy
- obesity
- old age
- polycythemia vera
- pregnancy
- recent surgery
- sickle cell disease
- thrombocytosis
- thrombophlebitis
- varicose veins
- vascular injury.

Pulmonary embolism may lead to infarction, especially if the person has chronic cardiac or pulmonary disease. Although pulmonary infarction (tissue death) may be mild and asymptomatic, massive embolism (more than 50% obstruction of pulmonary arterial flow) and infarction can be rapidly fatal.

alteplase
CONTRAINDICATIONS AND CAUTIONS
■ Contraindicated in patients with a history of cerebrovascular accident (CVA), patients who had a seizure at the onset of CVA (when used for acute ischemic CVA), patients with intraspinal or intracranial trauma or surgery within 2 months, and patients with active internal bleeding, aneurysm, arteriovenous malformation, bleeding diathesis, intracranial neoplasm, previous or current intracranial hemorrhage, severe uncontrolled hypertension, or possible subarachnoid hemorrhage.

■ Use cautiously in pregnant patients; patients who gave birth within 10 days; patients receiving anticoagulants; patients age 75 and older; patients having major surgery within 10 days (when bleeding is difficult to control because of its location); patients undergoing organ biopsy; patients with a systolic pressure of 180 mm Hg or higher or diastolic pressure of 110 mm Hg or higher; patients with mitral stenosis, atrial fibrillation, or other risks for left-heart thrombus; and patients who have acute pericarditis, cerebrovascular disease, diabetic hemorrhagic retinopathy, gastrointestinal (GI) bleeding, genitourinary (GU) bleeding, hemostatic defects from hepatic or renal impairment, septic thrombophlebitis, subacute bacterial endocarditis, or traumatic injury (including cardiopulmonary resuscitation).

KEY POINTS
■ Drug may be given to menstruating women.
■ Avoid invasive procedures during thrombolytic therapy. Closely monitor patient for evi-

dence of internal bleeding, and check all puncture sites frequently. Bleeding is the most common adverse effect and may occur internally and at external puncture sites.

■ If uncontrollable bleeding occurs, stop infusion and notify prescriber.

enoxaparin

CONTRAINDICATIONS AND CAUTIONS

■ Contraindicated in patients hypersensitive to drug, heparin, or pork products; patients with active major bleeding; and patients with thrombocytopenia and antiplatelet antibodies in presence of drug.

■ Use with extreme caution in patients who have a history of heparin-induced thrombocytopenia, aneurysms, cerebrovascular hemorrhage, spinal or epidural punctures (as with anesthesia), uncontrolled hypertension, or threatened abortion.

■ Use cautiously in elderly patients; patients who recently gave birth; patients with conditions that increase the risk of hemorrhage, such as angiodysplastic GI disease, bacterial endocarditis, congenital or acquired bleeding disorders, hemorrhagic CVA, ulcer disease, or recent spinal, ocular, or brain surgery; and patients with blood dyscrasias, pericardial effusion, pericarditis, regional or lumbar block anesthesia, renal insufficiency, or severe CNS trauma.

■ Enoxaparin isn't recommended for thromboprophylaxis in patients with prosthetic heart valves, because they may be at higher risk for thromboembolism.

KEY POINTS

■ Infants of women who received enoxaparin during pregnancy have an increased risk of congenital anomalies, including cerebral and limb anomalies, hypospadias, peripheral vascular malformation, fibrotic dysplasia, and cardiac defect.

ALERT Don't try to expel the air bubble from the 30- or 40-mg prefilled syringes. It may lead to drug loss and an incorrect dose.

■ With patient lying down, give by deep subcutaneous (S.C.) injection, alternating doses between left and right anterolateral and posterolateral abdominal walls. Never give drug I.M.

■ Don't massage the area after S.C. injection. Watch for bleeding at site. Rotate and document injection sites.

■ Enoxaparin isn't interchangeable with heparin or other low–molecular-weight heparins.

heparin
CONTRAINDICATIONS AND CAUTIONS

■ Contraindicated in patients hypersensitive to drug.

■ Conditionally contraindicated during or after brain, eye, or spinal cord surgery; during spinal tap, spinal anesthesia, or continuous tube drainage of stomach or small intestine; and in patients with active bleeding, advanced renal disease, ascorbic acid deficiency and other conditions that increase capillary permeability, bleeding tendencies (such as hemophilia, thrombocytopenia, or hepatic disease with hypoprothrombinemia), blood dyscrasias, extensive denuded skin, inaccessible ulcerative lesions (especially of the GI tract), open ulcerative wounds, severe hypertension, shock, subacute bacterial endocarditis, suspected intracranial hemorrhage, suppurative thrombophlebitis, or threatened abortion.

■ Use cautiously in women during menses or after childbirth and in patients with mild hepatic or renal disease, alcoholism, occupations with a high risk of physical injury, or a history of allergies, asthma, or GI ulcerations.

KEY POINTS

■ Check order and vial carefully; heparin comes in various concentrations. USP units and international units aren't equivalent for heparin.

■ Measure partial thromboplastin time (PTT) carefully and regularly. Anticoagulation is present when PTT values are 1½ to 2 times the control values.

■ Monitor patient for bleeding gums, bruising, petechiae, nosebleeds, melena, tarry stools, hematuria, and hematemesis.

streptokinase
CONTRAINDICATIONS AND CAUTIONS

■ Contraindicated in patients with recent cerebral embolism, thrombosis, or hemorrhage; within 10 days after intra-arterial diagnostic procedure or any surgery, including liver or kidney biopsy, lumbar puncture, thoracentesis, paracentesis, or extensive or multiple cutdowns; and in patients with active internal bleeding, acute or chronic hepatic or renal insufficiency, chronic pulmonary disease with cavitation, diverticulitis, previous severe allergic reaction to streptokinase, recent CVA, recent trauma with possible internal injuries, rheumatic valvular disease, severe hypertension, subacute bacterial endocarditis, ulcerative colitis, ulcerative wounds, uncontrolled hypoco-agulation, or visceral or intra-cranial malignancy.

■ I.M. injections and other in-vasive procedures are contra-indicated during streptokinase therapy.

■ Use cautiously when treating arterial embolism that origi-nates from the left side of the heart because of the danger of cerebral infarction.

KEY POINTS

■ To check for hypersensitivity reactions, give 100 international units intradermally; a wheal-and-flare response within 20 minutes means the patient is probably allergic. Monitor vital signs frequently.

■ Watch for signs of hypersen-sitivity and notify prescriber im-mediately if any occur. Antihist-amines or corticosteroids may be used to treat mild allergic re-actions. If a severe reaction oc-curs, stop infusion immediately and notify prescriber.

■ If patient has had either a re-cent streptococcal infection or recent treatment with streptoki-nase, a higher loading dose may be needed. Consider alternative thrombolytics.

tinzaparin
CONTRAINDICATIONS AND CAUTIONS

■ Contraindicated in patients hypersensitive to tinzaparin sodium or other low–molecular-weight heparins, heparin, sul-fites, benzyl alcohol, or pork products. Also contraindicated in patients with active major bleeding and in those with his-tory of heparin-induced throm-bocytopenia.

■ Use cautiously in breast-feeding women; elderly patients and those with renal insufficien-cy (because they may have re-duced elimination); patients who have recently undergone brain, spinal, or ophthalmic surgery; patients being treated with platelet inhibitors; and pa-tients with an increased risk of hemorrhage, such as those with bacterial endocarditis, congeni-tal or acquired bleeding disor-ders (including hepatic failure and amyloidosis), diabetic retinopathy, GI ulceration, he-morrhagic CVA, or uncon-trolled hypertension.

KEY POINTS

■ Drug isn't intended for I.M. or I.V. administration, and it shouldn't be mixed with other injections or infusions. Don't interchange drug (unit to unit) with heparin or other low–molecular-weight heparins.

■ When giving drug, have patient lie or sit down. Give by deep S.C. injection into abdominal wall. Introduce whole length of needle into skinfold held between thumb and forefinger. Make sure to hold skinfold throughout injection. Rotate injection sites between right and left anterolateral and posterolateral abdominal wall. To minimize bruising, don't rub injection site after administration.

■ Use an appropriate calibrated syringe to ensure correct withdrawal of drug volume from vials.

urokinase
CONTRAINDICATIONS AND CAUTIONS
■ Contraindicated in pregnant patients; patients who gave birth within 10 days; patients who had an intra-arterial diagnostic procedure or surgery (liver or kidney biopsy, lumbar puncture, thoracentesis, paracentesis, or extensive or multiple cutdowns) within 10 days; patients who had intracranial or intraspinal surgery within 2 months; patients with recent cerebral embolism, thrombosis, or hemorrhage; and patients with active internal bleeding, aneurysm, arteriovenous malformation, bleeding diathesis, chronic pulmonary disease with cavitation, diverticulitis, hemostatic defects (including those secondary to severe hepatic or renal insufficiency), history of CVA, recent trauma with possible internal injuries, rheumatic valvular disease, severe hypertension, subacute bacterial endocarditis, ulcerative colitis, uncontrolled hypocoagulation, or visceral or intracranial malignancy.

■ I.M. injections and other invasive procedures are contraindicated during therapy with urokinase.

KEY POINTS
■ Have typed and cross-matched red blood cells, whole blood, plasma expanders (other than dextran), and aminocaproic acid available to treat bleeding. Keep corticosteroids, epinephrine, and antihistamines available for allergic reactions.

■ Drug may be given to menstruating women.

■ Monitor patient for excessive bleeding every 15 minutes for first hour, every 30 minutes for second through eighth hours, and then once every 4 hours.

ALERT Pretreatment with drugs that affect platelets places patient at high risk of bleeding.

warfarin

CONTRAINDICATIONS AND CAUTIONS

■ Contraindicated in patients hypersensitive to drug; pregnant patients; patients with threatened abortion, eclampsia, or preeclampsia; patients with recent major regional or lumbar block anesthesia, spinal puncture, or diagnostic or therapeutic invasive procedures; patients with recent prostatectomy or surgery involving eye, brain, spinal cord, or large open areas; patients with bleeding from the GI, GU, or respiratory tract; and patients with aneurysm, blood dyscrasias, cerebrovascular hemorrhage, hemorrhagic tendencies, pericardial effusion, pericarditis, severe or malignant hypertension, severe renal or hepatic disease, or subacute bacterial endocarditis.

■ Avoid using drug in patients with a history of warfarin-induced necrosis; in unsupervised patients with senility, alcoholism, or psychosis; or in situations in which laboratory facilities are inadequate for coagulation testing.

■ Use cautiously in breast-feeding women, patients with drainage tubes in any orifice, patients with conditions that increase the risk of hemorrhage, and patients with colitis, diverticulitis, mild or moderate hepatic or renal disease, or mild or moderate hypertension.

■ Elderly patients and patients with renal or hepatic failure are especially sensitive to warfarin effect.

KEY POINTS

■ Draw blood to establish baseline coagulation parameters before therapy. Prothrombin time (PT) and international normalized ratio (INR) are essential for proper control.

■ Withhold drug and call prescriber at once if fever or rash (signs of severe adverse reaction) develops.

■ Half-life of warfarin's anticoagulant effect is 36 to 44 hours. Effect can be neutralized by parenteral or oral vitamin K.

RESPIRATORY SYNCYTIAL VIRUS INFECTION

A subgroup of the myxoviruses causes respiratory syncytial virus (RSV) infection, the leading cause of lower respiratory tract infection in infants and young children. It's the major cause of pneumonia, tracheobronchitis, and bronchiolitis in this age group and a suspected cause of fatal respiratory diseases of infancy. Each year, 125,000 infants are hospitalized with severe RSV; 1% to 2% die.

Few children younger than age 4 escape contracting some form of RSV, even if it's mild. In fact, RSV is the only viral disease that has its maximum impact during the first few months after birth (occurrence of RSV bronchiolitis peaks at age 2 months). The virus causes annual epidemics during late winter and early spring in temperate climates and during the rainy season in the tropics.

The organism is transmitted from person to person by respiratory secretions and has an incubation period of 4 to 5 days. Infants at higher risk include those who are exposed to tobacco smoke, attend day-care centers, live in crowded conditions, or have school-age siblings. Reinfection is common, producing milder symptoms than the primary infection. School-age children, adolescents, and young adults with mild reinfections are probably the source of infection for infants and young children.

RSV also causes repeated infections throughout life, usually with moderate-to-severe cold-like symptoms, and it may predispose a child to asthma. Severe lower respiratory tract disease can occur, especially among elderly people and those with compromised cardiac, pulmonary, or immune systems.

palivizumab

CONTRAINDICATIONS AND CAUTIONS

■ Contraindicated in children hypersensitive to drug or its components.

■ Use cautiously in patients with thrombocytopenia or other coagulation disorders.

KEY POINTS

■ Patients should receive monthly doses throughout RSV season, even if RSV infection develops. In the northern hemisphere, RSV season typically lasts from November to April.

✿ *CLINICAL TIP Give drug into anterolateral aspect of thigh. Don't use the gluteal muscle routinely as an injection site because of the risk of damaging the sciatic nerve. Divide injection volumes that are larger than 1 ml.*

■ Rarely, a patient may have an anaphylactoid reaction to the drug. If anaphylaxis or severe allergic reaction occurs, give epinephrine (1:1,000), and provide supportive care as needed. If the reaction is mild, use caution when giving again; if severe, stop therapy.

respiratory syncytial virus immune globulin intravenous, human

CONTRAINDICATIONS AND CAUTIONS

■ Contraindicated in patients severely hypersensitive to drug or other human immunoglobulin and patients with selective immunoglobulin A deficiency.

■ Children with fluid overload shouldn't receive drug.

KEY POINTS

■ First dose should be given before RSV season begins; later doses should be given monthly during RSV season to maintain protection. Children with RSV should continue to receive monthly doses for duration of RSV season.

■ Watch patient closely for evidence of fluid overload. Children with bronchopulmonary dysplasia may be more prone to this condition. Report increases in heart or respiratory rate, retractions, or crackles. Keep available a loop diuretic, such as furosemide or bumetanide.

■ If patient develops hypotension, anaphylaxis, or severe allergic reaction, stop infusion and give epinephrine 1:1,000. Patients with selective immunoglobulin A deficiency can develop antibodies to immunoglobulin A and have anaphylactic or allergic reactions to subsequent administration of blood products containing immunoglobulin A, including RSV-IGIV.

ribavirin

CONTRAINDICATIONS AND CAUTIONS

■ Contraindicated in patients hypersensitive to drug and in women who are or may become pregnant during treatment.

KEY POINTS

■ Give ribavirin aerosol only with the Viratek SPAG-2. Don't use any other aerosol-generating device.

■ The most frequent adverse effects in health care personnel exposed to aerosolized ribavirin include eye irritation and headache.

🌀 *ALERT Drug belongs to pregnancy risk category X; pregnant personnel should be advised of this status.*

■ Monitor ventilator function frequently. Ribavirin may precipitate in ventilator apparatus, causing equipment malfunction with serious consequences.

TUBERCULOSIS

An acute or chronic infection caused by *Mycobacterium tuber-*

culosis, tuberculosis (TB) is characterized by pulmonary infiltrates, formation of granulomas with caseation, fibrosis, and cavitation. TB is transmitted by droplet nuclei produced when an infected person coughs or sneezes and another person inhales the droplet. After exposure to *M. tuberculosis*, roughly 5% of infected people develop active TB within 1 year. In the rest, cell-mediated immunity to the mycobacteria, which develops about 3 to 6 weeks later, contains the infection and arrests the disease.

The host's immune system usually controls the tubercle bacillus by killing it or walling it up in a tiny nodule (tubercle). However, the bacillus may lie dormant within the tubercle for years and later reactivate and spread. Those at higher risk for disease progression or reactivation include infants, the elderly, and people who are immunocompromised (such as those with acquired immunodeficiency syndrome [AIDS], those undergoing chemotherapy, or transplant recipients taking antirejection drugs).

TB has become more common in the United States because of the increase in human immunodeficiency virus infection, the increasing number of homeless people, and the appearance of drug-resistant strains of TB. A person's risk of contracting TB increases if he has frequent contact with infected people, he lives in crowded or unsanitary living conditions, or he has poor nutrition.

Although the lungs are the primary infection site, mycobacteria commonly exist in other parts of the body. Sites of extrapulmonary TB include pleura, meninges, joints, lymph nodes, peritoneum, genitourinary tract, and bowel.

Several factors increase the risk of infection reactivation: gastrectomy, uncontrolled diabetes mellitus, Hodgkin's disease, leukemia, silicosis, AIDS, and corticosteroid or immunosuppressant therapy. If the infection reactivates, the body's response typically leads to caseation—the conversion of necrotic tissue to a cheeselike material. The caseum may localize, undergo fibrosis, or excavate and form cavities, the walls of which are studded with multiplying tubercle bacilli. If this happens, infected caseous debris may spread through the lungs by the tracheobronchial tree.

In patients with strains of *M. tuberculosis* that are sensitive to the usual antituberculotics, the prognosis is excellent with correct treatment. However, in those with strains that are resistant to two or more major antituberculotics, mortality is 50%.

bacillus Calmette-Guérin (BCG) vaccine

CONTRAINDICATIONS AND CAUTIONS

■ Contraindicated in patients hypersensitive to vaccine, pregnant women, patients with hypogammaglobulinemia, patients with immunosuppression and a positive tuberculin reaction (when meant for use as immunoprophylactic after exposure to TB), patients with fresh smallpox vaccinations, patients with burns, and patients receiving corticosteroid therapy.

■ Safety and efficacy for use in HIV-infected adults and children haven't been determined.

■ Use cautiously in patients with chronic skin disease. Inject only into healthy skin.

KEY POINTS

■ Give vaccine using a multipuncture disc. Don't inject it by the I.V., S.C., or intradermal route. Keep area dry for at least 24 hours after administration.

■ Expect lesions in 10 to 14 days. Papules reach a maximum diameter of 3 mm and then fade. Results occur more quickly when the patient has tuberculosis.

■ Allow at least 6 to 8 weeks between BCG and live-virus vaccines; give killed-virus vaccines 7 days before or 10 days after BCG.

cycloserine

CONTRAINDICATIONS AND CAUTIONS

■ Contraindicated in patients hypersensitive to drug, in those who use alcohol excessively, and in those with depression, psychosis, seizure disorders, severe anxiety, or severe renal insufficiency.

■ Use cautiously and at reduced dosage in patients with impaired renal function.

KEY POINTS

■ Cycloserine is considered a second-line drug in TB treatment and should always be given with other antituberculotics to prevent the development of resistant organisms.

■ Monitor cycloserine levels periodically, especially in patients receiving more than 500 mg daily, because toxic reactions may occur with blood levels above 30 mcg/ml.

■ Observe patient receiving more than 500 mg daily for evidence of central nervous system toxicity, such as seizures, anxiety, and tremor.

ethambutol

CONTRAINDICATIONS AND CAUTIONS

■ Contraindicated in children younger than age 13, patients hypersensitive to drug, and patients with optic neuritis.

■ Use cautiously in patients with cataracts, diabetic retinopathy, gout, impaired renal function, or recurrent eye inflammation.

KEY POINTS

■ Perform visual acuity and color discrimination tests before and during therapy.

■ Make sure any changes in vision don't result from an underlying condition.

■ Obtain aspartate transaminase and alanine transaminase levels before therapy, and monitor them every 3 to 4 weeks.

■ Always give ethambutol with other antituberculotics to prevent development of resistant organisms.

isoniazid

CONTRAINDICATIONS AND CAUTIONS

■ Contraindicated in patients with acute hepatic disease or isoniazid-related liver damage.

■ Use cautiously in elderly patients and patients with chronic non–isoniazid-related liver disease, chronic alcoholism, seizure disorders (especially those taking phenytoin), or severe renal impairment.

KEY POINTS

■ Isoniazid pharmacokinetics vary because drug is metabolized in the liver by genetically controlled acetylation. Fast acetylators metabolize it up to five times as fast as slow acetylators. About half of blacks and whites are slow acetylators; more than 80% of Chinese, Japanese, and Inuits are fast acetylators.

■ Peripheral neuropathy is more common in slow acetylators and patients who are malnourished, alcoholic, or diabetic. Give pyridoxine to prevent peripheral neuropathy, especially in malnourished patients.

■ Severe and sometimes fatal hepatitis may develop, even after many months of treatment. Risk increases with age. Monitor liver studies closely.

rifampin

CONTRAINDICATIONS AND CAUTIONS

■ Contraindicated in patients hypersensitive to rifampin or related drugs.

■ Use cautiously in patients with liver disease.

KEY POINTS

■ Give P.O. doses 1 hour before or 2 hours after meals for optimal absorption; if gastrointestinal irritation occurs, give with meals.

■ Monitor hepatic function, hematopoietic studies, and uric acid levels. Drug's systemic effects may cause asymptomatic elevation of liver function test results and uric acid level.

■ Drug may cause hemorrhage in neonates of rifampin-treated mothers.

rifapentine
CONTRAINDICATIONS AND CAUTIONS

■ Contraindicated in patients hypersensitive to rifamycins (rifapentine, rifampin, or rifabutin).

■ Use drug cautiously and with frequent monitoring in patients with liver disease.

KEY POINTS

■ Give drug with pyridoxine (vitamin B_6) in malnourished patients; those predisposed to neuropathy, such as alcoholics and diabetics; and adolescents.

■ Give drug with daily companion drugs. Compliance with all drugs, especially with companion drugs on the days when rifapentine isn't given, is crucial for early sputum conversion and protection from relapse.

■ If given during the last 2 weeks of pregnancy, drug may lead to postnatal hemorrhage in mother or infant. Monitor clotting parameters closely.

streptomycin
CONTRAINDICATIONS AND CAUTIONS

■ Contraindicated in patients hypersensitive to drug or other aminoglycosides.

■ Use cautiously in elderly patients and patients with impaired renal function or neuromuscular disorders.

KEY POINTS

■ Evaluate patient's hearing before therapy and for 6 months afterward. Notify prescriber if patient complains of hearing loss, roaring noises, or fullness in the ears.

■ Obtain blood for peak streptomycin level 1 to 2 hours after I.M. injection; for trough levels, draw blood just before next dose. Don't use a heparinized tube; heparin is incompatible with aminoglycosides.

■ Nephrotoxicity occurs less often with streptomycin than with other aminoglycosides.

20 / DRUGS FOR NEUROLOGIC DISORDERS

ALZHEIMER'S DISEASE

Also known as *primary degenerative dementia*, Alzheimer's disease accounts for more than half of all dementias. An estimated 5% of people older than age 65 have a severe form of this disease, and 12% suffer from mild to moderate dementia. The brain tissue of a patient with Alzheimer's disease typically shows cortical atrophy, the hallmark features being neurofibrillary tangles, neuritic plaques, and granulovascular degeneration.

Several factors contribute to the progression of Alzheimer's disease. They include neurochemical factors, such as deficiencies in acetylcholine (a neurotransmitter), somatostatin, substance P, and norepinephrine; environmental factors, such as aluminum and manganese; viral factors, such as slow-growing central nervous system (CNS) viruses; traumatic injury; and genetic immunologic factors.

Because Alzheimer's disease is a primary progressive dementia, the prognosis is poor.

donepezil

CONTRAINDICATIONS AND CAUTIONS

■ Contraindicated in patients hypersensitive to drug or to piperidine derivatives.

■ Use cautiously in patients who take nonsteroidal anti-inflammatory drugs (NSAIDs) or have asthma, cardiovascular (CV) disease, chronic obstructive pulmonary disease (COPD), impaired urine outflow, or a history of peptic ulcer disease.

KEY POINTS

■ Monitor patient for evidence of active or occult gastrointestinal (GI) bleeding.

🍀 *CLINICAL TIP Drug doesn't alter underlying degenerative disease but can temporarily stabilize or relieve symptoms. Ef-*

fectiveness depends on taking it regularly.

■ Give drug just before patient's bedtime.

galantamine
CONTRAINDICATIONS AND CAUTIONS

■ Contraindicated in patients hypersensitive to drug or its components.

■ Use cautiously in patients with a history of peptic ulcer disease; patients taking NSAIDs; patients with asthma, obstructed urine outflow, or seizures (because of possible cholinomimetic effects); patients with supraventricular cardiac conduction disorders; and patients taking drugs that significantly slow the heart rate.

■ Use cautiously before or during procedures involving succinylcholine-type or similar neuromuscular-blocking anesthesia.

KEY POINTS

■ Bradycardia and heart block may occur, whether or not the patient has cardiac conduction abnormalities. Consider all patients at risk for adverse effects on cardiac conduction.

■ Give drug with food and antiemetics, and ensure adequate fluid intake to decrease the risk of nausea and vomiting.

■ Use proper technique when dispensing oral solution with a pipette. Dispense measured amount in a nonalcoholic beverage and give right away.

■ If drug is stopped for several days or longer, restart at the lowest dose and gradually increase at 4-week or longer intervals to the previous dosage level.

memantine
CONTRAINDICATIONS AND CAUTIONS

■ Contraindicated in patients allergic to drug or its components.

■ Not recommended for patients with severe renal impairment.

■ Use cautiously in patients with hepatic impairment, moderate renal impairment, seizures, or an increased urine pH (from drugs, diet, renal tubular acidosis, or severe urinary tract infection, for example).

KEY POINTS

■ Memantine isn't indicated for mild Alzheimer's disease or other types of dementia.

■ Explain that memantine doesn't cure Alzheimer's disease but may improve the symptoms.

■ Advise against taking herbal or over-the-counter products

with this drug without consulting a health care provider.

rivastigmine

CONTRAINDICATIONS AND CAUTIONS

■ Contraindicated in patients hypersensitive to drug, other carbamate derivatives, or other components of the drug.

KEY POINTS

■ Expect significant GI adverse effects (such as nausea, vomiting, anorexia, and weight loss). These effects are less common during maintenance therapy.

■ Assess patient for evidence of active or occult GI bleeding. Carefully monitor a patient with a history of arrhythmias, GI bleeding, NSAID use, pulmonary conditions, or seizures for adverse effects.

■ Dramatic memory improvement is unlikely. As disease progresses, the benefits of rivastigmine may decline.

tacrine

CONTRAINDICATIONS AND CAUTIONS

■ Contraindicated in patients hypersensitive to drug or to acridine derivatives.

■ Contraindicated in patients for whom tacrine-related jaundice has previously been confirmed with a total bilirubin level of more than 3 mg/dl.

■ Use cautiously in patients with sick sinus syndrome or bradycardia, patients at risk for peptic ulcers (including those taking NSAIDs or those with a history of peptic ulcer), and in those with a history of hepatic disease.

■ Use cautiously in patients with asthma, prostatic hyperplasia, renal disease, or urine outflow impairment.

KEY POINTS

■ Drug should be given between meals if possible. If GI upset becomes a problem, drug may be taken with meals, although doing so may reduce plasma levels by 30% to 40%.

■ Monitor alanine transaminase (ALT) level weekly during first 18 weeks of therapy. If it's modestly elevated (twice the upper limit of normal range) after first 18 weeks, continue weekly monitoring. If no problems are detected, ALT tests may be decreased to once every 3 months. Each time dosage is increased, resume weekly monitoring for at least 6 weeks.

■ If drug is stopped for 4 weeks or longer, full dosage adjustment and monitoring schedule must be restarted.

ATTENTION DEFICIT HYPERACTIVITY DISORDER

A patient with attention deficit hyperactivity disorder (ADHD) has difficulty focusing his attention; engaging in quiet, passive activities; or both. Boys are three times more likely to be affected than girls. Although this disorder is present at birth, diagnosis before age 4 or 5 is unlikely unless the child has severe symptoms. Some patients aren't diagnosed until adulthood.

ADHD is commonly thought to be a physiologic brain disorder with a familial tendency. Some studies indicate that it may result from disturbances in neurotransmitter levels in the brain.

atomoxetine
CONTRAINDICATIONS AND CAUTIONS
■ Contraindicated in patients hypersensitive to atomoxetine or its components, patients who have taken a monoamine oxidase (MAO) inhibitor during the past 2 weeks, and patients with angle-closure glaucoma.

■ Use cautiously in pregnant women, breast-feeding women, and patients with cerebrovascular disease, cardiovascular (CV)

disease, hypertension, or tachycardia.

■ Safety and efficacy haven't been established in patients younger than age 6.

KEY POINTS
■ Patients taking drug for extended periods must be reevaluated periodically to determine drug's usefulness.

■ Monitor growth during treatment. If growth or weight gain is unsatisfactory, consider interrupting therapy

■ Assess blood pressure and pulse at baseline, after each dose increase, and periodically during treatment.

■ Patient can stop taking drug without tapering off.

■ Drug is the first nonstimulant drug approved for treating ADHD.

dexmethylphenidate
CONTRAINDICATIONS AND CAUTIONS
■ Contraindicated in patients hypersensitive to methylphenidate or its components; patients with agitation, glaucoma, motor tics, severe anxiety, severe tension, or Tourette syndrome (or family history of it); and patients who took an MAO inhibitor within 14 days.

■ Use in pregnant women only if the benefits outweigh the

risks; drug may delay skeletal ossification, suppress weight gain, and impair organ development in the fetus.

■ Use cautiously in patients with a history of drug abuse or alcoholism; patients with heart failure, hypertension, hyperthyroidism, psychosis, recent myocardial infarction (MI), or seizures.

KEY POINTS

■ Periodically reevaluate drug's long-term usefulness. Monitor patient for evidence of drug dependence or abuse.

■ Long-term stimulant use may temporarily suppress growth. Assess child's growth and weight gain. Stop treatment if growth slows or weight gain is lower than expected.

■ Check blood pressure and pulse routinely.

■ Stop drug if seizures occur.

dextroamphetamine
CONTRAINDICATIONS AND CAUTIONS

■ Contraindicated in patients hypersensitive to sympathomimetic amines, patients with idiosyncratic reactions to sympathomimetic amines, patients who took an MAO within 14 days, patients with a history of drug abuse, and patients with advanced arteriosclerosis, glaucoma, hyperthyroidism, moderate to severe hypertension, or symptomatic CV disease.

■ Use cautiously in agitated patients and patients with motor tics, phonic tics, or Tourette syndrome.

KEY POINTS

■ Dextroamphetamine has a paradoxical calming effect in children with ADHD.

ALERT Drug has a high abuse potential and may cause dependence.

■ Overdose may cause seizures.

methylphenidate
CONTRAINDICATIONS AND CAUTIONS

■ Contraindicated in patients hypersensitive to drug and patients with glaucoma, motor tics, Tourette syndrome (or a family history of it), or a history of marked anxiety, tension, or agitation.

■ Because it doesn't dissolve, Concerta is contraindicated in patients with severe gastrointestinal narrowing (such as small bowel inflammatory disease, short-gut syndrome caused by adhesions or decreased transit time, history of peritonitis, cystic fibrosis, chronic intestinal pseudo-obstruction, or Meckel's diverticulum).

■ Concerta, Metadate, Ritalin, Ritalin-SR, and Ritalin LA are contraindicated within 14 days of MAO inhibitor therapy.

■ Use cautiously in patients who are emotionally unstable; patients with a history of drug dependence or alcoholism; patients with a history of seizures, electroencephalogram abnormalities, or hypertension; and patients whose underlying medical condition may be compromised by increased blood pressure or heart rate (as in hypertension, heart failure, recent MI, or hyperthyroidism).

KEY POINTS

■ As with amphetamines, drug has a paradoxical calming effect in hyperactive children.

■ Drug may trigger Tourette syndrome in children. Monitor patient, especially at start of therapy.

■ Check results of periodic complete blood count, differential, and platelet counts with long-term use.

■ Assess height and weight in children on long-term therapy. Drug may delay growth spurt, but child will attain normal height when drug is stopped.

MIGRAINE

Migraine headaches, probably the most intensively studied type of headache, are throbbing, vascular headaches that usually begin in childhood or adolescence and recur throughout adulthood. Affecting up to 10% of Americans, they're more common in women and have a strong familial tendency.

The cause of migraine headaches is unknown, but they're associated with constriction and dilation of intracranial and extracranial arteries initiated by neurons in the brainstem. Certain biochemical abnormalities are thought to occur during a migraine as well. They include local leakage of a vasodilator polypeptide (neurokinin) through the dilated arteries as an inflammatory response and a decrease in the plasma level of serotonin.

Foods that may influence migraine headaches include aged or processed cheeses and meats, alcohol (particularly red wine), food additives (such as monosodium glutamate), chocolate, caffeine, and nuts. Changes in the weather, menstrual cycle, sleep pattern, and exercise may trigger a migraine headache, as may glaring lights and fatigue.

almotriptan
CONTRAINDICATIONS AND CAUTIONS
■ Contraindicated in patients hypersensitive to drug, patients who took a 5-HT$_1$ agonist or ergotamine drug within the previous 24 hours, patients with a history of coronary artery vasospasm, cardiovascular (CV) disease, myocardial infarction (MI), Prinzmetal's variant angina, or silent ischemia; and patients with angina pectoris, hemiplegic or basilar migraine, or uncontrolled hypertension.

■ Use cautiously in patients with renal or hepatic impairment, patients with cataracts (because of the risk of corneal opacities), and patients with risk factors for coronary artery disease (CAD), such as diabetes, obesity, and a family history of CAD.

KEY POINTS
■ Patients with poor renal or hepatic function should receive a reduced dosage.

■ Repeat dose after 2 hours, if needed, and don't give more than two doses in 24 hours.

■ Serious adverse CV effects include coronary artery vasospasm, MI, transient myocardial ischemia, ventricular fibrillation, and ventricular tachycardia.

dihydroergotamine
CONTRAINDICATIONS AND CAUTIONS
■ Contraindicated in pregnant women, breast-feeding women, patients hypersensitive to drug, patients taking CYP 3A4 inhibitors, and patients with CAD, coronary artery spasm (including Prinzmetal's angina), hemiplegic or basilar migraine, ischemic heart disease, malnutrition, peripheral and occlusive vascular disease, sepsis, severe hepatic or renal dysfunction, severe pruritus, or uncontrolled hypertension.

KEY POINTS
🔲 *CLINICAL TIP Drug is most effective when taken at first sign of migraine or soon after onset.*

■ Avoid prolonged use, and don't exceed recommended dosage. For best results, adjust to most effective minimal dosage.

■ Watch for ergotamine rebound (increase in frequency and duration of headache), which may occur when drug is stopped.

frovatriptan
CONTRAINDICATIONS AND CAUTIONS

- Contraindicated in patients hypersensitive to drug or its components; patients who took another $5\text{-}HT_1$ agonist, ergotamine drug, or ergot-type drug during the previous 24 hours; patients with risk factors for CAD (hypertension, hypercholesterolemia, smoking, obesity, strong family history, postmenopausal women, men older than age 40) unless patient has no underlying CV disease; patients with a history or symptoms of ischemic heart disease or coronary artery vasospasm (including Prinzmetal's variant angina); patients with cerebrovascular or peripheral vascular disease, including ischemic bowel disease; patients with uncontrolled hypertension; and patients with hemiplegic or basilar migraine.

- Use cautiously in breastfeeding patients. It isn't known whether drug appears in breast milk.

KEY POINTS

- Serious cardiac events include acute MI, life-threatening cardiac arrhythmias, and death within a few hours after taking a $5\text{-}HT_1$ agonist.

- Give drug only when patient has a clear diagnosis of migraine. If the patient has no response to drug when treating the first migraine attack, reconsider the migraine diagnosis.

- The safety of treating an average of more than four migraine headaches in a 30-day period hasn't been established.

- If drug is given to a patient with risk factors for CAD but no underlying CV disease, give first dose under close supervision. Consider obtaining an electrocardiogram after the first dose. Intermittent, long-term users of $5\text{-}HT_1$ agonists and patients with CAD risk factors should have periodic cardiac evaluation while taking frovatriptan.

naratriptan
CONTRAINDICATIONS AND CAUTIONS

- Contraindicated in elderly patients; patients hypersensitive to drug or its components; patients with creatinine clearance below 15 ml/minute; patients with Child-Pugh grade C hepatic impairment; patients who have taken ergot-containing, ergot-type, or other $5\text{-}HT_1$ agonists within 24 hours; patients with previous or current cardiac ischemia; patients with cerebrovascular or peripheral vascular syndromes; and patients with uncontrolled hypertension.

■ Use cautiously in patients with renal or hepatic impairment; patients with CAD risk factors, such as hypertension, hypercholesterolemia, obesity, diabetes, or a strong family history of CAD; and postmenopausal women, men older than age 40, and patients who smoke, unless patient is free from cardiac disease.

KEY POINTS

■ Use drug only if patient has a clear diagnosis of migraine. Drug isn't intended to prevent migraines or manage hemiplegic or basilar migraine.

■ Drug can cause coronary artery vasospasm and increased risk of cerebrovascular events.

■ Safety and effectiveness of treating cluster headaches or more than four headaches in a 30-day period haven't been established.

■ If patient has cardiac risk factors but satisfactory CV evaluation results, monitor him closely after first dose.

rizatriptan
CONTRAINDICATIONS AND CAUTIONS

■ Contraindicated in patients hypersensitive to drug or its components; patients with hemiplegic or basilar migraine; patients with uncontrolled hypertension; patients who took another 5-HT$_1$ agonist, ergotamine drug, or ergot-type drug, such as dihydroergotamine or methysergide, within 24 hours; patients who took a monoamine oxidase (MAO) inhibitor within 14 days; and patients with a history or symptoms of coronary artery vasospasm (Prinzmetal's variant angina), ischemic heart disease, or other significant underlying CV disease.

■ Use cautiously in patients with hepatic or renal impairment and patients with CAD risk factors (hypertension, hypercholesterolemia, smoking, obesity, diabetes, strong family history of CAD, postmenopausal women, or men older than age 40), unless patient is free from cardiac disease.

■ Safety of treating more than four headaches in a 30-day period hasn't been established.

KEY POINTS

■ If patient has CAD risk factors but no cardiac disease, monitor him closely after first dose.

■ Assess CV status in patients who develop CAD risk factors during treatment.

■ Give drug only when patient has a clear diagnosis of migraine.

■ Don't give drug to prevent migraines or to treat hemiplegic or basilar migraine or cluster headaches.

■ Orally disintegrating tablets contain phenylalanine.

sumatriptan

CONTRAINDICATIONS AND CAUTIONS

■ Contraindicated in patients hypersensitive to drug or its components; patients who took a 5-HT$_1$ agonist or ergotamine drug within 24 hours; patients who took an MAO inhibitor within 14 days; patients with a history or evidence of ischemic cardiac, cerebrovascular (such as stroke or transient ischemic attack), or peripheral vascular syndromes (such as ischemic bowel disease); patients with significant underlying CV diseases, including angina pectoris, MI, and silent myocardial ischemia; patients with uncontrolled hypertension; and patients with severe hepatic impairment.

■ Use cautiously in a patient who is or intends to become pregnant and in patients who may have unrecognized CAD (such as postmenopausal women, men older than age 40,

or patients with such risk factors as hypertension, hypercholesterolemia, obesity, diabetes, smoking, or family history of CAD).

KEY POINTS

■ When giving drug to patient at risk for unrecognized CAD, consider giving first dose with additional medical personnel. Serious adverse cardiac effects can follow administration, but they're rare.

■ After subcutaneous (S.C.) injection, most patients experience relief in 1 to 2 hours.

■ Redness or pain at injection site should subside within 1 hour after injection.

zolmitriptan

CONTRAINDICATIONS AND CAUTIONS

■ Contraindicated in pregnant women; breast-feeding women; patients hypersensitive to drug or its components; patients who took a 5-HT$_1$ agonist or ergot-containing drug within 24 hours; patients who took an MAO inhibitor within 14 days; patients with uncontrolled hypertension; and patients with coronary artery vasospasm (including Prinzmetal's variant angina), hemiplegic or basilar migraine, ischemic heart disease (angina pectoris, history of MI or documented silent ischemia), or other significant heart disease.

■ Use cautiously in patients with liver disease and patients who may be at risk for CAD (such as postmenopausal women and men over age 40) or those with such risk factors as hypertension, hypercholesterolemia, obesity, diabetes, smoking, or a family history.

KEY POINTS

■ Drug isn't intended for preventing migraines or treating hemiplegic or basilar migraines.
■ Safety of drug hasn't been established for cluster headaches.

PARKINSON'S DISEASE

Parkinson's disease (also known as *shaking palsy* and *paralysis agitans*) typically produces progressive muscle rigidity, akinesia, involuntary tremor, and progressive deterioration. Death may result from complications, such as aspiration pneumonia or another infection.

One of the most common crippling diseases in the United States, Parkinson's disease affects 2 of every 1,000 people older than age 50. It also occurs in younger adults and, rarely, in children. Although the cause of Parkinson's disease isn't known, study of extrapyramidal brain nuclei (corpus striatum, globus pallidus, substantia nigra) shows that dopamine deficiency prevents affected brain cells from performing their normal inhibitory function in the central nervous system.

benztropine

CONTRAINDICATIONS AND CAUTIONS

■ Contraindicated in children younger than age 3, patients hypersensitive to drug or its components, and patients who have angle-closure glaucoma.
■ Use cautiously in hot weather, patients with mental disorders, children age 3 and older, and patients with arrhythmias, prostatic hyperplasia, or seizure disorders.

KEY POINTS

■ Drug produces atropine-like adverse reactions and may aggravate tardive dyskinesia.

ALERT Watch for intermittent constipation and abdominal distention and pain, which may indicate onset of paralytic ileus.

■ Never stop drug abruptly. Reduce dosage gradually.

bromocriptine

CONTRAINDICATIONS AND CAUTIONS

■ Contraindicated in patients hypersensitive to ergot derivatives and in those with uncontrolled hypertension, toxemia of pregnancy, severe ischemic heart disease, or peripheral vascular disease.

■ Use cautiously in patients with impaired renal or hepatic function and in those with a history of myocardial infarction (MI) with residual arrhythmias.

KEY POINTS

■ Usually, drug is given with either levodopa or levodopa-carbidopa for patients with Parkinson's disease. The levodopa-carbidopa dose may need to be reduced.

■ Adverse reactions may be minimized if drug is given in the evening with food.

■ Watch for adverse reactions, which occur in 68% of patients, particularly when therapy starts. Most reactions are mild to moderate; nausea is most common. Minimize adverse reactions by gradually adjusting dosages to effective levels.

entacapone

CONTRAINDICATIONS AND CAUTIONS

■ Contraindicated in patients hypersensitive to drug.

■ Use cautiously in patients with hepatic impairment, biliary obstruction, or orthostatic hypotension.

KEY POINTS

■ Use drug only with levodopa-carbidopa; no antiparkinsonian effects occur when drug is given alone.

■ Diarrhea most often begins within 4 to 12 weeks after therapy starts but may begin as early as 1 week or as late as many months after therapy starts.

■ Rapid withdrawal or abrupt reduction in dose could lead to signs and symptoms of Parkinson's disease; it may also lead to hyperpyrexia and confusion, a group of symptoms resembling neuroleptic malignant syndrome. Stop drug gradually, and monitor patient closely. Adjust other dopaminergic treatments, as needed.

levodopa-carbidopa

CONTRAINDICATIONS AND CAUTIONS

■ Contraindicated in patients hypersensitive to drug, patients who took a monoamine oxidase (MAO) inhibitor within 14 days, and patients with angle-closure glaucoma, melanoma, or undiagnosed skin lesions.

■ Use cautiously in patients with severe cardiovascular, renal, hepatic, endocrine, or pulmonary disorders; a history of peptic ulcer; psychiatric illness; MI with residual arrhythmias; bronchial asthma; emphysema; and well-controlled, chronic open-angle glaucoma.

KEY POINTS

■ Levodopa-carbidopa typically decreases the amount of levodopa needed by 75%, reducing the risk of adverse reactions. If patient takes levodopa, stop drug at least 8 hours before starting levodopa-carbidopa.

■ Because of the risk of a symptom complex resembling neuroleptic malignant syndrome, observe patient closely if levodopa dosage is reduced abruptly or stopped.

■ Muscle twitching and blepharospasm may be early signs of drug overdose; report immediately.

pergolide
CONTRAINDICATIONS AND CAUTIONS

■ Contraindicated in patients hypersensitive to drug or to ergot alkaloids.

■ Use cautiously in patients prone to arrhythmias and patient with a history of pleuritis, pleural effusion, pleural fibrosis, pericarditis, pericardial effusion, cardiac valvulopathy, or retroperitoneal fibrosis.

KEY POINTS

■ Give drug with food.

■ Monitor blood pressure. Symptomatic orthostatic or sustained hypotension may occur, especially at start of therapy.

pramipexole
CONTRAINDICATIONS AND CAUTIONS

■ Contraindicated in patients hypersensitive to drug or its components.

■ It's unknown if drug appears in breast milk. Use cautiously in breast-feeding women.

KEY POINTS

■ If drug must be stopped, withdraw over 1 week.

■ Drug may cause orthostatic hypotension, especially during dosage increases. Monitor patient carefully.

■ Adjust dosage gradually to achieve maximum therapeutic effect, balanced against the main adverse effects of dyskinesia, hallucinations, somnolence, and dry mouth.

ropinirole

CONTRAINDICATIONS AND CAUTIONS

■ Contraindicated in patients hypersensitive to drug.

■ Use cautiously in patients with severe hepatic or renal impairment.

KEY POINTS

■ Drug may potentiate the dopaminergic adverse effects of levodopa and may cause or worsen dyskinesia. Dosage may be decreased.

ALERT *Monitor patient carefully for orthostatic hypotension, especially during dosage increases.*

■ Patient may have syncope, with or without bradycardia. Monitor patient carefully, especially for 4 weeks after start of therapy and with dosage increases.

selegiline

CONTRAINDICATIONS AND CAUTIONS

■ Contraindicated in patients hypersensitive to drug and in those receiving meperidine.

KEY POINTS

■ Some patients have increased adverse reactions to levodopa when it's given with selegiline and need a 10% to 30%

reduction of levodopa-carbidopa dosage.

■ Severe adverse reactions may occur if drug is given with antidepressants.

■ Patient should avoid foods high in tyramine because of risk of hypertensive crisis.

tolcapone

CONTRAINDICATIONS AND CAUTIONS

■ Contraindicated in patients hypersensitive to drug or its components, patients who were withdrawn from tolcapone because of drug-induced hepatocellular injury, and patients with elevated alanine transaminase or aspartate transaminase levels, hepatic disease, a history of drug-related confusion, and nontraumatic rhabdomyolysis or hyperpyrexia.

■ Use cautiously in patients with severe renal impairment and in breast-feeding women.

KEY POINTS

■ Make sure patient provides written informed consent before taking drug.

■ Because of risk of liver toxicity, stop treatment if patient shows no benefit within 3 weeks.

■ Because of risk of fatal hepatic failure, drug should be given only to patients taking levodopa-carbidopa who don't respond to or who aren't appropriate candidates for other adjunctive therapies.

■ Monitor liver function test results before starting drug, every 2 weeks for first year of therapy, every 4 weeks for next 6 months, and every 8 weeks thereafter. Stop drug if results are abnormal or patient appears jaundiced.

trihexyphenidyl
CONTRAINDICATIONS AND CAUTIONS

■ Contraindicated in patients hypersensitive to drug.

■ Use cautiously in patients with cardiac disorders, glaucoma, hepatic disorders, obstructive gastrointestinal or genitourinary disorders, prostatic hyperplasia, or renal disorders.

KEY POINTS

■ Dosage may need to be gradually increased in patients who develop tolerance to drug.

■ Drug may cause nausea if taken before meals.

■ Adverse reactions are dose-related and transient.

SEIZURES

Seizure disorder, or *epilepsy*, is a condition of the brain characterized by a susceptibility to recurrent seizures (paroxysmal events involving abnormal electrical discharges of neurons in the brain). It probably affects 1% to 2% of the population. In about half of people with seizure disorder, the cause is unknown. Possible causes include the following:
– anoxia
– birth trauma (inadequate oxygen to the brain, blood incompatibility, or hemorrhage)
– brain tumor
– cerebrovascular accident (hemorrhage, thrombosis, or embolism).
– head injury or trauma
– infectious diseases (meningitis, encephalitis, or brain abscess)
– ingestion of toxins (mercury, lead, or carbon monoxide)
– inherited disorders or degenerative disease, such as phenylketonuria or tuberous sclerosis
– metabolic disorders, such as hypoglycemia and hypoparathyroidism
– perinatal infection.

The prognosis is good if the patient adheres strictly to the prescribed treatment.

carbamazepine
CONTRAINDICATIONS AND CAUTIONS
■ Contraindicated in patients hypersensitive to carbamazepine or tricyclic antidepressants, patients with a history of bone marrow suppression, and patients who have taken a monoamine oxidase inhibitor within 14 days.

■ Use cautiously in patients with mixed seizure disorders (because they may have an increased risk of seizures) and patients with hepatic dysfunction.

KEY POINTS
■ Therapeutic carbamazepine level is 4 to 12 mcg/ml. Monitor level and effects closely. Ask patient when last dose was taken to better evaluate drug level.

CLINICAL TIP Capsules and tablets shouldn't be crushed or chewed unless labeled as chewable form. The contents of the extended-release capsules may be sprinkled over applesauce if patient has trouble swallowing them.

■ Watch for evidence of anorexia or subtle appetite changes, which may indicate excessive drug level.

fosphenytoin
CONTRAINDICATIONS AND CAUTIONS
■ Contraindicated in patients hypersensitive to drug or its components, patients hypersensitive to phenytoin or other hydantoins, and patients with sinus bradycardia, sinoatrial (SA) block, second- or third-degree atrioventricular (AV) block, or Adams-Stokes syndrome.

■ Use cautiously in patients with porphyria and patients with a history of hypersensitivity to similarly structured drugs, such as barbiturates, oxazolidinediones, and succinimides.

KEY POINTS
ALERT Fosphenytoin should always be prescribed and dispensed in phenytoin sodium equivalent (PE) units. Don't make adjustments in the recommended doses when substituting fosphenytoin for phenytoin, and vice versa.

■ Stop drug and notify prescriber if rash appears. If rash is exfoliative, purpuric, or bullous, or if lupus erythematosus, Stevens-Johnson syndrome, or toxic epidermal necrolysis is suspected, drug should be stopped and alternative therapy considered. If rash is mild (measles-like or scarlatiniform), therapy may resume after rash disappears. If rash recurs when therapy resumes, further fosphenytoin or phenytoin use is contraindicated. Document that patient is allergic to drug.

■ After administration, phenytoin levels shouldn't be checked until conversion to phenytoin is essentially complete—about 2 hours after the end of an I.V. infusion or 4 hours after I.M. administration.

gabapentin
CONTRAINDICATIONS AND CAUTIONS
■ Contraindicated in patients hypersensitive to drug.

KEY POINTS
■ First dose should be given at bedtime to minimize the effects of drowsiness, dizziness, fatigue, and ataxia.
■ If drug will be stopped or an alternative drug substituted, do so gradually over at least 1 week to minimize risk of seizures. Don't withdraw other anticonvulsants suddenly in patients starting gabapentin therapy.
■ Routine monitoring of drug levels isn't necessary. Drug doesn't appear to alter levels of other anticonvulsants.

lamotrigine
CONTRAINDICATIONS AND CAUTIONS
■ Contraindicated in patients hypersensitive to drug or its components.
■ Safety and efficacy of drug in children under age 16 (other than those with Lennox-Gastaut syndrome) haven't been established. Children who weigh less than 17 kg (37 lb) shouldn't receive drug because therapy can't follow dosing guidelines and currently available tablet strength.
■ Use cautiously in patients with renal, hepatic, or cardiac impairment.

KEY POINTS
■ Drug shouldn't be stopped abruptly because doing so may increase seizures. Instead, drug should be tapered over at least 2 weeks.
■ Stop drug at first sign of rash unless it clearly isn't drug-related.
■ Lamotrigine dose should be reduced if drug is added to a multidrug regimen that includes valproic acid.

levetiracetam
CONTRAINDICATIONS AND CAUTIONS
■ Contraindicated in patients hypersensitive to drug.

■ Leukopenia and neutropenia have been reported with drug use. Use cautiously in immuno-compromised patients, such as those with cancer or infection with human immunodeficiency virus.

■ Patients with poor renal function need dosage adjustment.

KEY POINTS

■ Give drug only with other anticonvulsants; it isn't recommended for monotherapy.

■ Seizures can occur if drug is stopped abruptly. Tapering is recommended.

■ Monitor patients closely for such adverse reactions as dizziness, which may lead to falls.

oxcarbazepine
CONTRAINDICATIONS AND CAUTIONS

■ Contraindicated in patients hypersensitive to drug or its components.

KEY POINTS

■■ *CLINICAL TIP* *Oral suspension and tablets may be interchanged at equal doses.*

■ Watch for evidence of hyponatremia, including nausea, malaise, headache, lethargy, confusion, and decreased sensation.

■ Oxcarbazepine use has been linked to several adverse nervous system reactions, including psychomotor slowing, difficulty concentrating, speech or language problems, somnolence, fatigue, and coordination abnormalities, such as ataxia and gait disturbances.

phenobarbital
CONTRAINDICATIONS AND CAUTIONS

■ Contraindicated in patients hypersensitive to barbiturates, patients with a history of manifest or latent porphyria, and patients with hepatic or renal dysfunction, respiratory disease with dyspnea or obstruction, or nephritis.

■ Use cautiously in elderly or debilitated patients, patients with a history of drug abuse, and patients with acute or chronic pain, blood pressure alterations, cardiovascular disease, depression, diabetes mellitus, fever, hyperthyroidism, severe anemia, shock, suicidal tendencies, or uremia.

KEY POINTS

■ Up to 30 minutes may be needed for maximum effect after I.V. use; allow time for anticonvulsant effect to develop to avoid overdose.

Alert *Watch for evidence of barbiturate toxicity: coma, cyanosis, asthmatic breathing, clammy skin, and hypotension. Overdose can be fatal.*

■ Therapeutic level is 15 to 40 mcg/ml.

phenytoin
CONTRAINDICATIONS AND CAUTIONS
■ Contraindicated in patients hypersensitive to hydantoin and in those with sinus bradycardia, SA block, second- or third-degree AV block, or Adams-Stokes syndrome.

■ Use cautiously in elderly or debilitated patients, patients receiving other hydantoin derivatives, and patients with diabetes, hepatic dysfunction, hypotension, myocardial insufficiency, or respiratory depression.

■ Elderly patients tend to metabolize phenytoin slowly and may need reduced dosages.

KEY POINTS
■ Stop drug if rash appears. If it's scarlatiniform or morbilliform, drug may be resumed after rash clears. If rash reappears, therapy should be stopped. If it's exfoliative, purpuric, or bullous, drug won't be resumed.

■ Doubling the dose doesn't produce twice the initial serum levels and may result in toxic serum levels. Consult pharmacist for specific dosing recommendations.

■ Monitor drug level in blood. Therapeutic level is 10 to 20 mcg/ml.

topiramate
CONTRAINDICATIONS AND CAUTIONS
■ Contraindicated in patients hypersensitive to drug or its components.

■ Use cautiously in pregnant women, breast-feeding women, patients with hepatic impairment, and patients taking other drugs that predispose to heat-related disorders (such as carbonic anhydrase inhibitors and anticholinergics).

KEY POINTS
■ If needed, withdraw drug gradually to minimize risk of increased seizure activity.

■ Topiramate level doesn't need monitoring.

■ Stop the drug if an ocular adverse event occurs, characterized by acute myopia and secondary angle-closure glaucoma.

valproate
CONTRAINDICATIONS AND CAUTIONS
■ Contraindicated in patients hypersensitive to drug, patients with a urea cycle disorder, and

KEY POINTS

■ Don't withdraw drug abruptly because withdrawal symptoms, including seizures, may occur. Abuse or addiction is possible.

■ Smoking may decrease drug's effectiveness.

■ Monitor hepatic, renal, and hematopoietic function periodically in patients receiving repeated or prolonged therapy.

buspirone
CONTRAINDICATIONS AND CAUTIONS

■ Contraindicated in patients hypersensitive to drug and patients who have taken a monoamine oxidase (MAO) inhibitor within 14 days.

■ Drug isn't recommended for patients with severe hepatic or renal impairment.

KEY POINTS

■ Before starting buspirone therapy in a patient already receiving a benzodiazepine, don't stop the benzodiazepine abruptly because a withdrawal reaction may occur.

■ Monitor patient closely for adverse central nervous system (CNS) reactions. Buspirone is less sedating than other anxiolytics, but CNS effects may be unpredictable.

■ Drug has shown no potential for abuse and hasn't been classified as a controlled substance.

chlordiazepoxide
CONTRAINDICATIONS AND CAUTIONS

■ Contraindicated in patients hypersensitive to drug. Don't give drug to pregnant women, especially during the first trimester.

■ Use cautiously in patients with depression, hepatic disease, porphyria, or renal disease.

KEY POINTS

ALERT Chlordiazepoxide 5-mg and 25-mg unit-dose capsules may look similar in color when viewed through the package. When using unit doses of this or any product, verify contents and read label carefully.

■ Injectable form (as hydrochloride) comes in two types of ampules — as diluent and as powdered drug. Read directions carefully.

■ The efficacy of long-term use hasn't been established.

clorazepate
CONTRAINDICATIONS AND CAUTIONS

■ Contraindicated in patients hypersensitive to drug and patients with acute angle-closure glaucoma.

■ Don't give drug to pregnant women, especially during the first trimester.

■ Use cautiously in patients with suicidal tendencies, renal or hepatic impairment, pulmonary disease, or a history of drug abuse.

KEY POINTS

■ Monitor hepatic, renal, and hematopoietic function periodically in patients receiving repeated or prolonged therapy.

■ Use of this drug may lead to abuse and addiction. Don't withdraw drug abruptly after prolonged use because withdrawal symptoms may occur.

■ Smoking decreases benzodiazepine effectiveness.

diazepam
CONTRAINDICATIONS AND CAUTIONS

■ Contraindicated in children younger than age 6 months (oral form), patients hypersensitive to drug or to soy protein, and patients experiencing acute alcohol intoxication, coma, or shock (parenteral form). Don't give drug to pregnant women, especially during the first trimester.

■ Use cautiously in elderly or debilitated patients and patients with chronic open-angle glau-

coma, depression, hepatic impairment, or renal impairment.

KEY POINTS

■ When using injectable diazepam, don't mix with other drugs, and don't store parenteral solution in plastic syringes.

■ When using oral concentrate solution, dilute dose just before giving.

■ Life-threatening adverse reactions include apnea, bradycardia, cardiovascular (CV) collapse, and respiratory depression.

lorazepam
CONTRAINDICATIONS AND CAUTIONS

■ Contraindicated in patients hypersensitive to drug or to other benzodiazepines and in patients with acute angle-closure glaucoma. Don't give drug to pregnant women, especially during the first trimester.

■ Use cautiously in elderly, acutely ill, or debilitated patients and in patients with pulmonary, renal, or hepatic impairment.

KEY POINTS

■ Monitor hepatic, renal, and hematopoietic function periodically in patients receiving repeated or prolonged therapy.

■ Use of this drug may lead to abuse and addiction. Don't stop drug abruptly after long-term use because withdrawal symptoms may occur.

■ Smoking may decrease drug's effectiveness.

oxazepam
CONTRAINDICATIONS AND CAUTIONS

■ Contraindicated in patients hypersensitive to the drug and in those with psychoses. Don't give drug to pregnant women, especially during the first trimester.

■ Use cautiously in elderly patients, patients with a history of drug abuse, and patients in whom decreased blood pressure could lead to cardiac problems.

KEY POINTS

■ Monitor hepatic, renal, and hematopoietic function periodically in patients receiving repeated or prolonged therapy.

■ Use of this drug may lead to abuse and addiction. Don't stop drug abruptly after long-term use because withdrawal symptoms may occur.

■ Serax tablets may contain tartrazine.

paroxetine
CONTRAINDICATIONS AND CAUTIONS

■ Contraindicated in patients hypersensitive to the drug and patients who took an MAO inhibitor within 14 days.

■ Use cautiously in patients at risk for volume depletion, patients with a history scizure disorders or mania, and patients with other severe, systemic illness.

KEY POINTS

■ If evidence of psychosis occurs or increases, expect prescriber to reduce dosage. Record mood changes. Monitor patient for suicidal tendencies, and allow only a minimum supply of drug.

■ Don't stop drug abruptly. Withdrawal or discontinuation syndrome may occur if drug is stopped abruptly. Symptoms include headache, myalgia, lethargy, and general flulike symptoms. Drug should be tapered slowly over 1 to 2 weeks.

■■ *CLINICAL TIP* *Don't cut, crush, or chew controlled-release formulation.*

■ If patient is at risk for volume depletion, monitor him closely.

trifluoperazine
CONTRAINDICATIONS AND CAUTIONS

■ Contraindicated in patients hypersensitive to phenothiazines and patients with bone marrow suppression, CNS depression, coma, or liver damage.

■ Use cautiously in elderly or debilitated patients, patients exposed to extreme heat, and patients with CV disease (may decrease blood pressure), glaucoma, prostatic hyperplasia, or seizure disorder.

KEY POINTS

■ Don't give drug longer than 12 weeks for anxiety.

■ Withhold dose and notify prescriber if jaundice, evidence of blood dyscrasia (fever, sore throat, infection, cellulitis, weakness), or persistent extrapyramidal reactions (longer than a few hours) develop, especially in children or pregnant women.

■ Watch for evidence of neuroleptic malignant syndrome (extrapyramidal effects, hyperthermia, autonomic disturbance), which is rare but commonly fatal. It may not be related to length of drug use or type of neuroleptic; more than 60% of patients are men.

DEPRESSION, MAJOR

Major depression is a syndrome of persistently sad, dysphoric mood with disturbed sleep and appetite, lethargy, and an inability to experience pleasure (anhedonia). Major depression occurs in 3% to 5% of adults and affects all racial, ethnic, and socioeconomic groups. It's more common in women than men.

About half of all depressed patients have a single episode and recover completely; the rest have at least one recurrence. Major depression can profoundly alter social, family, and occupational functioning. Suicide is the most serious complication. Nearly twice as many women as men attempt suicide, but men are far more likely to succeed.

The multiple causes of depression aren't completely understood and may include genetic, familial, biochemical, physical, psychological, and social aspects. Psychological factors may include feelings of helplessness, vulnerability, anger, hopelessness, pessimism, and low self-esteem; they may be related to abnormal character and behavior patterns and troubled personal relationships. In many patients, a specific personal loss or severe stressor interacts with the person's predisposition to provoke major depression.

Depression also may be secondary to a medical condition—for example, metabolic disturbances, such as hypoxia and hypercalcemia; endocrine disorders, such as diabetes and Cushing's disease; neurologic diseases, such as Parkinson's and Alzheimer's disease; and cancer, especially of the pancreas. Other medical conditions that may underlie depression include viral and bacterial infections, such as influenza and pneumonia; cardiovascular (CV) disorders, such as heart failure; pulmonary disorders, such as chronic obstructive pulmonary disease; musculoskeletal disorders, such as degenerative arthritis; gastrointestinal disorders, such as irritable bowel syndrome; genitourinary problems, such as incontinence; collagen vascular diseases, such as lupus; and anemias.

Drugs prescribed for medical and psychiatric conditions, as well as many abused substances, may also cause depression. Examples include antihypertensives, psychotropics, opioid and nonopioid analgesics, antiparkinsonian drugs, numerous CV medications, oral antidiabetics, antimicrobials, corticosteroids, chemotherapeutic drugs, cimetidine, and alcohol.

amitriptyline

CONTRAINDICATIONS AND CAUTIONS

■ Contraindicated in patients hypersensitive to drug, patients who have taken a monoamine oxidase (MAO) inhibitor within 14 days, and patients in the acute recovery phase of myocardial infarction (MI).

■ Use cautiously in patients with a history of angle-closure glaucoma, increased intraocular pressure, seizures, or urine retention; patients with CV disease, diabetes, hyperthyroidism, or impaired liver function; patients taking thyroid drugs; and patients undergoing electroconvulsive therapy.

KEY POINTS

■ Parenteral form of drug is for intramuscular (I.M.) use only.

■ Amitriptyline has strong anticholinergic effects and is one of the most sedating tricyclic antidepressants. Anticholinergic effects have rapid onset even though therapeutic effect is delayed for weeks.

ALERT *Because hypertensive episodes may occur during surgery in patients receiving tricyclic antidepressants, drug should be stopped gradually several days before surgery.*

amoxapine

CONTRAINDICATIONS AND CAUTIONS

■ Contraindicated in patients hypersensitive to drug, patients who have taken an MAO inhibitor within 14 days, and patients in the acute recovery phase of MI.

■ Use with extreme caution in patients who have a history of seizure disorders.

■ Use cautiously in patients with CV disease and patients with a history of angle-closure glaucoma, increased intraocular pressure, or urine retention.

■ Safe use of drug in patients younger than age 16 hasn't been determined.

KEY POINTS

■ Expect delay of 2 weeks or more before effect is noticeable. Full effect may take 4 weeks or longer. However, adverse anticholinergic effects can occur rapidly.

■ Monitor patient for nausea, headache, and malaise after abrupt withdrawal of long-term therapy; these symptoms don't indicate addiction. Avoid withdrawing drug abruptly.

■ Watch for evidence of tardive dyskinesia, especially in elderly women.

bupropion

CONTRAINDICATIONS AND CAUTIONS

■ Contraindicated in patients hypersensitive to drug, patients who have taken an MAO inhibitor within 14 days, patients with seizure disorders or a history of bulimia or anorexia nervosa (because of increased seizure risk), patients abruptly stopping alcohol or sedatives (including benzodiazepines), and patients taking Zyban or other bupropion-containing drugs used for smoking cessation.

■ Use cautiously in patients with a recent MI, unstable heart disease, or renal or hepatic impairment.

KEY POINTS

■ Many patients experience a period of increased restlessness, especially at start of therapy. This may include agitation, insomnia, and anxiety.

■ Patients who have seizures commonly have predisposing factors, including a history of head trauma, seizures, or central nervous system tumors; some may be taking a drug that lowers the seizure threshold.

■ Closely monitor patient with a history of bipolar disorder. Antidepressants can cause manic episodes during the depressed phase of bipolar disorder. However, this may be less likely to occur with bupropion than with other antidepressants.

citalopram

CONTRAINDICATIONS AND CAUTIONS

■ Contraindicated in patients hypersensitive to drug or its components and in patients who took an MAO inhibitor within 14 days.

■ Use cautiously in patients with a history of mania, seizures, suicidal ideation, or hepatic or renal impairment.

■ Safety and effectiveness of drug haven't been established in children.

KEY POINTS

■ Although drug hasn't been shown to impair psychomotor performance, any psychoactive drug may impair judgment, thinking, or motor skills.

■ The possibility of a suicide is inherent in depression and may persist until significant remission occurs. Closely supervise high-risk patients at start of drug therapy. Reduce risk of overdose by limiting amount of drug available per refill.

■ At least 14 days should elapse between MAO inhibitor therapy and citalopram therapy.

escitalopram

CONTRAINDICATIONS AND CAUTIONS

■ Contraindicated in patients hypersensitive to escitalopram, citalopram, or their components and in patients who took an MAO inhibitor within 14 days.

■ Use cautiously in elderly patients (because they may have greater sensitivity to drug), patients with diseases that alter metabolism or hemodynamic responses, and patients with a history of mania, seizure disorders, suicidal ideation, or renal or hepatic impairment.

KEY POINTS

■ Closely monitor patients at high risk of suicide.

■ Evaluate patient for history of drug abuse, and watch for evidence of misuse or abuse.

■ Periodically reassess patient to determine need for maintenance treatment and appropriate dosing.

fluoxetine

CONTRAINDICATIONS AND CAUTIONS

■ Contraindicated in patients hypersensitive to drug and in

those who took an MAO inhibitor within 14 days.

■ Use cautiously in patients at high risk for suicide and in those with a history of CV disease, diabetes mellitus, hepatic disease, mania, renal disease, or seizures.

KEY POINTS

■ Fluoxetine has may potential interactions with other drugs. Obtain a complete list of all prescription and over-the-counter drugs and supplements (including herbs) the patient takes.

■ Use antihistamines or topical corticosteroids to treat rashes or pruritus.

■ Record mood changes, and watch for suicidal tendencies.

■ Don't start an MAO inhibitor within 5 weeks of stopping fluoxetine.

■ Don't give thioridazine with fluoxetine or within 5 weeks of stopping fluoxetine.

nefazodone
CONTRAINDICATIONS AND CAUTIONS

■ Contraindicated in patients hypersensitive to drug or other phenylpiperazine antidepressants, patients who took an MAO inhibitor within 14 days, and patients who were withdrawn from nefazodone because of liver injury.

■ Use cautiously in patients with a history of mania, patients with CV or cerebrovascular disease that could be worsened by hypotension (such as history of angina, cerebrovascular accident, or MI), and patients with conditions that predispose them to hypotension (such as dehydration, hypovolemia, and treatment with antihypertensives).

KEY POINTS

■ Drug may cause hepatic failure. Don't start it in patients with active liver disease or elevated baseline transaminase levels. Although existing hepatic disease doesn't increase the likelihood of hepatic failure, baseline abnormalities can complicate patient monitoring. Stop drug if evidence of hepatic dysfunction appears, such as aspartate transaminase or alanine transaminase levels exceeding three times the upper limit of normal. Don't restart therapy.

■ Record mood changes. Monitor patient for suicidal tendencies, and allow only minimum supply of drug.

paroxetine

CONTRAINDICATIONS AND CAUTIONS

■ Contraindicated in patients hypersensitive to drug, patients who took an MAO inhibitor within 14 days, and patients taking thioridazine.

■ Use cautiously in patients with a history of seizure disorders or mania, patients at risk for volume depletion, and patients with other severe, systemic illness.

KEY POINTS

■ Drug isn't approved for treating major depression in children and adolescents under age 18. An increased risk of suicidal behavior has been reported but can't be attributed definitively to drug.

■ If evidence of psychosis occurs or increases, expect prescriber to reduce dosage. Record mood changes. Monitor patient for suicidal tendencies, and allow only a minimum supply of drug.

■ Don't stop drug abruptly; instead, taper it slowly over 1 to 2 weeks. Withdrawal syndrome may occur if drug is stopped abruptly. Symptoms include headache, myalgia, lethargy, and flulike symptoms.

■ If patient is at risk for volume depletion, monitor him closely.

sertraline

CONTRAINDICATIONS AND CAUTIONS

■ Contraindicated in patients hypersensitive to drug or its components, patients taking pimozide, and patients who took an MAO inhibitor within 14 days.

■ Use cautiously in patients at risk for suicide and those with seizure disorders, major affective disorder, or diseases or conditions that affect metabolism or hemodynamic responses.

KEY POINTS

■ Give sertraline once daily, either morning or evening, with or without food.

■ Make dosage adjustments no more often than weekly.

■ Record mood changes. Monitor patient for suicidal tendencies, and allow only a minimum supply of drug.

venlafaxine

CONTRAINDICATIONS AND CAUTIONS

■ Contraindicated in patients hypersensitive to drug and patient who took an MAO inhibitor within 14 days.

■ Use cautiously in patients with renal impairment, diseases or conditions that could affect hemodynamic responses or metabolism, or a history of mania or seizures.

KEY POINTS

■ Monitor patient for suicidal tendencies. Provide only a minimal supply of drug.

■ Carefully monitor blood pressure. Drug may cause sustained, dose-dependent increases in blood pressure. Greatest increases (average of 7 mm Hg above baseline) occur in patients taking 375 mg daily.

■ Monitor patient's weight, particularly if underweight.

OBSESSIVE–COMPULSIVE DISORDER

Obsessive thoughts and compulsive behaviors are recurring efforts to control overwhelming anxiety, guilt, or unacceptable impulses that persistently enter the consciousness. The word *obsession* refers to a recurrent idea, thought, impulse, or image that is intrusive and inappropriate and causes marked anxiety or distress. A *compulsion* is a ritualistic, repetitive, involuntary defensive behavior. Performing a compulsive behavior reduces the patient's anxiety and increases the probability that the behavior will recur. Compulsions are commonly associated with obsessions.

Patients with obsessive-compulsive disorder (OCD) are prone to abuse psychoactive substances, such as alcohol and anxiolytics, in an attempt to relieve their anxiety. In addition, other anxiety disorders and major depression commonly coexist with OCD. Typically, OCD is a chronic condition with remissions and flare-ups. Mild forms of the disorder are relatively common.

The cause of OCD isn't known. It may stem from brain lesions or other abnormalities, but most research suggests a psychological basis. Major depression, organic brain syndrome, and schizophrenia may contribute to the onset of OCD.

clomipramine

CONTRAINDICATIONS AND CAUTIONS

■ Contraindicated in patients hypersensitive to drug or other tricyclic antidepressants, patients who took a monoamine oxidase (MAO) inhibitor within 14 days, and patients in the acute recovery period after myocardial infarction.

■ Use cautiously in patients with a history of seizure disorders or brain damage, patients taking drugs that lower the seizure threshold, patients at risk for suicide, patients with a history of urine retention, patients with tumors of the adrenal medulla, patients taking thyroid drugs, patients undergoing electroconvulsive therapy or elective surgery, and patients with angle-closure glaucoma, cardiovascular (CV) disease, hyperthyroidism, impaired hepatic or renal function, or increased intraocular pressure.

KEY POINTS

■ Monitor mood, and watch for suicidal tendencies. Allow patient only a minimal amount of drug.

■ Don't stop drug abruptly.

🌀 *ALERT Because hypertensive episodes may occur during surgery in patients receiving tricyclic antidepressants, drug should be gradually discontinued several days before surgery.*

fluoxetine
CONTRAINDICATIONS AND CAUTIONS

■ Contraindicated in patients hypersensitive to drug and patients who took an MAO inhibitor within 14 days.

■ Use cautiously in patients at high risk for suicide, patients with a history of diabetes mellitus, and patients with seizures, mania, or hepatic, renal, or CV disease.

KEY POINTS

■ Be alert for drug interactions.

■ Watch for weight change during therapy.

■ Record mood changes. Watch for suicidal tendencies.

■ Don't start an MAO inhibitor within 5 weeks of stopping fluoxetine. Don't give thioridazine with fluoxetine or within 5 weeks after stopping fluoxetine.

fluvoxamine
CONTRAINDICATIONS AND CAUTIONS

■ Contraindicated in patients hypersensitive to drug or to other phenyl piperazine antidepressants, patients taking pimozide or thioridazine, and patients who took an MAO inhibitor within 14 days.

■ Use cautiously in patients with hepatic dysfunction, other conditions that may affect hemodynamic responses or metabolism, or a history of mania or seizures.

KEY POINTS

■ Record mood changes. Monitor patient for suicidal tendencies.

■ Abruptly stopping drug may cause withdrawal syndrome; symptoms include headache, muscle ache, and flulike symptoms.

paroxetine

CONTRAINDICATIONS AND CAUTIONS

■ Contraindicated in patients hypersensitive to drug, patients who took an MAO inhibitor within 14 days, and patients taking thioridazine.

■ Use cautiously in patients with a history of seizure disorders or mania, patients at risk for volume depletion, and patients with other severe, systemic illness.

KEY POINTS

■ Controlled-release form isn't approved for patients with OCD.

■ If evidence of psychosis occurs or increases, expect prescriber to reduce dosage. Record mood changes. Monitor patient for suicidal tendencies, and allow only a minimum supply of drug.

■ Don't stop drug abruptly; instead, taper it slowly over 1 to 2 weeks. Withdrawal syndrome may occur if drug is stopped abruptly. Symptoms include headache, myalgia, lethargy, and general flulike symptoms.

■ If patient is at risk for volume depletion, monitor him closely.

sertraline

CONTRAINDICATIONS AND CAUTIONS

■ Contraindicated in patients hypersensitive to drug or its components, patients taking pimozide, and patients who took an MAO inhibitor within 14 days.

■ Use cautiously in patients at risk for suicide and patients with seizure disorders, major affective disorder, or conditions that affect metabolism or hemodynamic responses.

KEY POINTS

■ Give sertraline once daily, morning or evening, with or without food. Don't use the oral concentrate dropper, which is made of rubber, for a patient with latex allergy.

■ Adjust dosage no more often than weekly.

■ Record mood changes. Monitor patient for suicidal tendencies, and allow only a minimum supply of drug.

PANIC DISORDER

Panic disorder represents anxiety in its most severe form and is characterized by recurrent episodes of intense apprehension, terror, and impending doom. Initially unpredictable, these panic attacks may come to be associated with specific situations or tasks. The disorder commonly exists with agoraphobia. Men and women are affected equally by panic disorder alone, whereas panic disorder with agoraphobia occurs about twice as often in women.

Panic disorder typically starts in late adolescence or early adulthood and probably stems from both physiologic and psychological factors. Evidence implicates hereditary and temporal lobe dysfunction, and many theorists point to the role of stressful events—such as sudden loss—or unconscious conflicts in early childhood. The disorder may also develop as a persistent pattern of maladaptive behavior acquired by learning. Altered brain biochemistry, especially involving norepinephrine, serotonin, and gamma-aminobutyric acid activity, may also contribute to panic disorder.

Without treatment, panic disorder can persist for years, with alternating exacerbations and remissions. A patient with panic disorder is at high risk for a psychoactive substance abuse disorder and may resort to alcohol or anxiolytics in an attempt to relieve the panic.

alprazolam

CONTRAINDICATIONS AND CAUTIONS

■ Contraindicated in patients hypersensitive to drug or other benzodiazepines and patients with acute angle-closure glaucoma.

■ Use cautiously in patients with hepatic, renal, or pulmonary disease.

KEY POINTS

■ Don't withdraw drug abruptly; withdrawal symptoms, including seizures, may occur. Abuse or addiction is possible.

■ Smoking may decrease drug's effectiveness.

■ Monitor hepatic, renal, and hematopoietic function periodically in patients receiving repeated or prolonged therapy.

clomipramine

CONTRAINDICATIONS AND CAUTIONS

■ Contraindicated in patients hypersensitive to drug or other tricyclic antidepressants, patients who took a monoamine oxidase (MAO) inhibitor within 14 days, and patients in acute recovery period after myocardial infarction.

■ Use cautiously in patients with a history of a seizure disorders or brain damage, patients taking drugs that lower the seizure threshold, patients at risk for suicide, patients with tumors of the adrenal medulla, patients taking thyroid drugs, patients undergoing electroconvulsive therapy or elective surgery, patients with a history of urine retention or angle-closure glaucoma, and patients with cardiovascular (CV) disease, hyperthyroidism, impaired hepatic or renal function, or increased intraocular pressure.

KEY POINTS

■ Monitor patient's mood, and watch for suicidal tendencies. Allow patient only a minimal amount of drug.

■ Don't stop drug abruptly.

ALERT Because hypertensive episodes may occur during surgery in patients receiving tricyclic antidepressants, drug should be gradually discontinued several days before surgery.

clonazepam

CONTRAINDICATIONS AND CAUTIONS

■ Contraindicated in patients hypersensitive to benzodiazepines and patients with significant hepatic disease or acute angle-closure glaucoma.

■ Use cautiously in patients with mixed-type seizures because drug may cause generalized tonic-clonic seizures, in children, and in patients with chronic respiratory disease or open-angle glaucoma.

KEY POINTS

■ To reduce the inconvenience of somnolence when drug is used for panic disorder, taking one dose at bedtime may be desirable.

■ Assess elderly patient's response closely because these patients are more sensitive to central nervous system effects.

■ Monitor patient for oversedation.

fluoxetine

CONTRAINDICATIONS AND CAUTIONS

■ Contraindicated in patients hypersensitive to drug and patients who took an MAO inhibitor within 14 days.

■ Use cautiously in patients at high risk for suicide, patients with a history of diabetes mellitus, and patients with seizures, mania, or hepatic, renal, or CV disease.

KEY POINTS
- Be alert for drug interactions.
- Watch for weight change during therapy.
- Record mood changes, and watch for suicidal tendencies.
- Don't start an MAO inhibitor within 5 weeks of stopping fluoxetine. Don't give thioridazine with fluoxetine or within 5 weeks after stopping fluoxetine.

paroxetine
CONTRAINDICATIONS AND CAUTIONS
- Contraindicated in patients hypersensitive to drug, patients taking thioridazine, and patients who took an MAO inhibitor within 14 days.
- Use cautiously in patients at risk for volume depletion, patients with a history of seizure disorders or mania, and patients with other severe, systemic illness.

KEY POINTS
- If evidence of psychosis occurs or increases, expect prescriber to reduce dosage. Record mood changes. Monitor patient for suicidal tendencies, and allow only a minimum supply of drug.
- Don't stop drug abruptly; instead, taper it gradually over 1 to 2 weeks. Withdrawal syndrome may occur if drug is stopped abruptly. Symptoms include headache, myalgia, lethargy, and general flulike symptoms.
- Monitor patient for complaints of sexual dysfunction. In men, they include anorgasmy, erectile difficulties, delayed ejaculation or orgasm, or impotence; in women, they include anorgasmy or difficulty with orgasm.
- If patient is at risk for volume depletion, monitor him closely.

sertraline
CONTRAINDICATIONS AND CAUTIONS
- Contraindicated in patients hypersensitive to drug or its components, patients taking pimozide, and patients who took an MAO inhibitor within 14 days.
- Use cautiously in patients at risk for suicide and those with seizure disorders, major affective disorder, or conditions that affect metabolism or hemodynamic responses.

KEY POINTS

■ Give sertraline once daily, morning or evening, with or without food.

■ Adjust dosage no more often than weekly.

■ Record mood changes. Monitor patient for suicidal tendencies, and allow only a minimum supply of drug.

SCHIZOPHRENIA

Schizophrenia comes in paranoid, disorganized, catatonic, undifferentiated, and residual forms and is characterized by at least 6 months of disturbances in thought content and form, perception, affect, sense of self, volition, interpersonal relationships, and psychomotor behavior. The disorder affects 1% of people worldwide and occurs equally often in men and women. It may result from a combination of genetic, biological, cultural, and psychological factors.

Close relatives of persons with schizophrenia are up to 50 times more likely to develop it themselves; the closer the degree of relation, the higher the risk. The most widely accepted biochemical hypothesis holds that schizophrenia results from excessive activity at dopaminergic synapses. Other neurotransmitter alterations may contribute as well. People with schizophrenia also have structural abnormalities of the frontal and temporolimbic systems.

Numerous psychological and sociocultural causes have been proposed, including disturbed family and interpersonal patterns, lower socioeconomic status, downward social drift, lack of upward socioeconomic mobility, low birth weight, and high stress levels related to poverty, social failure, illness, and inadequate social resources.

Symptoms of schizophrenia typically begin during adolescence or early adulthood and produce varying degrees of impairment. Up to one-third of patients have only one psychotic episode and no more. Some patients have no disability between periods of exacerbation, although the prognosis worsens with each episode. Some patients need continuous institutional care.

aripiprazole
CONTRAINDICATIONS AND CAUTIONS

■ Contraindicated in patients hypersensitive to aripiprazole.

■ Give drug to pregnant patients only if benefits outweigh risks.

■ Use cautiously in patients with cardiovascular (CV) disease, cerebrovascular disease, or conditions that could predispose the patient to hypotension, such as dehydration or hypovolemia; patients with a history of seizures or with conditions that lower the seizure threshold; patients who engage in strenuous exercise, are exposed to extreme heat, take anticholinergic drugs, or are susceptible to dehydration; and patients at risk for aspiration pneumonia, such as those with Alzheimer's disease.

KEY POINTS

■ Patients should be treated with the smallest dose for the shortest time and periodically re-evaluated for continued treatment.

■ Neuroleptic malignant syndrome may occur. Monitor patient for hyperpyrexia, muscle rigidity, altered mental status, irregular pulse or blood pressure, tachycardia, diaphoresis, and cardiac arrhythmias. If evidence of neuroleptic malignant syndrome occurs, immediately stop drug and notify prescriber.

■ Hyperglycemia may develop. Regularly monitor patients with diabetes. For patients at risk for diabetes, obtain baseline fasting blood glucose level and monitor it periodically. Monitor all patients for signs and symptoms of hyperglycemia, including excessive hunger or thirst, increased urination, and weakness.

■ Monitor patient for evidence of tardive dyskinesia. Elderly patients, especially women, are at highest risk.

clozapine
CONTRAINDICATIONS AND CAUTIONS

■ Contraindicated in patients with uncontrolled epilepsy, patients taking drugs that suppress bone marrow function, patients with a history of clozapine-induced agranulocytosis, and patients with a white blood cell (WBC) count that falls below 3,500/mm³, coma, severe central nervous system (CNS) depression, or myelosuppressive disorders.

■ Use cautiously in patients with prostatic hyperplasia or angle-closure glaucoma because drug has potent anticholinergic effects.

KEY POINTS

■ Clozapine carries significant risk of agranulocytosis. If possible, patient should receive at least two trials of therapy with a standard antipsychotic before clozapine therapy begins. Baseline WBC and differential counts are needed before therapy. Monitor WBC counts weekly for at least 4 weeks after clozapine therapy ends.

■ When giving clozapine, make sure WBC counts and blood tests are performed weekly and that no more than a 1-week supply of drug is dispensed at a time for the first 6 months of therapy. If WBC count stays at 3,000/mm³ or more and absolute neutrophil count stays at 1,500/mm³ or more during first 6 months of continuous therapy, monitoring of blood counts may be reduced to every other week.

■ Clozapine increases the risk of fatal myocarditis, especially during the first month of therapy. If you suspect myocarditis (unexplained fatigue, dyspnea, tachypnea, chest pain, tachycardia, fever, palpitations, and evidence of heart failure or such electrocardiogram [ECG] abnormalities as ST-T wave abnormalities or arrhythmias), clozapine should be stopped immediately and not restarted.

■ Severe hyperglycemia leading to ketoacidosis may develop. Monitor patients for signs and symptoms of hyperglycemia, including excessive hunger or thirst, increased urination, and weakness.

mesoridazine

CONTRAINDICATIONS AND CAUTIONS

■ Contraindicated in patients hypersensitive to drug and in those with severe CNS depression or coma.

■ Don't give this drug with other drugs known to prolong the QTc interval and in patients with congenital long-QT syndrome or a history of cardiac arrhythmias.

KEY POINTS

■ Before treatment, obtain baseline ECG and measure potassium levels. Potassium should be normalized before starting drug.

■ Patient with a QTc interval above 450 msec shouldn't receive drug. Patient with a QTc interval above 500 msec should discontinue use.

■ Obtain baseline blood pressure measurements before starting therapy, and check them regularly. Watch for orthostatic hypotension, especially with parenteral administration.

CLINICAL TIP Protect drug from light. Slight yellowing of injection or concentrate is common and doesn't affect potency.

tions develop, especially in children or pregnant women.

trifluoperazine

CONTRAINDICATIONS AND CAUTIONS

■ Contraindicated in patients hypersensitive to phenothiazines and in those with bone marrow suppression, CNS depression, coma, or liver damage.

■ Use cautiously in elderly or debilitated patients, patients exposed to extreme heat, and patients with CV disease (may decrease blood pressure), glaucoma, prostatic hyperplasia, or seizure disorder.

■ Use in children should be reserved for those who are hospitalized or under close supervision.

KEY POINTS

■ Wear gloves when preparing liquid forms.

■ Dilute liquid concentrate with 60 ml of tomato or fruit juice, carbonated beverage, coffee, tea, milk, water, or semisolid food just before giving.

CLINICAL TIP *Protect drug from light. Slight yellowing of injection or concentrate is common and doesn't affect potency. Discard markedly discolored solutions.*

■ Monitor therapy with weekly bilirubin tests during first month, periodic blood tests (CBC and liver function tests), and ophthalmic tests (long-term use). Withhold dose and notify prescriber if jaundice, symptoms of blood dyscrasia (fever, sore throat, infection, cellulitis, weakness), or persistent extrapyramidal reactions (longer than a few hours) develop, especially in children or pregnant women.

ziprasidone

CONTRAINDICATIONS AND CAUTIONS

■ Contraindicated in patients hypersensitive to drug; patients with a history of prolonged QT interval, congenital long-QT syndrome, recent myocardial infarction, or uncompensated heart failure; patients with a QTc interval more than 500 msec; and patients taking other drugs that prolong the QT interval, such as arsenic trioxide, class Ia and III antiarrhythmics, chlorpromazine, dofetilide, dolasetron mesylate, droperidol, gatifloxacin, halofantrine, levomethadyl acetate, mefloquine, mesoridazine, moxifloxacin, pentamidine, pimozide, probucol, quinidine, sotalol, sparfloxacin, tacrolimus, and thioridazine.

■ Use cautiously in patients with acute diarrhea, patients

with a history of seizures or conditions that could lower the seizure threshold (such as Alzheimer's dementia), patients at risk for aspiration pneumonia, patients with impaired renal function, and patients with a history of bradycardia, hypokalemia, or hypomagnesemia.

KEY POINTS

▪ Dizziness, palpitations, or syncope may be symptoms of a life-threatening arrhythmia such as torsades de pointes. Further CV evaluation and monitoring are needed in patients with these symptoms.

▪ Hyperglycemia may develop. Regularly monitor patients with diabetes. For patients at risk for diabetes, obtain baseline fasting blood glucose level and monitor it periodically. Monitor all patients for signs and symptoms of hyperglycemia, including excessive hunger or thirst, increased urination, and weakness.

▪ Electrolyte disturbances, such as hypokalemia or hypomagnesemia, increase the risk of developing an arrhythmia. Don't give drug under these circumstances.

▪ Symptoms may not improve for 4 to 6 weeks.

22 / DRUGS FOR NEOPLASTIC DISORDERS

BLADDER CANCER

Bladder tumors can develop on the surface of the bladder wall or grow in the bladder wall and quickly invade underlying muscles. Most bladder tumors (90%) are transitional cell carcinomas, arising from the transitional epithelium of mucous membranes. Less common are adenocarcinomas, epidermoid carcinomas, squamous cell carcinomas, sarcomas, tumors in bladder diverticula, and carcinoma in situ.

Certain environmental carcinogens—such as 2-naphthylamine, benzidine, tobacco, and nitrates—predispose people to transitional cell tumors. Thus, workers in certain industries (rubber workers, weavers, leather finishers, aniline dye workers, hairdressers, petroleum workers, and spray painters) are at high risk for such tumors. The period between exposure to the carcino-gen and development of symptoms is about 18 years.

Squamous cell carcinoma of the bladder is most common in geographic areas where schistosomiasis is endemic. It's also associated with chronic bladder irritation and infection (for example, from kidney stones, indwelling urinary catheters, and cystitis caused by cyclophosphamide).

Bladder tumors are most common in men older than age 50 and in densely populated industrial areas; however, women are diagnosed at more advanced stages.

bacillus Calmette-Guérin (BCG), live intravesical

CONTRAINDICATIONS AND CAUTIONS

■ Contraindicated in immunocompromised patients, asymptomatic carriers positive for human immunodeficiency virus (HIV), patients receiving immunosuppressive therapy, patients with active tuberculosis, patients with stage TaG1 papillary tumors (unless they're judged to be at high risk of tumor recurrence), and patients with urinary tract infection, gross hematuria, or fever of unknown origin.

KEY POINTS

■ BCG intravesical shouldn't be given within 7 to 14 days of transurethral resection or biopsy. Fatal disseminated BCG infection has occurred after traumatic catheterization.

ALERT Handle drug and material used for instillation as infectious because it contains live, attenuated mycobacteria. Dispose of equipment (syringes, catheters, and containers) as biohazardous waste.

■ Closely monitor patient for evidence of systemic BCG infection (short-term temperature higher than 103° F [39° C] or persistent temperature higher than 101° F [38° C] for longer than 2 days or with severe malaise). BCG infections are rarely detected by positive cultures. Withhold therapy if systemic infection is suspected. Contact an infectious disease specialist for initiation of fast-acting antituberculosis therapy.

cisplatin

CONTRAINDICATIONS AND CAUTIONS

■ Contraindicated in patients hypersensitive to drug or other platinum-containing compounds and in those with severe renal disease, hearing impairment, or myelosuppression.

■ Use cautiously in patients previously treated with radiation or cytotoxic drugs, patients with peripheral neuropathies, and patients taking other ototoxic and nephrotoxic drugs.

KEY POINTS

■ Therapeutic effects are commonly accompanied by toxicity. Check current protocol. Some prescribers use I.V. sodium thiosulfate or amifostine to minimize toxicity.

■ Patients may develop vomiting 3 to 5 days after treatment, requiring prolonged antiemetic therapy. Some prescribers combine metoclopramide with dexamethasone and antihistamines, or ondansetron or granisetron with dexamethasone to control vomiting. Monitor intake and output. Continue I.V. hydration until patient can tolerate adequate oral intake.

■ Renal toxicity is cumulative; renal function must return to normal before next dose can be given.

- Don't repeat dose unless platelet count is greater than 100,000/mm³, white blood cell (WBC) count is greater than 4,000/mm³, creatinine level is less than 1.5 mg/dl, creatinine clearance is 50 ml/minute or more, and blood urea nitrogen level is less than 25 mg/dl.

doxorubicin

CONTRAINDICATIONS AND CAUTIONS

- Contraindicated in patients hypersensitive to doxorubicin or its components, patients with marked myelosuppression induced by previous treatment with antitumor drugs or radiotherapy, and patients who have received a lifetime cumulative dose of 550 mg/m² of doxorubicin or daunorubicin.
- Dosage adjustment may be needed in elderly patients and patients with myelosuppression or impaired cardiac or hepatic function.

KEY POINTS

- Monitor electrocardiogram for changes such as sinus tachycardia, T-wave flattening, ST-segment depression, and voltage reduction. Be prepared to stop drug or slow rate of infusion, and notify prescriber if tachycardia develops.

- If signs of heart failure develop, stop drug and notify prescriber. Heart failure often can be prevented by limiting cumulative dose to 550 mg/m² (400 mg/m² when patient is also receiving or has received cyclophosphamide or radiation therapy to cardiac area).
- Reddish color of drug is similar to that of daunorubicin; don't confuse the two drugs.

thiotepa

CONTRAINDICATIONS AND CAUTIONS

- Contraindicated in breast-feeding women, patients hypersensitive to drug, and patients with severe bone marrow, hepatic, or renal dysfunction.
- Use in pregnant women only when benefits to mother outweigh risk of teratogenicity.
- Use cautiously in patients with mild bone marrow suppression and renal or hepatic dysfunction.

KEY POINTS

- For bladder instillation, dehydrate patient 8 to 10 hours before therapy. Instill drug into bladder by catheter; ask patient to retain solution for 2 hours. Volume may be reduced to 30 ml if discomfort is too great with 60 ml. Reposition patient

of bladder toxicity. Test urine for blood.

■ Use caution to ensure correct dose and decrease risk of cardiac toxicity.

■ Monitor patient for cyclophosphamide toxicity (leukopenia, thrombocytopenia, cardiotoxicity) if patient's corticosteroid therapy is stopped.

docetaxel

CONTRAINDICATIONS AND CAUTIONS

■ Contraindicated in patients severely hypersensitive to drug or other forms containing polysorbate 80 and in patients with neutrophil counts below 1,500 cells/mm³.

■ Don't give drug to patients with bilirubin levels exceeding upper limit of normal. Also, avoid use of drug in patients with alanine transaminase or aspartate transaminase levels above 1.5 times the upper limit of normal, alkaline phosphatase levels more than 2.5 times the upper limit of normal, or baseline neutrophil count less than 1,500/mm³.

KEY POINTS

■ Give oral corticosteroid such as dexamethasone 16 mg P.O. (8 mg b.i.d.) daily for 3 days starting 1 day before docetaxel administration, to reduce risk

and severity of fluid retention and hypersensitivity reactions.

■ Bone marrow toxicity is the most common and dose-limiting toxicity. Frequent blood count monitoring is needed during therapy.

■ Monitor patient closely for hypersensitivity reactions, especially during first and second infusions.

doxorubicin

CONTRAINDICATIONS AND CAUTIONS

■ Contraindicated in patients with a history of sensitivity reactions to doxorubicin or its components, patients with marked myelosuppression from previous treatment with antitumor drugs or radiotherapy, and patients who have received a lifetime cumulative dose of 550 mg/m² of doxorubicin or daunorubicin.

■ Dosage adjustment may be needed in elderly patients and patients with myelosuppression or impaired cardiac or hepatic function.

KEY POINTS

■ Monitor electocardiogram (ECG) for changes such as sinus tachycardia, T-wave flattening, ST-segment depression, and voltage reduction. Be prepared to stop drug or slow rate of infusion, and notify prescriber if tachycardia develops.

■ If signs of heart failure develop, stop drug and notify prescriber. Heart failure often can be prevented by limiting cumulative dose to 550 mg/m^2 (400 mg/m^2 when patient is also receiving or has received cyclophosphamide or radiation therapy to cardiac area).

■ Reddish color of drug is similar to that of daunorubicin; don't confuse the two.

epirubicin
CONTRAINDICATIONS AND CAUTIONS

■ Contraindicated in patients hypersensitive to drug, anthracyclines, or anthracenediones; patients with baseline neutrophil counts that are below 1,500 cells/mm^3; patients who have had previous treatment with anthracyclines to total cumulative doses; and patients with severe myocardial insufficiency, recent myocardial infarction, serious arrhythmias, or severe hepatic dysfunction.

■ Use cautiously in patients receiving other cardiotoxic drugs, patients with active or dormant cardiac disease, patients with previous or current radiotherapy to the mediastinal and pericardial areas, and patients who have had previous therapy with other anthracyclines or anthracenediones.

KEY POINTS

■ Obtain total and differential white blood cell (WBC) counts, complete blood counts (CBCs), platelet counts, and liver function tests before and during each therapy cycle.

■ Monitor left ventricular ejection fraction (LVEF) regularly during therapy. Stop drug at first sign of impaired cardiac function. Early signs of cardiac toxicity include sinus tachycardia, ECG abnormalities, tachyarrhythmias, bradycardia, atrioventricular block, and bundle-branch block.

■ Delayed cardiac toxicity may occur 2 to 3 months after treatment ends; indications include reduced LVEF and evidence of heart failure (tachycardia, dyspnea, pulmonary edema, dependent edema, hepatomegaly, ascites, pleural effusion, and gallop rhythm). Delayed cardiac toxicity depends on cumulative dose of epirubicin. Don't exceed cumulative dose of 900 mg/m^2.

■ Monitor uric acid, potassium, calcium phosphate, and creatinine levels immediately after initial chemotherapy in patients susceptible to tumor lysis syndrome. Hydration, urine alkalinization, and prophylaxis with allopurinol may prevent hyperuricemia and minimize complications of tumor lysis syndrome.

fluorouracil

CONTRAINDICATIONS AND CAUTIONS

■ Contraindicated in pregnant women, patients hypersensitive to drug, patients in a poor nutritional state, patients who have had major surgery within the previous month, and patients with potentially serious infections or bone marrow suppression (WBC counts of 5,000/mm³ or less or platelet counts of 100,000/mm³ or less).

■ Use cautiously in patients who have received high-dose pelvic radiation or alkylating drugs and in those with impaired hepatic or renal function or widespread neoplastic infiltration of bone marrow.

KEY POINTS

■ Fluorouracil toxicity may be delayed for 1 to 3 weeks.

■ The WBC count nadir occurs 9 to 14 days after first dose; the platelet count nadir occurs in 7 to 14 days.

■ Watch for stomatitis or diarrhea (signs of toxicity). Use topical oral anesthetic to soothe lesions. Stop drug and notify prescriber if diarrhea occurs.

■ Long-term use of drug may cause erythematous, desquamative rash of the hands and feet.

■ Dermatologic adverse effects are reversible when drug is stopped.

paclitaxel

CONTRAINDICATIONS AND CAUTIONS

■ Contraindicated in patients hypersensitive to drug or polyoxyethylated castor oil (a vehicle used in drug solution), patients with baseline neutrophil counts below 1,500/mm³, and patients with acquired immunodeficiency syndrome–related Kaposi's sarcoma and baseline neutrophil counts that are below 1,000/mm³.

■ Use cautiously in patients with hepatic impairment.

KEY POINTS

■ Some patients experience peripheral neuropathies, which may be cumulative and dose-related. Patients with severe symptoms may need dosage reduction.

■ To reduce risk or severity of hypersensitivity, patients must receive pretreatment with corticosteroids, such as dexamethasone, and antihistamines. Both H_1-receptor antagonists, such as diphenhydramine, and H_2-receptor antagonists, such as cimetidine or ranitidine, may be used. Severe hypersensitivity reactions have occurred in as many as 2% of patients.

- Monitor blood counts often during therapy. Bone marrow toxicity is the most common and dose-limiting toxicity. Packed red blood cell or platelet transfusions may be needed in severe cases. Take bleeding precautions as appropriate.

tamoxifen

CONTRAINDICATIONS AND CAUTIONS

- Contraindicated in pregnant women, patients hypersensitive to drug, women with a history of deep vein thrombosis or pulmonary embolism, and as therapy to reduce the risk of breast cancer in high-risk women who also need coumarin-type anticoagulant therapy.
- Use cautiously in patients with leukopenia or thrombocytopenia. Monitor CBC closely.

KEY POINTS

- Monitor lipid levels during long-term therapy in patients with hyperlipidemia.
- Monitor calcium levels. At start of therapy, drug may compound hypercalcemia related to bone metastases.
- Women at high risk for breast cancer or who have duc-tal carcinoma in situ and are taking tamoxifen to reduce risk may experience serious, life-threatening, or fatal endometrial cancer, uterine sarcoma, cerebrovascular accident, and pulmonary embolism. Prescriber should discuss with patients the benefits of drug and risks of these serious events. The benefits of tamoxifen outweigh its risks in women already diagnosed with breast cancer.

- Symptoms may worsen initially.

trastuzumab

CONTRAINDICATIONS AND CAUTIONS

- Contraindicated in patients hypersensitive to drug.
- Use extreme caution in patients with pulmonary compromise, symptomatic intrinsic pulmonary disease (such as asthma and chronic obstructive pulmonary disease), or extensive tumor involvement of the lungs.
- Use cautiously in elderly patients, patients hypersensitive to drug or its components, and patients with cardiac dysfunction.

KEY POINTS

- Drug should be used only for patients with metastatic breast cancer whose tumors have HER2 protein overexpression.

■ Check for first-infusion symptom complex, commonly consisting of chills or fever. Treat with acetaminophen, diphenhydramine, and meperidine (with or without reducing infusion rate). Other effects include nausea, vomiting, pain, rigors, headache, dizziness, dyspnea, hypotension, rash, and asthenia. These symptoms occur infrequently with subsequent infusions.

■ Check for dyspnea, increased cough, paroxysmal nocturnal dyspnea, peripheral edema, or S_3 gallop. Treatment may be stopped if patient develops a significant decrease in left ventricular function.

vinblastine

CONTRAINDICATIONS AND CAUTIONS

■ Contraindicated in patients hypersensitive to drug and patients with severe leukopenia or bacterial infection.

■ Use cautiously in patients with hepatic dysfunction.

KEY POINTS

■ After giving drug, watch for life-threatening acute bronchospasm. If it occurs, notify prescriber immediately. It's most likely in patients who also receive mitomycin.

■ Dose shouldn't be repeated more often than every 7 days or severe leukopenia will occur. Nadir occurs on days 4 to 10 and lasts another 7 to 14 days.

■ Assess patient for numbness and tingling in hands and feet. Assess gait for early evidence of footdrop. Drug is less neurotoxic than vincristine.

COLORECTAL CANCER

In the United States and Europe, colorectal cancer is the second most common visceral neoplasm. Colon cancer is more than twice as common as rectal cancer. Malignant colorectal tumors are almost always adenocarcinomas. About half are sessile lesions of the rectosigmoid area; the rest are polypoid lesions.

The exact cause of colorectal cancer is unknown, but it may relate most to diet (especially excess animal fat, particularly beef, and low fiber). Other factors that increase the risk include:

– other diseases of the digestive tract, especially chronic inflammatory diseases
– age (older than age 40)

– history of ulcerative colitis (the average interval before onset of cancer is 11 to 17 years)
– familial polyposis (cancer almost always develops by age 50).

Colorectal cancer tends to progress slowly and remain localized for a long time. Consequently, it's potentially curable in 75% of patients if early diagnosis allows resection before nodal involvement. With early diagnosis, the overall 5-year survival rate is about 50%.

capecitabine

CONTRAINDICATIONS AND CAUTIONS

■ Contraindicated in patients hypersensitive to 5-fluorouracil (5-FU) and in those with severe renal impairment.

■ Use cautiously in elderly patients and patients with a history of coronary artery disease, mild to moderate hepatic dysfunction from liver metastases, hyperbilirubinemia, or renal insufficiency.

■ Safety and efficacy of drug in patients age 18 and younger haven't been established.

KEY POINTS

■ Assess patient for severe diarrhea, and notify prescriber if it occurs. Replace fluids and electrolytes if patient becomes dehydrated. Drug may need to be immediately interrupted until diarrhea resolves or becomes less intense.

■ Monitor patient for hand-and-foot syndrome (numbness, paresthesia, painless or painful swelling, erythema, desquamation, blistering, and severe pain of hands or feet), hyperbilirubinemia, and severe nausea. Drug must be immediately adjusted. Hand-and-foot syndrome is staged from 1 to 4; drug may be stopped if severe or recurrent episodes occur.

■ Hyperbilirubinemia may require stopping drug.

fluorouracil

CONTRAINDICATIONS AND CAUTIONS

■ Contraindicated in patients hypersensitive to drug, patients in a poor nutritional state, patients who have had major surgery within the previous month, patients with potentially serious infections, and patients with bone marrow suppression (white blood cell [WBC] counts of 5,000/mm³ or less or platelet counts of 100,000/mm³ or less).

■ Use cautiously in patients who have received high-dose pelvic radiation or alkylating drugs and in those with impaired hepatic or renal function or widespread neoplastic infiltration of bone marrow.

KEY POINTS

■ Fluorouracil toxicity may be delayed for 1 to 3 weeks.

■ The WBC count nadir occurs 9 to 14 days after first dose; the platelet count nadir occurs in 7 to 14 days.

■ Watch for stomatitis or diarrhea (signs of toxicity). Use topical oral anesthetic to soothe lesions. Stop drug and notify prescriber if diarrhea occurs.

■ Long-term use of drug may cause erythematous, desquamative rash of the hands and feet, which may be treated with pyridoxine 50 to 150 mg P.O. daily for 5 to 7 days.

■ Dermatologic adverse effects are reversible when drug is stopped.

irinotecan

CONTRAINDICATIONS AND CAUTIONS

■ Contraindicated in patients hypersensitive to drug.

■ Safety and effectiveness of drug in children haven't been established.

■ Use cautiously in elderly patients.

KEY POINTS

■ Drug can induce severe diarrhea. Diarrhea occurring within 24 hours of administration may be preceded by diaphoresis and abdominal cramping and may be relieved by 0.25 to 1 mg atropine I.V., unless contraindicated.

■ Diarrhea occurring more than 24 hours after drug administration may be prolonged, leading to dehydration and electrolyte imbalances; it may be life threatening and should be treated promptly with loperamide. Watch for dehydration, electrolyte imbalance, or sepsis, and treat appropriately. Delay subsequent irinotecan treatments until normal bowel function returns for at least 24 hours without anti-diarrhea treatment. If grade 2, 3, or 4 late diarrhea occurs, later doses of irinotecan should be decreased in the current cycle.

■ Temporarily stop therapy if neutropenic fever occurs or absolute neutrophil count drops below 500/mm^3. Dosage should be reduced, especially if WBC count falls below 2,000/mm^3, neutrophil count falls below 1,000/mm^3, hemoglobin level is below 8 g/dl, or platelet count is below 100,000/mm^3.

oxaliplatin

CONTRAINDICATIONS AND CAUTIONS

■ Contraindicated in pregnant women, breast-feeding women, and patients allergic to drug or other platinum-containing compounds.

■ Use cautiously in patients with renal impairment or peripheral sensory neuropathy.

KEY POINTS

■ Monitor patient for hypersensitivity reactions, which may occur within minutes of administration.

■ Monitor patient for neuropathy and pulmonary toxicity. Peripheral neuropathy may be acute or persistent. Acute neuropathy is reversible; it occurs within 2 days of dosing and resolves within 14 days. Persistent peripheral neuropathy occurs more than 14 days after dosing and causes paresthesias, dysesthesias, hypoesthesias, and deficits in proprioception that can interfere with daily activities (such as walking or swallowing).

■ Avoid ice and cold exposure during infusion of drug because cold temperatures can worsen acute neurologic symptoms. Cover patient with a blanket during infusion.

HODGKIN'S DISEASE

A neoplastic disease, Hodgkin's disease is characterized by painless, progressive enlargement of lymph nodes, spleen, and other lymphoid tissue resulting from proliferation of lymphocytes, histiocytes, eosinophils, and Reed-Sternberg giant cells. The latter cells are its special histologic feature.

The cause of Hodgkin's disease is unknown. It's most common in young adults and more common in men than women. It occurs in all races but is slightly more common in whites and in two age-groups: ages 15 to 38 and after age 50 (except in Japan, where it occurs only among people older than age 50).

Treatment of Hodgkin's disease depends on its stage. (See *Staging Hodgkin's disease*, page 570.) Untreated, the disease follows a variable but relentlessly progressive and ultimately fatal course. Advances in therapy have made Hodgkin's disease potentially curable, even in advanced stages, and appropriate treatment yields a 5-year survival rate of about 90%.

STAGING HODGKIN'S DISEASE

Treatment of Hodgkin's disease depends on the stage—that is, the number, location, and degree of involved lymph nodes. The Ann Arbor Classification System, adopted in 1971, divides Hodgkin's disease into four stages, which are then subdivided into categories.

Category A includes patients with undefined signs and symptoms, and category B includes patients who experience such defined signs as recent unexplained weight loss, fever, and night sweats.

Stage I
Hodgkin's disease appears in a single lymph node region (I) or a single extralymphatic organ (IE).

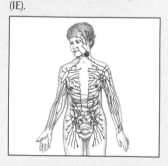

Stage II
The disease appears in two or more nodes on the same side of the diaphragm (II) and in an extralymphatic organ (IIE).

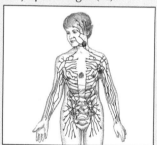

Stage III
Hodgkin's disease spreads to both sides of the diaphragm (III) and perhaps to an extralymphatic organ (IIIE), the spleen (IIIS), or both (IIIES).

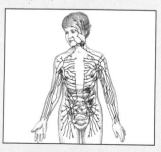

Stage IV
The disease disseminates, involving one more extralymphatic organs or tissues, with or without associated lymph node involvement.

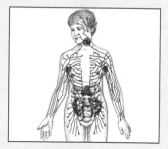

bleomycin

CONTRAINDICATIONS AND CAUTIONS

- Contraindicated in patients hypersensitive to drug.
- Use cautiously in patients with renal or pulmonary impairment.

KEY POINTS

- Pulmonary toxicity appears to be dose-related, with an increase when total dose is more than 400 units. Give total doses of more than 400 units cautiously.
- Adverse pulmonary reactions are more common in patients older than age 70. Pulmonary fibrosis is fatal in 1% of patients, especially when cumulative dosage exceeds 400 units. Also, toxic pulmonary effects may be increased in patients receiving radiation therapy, patients with lung disease, and patients requiring oxygen therapy.
- Watch for fever, which may be treated with antipyretics. Fever usually occurs within 3 to 6 hours of administration.

carmustine

CONTRAINDICATIONS AND CAUTIONS

- Contraindicated in patients hypersensitive to drug.

KEY POINTS

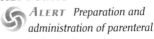 ALERT Preparation and administration of parenteral form can be carcinogenic, mutagenic, and teratogenic. Follow facility policy to reduce risks to staff.

- Pulmonary toxicity appears to be dose-related and may occur 9 days to 15 years after treatment. Obtain pulmonary function tests before and during therapy.
- Bone marrow suppression is delayed with carmustine. Drug shouldn't be given more often than every 6 weeks.
- Monitor complete blood count (CBC) with differential. The absolute neutrophil count may be used to better calculate the patient's immunosuppressive state.

chlorambucil

CONTRAINDICATIONS AND CAUTIONS

- Contraindicated in patients hypersensitive to drug or other alkylating drugs and in patients resistant to previous therapy.
- Use cautiously in patients with a history of head trauma or seizures, patients receiving drugs that lower the seizure threshold, and patients who have had a full course of radiation or chemotherapy within 4 weeks.

layed, usually occurring 4 to 6 weeks after drug administration.

mechlorethamine

CONTRAINDICATIONS AND CAUTIONS

■ Contraindicated in patients hypersensitive to drug and in those with infectious diseases.

■ Use cautiously in patients with severe anemia or depressed neutrophil or platelet count and in patients who have recently undergone radiation therapy or chemotherapy. Monitor CBC.

KEY POINTS

■ Monitor uric acid level. To prevent hyperuricemia and uric acid or nephropathy, mechlorethamine may be used with adequate hydration.

■ Neurotoxicity increases with dosage and patient age.

■ Monitor patient closely for bone marrow suppression (nadir of myelosuppression occurs between days 4 and 10 and lasts 10 to 21 days).

vinblastine

CONTRAINDICATIONS AND CAUTIONS

■ Contraindicated in patients hypersensitive to drug and patients with severe leukopenia or bacterial infection.

■ Use cautiously in patients with hepatic dysfunction.

KEY POINTS

■ After giving drug, monitor patient for life-threatening acute bronchospasm. If it occurs, notify prescriber immediately. Reaction is most likely in patients who also receive mitomycin.

■ Dosage shouldn't be repeated more often than every 7 days or severe leukopenia will occur. Nadir occurs on days 4 to 10 and lasts another 7 to 14 days.

■ Assess patient for numbness and tingling in hands and feet. Assess gait for early evidence of footdrop. Drug is less neurotoxic than vincristine.

vincristine

CONTRAINDICATIONS AND CAUTIONS

■ Contraindicated in patients hypersensitive to drug, patients who are receiving radiation therapy through ports that include the liver, and patients with demyelinating form of Charcot-Marie-Tooth syndrome.

■ Use cautiously in patients with hepatic dysfunction, neuromuscular disease, or infection.

KEY POINTS

■ After giving drug, monitor patient for life-threatening acute bronchospasm. If it occurs, notify prescriber immediately. This reaction is most likely in patients receiving mitomycin.

■ Because of risk of neurotoxicity, drug shouldn't be given more often than once weekly. Neurotoxicity is dose-related and usually reversible. Some neurotoxicities may be permanent. Elderly patients and those with underlying neurologic disease may be more susceptible to neurotoxic effects. Children are more resistant to it than adults.

■ Check for depression of Achilles tendon reflex, numbness, tingling, footdrop or wristdrop, difficulty in walking, ataxia, and slapping gait. Also check ability to walk on heels. Support patient when walking.

KAPOSI'S SARCOMA

Kaposi's sarcoma, a cancer of the lymphatic cell wall, affects tissues under the skin or mucous membranes that line the mouth, nose, and anus. It causes structural and functional damage and progresses aggressively, involving the lymph nodes, viscera, and possibly gastrointestinal (GI) structures. In recent years, Kaposi's sarcoma has become much more common because of the increased numbers of people infected with human immunodeficiency virus (HIV); it's now the most common HIV-related cancer. The exact cause of Kaposi's sarcoma is unknown, but the disease may be related to immunosuppression. Genetic or hereditary predisposition also may play a role.

daunorubicin citrate liposomal
CONTRAINDICATIONS AND CAUTIONS

■ Contraindicated in patients who have had a severe hypersensitivity reaction to drug or its components.

■ Use cautiously in patients with myelosuppression, cardiac disease, previous radiotherapy around the heart, previous anthracycline use (doxorubicin at 300 mg/m^2 or above), or hepatic or renal dysfunction.

KEY POINTS

■ Liposomal daunorubicin causes less nausea, vomiting, alopecia, neutropenia, thrombocytopenia, and cardiotoxicity than conventional daunorubicin.

■ Monitor cardiac function regularly. Assess patient before giving each dose because of risk of cardiac toxicity and heart failure. Determine left ventricular ejection fraction at total cumulative doses of 320 mg/m^2

and every 160 mg/m^2 thereafter. Total cumulative doses typically shouldn't exceed 550 mg/m^2.

■ Careful hematologic monitoring is needed because severe myelosuppression may occur. Repeat blood counts and evaluate before giving each dose. Withhold treatment if absolute granulocyte count is below 750 cells/mm^3.

doxorubicin hydrochloride liposomal
CONTRAINDICATIONS AND CAUTIONS

■ Contraindicated in patients hypersensitive to conventional form of doxorubicin hydrochloride or any component in the liposomal form, patients with marked myelosuppression, and patients who have received a lifetime cumulative dose of 550 mg/m^2 (400 mg/m^2 in patients who have received radiotherapy to the mediastinal area or therapy with other cardiotoxic drugs such as cyclophosphamide).

■ Use cautiously in patients who have received other anthracyclines.

KEY POINTS

■ Monitor patient for evidence of palmar-plantar erythrodysesthesia, hematologic toxicity, or stomatitis. These adverse reactions may be managed with dosage delays and adjustments.

■ Consider previous or current therapy with related compounds such as daunorubicin when calculating total dose of drug. Heart failure and cardiomyopathy may occur after therapy stops. Give drug to patient with history of cardiovascular (CV) disease only when benefit outweighs risk to patient.

■ Drug has pharmacokinetic properties different from those of conventional doxorubicin hydrochloride and shouldn't be substituted mg per mg.

interferon alfa-2a, recombinant
CONTRAINDICATIONS AND CAUTIONS

■ Contraindicated in neonates (injection contains benzyl alcohol); patients hypersensitive to drug, murine (mouse) immunoglobulin, or other drug components; patients with a history of autoimmune hepatitis or autoimmune disease; immunocompromised transplant patients; and patients with severe visceral AIDS-related Kaposi's sarcoma, severe depression, or suicidal behavior.

■ Use cautiously in patients with severe hepatic or renal function impairment, seizure disorders, compromised central nervous system (CNS) function, cardiac disease, or myelosuppression.

KEY POINTS

■ Alpha interferons cause or aggravate fatal or life-threatening neuropsychiatric, autoimmune, ischemic, and infectious disorders. Monitor patient closely with periodic clinical and laboratory evaluations. Patients with persistently severe or worsening evidence of these conditions should be withdrawn from therapy.

■ Give drug at bedtime to minimize daytime drowsiness.

■ Different brands of interferon may not be equivalent and may need different dosages.

■ Depression and suicidal behavior have been linked to treatment.

■ Neurotoxicity and cardiotoxicity are more common in elderly patients, especially those with underlying CNS or cardiac impairment.

interferon alfa-2b, recombinant
CONTRAINDICATIONS AND CAUTIONS

■ Contraindicated in patients hypersensitive to drug or its components.

■ Use cautiously in patients with a history of CV disease, pulmonary disease, diabetes mellitus, coagulation disorders, and severe myelosuppression.

■ Patients with psychotic disorders, especially depression, shouldn't continue treatment because depression and suicidal behavior have been linked to drug use.

KEY POINTS

■ Alpha interferons cause or aggravate fatal or life-threatening neuropsychiatric, autoimmune, ischemic, and infectious disorders. Monitor patient closely with periodic clinical and laboratory evaluations. Patients with persistently severe or worsening evidence of these conditions should be withdrawn from therapy.

■ Make sure patient is well hydrated, especially during initial treatment.

■ At start of treatment, watch for flulike signs and symptoms, which tend to diminish with continued therapy. Premedicate patient with acetaminophen to minimize these symptoms.

■ Neurotoxicity and cardiotoxicity are more common in elderly patients, especially those with underlying CNS or cardiac impairment.

paclitaxel

CONTRAINDICATIONS AND CAUTIONS

■ Contraindicated in patients hypersensitive to drug or poly-oxyethylated castor oil (a vehicle used in drug solution) and in those with baseline neutrophil counts below 1,000/mm^3.

■ Use cautiously in patients with hepatic impairment.

KEY POINTS

■ Some patients develop peripheral neuropathies, which may be cumulative and dose-related. Patients with severe symptoms may need dosage reduction.

■ To reduce risk or severity of hypersensitivity, patients must be pretreated with corticosteroids, such as dexamethasone, and antihistamines. Both H$_1$-receptor antagonists, such as diphenhydramine, and H$_2$-receptor antagonists, such as cimetidine or ranitidine, may be used. Severe hypersensitivity reactions affect as many as 2% of patients.

■ Monitor blood counts often during therapy. Bone marrow toxicity is the most common and dose-limiting toxicity. Packed red blood cell or platelet transfusions may be needed in severe cases. Take bleeding precautions as appropriate.

vinblastine

CONTRAINDICATIONS AND CAUTIONS

■ Contraindicated in patients hypersensitive to drug and patients with severe leukopenia or bacterial infection.

■ Use cautiously in patients with hepatic dysfunction.

KEY POINTS

■ After giving drug, monitor patient for life-threatening acute bronchospasm. If it occurs, notify prescriber immediately. Reaction is most likely in patients also receiving mitomycin.

■ Dosage shouldn't be repeated more often than every 7 days or severe leukopenia will occur. Nadir occurs on days 4 to 10 and lasts another 7 to 14 days.

■ Monitor patient for stomatitis. Stop drug if stomatitis occurs, and notify prescriber.

■ Drug is less neurotoxic than vincristine.

LEUKEMIA, ACUTE

Acute leukemia is a malignant proliferation of white blood cell (WBC) precursors (blasts) in bone marrow or lymph tissue and their accumulation in peripheral blood, bone marrow, and body tissues. The most common forms are acute lym-

WHAT HAPPENS IN LEUKEMIA

This illustration shows how white blood cells (agranulocytes and granulocytes) proliferate in the bloodstream in leukemia, overwhelming red blood cells (RBCs) and platelets.

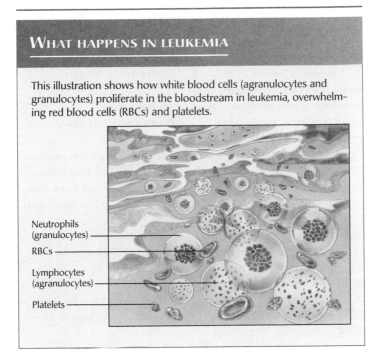

Neutrophils (granulocytes)

RBCs

Lymphocytes (agranulocytes)

Platelets

phoblastic (lymphocytic) leukemia (ALL), characterized by abnormal growth of lymphocyte precursors (lymphoblasts); acute myeloblastic (myelogenous) leukemia (AML), in which myeloid precursors (myeloblasts) rapidly accumulate; and acute monoblastic (monocytic) leukemia, or Schilling's type, characterized by a marked increase in monocyte precursors (monoblasts). Other variants include acute myelomonocytic leukemia and acute erythroleukemia.

Research on predisposing factors is inconclusive but points to some combination of viruses (viral remnants have been found in leukemic cells), genetic and immunologic factors, and exposure to radiation and certain chemicals.

Pathogenesis isn't clearly understood, but immature, nonfunctioning WBCs appear to accumulate first in the tissue where they originate (lymphocytes in lymph tissue, granulocytes in bone marrow) and then in the bloodstream, eventually infiltrating other tissues and causing organ malfunction from encroachment or hemorrhage. (See *What happens in leukemia*.)

Acute leukemia is more common in males than in females, in whites (especially people of Jewish descent), in children ages 2 to 5 (80% of all leukemias in this age group are ALL), and in people who live in urban and industrialized areas. Acute leukemia ranks 20th in overall cancer-related deaths. Among children, it's the most common form of cancer.

Untreated, acute leukemia is invariably fatal, usually because of complications from leukemic cell infiltration of bone marrow or vital organs. With treatment, the prognosis varies. With ALL, treatment induces remissions in 90% of children (average survival time is 5 years) and in 65% of adults (average survival time is 1 to 2 years). Children ages 2 to 8 have the best survival rate with intensive therapy. With AML, the average survival time is only 1 year after diagnosis, even with aggressive treatment. With acute monoblastic leukemia, treatment induces remissions lasting 2 to 10 months in 50% of children; adults survive only about 1 year after diagnosis, even with treatment.

LEUKEMIA, ACUTE LYMPHOBLASTIC (LYMPHOCYTIC)

asparaginase

CONTRAINDICATIONS AND CAUTIONS

■ Contraindicated in patients hypersensitive to drug (unless desensitized) and in those with pancreatitis or a history of pancreatitis.

■ Use cautiously in patients with hepatic dysfunction.

KEY POINTS

■ Drug should first be given in a hospital under close supervision.

■ Risk of hypersensitivity increases with repeated doses. An intradermal skin test should be performed before initial dose and after an interval of 1 week or more between doses. Give 2 international units asparaginase as an intradermal (I.D.) injection and observe site for a positive response (erythema or wheal) for at least 1 hour. Patient with negative skin test may still develop allergic reaction to drug.

■ Desensitization may be needed before first treatment dose is given and with retreatment. One international unit of drug may be ordered I.V. Dose is then doubled every 10 minutes, provided no reaction occurs, until total amount given equals patient's total dose for that day.

■ Keep epinephrine, diphenhydramine, and I.V. corticosteroids available for treating anaphylaxis.

■ Help prevent tumor lysis (which can result in uric acid nephropathy) by increasing patient's fluid intake.

cyclophosphamide
CONTRAINDICATIONS AND CAUTIONS

■ Contraindicated in patients hypersensitive to drug and in those with severe bone marrow suppression.

■ Use cautiously in patients who have recently undergone radiation therapy or chemotherapy and patients with hepatic disease, leukopenia, malignant cell infiltration of bone marrow, thrombocytopenia, or renal disease.

KEY POINTS

■ Don't give drug at bedtime; infrequent urination during the night may increase risk of cystitis. If it occurs, stop drug and notify prescriber. Cystitis can occur months after therapy ceases. Mesna may be given to reduce frequency and severity of bladder toxicity. Test urine for blood.

■ Use caution to ensure correct dose and decrease risk of cardiac toxicity.

■ Monitor patient for cyclophosphamide toxicity (leukopenia, thrombocytopenia, cardiotoxicity) if corticosteroid therapy is stopped.

cytarabine
CONTRAINDICATIONS AND CAUTIONS

■ Contraindicated in patients hypersensitive to drug.

■ Use cautiously in patients with hepatic or renal compromise, gout, or myelosuppression.

KEY POINTS

■ Monitor fluid intake and output carefully. Maintain high fluid intake, and give allopurinol to avoid urate nephropathy in leukemia-induction therapy. Monitor uric acid level.

■ Therapy may be modified or stopped if granulocyte count is below 1,000/mm^3 or platelet count is below 50,000/mm^3.

■ Assess patient receiving high doses for neurotoxicity, which may first appear as nystagmus but can progress to ataxia and cerebellar dysfunction.

daunorubicin

CONTRAINDICATIONS AND CAUTIONS

- Contraindicated in patients hypersensitive to the drug.
- Use cautiously in patients with myelosuppression or impaired cardiac, renal, or hepatic function.

KEY POINTS

- Take preventive measures (including adequate hydration) before starting treatment. Hyperuricemia may result from rapid lysis of leukemic cells. Allopurinol may be ordered.
- Check cardiac function studies, including electrocardiogram (ECG) and ejection fraction, before treatment and then periodically throughout therapy.
- Stop drug immediately and notify prescriber if evidence of heart failure, cardiomyopathy, or arrhythmia develops.
- Reddish color of drug is similar to that of doxorubicin; don't confuse the two.

doxorubicin

CONTRAINDICATIONS AND CAUTIONS

- Contraindicated in patients with a history of sensitivity reactions to doxorubicin or its components, patients with marked myelosuppression induced by previous treatment

with other antitumor drugs or radiotherapy, and patients who have received a lifetime cumulative dose of 550 mg/m² of doxorubicin or daunorubicin.

- Dosage adjustment may be needed in elderly patients and patients with myelosuppression or impaired cardiac or hepatic function.

KEY POINTS

- Monitor ECG for changes such as sinus tachycardia, T-wave flattening, ST-segment depression, and voltage reduction. Be prepared to stop drug or slow infusion rate, and notify prescriber if tachycardia develops.
- If signs of heart failure develop, stop drug and notify prescriber. Heart failure often can be prevented by limiting cumulative dose to 550 mg/m² (400 mg/m² when patient is also receiving or has received cyclophosphamide or radiation therapy to cardiac area).
- Reddish color of drug is similar to that of daunorubicin; don't confuse the two.

methotrexate

CONTRAINDICATIONS AND CAUTIONS

- Contraindicated in pregnant women, breast-feeding women, patients hypersensitive to drug, and patients with psoriasis or rheumatoid arthritis who also have alcoholism, alcoholic liver, chronic liver disease, immunodeficiency syndromes, or blood dyscrasias.

■ Use cautiously and at modified dosage in very young, elderly, or debilitated patients; patients with infection, peptic ulceration, or ulcerative colitis; and patients with anemia, aplasia, bone marrow suppression, impaired hepatic or renal function, leukopenia, or thrombocytopenia.

KEY POINTS

■ Methotrexate may be given daily or once weekly, depending on the disease. To avoid errors, confirm which disease the patient has.

■ Monitor pulmonary function tests periodically and fluid intake and output daily. Encourage fluid intake of 2 to 3 L daily.

■ Alkalinize urine by giving sodium bicarbonate tablets or I.V. fluids containing sodium bicarbonate to prevent precipitation of drug, especially at high doses. Maintain urine pH above 7. Reduce dosage if blood urea nitrogen (BUN) level is 20 to 30 mg/dl or creatinine level is 1.2 to 2 mg/dl. Stop drug and notify prescriber if BUN level exceeds 30 mg/dl or creatinine level is higher than 2 mg/dl.

pegaspargase
CONTRAINDICATIONS AND CAUTIONS

■ Contraindicated in patients with pancreatitis or history of pancreatitis, patients who have had significant hemorrhagic events from previous treatment with L-asparaginase, and patients with a history of serious allergic reactions to drug, such as generalized urticaria, bronchospasm, laryngeal edema, hypotension, or other unacceptable adverse reactions.

■ Use cautiously in patients with liver dysfunction, and use only when clearly indicated in pregnant women.

KEY POINTS

■ Take preventive measures (including adequate hydration) before starting treatment. Hyperuricemia may result from rapid lysis of leukemic cells. Allopurinol may be ordered.

■ I.M. route is preferred because it has the lowest risk of hepatotoxicity, coagulopathy, and GI and renal disorders.

■ Monitor patient closely for hypersensitivity (including life-threatening anaphylaxis), especially if hypersensitive to other forms of L-asparaginase. Keep patient under observation for 1 hour, with resuscitation equipment and other drugs needed to treat anaphylaxis (such as epinephrine, oxygen, and I.V. corticosteroids) readily available. Moderate to life-threatening hypersensitivity requires stopping L-asparaginase.

vincristine

CONTRAINDICATIONS AND CAUTIONS

■ Contraindicated in patients hypersensitive to drug, patients receiving radiation therapy through ports that include the liver, and patients with demyelinating form of Charcot-Marie-Tooth syndrome.

■ Use cautiously in patients with hepatic dysfunction, neuromuscular disease, or infection.

KEY POINTS

■ After giving drug, check for life-threatening acute bronchospasm. If it occurs, notify prescriber immediately. This reaction is most likely in patients receiving mitomycin.

■ Because of risk of neurotoxicity, drug shouldn't be given more than once weekly. Neurotoxicity is dose-related and usually reversible. Some neurotoxicities may be permanent. Elderly patients and those with underlying neurologic disease

may be more susceptible to neurotoxic effects. Children are more resistant to neurotoxicity than adults.

■ Check for hyperuricemia, especially in patients with leukemia or lymphoma. Maintain hydration, and give allopurinol to prevent uric acid nephropathy. Check for toxicity.

LEUKEMIA, ACUTE MYELOID

cyclophosphamide

CONTRAINDICATIONS AND CAUTIONS

■ Contraindicated in patients hypersensitive to drug and in those with severe bone marrow suppression.

■ Use cautiously in patients who have recently undergone radiation therapy or chemotherapy and patients with hepatic disease, leukopenia, malignant cell infiltration of bone marrow, thrombocytopenia, or renal disease.

KEY POINTS

■ Don't give drug at bedtime; infrequent urination during the night may increase risk of cystitis. If it occurs, stop drug and notify prescriber. Cystitis can occur months after therapy ceases. Mesna may be given to reduce frequency and severity of bladder toxicity. Test urine for blood.

■ Use caution to ensure correct dose and decrease risk of cardiac toxicity.

■ Monitor patient for cyclophosphamide toxicity (leukopenia, thrombocytopenia, cardiotoxicity) if corticosteroid therapy is stopped.

daunorubicin
CONTRAINDICATIONS AND CAUTIONS

■ Contraindicated in patients hypersensitive to the drug.

■ Use cautiously in patients with myelosuppression or impaired cardiac, renal, or hepatic function.

KEY POINTS

■ Take preventive measures (including adequate hydration) before starting treatment. Hyperuricemia may result from rapid lysis of leukemic cells. Allopurinol may be ordered.

■ Perform cardiac function studies, including electrocardiogram (ECG) and ejection fraction, before and periodically during treatment.

■ Stop drug immediately and notify prescriber if signs of heart failure, cardiomyopathy, or arrhythmia develop.

■ Reddish color of drug is similar to that of doxorubicin; don't confuse the two.

doxorubicin
CONTRAINDICATIONS AND CAUTIONS

■ Contraindicated in patients with a history of sensitivity reactions to doxorubicin or its components, patients with marked myelosuppression from previous treatment with other antitumor drugs or radiotherapy, and patients who have received a lifetime cumulative dose of 550 mg/m^2 of doxorubicin or daunorubicin.

■ Dosage adjustment may be needed in elderly patients and patients with myelosuppression or impaired cardiac or hepatic function.

KEY POINTS

■ Monitor ECG for changes such as sinus tachycardia, T-wave flattening, ST-segment depression, and voltage reduction. Be prepared to stop drug or slow infusion rate, and notify prescriber if tachycardia occurs.

■ If signs of heart failure develop, stop drug and notify prescriber. Heart failure often can be prevented by limiting cumulative dose to 550 mg/m^2 (400 mg/m^2 when patient is also receiving or has received cyclophosphamide or radiation therapy to cardiac area).

- Reddish color of drug is similar to that of daunorubicin; don't confuse the two.

gemtuzumab

Contraindications and cautions

- Contraindicated in patients hypersensitive to drug or its components.
- Use cautiously in patients with hepatic impairment.

Key points

- Monitor vital signs during infusion and for 4 hours after infusion.
- Watch for postinfusion symptom complex of chills, fever, hypotension, hypertension, hyperglycemia, hypoxia, and dyspnea that may occur during the first 24 hours after administration.
- Fatal hepatic reno-occlusive disease may occur after treatment with gemtuzumab and subsequent chemotherapy.

idarubicin

Contraindications and cautions

- Use with extreme caution in patients with bone marrow suppression induced by previous drug therapy or radiotherapy, impaired hepatic or renal function, previous treatment with anthracyclines or cardiotoxic drugs, or a cardiac condition.

Key points

- Cardiotoxicity is the dose-limiting toxicity.
- Take preventive measures, including adequate hydration, before starting treatment. Hyperuricemia may result from rapid lysis of leukemic cells. Allopurinol may be ordered.
- Assess patient for systemic infection, and make sure it's controlled before therapy begins.

mercaptopurine

Contraindications and cautions

- Contraindicated in patients hypersensitive to drug and patients whose disease has shown resistance to drug.

Key points

Clinical tip *Drug is sometimes ordered as 6-mercaptopurine, or 6-MP. The numeral 6 is part of drug name and doesn't signify number of dosage units.*

- Dosage adjustment may be needed after chemotherapy or radiation therapy in patients with depressed neutrophil or platelet counts and in those with impaired hepatic or renal function.

■ Watch for jaundice, clay-colored stools, and frothy, dark urine. Hepatic dysfunction is reversible when drug is stopped. If right-sided abdominal tenderness occurs, stop drug and notify prescriber.

LEUKEMIA, CHRONIC GRANULOCYTIC

Chronic granulocytic leukemia (CGL) is also known as chronic myelogenous (or myelocytic) leukemia. The disease is characterized by the abnormal overgrowth of granulocytic precursors (myeloblasts, promyelocytes, metamyelocytes, and myelocytes) in bone marrow, peripheral blood, and body tissues.

CGL is most common in young and middle-age adults and is slightly more common in men than in women; it's rare in children. In the United States, 3,000 to 4,000 cases of CGL occur annually, accounting for roughly 20% of all leukemias.

The exact cause of this disease isn't known. However, almost 90% of patients with CGL have the Philadelphia (Ph[1]) chromosome, an abnormality discovered in 1960 in which the long arm of chromosome 22 is translocated, usually to chromosome 9. Radiation and carcinogenic chemicals may cause this abnormality. Myeloproliferative diseases also seem to increase the likelihood of CGL, and an unidentified virus may play a role as well.

CGL proceeds in two distinct phases: the insidious chronic phase, with anemia and bleeding abnormalities, and the acute phase (blastic crisis), in which myeloblasts, the most primitive granulocytic precursors, proliferate rapidly. This disease is invariably fatal. Average survival time is 3 to 4 years after onset of the chronic phase and 3 to 6 months after onset of the acute phase.

busulfan
CONTRAINDICATIONS AND CAUTIONS

■ Contraindicated in patients with chronic myelogenous leukemia resistant to drug and in those with chronic lymphocytic or acute leukemia or in the blastic crisis of chronic myelogenous leukemia.

■ Use cautiously in patients with a history of head trauma or seizures, patients receiving other drugs that lower the seizure threshold, patients recently given other myelosuppressives or radiation treatment, and patients with depressed neutrophil or platelet count.

KEY POINTS

■ Give antiemetic before first dose of busulfan injection and then on a fixed schedule during therapy; give phenytoin to prevent seizures.

■ Monitor patient for jaundice and liver function abnormalities if giving high doses.

■ Pulmonary fibrosis may occur as late as 8 months to 10 years after treatment with busulfan. (Average duration of therapy is 4 years.)

cyclophosphamide
CONTRAINDICATIONS AND CAUTIONS

■ Contraindicated in patients hypersensitive to drug and in those with severe bone marrow suppression.

■ Use cautiously in patients who have recently undergone radiation therapy or chemotherapy and patients with hepatic disease, leukopenia, malignant cell infiltration of bone marrow, renal disease, or thrombocytopenia.

KEY POINTS

■ Don't give drug at bedtime; infrequent urination during the night may increase risk of cystitis. If it occurs, stop drug and notify prescriber. Cystitis can occur months after therapy ceases. Mesna may be given to reduce frequency and severity of bladder toxicity. Test urine for blood.

■ Use caution to ensure correct dose and decrease risk of cardiac toxicity.

■ Monitor patient for cyclophosphamide toxicity (leukopenia, thrombocytopenia, cardiotoxicity) if corticosteroid therapy is stopped.

hydroxyurea
CONTRAINDICATIONS AND CAUTIONS

■ Contraindicated in patients hypersensitive to drug, patients with severe anemia, and patients with white blood cell (WBC) counts below 2,500/mm^3 or platelets below 100,000/mm^3.

■ Use cautiously in patients with renal dysfunction.

KEY POINTS

■ Acceptable blood counts during dosage adjustment are neutrophil count 2,500 cells/mm^3 or more; platelet count 95,000/mm^3 or more; hemoglobin more than 5.3 g/dl; and reticulocyte count (if hemoglobin is below 9 g/dl), more than 95,000/mm³.

■ Toxic levels are neutrophil count below 2,000 cells/mm³, platelet count that falls below 80,000/mm³, hemoglobin less than 4.5 g/dl, and reticulocyte count (if hemoglobin is below 9 g/dl) below 80,000/mm³.

■ Hydroxyurea may dramatically lower the WBC count in 24 to 48 hours.

■ Auditory and visual hallucinations and hematologic toxicity increase when renal function decreases.

imatinib
CONTRAINDICATIONS AND CAUTIONS
■ Contraindicated in patients hypersensitive to drug or its components.

■ Use cautiously in patients with hepatic impairment.

KEY POINTS
■ Monitor patients closely for fluid retention, which can be severe.

■ Elderly patients may have an increased risk of edema when taking this drug.

■ Monitor liver function tests carefully because hepatotoxicity (occasionally severe) may occur; decrease dosage as needed.

■ Consider dosage increases only if there are no severe adverse reactions or severe non–leukemia-related neutropenia or thrombocytopenia in the following circumstances: disease progression (at any time), failure to achieve a satisfactory hematologic response after at least 3 months of treatment, or loss of a previously achieved hematologic response.

mechlorethamine
CONTRAINDICATIONS AND CAUTIONS
■ Contraindicated in patients hypersensitive to drug and in those with infectious diseases.

■ Use cautiously in patients who have recently undergone radiation therapy or chemotherapy and patient with severe anemia or depressed neutrophil or platelet count. Monitor complete blood count.

KEY POINTS
■ Monitor uric acid level. To prevent hyperuricemia and uric acid nephropathy, mechlorethamine may be used with adequate hydration.

■ Neurotoxicity increases with dosage and patient age.

■ Monitor patient closely for bone marrow suppression (nadir of myelosuppression occurring between days 4 and 10 and lasting 10 to 21 days).

LEUKEMIA, CHRONIC LYMPHOCYTIC

A generalized, progressive disease that's common in elderly people, chronic lymphocytic leukemia is marked by the uncontrollable spread of abnormal, small lymphocytes in lymphoid tissue, blood, and bone marrow. Nearly all patients with chronic lymphocytic leukemia are men older than age 50. According to the American Cancer Society, chronic lymphocytic leukemia accounts for almost one-third of new leukemia cases annually.

Although the cause of chronic lymphocytic leukemia is unknown, researchers suspect genetic factors, still-undefined chromosome abnormalities, and certain immunologic defects (such as ataxia-telangiectasia or acquired agammaglobulinemia). The disease doesn't seem to be related to radiation exposure.

The prognosis for chronic lymphocytic leukemia is poor if the patient has anemia, thrombocytopenia, neutropenia, bulky lymphadenopathy, or severe lymphocytosis.

alemtuzumab
CONTRAINDICATIONS AND CAUTIONS
■ Contraindicated in patients with active systemic infections, underlying immunodeficiency (such as human immunodeficiency virus infection), or type I hypersensitivity or anaphylactic reactions to alemtuzumab or its components.

KEY POINTS
■ Monitor blood pressure and hypotensive symptoms during administration.
■ Don't give drug if patient has systemic infection at scheduled dose time.
■ If therapy is interrupted for 7 days or longer, restart with gradual dose increase.

chlorambucil
CONTRAINDICATIONS AND CAUTIONS
■ Contraindicated in patients hypersensitive to previous therapy or to other alkylating drugs and in patients resistant to drug.
■ Use cautiously in patients with a history of head trauma or seizures, in patients receiving other drugs that lower the seizure threshold, and within 4 weeks of a full course of radiation or chemotherapy.

KEY POINTS

■ Monitor patient for neutropenia, which may not appear until after the third week of treatment. The neutrophil count may continue to decrease for up to 10 days after treatment ends.

■ Absolute neutrophil count may be used to better calculate the patient's immunosuppressive state.

■ Monitor uric acid level. To prevent hyperuricemia and uric acid nephropathy, allopurinol may be used with adequate hydration.

■ If white blood cell (WBC) count falls below 2,000/mm^3 or granulocyte count falls below 1,000/mm^3, follow facility policy for infection control in immunocompromised patients. Patients may receive injections of WBC colony-stimulating factor to increase WBC count recovery. Severe neutropenia is reversible up to cumulative dose of 6.5 mg/kg in a single course.

■ Therapeutic effects often are accompanied by toxicity.

cyclophosphamide
CONTRAINDICATIONS AND CAUTIONS

■ Contraindicated in patients hypersensitive to drug and in those with severe bone marrow suppression.

■ Use cautiously in patients who have recently undergone radiation therapy or chemotherapy and in patients with hepatic disease, leukopenia, malignant cell infiltration of bone marrow, renal disease, or thrombocytopenia.

KEY POINTS

■ Don't give drug at bedtime; infrequent urination during the night may increase risk of cystitis. If it occurs, stop drug and notify prescriber. Cystitis can occur months after therapy ceases. Mesna may be given to reduce frequency and severity of bladder toxicity. Test urine for blood.

■ Use caution to ensure correct dose and decrease risk of cardiac toxicity.

■ Monitor patient for cyclophosphamide toxicity (leukopenia, thrombocytopenia, cardiotoxicity) if corticosteroid therapy is stopped.

fludarabine
CONTRAINDICATIONS AND CAUTIONS

■ Contraindicated in patients hypersensitive to drug or its components and in those with creatinine clearance less than 30 ml/minute.

- Use cautiously in patients with renal insufficiency.

KEY POINTS

- Monitor patient closely and expect modified dosage based on toxicity. Most toxic effects are dose-dependent. Advanced age, renal insufficiency, and bone marrow impairment may predispose patients to increased or excessive toxicity.
- Careful hematologic monitoring is needed, especially of neutrophil and platelet counts. Bone marrow suppression can be severe.
- Take preventive measures before starting treatment. Hyperuricemia, hypocalcemia, hyperkalemia, and renal failure may result from rapid lysis of tumor cells.

mechlorethamine
CONTRAINDICATIONS AND CAUTIONS

- Contraindicated in patients hypersensitive to drug and in those with infectious diseases.
- Use cautiously in patients with severe anemia or depressed neutrophil or platelet count. Also use cautiously in those who have recently undergone radiation therapy or chemother-

apy. Monitor complete blood count.

KEY POINTS

- Monitor uric acid level. To prevent hyperuricemia and uric acid nephropathy, mechlorethamine may be used with adequate hydration.
- Neurotoxicity increases with dosage and patient age.
- Monitor patient closely for bone marrow suppression (nadir of myelosuppression occurring between days 4 and 10 and lasting 10 to 21 days).

LUNG CANCER

Lung cancer usually develops in the wall or epithelium of the bronchial tree. The most common types are epidermoid (squamous cell) carcinoma, small cell (oat cell) carcinoma, adenocarcinoma, and large cell (anaplastic) carcinoma. Lung cancer is the most common cause of cancer death in men and is fast becoming the most common cause in women, even though it's largely preventable. It causes more cancer deaths per year than heart, colon, and prostate cancer combined.

Most experts agree that lung cancer is attributable to inhalation of carcinogenic pollutants by a susceptible host. Most susceptible are people who smoke or who work with or near asbestos. Pollutants in tobacco smoke cause progressive degeneration of lung cells. Lung cancer is 10 times more common in smokers than in nonsmokers; indeed, 80% of lung cancer patients are or were smokers.

Cancer risk is determined by the number of cigarettes smoked daily, the depth of inhalation, how early in life smoking began, and the nicotine content of the cigarettes. Two other factors also increase susceptibility: exposure to carcinogenic industrial and air pollutants (asbestos, uranium, arsenic, nickel, iron oxides, chromium, radioactive dust, and coal dust), and familial susceptibility.

Although the prognosis is usually poor, it varies with the extent of spread at the time of diagnosis and the growth rate of the specific cell type. (See *Staging lung cancer*, page 594.) Only about 13% of patients with lung cancer survive 5 years after diagnosis.

docetaxel

CONTRAINDICATIONS AND CAUTIONS

■ Contraindicated in patients severely hypersensitive to drug or to other forms containing polysorbate 80 and in patients with neutrophil counts below 1,500 cells/mm^3.

■ Don't give drug to patients with bilirubin levels exceeding upper limit of normal, patients with alanine transaminase or aspartate transaminase levels above 1.5 times upper limit of normal and alkaline phosphatase levels over 2.5 times upper limit of normal, or patients with baseline neutrophil count less than 1,500/mm^3.

■ Safety and efficacy of drug in children haven't been established.

KEY POINTS

■ Give oral corticosteroid such as dexamethasone 16 mg P.O. (8 mg b.i.d.) daily for 3 days starting 1 day before docetaxel administration, to reduce risk and severity of fluid retention and hypersensitivity reactions.

■ Bone marrow toxicity is the most frequent and dose-limiting toxicity. Check blood count often during therapy.

■ Monitor patient closely for hypersensitivity reactions, espe-

STAGING LUNG CANCER

Using the TNM (tumor, node, metastasis) classification system, the American Joint Committee on Cancer stages lung cancer as follows:

Primary tumor

TX – primary tumor can't be assessed, or malignant tumor cells detected in sputum or bronchial washings but undetected by X-ray or bronchoscopy

T0 – no evidence of primary tumor

Tis – carcinoma in situ

T1 – tumor 3 cm or less in greatest dimension, surrounded by normal lung or visceral pleura; no bronchoscopic evidence of cancer closer to the center of the body than the lobar bronchus

T2 – tumor larger than 3 cm; or one that involves the main bronchus and is ¾" (2 cm) or more from the carina; or one that invades the visceral pleura; or one that's accompanied by atelectasis or obstructive pneumonitis that extends to the hilar region but doesn't involve the entire lung

T3 – tumor of any size that extends into neighboring structures, such as the chest wall, diaphragm, or mediastinal pleura; or a tumor in the main bronchus that doesn't involve but is less than ¾" from the carina; or a tumor that's accompanied by atelectasis or obstructive pneumonitis of the entire lung

T4 – tumor of any size that invades the mediastinum, heart, great vessels, trachea, esophagus, vertebral body, or carina; or a tumor with malignant pleural effusion

Regional lymph nodes

NX – regional lymph nodes can't be assessed

N0 – no detectable metastasis to lymph nodes

N1 – metastasis to the ipsilateral peribronchial or hilar lymph nodes or both

N2 – metastasis to the ipsilateral mediastinal or subcarinal lymph nodes or both

N3 – metastasis to the contralateral mediastinal or hilar lymph nodes, the ipsilateral or contralateral scalene lymph nodes, or the supraclavicular lymph nodes

Distant metastasis

MX – distant metastasis can't be assessed

M0 – no evidence of distant metastasis

M1 – distant metastasis

Staging categories

Lung cancer progresses from mild to severe as follows:

Occult carcinoma – TX, N0, M0

Stage 0 – Tis, N0, M0

Stage I – T1, N0, M0; T2, N0, M0

Stage II – T1, N1, M0; T2, N1, M0

Stage IIIA – T1, N2, M0; T2, N2, M0; T3, N0, M0; T3, N1, M0; T3, N2, M0

Stage IIIB – any T, N3, M0; T4, any N, M0

Stage IV – any T, any N, M1

cially during first and second infusions.

doxorubicin
CONTRAINDICATIONS AND CAUTIONS
■ Contraindicated in patients with a history of sensitivity reactions to doxorubicin or its components, patients with marked myelosuppression from previous treatment with other antitumor drugs or radiotherapy, and patients who have received a lifetime cumulative dose of 550 mg/m^2 of doxorubicin or daunorubicin.

■ Dosage adjustment may be needed in elderly patients and patients with myelosuppression or impaired cardiac or hepatic function.

KEY POINTS
■ Monitor electrocardiogram for changes such as sinus tachycardia, T-wave flattening, ST-segment depression, and voltage reduction. Be prepared to stop drug or slow infusion rate, and notify prescriber if tachycardia develops.

■ If signs of heart failure develop, stop drug and notify prescriber. Heart failure often can be prevented by limiting cumulative dose to 550 mg/m^2 (400 mg/m^2 when patient is also receiving or has received cy-

clophosphamide or radiation therapy to cardiac area).

■ Reddish color of drug is similar to that of daunorubicin; don't confuse the two.

etoposide
CONTRAINDICATIONS AND CAUTIONS
■ Contraindicated in patients hypersensitive to drug.

■ Use cautiously in patients who have had cytotoxic or radiation therapy and in patients with hepatic impairment.

KEY POINTS
■ Obtain baseline blood pressure before starting therapy.

■ Keep diphenhydramine, hydrocortisone, epinephrine, and emergency equipment available to establish an airway in case anaphylaxis occurs.

■■ *CLINICAL TIP* *Dose of etoposide phosphate is expressed as etoposide equivalents; 119.3 mg of etoposide phosphate is equivalent to 100 mg of etoposide.*

gemcitabine
CONTRAINDICATIONS AND CAUTIONS
■ Contraindicated in patients hypersensitive to drug and in pregnant or breast-feeding women.

- Use cautiously in patients with renal or hepatic impairment.
- Safety and effectiveness of drug in children haven't been determined.

KEY POINTS

- Monitor patient closely. Expect dosage adjustment according to toxicity and degree of myelosuppression. Age, sex, and renal impairment may predispose patient to toxicity.
- Carefully monitor hematologic values, especially of neutrophil and platelet counts.
- Obtain baseline and periodic renal and hepatic laboratory tests.
- Prolonging infusion time beyond 60 minutes or giving drug more than once weekly may increase toxicity.

paclitaxel
CONTRAINDICATIONS AND CAUTIONS

- Contraindicated in patients hypersensitive to drug or polyoxyethylated castor oil (a vehicle used in drug solution) and in those with baseline neutrophil counts below $1,500/mm^3$.
- Use cautiously in patients with hepatic impairment.

KEY POINTS

- Some patients experience peripheral neuropathies, which may be cumulative and dose-related. Patients with severe symptoms may need dosage reduction.
- To reduce risk or severity of hypersensitivity, patients must be pretreated with corticosteroids, such as dexamethasone, and antihistamines. Both H_1-receptor antagonists, such as diphenhydramine, and H_2-receptor antagonists, such as cimetidine or ranitidine, may be used. Severe hypersensitivity reactions occur in as many as 2% of patients.
- Monitor blood counts often during therapy. Bone marrow toxicity is the most common and dose-limiting toxicity. Packed red blood cell or platelet transfusions may be needed in severe cases. Take bleeding precautions as appropriate.

topotecan
CONTRAINDICATIONS AND CAUTIONS

- Contraindicated in pregnant women, breast-feeding women, patients hypersensitive to drug or its components, and patients with severe bone marrow depression.

■ Safety and effectiveness of drug in children haven't been established.

KEY POINTS

■ Before first course of therapy, patient must have baseline neutrophil count that's over 1,500 cells/mm³ and platelet count over 100,000 cells/mm³.

■ Bone marrow suppression (primarily neutropenia) indicates toxic levels of topotecan. The nadir occurs at about 11 days. Neutropenia isn't cumulative over time

■ Duration of thrombocytopenia is about 5 days, with nadir at 15 days. The nadir for anemia is 15 days. Blood or platelet transfusions may be needed.

■ Monitor peripheral blood cell counts frequently. Don't give subsequent courses of topotecan until neutrophil count recovers to more than 1,000 cells/mm³, platelet count to exceed 100,000 cells/mm³, and hemoglobin level to more than 9 mg/dl (with transfusion, if needed).

vinorelbine

CONTRAINDICATIONS AND CAUTIONS

■ Contraindicated in patients with pretreatment granulocyte counts below 1,000 cells/mm³ and in patients hypersensitive to drug.

■ Use with extreme caution in patients whose bone marrow may have been compromised by previous exposure to radiation therapy or chemotherapy or whose bone marrow is still recovering from chemotherapy.

■ Use cautiously in patients with hepatic impairment. Monitor liver enzyme levels.

KEY POINTS

■ Check patient's granulocyte count before giving drug; it should be 1,000 cells/mm³ or more. Withhold drug and notify prescriber if count is lower. Granulocyte nadirs occur between days 7 and 10. As a guide to the effects of therapy, monitor patient's peripheral blood count and bone marrow.

ALERT Drug is fatal if given intrathecally; it's for I.V. use only.

■ Dosage is adjusted according to hematologic toxicity or hepatic insufficiency, whichever results in the lower dosage. Expect dosage reduction of 50% if granulocyte count falls below 1,500 cells/mm³ but is greater than 1,000 cells/mm³. If three consecutive doses are skipped because of agranulocytosis, don't resume vinorelbine.

LYMPHOMAS, MALIGNANT

Also known as *non-Hodgkin's lymphomas* and *lymphosarcomas*, malignant lymphomas are a heterogeneous group of malignant diseases originating in lymph glands and other lymphoid tissue. They may be nodular or diffuse.

The cause of malignant lymphomas is unknown, although some theories suggest a viral source. They're two to three times more common in males than in females and occur in all age groups. Up to 35,000 new cases occur annually in the United States. Although rare in children, these lymphomas occur one to three times more often and cause twice as many deaths as Hodgkin's disease in children under age 15. Occurrence rises with age, and the median age is 50. Malignant lymphomas seem linked to certain races and ethnic groups, with increased risk in whites and people of Jewish ancestry.

Nodular lymphomas have a better prognosis than the diffuse form of the disease, but both have a worse prognosis than Hodgkin's disease.

bleomycin

CONTRAINDICATIONS AND CAUTIONS
■ Contraindicated in patients hypersensitive to drug.
■ Use cautiously in patients with renal or pulmonary impairment.

KEY POINTS
■ Obtain pulmonary function tests and chest X-rays before each course of therapy. Stop drug if tests show a marked decline. Monitor chest X-ray and listen to lungs regularly.
■ Adverse pulmonary reactions are more common in patients older than age 70. Pulmonary fibrosis is fatal in 1% of patients, especially when cumulative dosage exceeds 400 units. Also, pulmonary toxic adverse effects may increase in patients receiving radiation therapy, patients with lung disease, and patients who need oxygen therapy.
■ Watch for hypersensitivity reactions, which may be delayed for several hours, especially in patients with lymphoma. (Give test dose of 1 to 2 units before first two doses in these patients. If no reaction occurs, follow regular dosage.)

carmustine

CONTRAINDICATIONS AND CAUTIONS

■ Contraindicated in patients hypersensitive to drug.

KEY POINTS

■ Pulmonary toxicity appears to be dose-related and may occur 9 days to 15 years after treatment. Obtain pulmonary function tests before and during therapy.

■ Bone marrow suppression is delayed with carmustine. Don't give drug more often than every 6 weeks.

■ Monitor complete blood count with differential. Absolute neutrophil count may be used to better calculate the patient's immunosuppressive state.

chlorambucil

CONTRAINDICATIONS AND CAUTIONS

■ Contraindicated in patients hypersensitive to drug or to other alkylating drugs and in patients resistant to previous therapy.

■ Use cautiously in patients with a history of head trauma or seizures, patients taking drugs that lower the seizure threshold, and patients within 4 weeks of a full course of radiation or chemotherapy.

KEY POINTS

■ Monitor patient for neutropenia, which may not appear until after the third week of treatment. The neutrophil count may continue to decrease for up to 10 days after treatment ends.

■ Absolute neutrophil count may be used to better calculate the patient's immunosuppressive state.

■ Monitor uric acid level. To prevent hyperuricemia and uric acid nephropathy, allopurinol may be used with adequate hydration.

■ If white blood cell (WBC) count falls below $2,000/mm^3$ or granulocyte count falls below $1,000/mm^3$, follow facility policy for infection control in immunocompromised patients. Patients may receive injections of WBC colony-stimulating factor to increase WBC count recovery. Severe neutropenia is reversible up to cumulative dose of 6.5 mg/kg in a single course.

■ Therapeutic effects often are accompanied by toxicity.

cyclophosphamide

CONTRAINDICATIONS AND CAUTIONS

■ Contraindicated in patients hypersensitive to drug and in those with severe bone marrow suppression.

■ Use cautiously in patients who have recently undergone radiation therapy or chemotherapy and patients with hepatic disease, leukopenia, malignant cell infiltration of bone marrow, renal disease, or thrombocytopenia.

KEY POINTS

■ Don't give drug at bedtime; infrequent urination during the night may increase risk of cystitis. If it occurs, stop drug and notify prescriber. Cystitis can occur months after therapy ceases. Mesna may be given to reduce frequency and severity of bladder toxicity. Test urine for blood.

■ Use caution to ensure correct dose and decrease risk of cardiac toxicity.

■ Monitor patient for cyclophosphamide toxicity (leukopenia, thrombocytopenia, cardiotoxicity) if corticosteroid therapy is stopped.

doxorubicin
CONTRAINDICATIONS AND CAUTIONS

■ Contraindicated in patients with a history of sensitivity reactions to doxorubicin or its components, patients with marked myelosuppression from previous treatment with other antitumor drugs or radiotherapy, and patients who have received a lifetime cumulative dose of 550 mg/m² of doxorubicin or daunorubicin.

■ Dosage adjustment may be needed in elderly patients and patients with myelosuppression or impaired cardiac or hepatic function.

KEY POINTS

■ Monitor electrocardiogram for changes such as sinus tachycardia, T-wave flattening, ST-segment depression, and voltage reduction. Be prepared to stop drug or slow infusion rate, and notify prescriber if tachycardia develops.

■ If signs of heart failure develop, stop drug and notify prescriber. Heart failure often can be prevented by limiting cumulative dose to 550 mg/m² (400 mg/m² when patient is also receiving or has received cyclophosphamide or radiation therapy to cardiac area).

■ Reddish color of drug is similar to that of daunorubicin; don't confuse the two.

ibritumomab
CONTRAINDICATIONS AND CAUTIONS

■ Contraindicated in patients with hypersensitivity or anaphylactic reactions to murine proteins or to any component of the drug, including rituximab, yttrium chloride, and indium chloride; patients with at least 25% lymphoma marrow involvement or impaired bone marrow reserve; patients with a history of failed stem-cell collection; and patients with platelet counts below 100,000/mm³.

■ Use cautiously in patients with evidence of human anti-mouse antibodies and in those receiving live-virus vaccines.

KEY POINTS

■ Drug may cause severe, possibly fatal infusion reactions, which typically occur during the first 30 to 120 minutes of rituximab infusion. Signs and symptoms include angioedema, hypotension, hypoxia, or bronchospasm; interruption of rituximab, In-111 ibritumomab tiuxetan, and Y-90 ibritumomab tiuxetan may be required. Keep drugs to treat hypersensitivity reactions available during administration.

■ Don't use In-111 and Y-90 without the rituximab pre-dose. Don't give rituximab as I.V. push or bolus.

■ Y-90 ibritumomab tiuxetan shouldn't be given to patients with altered biodistribution as determined by imaging with In-111 ibritumomab tiuxetan.

■ Advise women of childbearing age to avoid pregnancy during therapy. If patient becomes pregnant during therapy, she should be informed of risks to fetus.

interferon alfa-2b, recombinant
CONTRAINDICATIONS AND CAUTIONS

■ Contraindicated in patients hypersensitive to drug or its components.

■ Use cautiously in patients with history of cardiovascular disease, pulmonary disease, diabetes mellitus, coagulation disorders, and severe myelosuppression.

■ Depression and suicidal behavior have been linked to drug use; patients with psychotic disorders, especially depression, shouldn't continue drug treatment.

■ Neurotoxicity and cardiotoxicity are more common in elderly patients, especially those with underlying central nervous system or cardiac impairment.

KEY POINTS

■ Alpha interferons cause or aggravate fatal or life-threatening neuropsychiatric, autoimmune, ischemic, and infectious disorders. Monitor patients closely with periodic clinical and laboratory evaluations. Patients with persistently severe or worsening evidence of these conditions should be withdrawn from therapy.

■ Make sure patient is well hydrated, especially during initial treatment.

■ At beginning of treatment, assess patient for flulike signs and symptoms, which tend to diminish with continued therapy. Premedicate patient with acetaminophen to minimize these symptoms.

rituximab
CONTRAINDICATIONS AND CAUTIONS

■ Contraindicated in patients with type I hypersensitivity or anaphylactic reactions to murine proteins or components of rituximab.

KEY POINTS

■ Monitor patient closely for evidence of hypersensitivity. Keep drugs, such as epinephrine, antihistamines, and corticosteroids, available to immediately treat such a reaction. Premedicate with acetaminophen and diphenhydramine before each infusion.

■ Severe mucocutaneous reactions—including toxic epidermal necrosis, Stevens-Johnson syndrome, paraneoplastic pemphigus, and lichenoid or vesiculobullous dermatitis) may occur 1 to 13 weeks after rituximab administration. Further infusions should be avoided, and treatment of the skin reaction should start promptly.

■ Infusion-related reactions are most severe with the first infusion. Subsequent infusions are generally well tolerated.

MELANOMA, MALIGNANT

Malignant melanoma arises from melanocytes, and cases have increased by 50% in the last 20 years, probably in part from earlier detection. The disorder is about 10 times more common in white than in nonwhite people and has four types: superficial spreading melanoma, nodular malignant melanoma, lentigo maligna melanoma, and acral-lentiginous melanoma.

Several factors may influence the development of melanoma:

■ *Excessive exposure to ultraviolet light.* Melanoma is most common in sunny, warm areas and commonly develops on parts of the body exposed to the sun. A person who has a blistering sunburn before age 20 has twice the risk of melanoma.

■ *Skin type.* Most persons with melanoma have blond or red hair, fair skin, and blue eyes; are prone to sunburn; and are of Celtic or Scandinavian descent. Melanoma is rare among blacks; when it does develop, it usually arises in lightly pigmented areas (the palms, plantar surface of the feet, or mucous membranes).

■ *Autoimmune factors.* Genetic and autoimmune factors may influence the development of melanoma.

■ *Hormonal factors.* Pregnancy may increase the risk and the growth of melanoma.

■ *Family history.* A person with a family history of melanoma has eight times the risk of developing the disorder.

■ *History of melanoma.* A person who has had one melanoma has 10 times the risk of developing a second.

Melanoma spreads through the lymphatic and vascular systems and metastasizes to regional lymph nodes, skin, liver, lungs, and central nervous system (CNS). Its course is unpredictable, and it may recur or metastasize more than 5 years after resection of the primary lesion. If it spreads to regional lymph nodes, the patient has a 50% chance of survival.

The prognosis also varies with tumor thickness. Usually, superficial lesions are curable, whereas deeper lesions tend to metastasize. The Breslow Level Method measures tumor depth from the granular level of the epidermis to the deepest melanoma cell. Lesions less than 0.76 mm deep have an excellent prognosis; deeper lesions (more than 0.76 mm deep) may metastasize. The prognosis is better for a tumor on a limb (which is drained by one lymphatic network) than for one on the head, neck, or trunk (which are drained by several networks).

dacarbazine

CONTRAINDICATIONS AND CAUTIONS

■ Contraindicated in patients hypersensitive to drug.

■ Use cautiously in patients with impaired bone marrow function and those with severe renal or hepatic dysfunction.

KEY POINTS

■ Therapeutic effects commonly are accompanied by toxicity. Monitor complete blood count and platelet count.

■ Flu syndrome (fever, malaise, and muscle pain starting 7 days after treatment ends and possibly lasting 7 to 21 days) may be treated with mild fever reducers, such as acetamino-phen.

■ Drug may cause a photosen-sitivity reaction, especially dur-ing the first 2 days of therapy. Advise patient to avoid excessive sunlight exposure.

hydroxyurea
CONTRAINDICATIONS AND CAUTIONS

■ Contraindicated in patients hypersensitive to drug and in those with severe anemia, fewer than 2,500/mm³ white blood cells (WBCs), or fewer than 100,000/mm³ platelets.

■ Use cautiously in patients with renal dysfunction.

KEY POINTS

■ Acceptable blood counts during dosage adjustment are neutrophil count 2,500 cells/mm³ or more; platelet count 95,000/mm³ or more; hemoglo-bin more than 5.3 g/dl; and reticulocyte count (if hemoglo-bin is below 9 g/dl), more than 95,000/mm³.

■ Toxic levels are neutrophil count below 2,000 cells/mm³, platelet count below 80,000/mm³, hemoglobin less than 4.5 g/dl, and reticulocyte count (if hemoglobin is below 9 g/dl) below 80,000/mm³.

■ Hydroxyurea may dramati-cally lower the WBC count in 24 to 48 hours.

■ Auditory and visual halluci-nations and hematologic toxici-ty increase when renal function decreases.

interferon alfa-2b, recombinant
CONTRAINDICATIONS AND CAUTIONS

■ Contraindicated in patients hypersensitive to drug or its components.

■ Use cautiously in patients with a history of coagulation disorders and patients with car-diovascular disease, diabetes mellitus, pulmonary disease, or severe myelosuppression.

KEY POINTS

■ Alpha interferons cause or aggravate fatal or life-threaten-ing neuropsychiatric, autoim-mune, ischemic, and infectious disorders. Patients should be monitored closely with periodic clinical and laboratory evalua-tions. Patients with persistently severe or worsening evidence of these conditions should be withdrawn from therapy.

■ Depression and suicidal be-havior have been linked to drug use; patients with psychotic dis-orders, especially depression, shouldn't continue treatment.

- Make sure patient is well hydrated, especially during initial treatment.
- At start of treatment, monitor patient for flulike signs and symptoms, which tend to diminish with continued therapy. Premedicate patient with acetaminophen to minimize these symptoms.
- Neurotoxicity and cardiotoxicity are more common in elderly patients, especially those with CNS or cardiac impairment.

MYELOMA, MULTIPLE

Multiple myeloma is also known as *malignant plasmacytoma*, *plasma cell myeloma*, and *myelomatosis*. It's a disseminated neoplasm of marrow plasma cells that infiltrates bone to produce osteolytic lesions throughout the skeleton (flat bones, vertebrae, skull, pelvis, ribs); in late stages, it infiltrates the body organs (liver, spleen, lymph nodes, lungs, adrenal glands, kidneys, skin, and gastrointestinal tract). Multiple myeloma strikes mostly men older than age 40.

The prognosis is usually poor because the disease is commonly diagnosed after it has already infiltrated the vertebrae, pelvis, skull, ribs, clavicles, and sternum. By then, skeletal destruction is widespread and, without treatment, leads to vertebral collapse. Early diagnosis and treatment prolong the lives of many patients by 3 to 5 years. Death usually follows complications, such as infection, renal failure, hematologic disorders, fractures, hypercalcemia, hyperuricemia, or dehydration.

carmustine
CONTRAINDICATIONS AND CAUTIONS
- Contraindicated in patients hypersensitive to drug.

KEY POINTS
- Pulmonary toxicity appears to be dose-related and may occur 9 days to 15 years after treatment. Obtain pulmonary function tests before and during therapy.
- Bone marrow suppression is delayed with carmustine. Drug shouldn't be given more often than every 6 weeks.
- Monitor complete blood count with differential. Absolute neutrophil count may be used to better calculate the patient's immunosuppressive state.

cyclophosphamide

CONTRAINDICATIONS AND CAUTIONS

■ Contraindicated in patients hypersensitive to drug and in those with severe bone marrow suppression.

■ Use cautiously in patients who have recently undergone radiation therapy or chemotherapy and patients with hepatic disease, leukopenia, tumor cell infiltration of bone marrow, renal disease, or thrombocytopenia.

KEY POINTS

■ Don't give drug at bedtime; infrequent urination during the night may increase risk of cystitis. If cystitis occurs, stop drug and notify prescriber. Cystitis can occur months after therapy ceases. Mesna may be given to reduce frequency and severity of bladder toxicity. Test urine for blood.

■ Use caution to ensure correct dose and decrease risk of cardiac toxicity.

■ Monitor patient for cyclophosphamide toxicity (leukopenia, thrombocytopenia, cardiotoxicity) if corticosteroid therapy is stopped.

melphalan

CONTRAINDICATIONS AND CAUTIONS

■ Contraindicated in patients hypersensitive to drug or chlorambucil, patients whose disease is resistant to drug, patients with chronic lymphocytic leukemia, and patients with severe leukopenia, thrombocytopenia, or anemia.

■ Use cautiously in patients receiving radiation and chemotherapy.

■ Dosage may need to be reduced in patients with renal impairment.

KEY POINTS

■ Melphalan is drug of choice with prednisone in patients with multiple myeloma.

■ Give oral form on empty stomach because food decreases drug absorption.

■ Anaphylaxis may occur. Keep antihistamines and corticosteroids readily available to give if needed.

OVARIAN CANCER

After cancer of the lung, breast, and colon, primary ovarian cancer ranks as the most common cause of cancer deaths among American women. In women with previously treated breast cancer, metastatic ovarian cancer is more common than cancer at any other site. There are three main types of ovarian cancer:

■ *Primary epithelial tumors* account for 90% of ovarian cancers and include serous cystadenocarcinoma, mucinous cyst-adenocarcinoma, and endometrioid and mesonephric malignancies. Serous cystadenocarcinoma is the most common type and accounts for 50% of all cases.

■ *Germ cell tumors* include endodermal sinus malignancies, embryonal carcinoma (a rare ovarian cancer that appears in children), immature teratomas, and dysgerminoma.

■ *Sex cord (stromal) tumors* include granulosa cell tumors (which produce estrogen and may have feminizing effects), granulosa-theca cell tumors, and the rare arrhenoblastomas (which produce androgen and have virilizing effects).

The exact cause of ovarian cancer is unknown, but it's noticeably more common among women of upper socioeconomic levels between ages 20 and 54. Certain genes, including BRCA1 and BRCA2, may increase the risk. Other contributing factors include age at menopause; infertility; celibacy; a high-fat diet; exposure to asbestos, talc, and industrial pollutants; nulliparity; familial risk; and a history of breast or uterine cancer.

Ovarian tumors spread rapidly intraperitoneally by local extension or surface seeding and, occasionally, through the lymphatics and the bloodstream. Usually, extraperitoneal spread is through the diaphragm into the chest cavity, which may cause pleural effusions. Other types of metastasis are rare.

The prognosis varies with the histologic type and stage of the disease but usually is poor because ovarian tumors produce few early signs and usually are advanced at diagnosis.

carboplatin

CONTRAINDICATIONS AND CAUTIONS

■ Contraindicated in patients with severe bone marrow suppression, bleeding, or a history of hypersensitivity to cisplatin, platinum-containing compounds, or mannitol.

■ Bone marrow suppression may be more severe in patients with creatinine clearance below 60 ml/minute, and dosage should be adjusted for these patients.

KEY POINTS

■ Check complete blood count (CBC), creatinine clearance, and electrolyte, creatinine, and blood urea nitrogen (BUN) levels before first infusion and each course of treatment. Carefully check ordered dose against laboratory test results. Only one increase in dosage is recommended. Subsequent doses shouldn't exceed 125% of starting dose.

■ Monitor CBC and platelet count frequently during therapy and, when indicated, until recovery. White blood cell (WBC) and platelet count nadirs usually occur by day 21 and return to baseline by day 28. Dose shouldn't be repeated unless platelet count exceeds 100,000/mm³.

■ Carboplatin has less nephrotoxicity and neurotoxicity than cisplatin, but it causes more severe myelosuppression.

■ Patients older than age 65 are at greater risk for neurotoxicity.

cisplatin

CONTRAINDICATIONS AND CAUTIONS

■ Contraindicated in patients hypersensitive to drug or other platinum-containing compounds and in those with severe renal disease, hearing impairment, or myelosuppression.

■ Use cautiously in patients previously treated with radiation or cytotoxic drugs, patients with peripheral neuropathies, and patients receiving other ototoxic and nephrotoxic drugs.

KEY POINTS

■ Therapeutic effects often are accompanied by toxicity. Check current protocol. Some prescribers use I.V. sodium thiosulfate or amifostine to minimize toxicity.

■ Patients may experience vomiting 3 to 5 days after treatment, requiring prolonged antiemetic treatment. Some prescribers combine metoclopramide with dexamethasone and antihistamines, or ondansetron or granisetron with dexamethasone to control vomiting. Monitor intake and output. Continue I.V. hydration until patient can tolerate adequate oral intake.

■ Renal toxicity is cumulative; renal function must return to normal before next dose can be given.

■ Don't repeat dose unless platelet count is greater than 100,000/mm³, WBC count is greater than 4,000/mm³, creatinine level is less than 1.5 mg/dl, creatinine clearance equals or exceeds 50 ml/minute or more, and BUN level is less than 25 mg/dl.

doxorubicin hydrochloride
CONTRAINDICATIONS AND CAUTIONS
■ Contraindicated in patients with a history of sensitivity reactions to doxorubicin or its components, patients with marked myelosuppression from previous treatment with other antitumor drugs or radiotherapy, and patients who have received a lifetime cumulative dose of 550 mg/m^2 of doxorubicin or daunorubicin.
■ Dosage adjustment may be needed in elderly patients and patients with myelosuppression or impaired cardiac or hepatic function.

KEY POINTS
■ Monitor electrocardiogram for changes such as sinus tachycardia, T-wave flattening, ST-segment depression, and voltage reduction. Be prepared to stop drug or slow infusion rate, and notify prescriber if tachycardia develops.
■ If signs of heart failure develop, stop drug and notify prescriber. Heart failure often can be prevented by limiting cumulative dose to 550 mg/m^2

(400 mg/m^2 when patient is also receiving or has received cyclophosphamide or radiation therapy to cardiac area).
■ Reddish color of drug is similar to that of daunorubicin; don't confuse the two.

melphalan
CONTRAINDICATIONS AND CAUTIONS
■ Contraindicated in patients hypersensitive to drug or to chlorambucil, patients whose disease is resistant to drug, patients with chronic lymphocytic leukemia, and patients with severe leukopenia, thrombocytopenia, or anemia.
■ Use cautiously in patients receiving radiation and chemotherapy.
■ Dosage may need to be reduced in patients with renal impairment.

KEY POINTS
■ Give oral form on empty stomach because food decreases drug absorption.
■ Anaphylaxis may occur. Keep antihistamines and corticosteroids readily available to give if needed.
■ Monitor uric acid level and CBC.

paclitaxel

CONTRAINDICATIONS AND CAUTIONS

■ Contraindicated in patients hypersensitive to drug or polyoxyethylated castor oil (a vehicle used in drug solution), patients with baseline neutrophil counts below $1,500/mm^3$, and patients with acquired immunodeficiency syndrome–related Kaposi's sarcoma and baseline neutrophil counts below $1,000/mm^3$.

■ Use cautiously in patients with hepatic impairment.

KEY POINTS

■ Some patients experience peripheral neuropathies, which may be cumulative and dose-related. Patients with severe symptoms may need dosage reduction.

■ To reduce risk and severity of hypersensitivity, patients must be pretreated with corticosteroids, such as dexamethasone, and antihistamines. Both H_1-receptor antagonists, such as diphenhydramine, and H_2-receptor antagonists, such as cimetidine or ranitidine, may be used. Severe hypersensitivity reactions occur in as many as 2% of patients.

■ Monitor blood counts often during therapy. Bone marrow toxicity is the most common and dose-limiting toxicity. Packed red blood cell or platelet transfusions may be needed in severe cases. Take bleeding precautions as appropriate.

PROSTATIC CANCER

One in 11 men will develop prostatic cancer, the most common neoplasm in black men and the second most common in all men over age 55. Adenocarcinoma is the most common form; sarcoma occurs only rarely. Although androgens regulate prostate growth and function and may also speed tumor growth, no definite link has been found between increased androgen levels and prostatic cancer.

Most prostatic cancers originate in the posterior prostate gland; the rest, near the urethra. They seldom result from the benign hyperplastic enlargement common in older men; they seldom produce symptoms until advanced. When primary prostatic lesions metastasize, they typically invade the prostatic capsule and spread along the ejaculatory ducts in the space between the seminal vesicles or perivesicular fascia.

estramustine

CONTRAINDICATIONS AND CAUTIONS

■ Contraindicated in patients hypersensitive to estradiol or nitrogen mustard and in those with active thrombophlebitis or thromboembolic disorders, except when the actual tumor mass is causing the thromboembolic phenomenon.

■ Use cautiously in patients with a history of thrombophlebitis, thromboembolic disorders, or cerebrovascular or coronary artery disease. Monitor weight regularly in these patients. Drug may worsen peripheral edema or heart failure.

■ Also use cautiously in patients with impaired liver function. Monitor liver function periodically during therapy.

KEY POINTS

■ Drug may increase blood pressure and decrease glucose level. Check these characteristics periodically during therapy.

■ Drug is a combination of estrogen estradiol and a nitrogen mustard and may be effective in patients refractory to estrogen therapy alone.

■ Patient may continue therapy as long as response is favorable. Some patients have taken drug for more than 3 years.

flutamide

CONTRAINDICATIONS AND CAUTIONS

■ Contraindicated in patients hypersensitive to drug and in patients with severe liver dysfunction.

KEY POINTS

■ Flutamide must be taken continuously with a drug used for medical castration (such as leuprolide) to allow full benefit of therapy. Leuprolide suppresses testosterone production, whereas flutamide inhibits testosterone action at the cellular level; together, they can impair growth of androgen-responsive tumors.

■ Monitor liver function tests and complete blood count periodically.

■ Drug may cause photosensitivity reactions. Advise patient to avoid excessive sunlight exposure.

goserelin

CONTRAINDICATIONS AND CAUTIONS

■ Contraindicated in patients with obstructive uropathy or vertebral metastases and patients hypersensitive to luteinizing hormone–releasing hormone (LH-RH), LH-RH agonist analogues, or goserelin acetate.

■ Use cautiously in patients with risk factors for osteoporosis, such as a family history of osteoporosis, chronic alcohol or tobacco abuse, or use of drugs that affect bone density, such as corticosteroids or anticonvulsants.

KEY POINTS

■ Symptoms of prostate cancer may initially worsen, and some patients may have increased bone pain, because drug first increases testosterone levels. Rarely, the disease has been worsened, either through spinal cord compression or ureteral obstruction.

ALERT The implant comes in a preloaded syringe. If the package is damaged, don't use the syringe. Make sure drug is visible in the translucent chamber of the syringe.

■ Give drug into the upper abdominal wall using aseptic technique. After cleaning the area with an alcohol swab and injecting a local anesthetic, stretch patient's skin with one hand while grasping barrel of syringe with the other. Insert needle into the subcutaneous fat; then change direction of needle so that it parallels the abdominal wall. Push needle in until hub touches patient's skin; withdraw about 1 cm (to create a gap for drug to be injected) before depressing plunger completely.

leuprolide
CONTRAINDICATIONS AND CAUTIONS

■ Contraindicated in patients hypersensitive to drug or other gonadotropin-releasing hormone analogues.

■ Use cautiously in patients hypersensitive to benzyl alcohol.

KEY POINTS

■ A fractional dose of drug formulated to give every 3 months isn't equivalent to the same dose of once-a-month formulation.

■ During the first few weeks of therapy, drug may increase signs and symptoms being treated (flare).

nilutamide
CONTRAINDICATIONS AND CAUTIONS

■ Contraindicated in patients hypersensitive to drug and in those with severe hepatic or respiratory disease.

KEY POINTS

■ Drug is used with surgical castration; for maximum benefit, treatment should begin on the same day or the day after surgery.

■ Obtain baseline liver enzyme levels, and repeat at 3-month intervals. Stop drug if transaminase level exceeds three times the upper limit of normal.

■ Obtain a baseline chest X-ray before therapy starts. Monitor patient (especially if Asian) for evidence of interstitial pneumonitis, and notify prescriber if it occurs.

triptorelin
CONTRAINDICATIONS AND CAUTIONS

■ Contraindicated in patients hypersensitive to triptorclin, its components, other LH-RH agonists, or LH-RH.

■ Use cautiously in patients with metastatic vertebral lesions or upper or lower urinary tract obstruction during the first few weeks of therapy.

KEY POINTS

■ Initially, triptorelin causes a transient increase in testosterone levels. As a result, signs and symptoms of prostate cancer may worsen during the first few weeks of treatment. Monitor testosterone and prostate specific antigen levels.

■ Patients may have worsening symptoms or new symptoms, including bone pain, neuropathy, hematuria, or urethral or bladder outlet obstruction.

■ Spinal cord compression may occur, which can lead to paralysis and possibly death. If spinal cord compression or renal impairment develops, standard treatment should be given. In extreme cases, immediate orchiectomy is considered.

■ Patients with renal or hepatic impairment may retain the drug longer and have a twofold to fourfold higher exposure to the drug than young healthy men.

TESTICULAR CANCER

Malignant testicular tumors affect mainly young to middle-aged men and rank first in cancer deaths among men ages 20 to 35; they are the most common solid tumor in this group. (In children, testicular tumors are rare.) Most testicular tumors originate in gonadal cells. About 40% are seminomas—uniform, undifferentiated cells resembling primitive gonadal cells. The rest are nonseminomas—tumor cells showing various degrees of differentiation.

The cause of testicular cancer isn't known, but it's more common in men with cryptorchidism (even when surgically corrected) and men whose mothers took diethylstilbestrol during pregnancy. Exposure to certain chemicals, infection with human immunodeficiency virus, and a family history of testicular cancer increase the risk.

Testicular cancer spreads through the lymphatic system to the para-aortic, iliac, and mediastinal lymph nodes and may metastasize to the lungs, liver, viscera, and bone. The prognosis varies with the cell type and disease stage. When treated with surgery and radiation, almost all patients with localized disease survive beyond 5 years.

bleomycin

CONTRAINDICATIONS AND CAUTIONS

■ Contraindicated in patients hypersensitive to drug.

■ Use cautiously in patients with renal or pulmonary impairment.

KEY POINTS

■ Obtain pulmonary function tests and chest X-rays before each course of therapy. Stop drug if tests show a marked decline. Monitor chest X-ray and listen to lungs regularly.

■ Adverse pulmonary reactions are more common in patients over age 70. Pulmonary fibrosis is fatal in 1% of patients, especially when cumulative dosage exceeds 400 units. Also, toxic pulmonary effects may be increased in patients receiving radiation therapy, patients with lung disease, and patients who need oxygen therapy.

■ Watch for hypersensitivity reactions, which may be delayed for several hours, especially in patients with lymphoma. (Give test dose of 1 to 2 units before first two doses in these patients. If no reaction occurs, follow regular dosage.)

cisplatin

CONTRAINDICATIONS AND CAUTIONS

■ Contraindicated in patients hypersensitive to drug or other platinum-containing compounds and in those with severe renal disease, hearing impairment, or myelosuppression.

■ Use cautiously in patients previously treated with radiation or cytotoxic drugs, patients with peripheral neuropathies, and patients taking other ototoxic and nephrotoxic drugs.

KEY POINTS

■ Therapeutic effects often are accompanied by toxicity. Check current protocol. Some prescribers use I.V. sodium thiosulfate or amifostine to minimize toxicity.

■ Patients may develop vomiting 3 to 5 days after treatment, requiring prolonged antiemetic treatment. Some prescribers combine metoclopramide with dexamethasone and antihistamines, or ondansetron or granisetron with dexamethasone to control vomiting. Monitor intake and output. Continue I.V. hydration until patient can tolerate adequate oral intake.

■ Renal toxicity is cumulative; renal function must return to normal before next dose can be given.

■ Don't repeat dose unless platelet count is greater than 100,000/mm^3, white blood cell count is more than 4,000/mm^3, creatinine level is less than 1.5 mg/dl, creatinine clearance is 50 ml/minute or more, and blood urea nitrogen level is less than 25 mg/dl.

etoposide

CONTRAINDICATIONS AND CAUTIONS

■ Contraindicated in patients hypersensitive to drug.

■ Use cautiously in patients with hepatic impairment and patients who have had cytotoxic or radiation therapy.

KEY POINTS

■ Obtain baseline blood pressure before starting therapy.

■ Have diphenhydramine, hydrocortisone, epinephrine, and emergency equipment available to establish an airway in case anaphylaxis occurs.

CLINICAL TIP Dose of etoposide phosphate is expressed as etoposide equivalents; 119.3 mg of etoposide phosphate is equivalent to 100 mg of etoposide.

ifosfamide

CONTRAINDICATIONS AND CAUTIONS

■ Contraindicated in patients hypersensitive to drug and in those with severe bone marrow suppression.

■ Use cautiously in patients with renal impairment or compromised bone marrow reserve as indicated by leukopenia, granulocytopenia, extensive bone marrow metastases, previous radiation therapy, or previous therapy with cytotoxic drugs.

KEY POINTS

■ Give antiemetic before drug to reduce nausea.

■ Don't give drug at bedtime; infrequent urination during the night may increase risk of cystitis. If it develops, stop drug and notify prescriber.

■ Bladder may be irrigated with normal saline solution to treat cystitis.

- Assess patient for mental status changes; dosage may have to be decreased.

vinblastine

CONTRAINDICATIONS AND CAUTIONS

- Contraindicated in patients hypersensitive to the drug and patients with severe leukopenia or bacterial infection.
- Use cautiously in patients with hepatic dysfunction.

KEY POINTS

- After giving drug, check for development of life-threatening acute bronchospasm. If it occurs, notify prescriber immediately. Reaction is most likely to occur in patients receiving mitomycin.
- Dosage shouldn't be repeated more often than every 7 days or severe leukopenia will occur. Nadir occurs on days 4 to 10 and lasts another 7 to 14 days.
- Assess patient for numbness and tingling in hands and feet. Assess gait for early evidence of footdrop. Drug is less neurotoxic than vincristine.

PART V

SPECIAL SKILLS

23 / CHEMOTHERAPY

Managing a patient's chemotherapy takes special skills and meticulous attention to safety. In this chapter, you'll find eight important resources to help you understand and manage this complex therapy:

- The cell cycle and chemotherapy
- Selected chemotherapy drugs
- Chemotherapy acronyms and protocols
- Guidelines for handling chemotherapeutic drugs
- Risks of tissue damage
- Preventing errors
- Preventing infiltration
- Managing complications of chemotherapy

THE CELL CYCLE AND CHEMOTHERAPY

All cells cycle through five phases. Chemotherapy drugs that act on cells during one or more of these phases are called cycle-specific drugs. The illustration below shows what happens at each phase of the cell cycle and gives examples of cycle-specific drugs for each phase.

G₂ phase
Deoxyribonucleic acid (DNA) synthesis halts. Ribonucleic acid (RNA) and protein synthesis continues in preparation for mitosis.

M phase
Mitosis occurs. Daughter cells may repeat the cell cycle or enter the G₀ phase.

G₀ phase
The resting phase. Some cells will replicate while others will remain inactive.

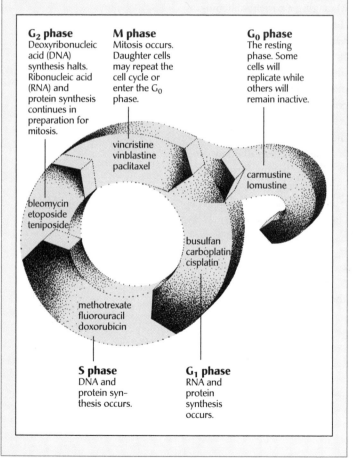

vincristine
vinblastine
paclitaxel

carmustine
lomustine

bleomycin
etoposide
teniposide

busulfan
carboplatin
cisplatin

methotrexate
fluorouracil
doxorubicin

S phase
DNA and protein synthesis occurs.

G₁ phase
RNA and protein synthesis occurs.

SELECTED CHEMOTHERAPY DRUGS

Compare the characteristics and toxic effects of chemotherapy drugs.

CATEGORY	CHARACTERISTICS	TOXIC EFFECTS
Cycle-specific		
Antimetabolites cytarabine, floxuridine, fluorouracil, hydroxy-urea, methotrexate, thioguanine	■ Interfere with nucleic acid synthesis ■ Attack during S phase of cell cycle	■ Effects on bone marrow (myelosuppression), central nervous system (CNS), and gastrointestinal (GI) system
Plant alkaloids vinblastine, vincristine	■ Prevent mitotic spindle formation ■ Cycle-specific to M phase	■ Effects on CNS, GI system ■ Myelosuppression ■ Tissue damage
Enzyme asparaginase	■ Useful only for leukemias	■ Hypersensitivity reactions
Cycle-nonspecific		
Alkylating agents carboplatin, cisplatin, cyclophosphamide, ifosfamide, thiotepa	■ Disrupt deoxyribonucleic acid (DNA) replication	■ Infertility ■ Secondary carcinoma ■ Renal system
Antibiotics bleomycin, doxorubicin, idarubicin, mitoxantrone, mitomycin	■ Bind with DNA to inhibit synthesis of DNA and ribonucleic acid	■ Effects on GI, renal, and hepatic systems ■ Effects on bone marrow
Hormones and hormone inhibitors		
Androgen testolactone **Antiandrogen** flutamide **Antiestrogen** tamoxifen **Estrogen** estramustine **Gonadotropin** leuprolide **Progestin** megestrol	■ Interfere with binding of normal hormones to receptor proteins, manipulate hormone levels, and alter hormone environment ■ Mechanism of action not always clear ■ Usually palliative, not curative	■ No known toxic effect

(continued)

SELECTED CHEMOTHERAPY DRUGS *(continued)*

CATEGORY	CHARACTERISTICS	TOXIC EFFECTS
Folic acid analog		
leucovorin	■ Antidote for methotrexate toxicity	■ Hypersensitivity reaction possible
Cytoprotective agents		
dexrazoxane, mesna	■ Protect normal tissue by binding with metabolites of other cytotoxic drugs	■ None

CHEMOTHERAPY ACRONYMS AND PROTOCOLS

This table lists commonly used chemotherapy acronyms and protocols, including standard dosages for specific cancers.

INDICATION AND ACRONYM	GENERIC DRUG NAME	TRADE DRUG NAME	DOSAGE
Adenocarcinoma			
FAM	fluorouracil (5-FU)	Adrucil	600 mg/m² I.V., days 1, 8, 29, and 36
	doxorubicin	Adriamycin	30 mg/m² I.V., days 1 and 29
	mitomycin	Mutamycin	10 mg/m² I.V., day 1 *Repeat cycle q 8 wk.*
Bladder cancer			
CISCA	cisplatin	Platinol	100 mg/m² I.V., day 2
	cyclophosphamide	Cytoxan	650 mg/m² I.V., day 1
	doxorubicin	Adriamycin	50 mg/m² I.V., day 1 *Repeat cycle q 21-28 days*
GC	gemcitabine	Gemzar	1 g/m² I.V. over 30-60 min, days 1, 8, and 15
	cisplatin	Platinol	70 mg/m² I.V., day 2 *Repeat cycle q 28 days.*
MVAC	methotrexate		30 mg/m² I.V., days 1, 15, and 22
	vinblastine	Velban	3 mg/m² I.V., days 2, 15, and 22
	doxorubicin	Adriamycin	30 mg/m² I.V., day 2
	cisplatin	Platinol	70 mg/m² I.V., day 2 *Repeat cycle q 28 days.*
Bony sarcoma			
AC	doxorubicin	Adriamycin	75-90 mg/m² (total dose) by 96-hr continuous I.V. infusion

(continued)

INDICATION AND ACRONYM	GENERIC DRUG NAME	TRADE DRUG NAME	DOSAGE
Bony sarcoma *(continued)*			
AC *(continued)*	cisplatin	Platinol	90-120 mg/m^2 intra-arterial or I.V., day 6 *Repeat cycle q 28 days.*
HDMTX (high–dose methotrexate)	methotrexate		8-12 g/m^2 I.V. weekly for 2-12 wk
	leucovorin calcium		15-25 mg/m^2 I.V. or P.O. q 6 hr for 10 doses, beginning 24 hr after methotrexate dose (monitor methotrexate levels) *Repeat cycle q 7 days for 2-4 wk.*
Brain tumors			
PCV	procarbazine	Matulane	60 mg/m^2 P.O., days 8-21
	lomustine (CCNU)	CeeNu	110 mg/m^2 P.O., day 1
	vincristine	Oncovin	1.4 mg/m^2 (2 mg maximum) I.V., days 8 and 29 *Repeat cycle q 6-8 wk.*
Breast cancer			
AC	doxorubicin	Adriamycin	60 mg/m^2 I.V., day 1
	cyclophosphamide	Cytoxan	600 mg/m^2 I.V., day 1 *Repeat cycle q 21 days.*
CAF	cyclophosphamide	Cytoxan	100 mg/m^2 P.O., days 1-14
	doxorubicin	Adriamycin	30 mg/m^2 I.V., days 1 and 8
	fluorouracil (5-FU)	Adrucil	500 mg/m^2 I.V., days 1 and 8 *Repeat cycle q 28 days.*

CHEMOTHERAPY ACRONYMS AND PROTOCOLS *(continued)*

INDICATION AND ACRONYM	GENERIC DRUG NAME	TRADE DRUG NAME	DOSAGE
Breast cancer *(continued)*			
CAF *(continued)*	*or*		
	cyclophos-phamide	Cytoxan	500 mg/m² I.V., day 1
	doxorubicin	Adriamycin	50 mg/m² I.V., day 1
	fluorouracil (5-FU)	Adrucil	500 mg/m² I.V., day 1 *Repeat cycle q 21 days.*
CEF	cyclophos-phamide	Cytoxan	75 mg/m² P.O., days 1-14
	epirubicin	Ellence	60 mg/m² I.V., days 1 and 8
	fluorouracil (5-FU)	Adrucil	500 mg/m² I.V., days 1 and 8
	co-trimoxazole	Bactrim	2 tablets (single-strength) P.O. twice daily, days 1-28 *Repeat cycle q 28 days.*
CMF	cyclophos-phamide	Cytoxan	100 mg/m² P.O., days 1-14; or 400-600 mg/m² I.V., day 1
	methotrexate		40 mg/m² I.V., days 1 and 8
	fluorouracil (5-FU)	Adrucil	400-600 mg/m² I.V., days 1 and 8 *Repeat cycle q 28 days.*
Dox-CMF, Sequential	doxorubicin	Adriamycin	75 mg/m² I.V., day 1 for 4 cycles, fol-lowed by CMF regi-men for 8 cycles *Repeat cycle q 21 days.*
FAC (CAF)	fluorouracil (5-FU)	Adrucil	500 mg/m² I.V., day 1
	doxorubicin	Adriamycin	50 mg/m² I.V., day 1
	cyclophos-phamide	Cytoxan	500 mg/m² I.V., day 1 *Repeat cycle q 21 days.*

(continued)

CHEMOTHERAPY ACRONYMS AND PROTOCOLS *(continued)*

INDICATION AND ACRONYM	GENERIC DRUG NAME	TRADE DRUG NAME	DOSAGE
Breast cancer *(continued)*			
FEC	fluorouracil (5-FU)	Adrucil	500 mg/m² I.V., day 1
	epirubicin	Ellence	100 mg/m² I.V., day 1
	cyclophos- phamide	Cytoxan	500 mg/m² I.V., day 1 *Repeat cycle q 21 days.*
Trastuzumab– paclitaxel	trastuzumab	Herceptin	4 mg/kg I.V. over 90 min as loading dose, day 1; then 2 mg/kg I.V. over 30 min weekly, days 1, 8, and 15, except for day 1 of first cycle
	paclitaxel	Taxol	175 mg/m² I.V. over 3 hr, day 1 *Repeat cycle q 21 days.*
Colorectal cancer			
F–CL (FU/LV)	fluorouracil (5-FU)	Adrucil	370–425 mg/m² I.V., days 1–5, after starting leucovorin
	leucovorin calcium		20 mg/m² I.V., days 1–5 *Repeat cycle q 28-56 days.*
	or		
	fluorouracil (5-FU)	Adrucil	600 mg/m² I.V., 1 hr after starting leu- covorin infusion, weekly for 6 wk; then 2-wk rest pe- riod
	leucovorin calcium		500 mg/m² over 2 hr weekly for 6 wk; then 2-wk rest pe- riod *Repeat cycle q 28-56 days.*

CHEMOTHERAPY ACRONYMS AND PROTOCOLS *(continued)*

INDICATION AND ACRONYM	GENERIC DRUG NAME	TRADE DRUG NAME	DOSAGE
Colorectal cancer *(continued)*			
FU/LV/CPT-11	irinotecan	Camptosar	125 mg/m² I.V. over 90 min, days 1, 8, 15, and 22
	fluorouracil (5-FU)	Adrucil	500 mg/m² I.V., days 1, 8, 15, and 22
	leucovorin calcium		20 mg/m² I.V., days 1, 8, 15, and 22 *Repeat cycle q 42 days.*
Endometrial cancer			
AP	doxorubicin	Adriamycin	50-60 mg/m² I.V., day 1
	cisplatin	Platinol	50-60 mg/m² I.V., day 1 *Repeat q 21-28 days.*
Gastric cancer			
FAM	fluorouracil (5-FU)	Adrucil	600 mg/m² I.V., days 1, 8, 29, and 36
	doxorubicin	Adriamycin	30 mg/m² I.V., days 1 and 29
	mitomycin	Mutamycin	10 mg/m² I.V., day 1 *Repeat cycle q 8 wk.*
Head and neck cancer			
CF	cisplatin	Platinol	100 mg/m² I.V., day 1
	fluorouracil (5-FU)	Adrucil	1,000 mg/m² daily by continuous I.V. infusion, days 1-5 *Repeat cycle q 21-28 days.*
	or carboplatin	Paraplatin	300 mg/m² I.V., day 1
	fluorouracil (5-FU)	Adrucil	1,000 mg/m² daily by continuous I.V. infusion, days 1-5 *Repeat cycle q 21-28 days.*

(continued)

CHEMOTHERAPY ACRONYMS AND PROTOCOLS *(continued)*

INDICATION AND ACRONYM	GENERIC DRUG NAME	TRADE DRUG NAME	DOSAGE
Hodgkin's disease			
ABVD	doxorubicin	Adriamycin	25 mg/m² I.V., days 1 and 15
	bleomycin	Blenoxane	10 units/m² I.V., days 1 and 15
	vinblastine	Velban	6 mg/m² I.V., days 1 and 15
	dacarbazine	DTIC-Dome	350-375 mg/m² I.V., days 1 and 15 *Repeat cycle q 28 days.*
MOPP	mechloretha-mine (nitro-gen mustard)	Mustargen	6 mg/m² I.V., days 1 and 8
	vincristine	Oncovin	1.4 mg/m² (2 mg maximum) I.V., days 1 and 8
	procarbazine	Matulane	100 mg/m² P.O., days 1-14
	prednisone	Deltasone	40 mg/m² P.O., days 1-14 *Repeat cycle q 28 days.*
MVPP	mechloretha-mine (nitro-gen mustard)	Mustargen	6 mg/m² I.V., days 1 and 8
	vinblastine	Velban	4 mg/m² I.V., days 1 and 8
	procarbazine	Matulane	100 mg/m² P.O., days 1-14
	prednisone	Deltasone	40 mg/m² P.O., days 1-14 *Repeat cycle q 4-6 wk.*
Stanford V	mechloretha-mine (nitro-gen mustard)	Mustargen	6 mg/m² I.V., day 1
	doxorubicin	Adriamycin	25 mg/m² I.V., days 1 and 15
	vinblastine	Velban	6 mg/m² I.V., days 1 and 15

CHEMOTHERAPY ACRONYMS AND PROTOCOLS *(continued)*

INDICATION AND ACRONYM	GENERIC DRUG NAME	TRADE DRUG NAME	DOSAGE
Hodgkin's disease *(continued)*			
Stanford V *(continued)*	vincristine	Oncovin	1.4 mg/m^2 (2 mg maximum) I.V., days 8 and 22
	bleomycin	Blenoxane	5 units/m^2 I.V., days 8 and 22
	etoposide	VePesid	60 mg/m^2 I.V., days 15 and 16
	prednisone	Deltasone	40 mg/m^2 P.O., every other day for 10 wk; then taper off by 10 mg every other day for next 14 days *Repeat cycle q 28 days.*
Leukemia—ALL, adult induction			
Hyper-CVAD	cyclophos-phamide	Cytoxan	300 mg/m^2 I.V. over 3 hr q 12 hr, days 1–3
	mesna	Mesnex	600 mg/m^2 continu-ous I.V. infusion, days 1–3
	vincristine	Oncovin	2 mg I.V., days 4 and 11
	doxorubicin	Adriamycin	50 mg/m^2 I.V., day 4
	dexamethasone	Decadron	40 mg P.O. daily, days 1–4 and 11–14
	filgrastim	Neupogen	5 mcg/kg S.C. b.i.d., day 5, until ANC recovery *Alternate cycles with HD MTX–Ara-C regimen q 3-4 wk.*
HD MTX–Ara-C	methotrexate		200 mg/m^2 I.V. over 2 hr, day 1, fol-lowed by 800 mg/m^2 over 24 hr, day 1

(continued)

CHEMOTHERAPY ACRONYMS AND PROTOCOLS *(continued)*

INDICATION AND ACRONYM	GENERIC DRUG NAME	TRADE DRUG NAME	DOSAGE
Leukemia—ALL, adult induction *(continued)*			
HD MTX–Ara-C (continued)	cytarabine (ara-C)	Cytosar-U	3 g/m² I.V. over 2 hr q 12 hr, days 2 and 3
	methylpred- nisolone	Solu-Medrol	50 mg I.V. b.i.d., days 1-3
	filgrastim	Neupogen	5 mcg/kg S.C. b.i.d., day 4, until ANC recovery
	leucovorin calcium		15 mg P.O. q 6 hr for eight doses, start- ing 24 hr after completion of methotrexate infu- sion *Alternate cycles with Hyper-CVAD regi- men for a total of 8 cycles.*
Leukemia—AML, induction			
5 + 2	cytarabine (ara-C)	Cytosar-U	100-200 mg/m² by continuous I.V. in- fusion, days 1-5
	daunorubicin	Cerubidine	45 mg/m² I.V., days 1 and 2 *Repeat cycle q 7 days.*
	or cytarabine (ara-C)	Cytosar-U	100-200 mg/m² by continuous I.V. in- fusion, days 1-5
	mitoxantrone	Novantrone	12 mg/m² I.V. daily, days 1 and 2 *Repeat cycle q 7 days.*
7 + 3 (with mitoxantrone)	mitoxantrone	Novantrone	12 mg/m² I.V. daily, days 1-3
	cytarabine (ara-C)	Cytosar-U	100-200 mg/m² daily by continuous I.V. infusion, days 1-7 *Give 1 cycle only.*

CHEMOTHERAPY ACRONYMS AND PROTOCOLS (continued)

INDICATION AND ACRONYM	GENERIC DRUG NAME	TRADE DRUG NAME	DOSAGE
Leukemia—AML, induction (continued)			
7 + 3 (with daunorubicin)	cytarabine (ara-C)	Cytosar-U	100-200 mg/m² daily by continuous I.V. infusion, days 1-7
	daunorubicin	Cerubidine	30 or 45 mg/m² I.V., days 1-3 *Give 1 cycle only.*
Leukemia—CLL			
CVP	cyclophosphamide	Cytoxan	300-400 mg/m² P.O., days 1-5
	vincristine	Oncovin	1.4 mg/m² (2 mg maximum) I.V., day 1
	prednisone	Deltasone	100 mg/m² P.O., days 1-5 *Repeat cycle q 21 days.*
Melanoma			
DTIC/Tamoxifen	dacarbazine	DTIC–Dome	250 mg/m² I.V., days 1-5
	tamoxifen	Nolvadex	20 mg/m² P.O., days 1-5 *Repeat cycle q 21 days.*
VDP	vinblastine	Velban	5 mg/m² I.V., days 1 and 2
	dacarbazine	DTIC–Dome	150 mg/m² I.V., days 1-5
	cisplatin	Platinol	75 mg/m² I.V., day 5 *Repeat cycle q 21-28 days.*
Multiple myeloma			
MP	melphalan (phenylalanine mustard)	Alkeran	8 mg/m² P.O., days 1-4
	prednisone	Deltasone	60 mg/² P.O., days 1-4 *Repeat cycle q 21-28 days.*

(continued)

CHEMOTHERAPY ACRONYMS AND PROTOCOLS *(continued)*

INDICATION AND ACRONYM	GENERIC DRUG NAME	TRADE DRUG NAME	DOSAGE
Multiple myeloma *(continued)*			
VAD	vincristine	Oncovin	0.4 mg by continuous I.V. infusion, days 1–4
	doxorubicin	Adriamycin	9 mg/m^2 by continuous I.V. infusion, days 1–4
	dexamethasone	Decadron	40 mg P.O. on days 1–4, 9–12, and 17–20 *Repeat cycle q 4-5 wk.*
Non-Hodgkin's lymphoma			
CHOP	cyclophosphamide	Cytoxan	750 mg/m^2 I.V., day 1
	doxorubicin	Adriamycin	50 mg/m^2 I.V., day 1
	vincristine	Oncovin	1.4 mg/m^2 (2 mg maximum) I.V., day 1
	prednisone	Deltasone	100 mg P.O., days 1–5 *Repeat cycle q 21-28 days.*
CHOP-BLEO	bleomycin	Blenoxane	15 units/day I.V., days 1–5 Add to CHOP regimen. *Repeat cycle q 21-28 days.*
CHOP-rituximab	rituximab	Rituxan	375 mg/m^2 I.V., day 1 Add to CHOP regimen. *Repeat cycle q 21 days.*

CHEMOTHERAPY ACRONYMS AND PROTOCOLS *(continued)*

INDICATION AND ACRONYM	GENERIC DRUG NAME	TRADE DRUG NAME	DOSAGE
Non-Hodgkin's lymphoma *(continued)*			
CNOP	cyclophos-phamide	Cytoxan	750 mg/m^2 I.V., day 1
	mitoxantrone	Novantrone	12 mg/m^2 I.V., day 1
	vincristine	Oncovin	1.4 mg/m^2 (2 mg maximum) I.V., day 1
	prednisone	Deltasone	50 mg/m^2/day P.O., days 1-5 *Repeat cycle q 21-28 days.*
COPP	cyclophos-phamide	Cytoxan	450-600 mg/m^2 I.V., days 1 and 8
	vincristine	Oncovin	1.4 mg/m^2 (2 mg maximum) I.V., days 1 and 8
	procarbazine	Matulane	100 mg/m^2 P.O., days 1-14
	prednisone	Deltasone	40 mg/m^2 P.O., days 1-14 *Repeat cycle q 28 days.*
CVP	cyclophos-phamide	Cytoxan	300-400 mg/m^2 P.O., days 1-5
	vincristine	Oncovin	1.4 mg/m^2 (2 mg maximum) I.V., day 1
	prednisone	Deltasone	100 mg/m^2 P.O., days 1-5 *Repeat cycle q 21 days.*
ESHAP	etoposide	VePesid	40-60 mg/m^2/day I.V., days 1-4
	methylpred-nisolone	Solu-Medrol	250-500 mg I.V., days 1-4 or 15
	cisplatin	Platinol	25 mg/m^2 by contin-uous I.V. infusion, days 1-4
	cytarabine	Cytosar-U	2 g/m^2 I.V., day 5 *Repeat cycle q 21-28 days.*

(continued)

CHEMOTHERAPY ACRONYMS AND PROTOCOLS *(continued)*

INDICATION AND ACRONYM	GENERIC DRUG NAME	TRADE DRUG NAME	DOSAGE
Non-Hodgkin's lymphoma *(continued)*			
MACOP-B	methotrexate		400 mg/m² I.V., wk 2, 6, and 10
	leucovorin calcium		15 mg/m² P.O. q 6 hr for six doses, beginning 24 hr after methotrexate dose
	doxorubicin	Adriamycin	50 mg/m² I.V., wk 1, 3, 5, 7, 9, and 11
	cyclophosphamide	Cytoxan	350 mg/m² I.V., wk 1, 3, 5, 7, 9, and 11
	vincristine	Oncovin	1.4 mg/m² (2 mg maximum) I.V., wk 2, 4, 6, 8, 10, and 12
	bleomycin	Blenoxane	10 units/m² I.V. weekly, wk 4, 8, and 12
	prednisone	Deltasone	75 mg P.O., daily for 12 wk; taper dose over last 2 wk *Give only 1 cycle.*
ProMACE	prednisone	Deltasone	60 mg/m² P.O., days 1-14
	methotrexate		750 mg/m² I.V., day 14
	leucovorin calcium		50 mg/m² I.V. q 6 hr for five to six doses, beginning 24 hr after methotrexate dose
	doxorubicin	Adriamycin	25 mg/m² I.V., days 1 and 8
	cyclophosphamide	Cytoxan	650 mg/m² I.V., days 1 and 8
	etoposide (VP-16)	VePesid	120 mg/m² I.V., days 1 and 8 *Repeat cycle q 28 days.*

CHEMOTHERAPY ACRONYMS AND PROTOCOLS *(continued)*

INDICATION AND ACRONYM	GENERIC DRUG NAME	TRADE DRUG NAME	DOSAGE
Non-Hodgkin's lymphoma *(continued)*			
ProMACE/ cytaBOM	cyclophos- phamide	Cytoxan	650 mg/m² I.V., day 1
	doxorubicin	Adriamycin	25 mg/m² I.V., day 1
	etoposide (VP-16)	VePesid	120 mg/m² I.V., day 1
	prednisone	Deltasone	60 mg/m² P.O., days 1-14
	cytarabine (ara-C)	Cytosar-U	300 mg/m² I.V., day 8
	bleomycin	Blenoxane	5 units/m² I.V., day 8
	vincristine	Oncovin	1.4 mg/m² (2 mg maximum) I.V., day 8
	methotrexate		120 mg/m² I.V., day 8
	leucovorin calcium		25 mg/m² P.O. q 6 hr for six doses, be- ginning 24 hr after methotrexate dose
	co-trimoxazole	Bactrim DS	2 tablets (double- strength) P.O. b.i.d., days 1-28 *Repeat cycle q 21-28 days.*
Non–small-cell lung cancer			
CP	carboplatin	Paraplatin	Area under the curve 6 I.V., day 1
	paclitaxel	Taxol	225 mg/m² I.V. over 3 hr, day 1 *Repeat cycle q 21 days.*
CG	cisplatin	Platinol	100 mg/m² I.V. over 30-120 min, day 1
	gemcitabine	Gemzar	1-1.2 g/m² I.V. over 30-60 min, days 1, 8, and 15 *Repeat cycle q 28 days.*

(continued)

CHEMOTHERAPY ACRONYMS AND PROTOCOLS *(continued)*

INDICATION AND ACRONYM	GENERIC DRUG NAME	TRADE DRUG NAME	DOSAGE
Non–small-cell lung cancer *(continued)*			
EP	cisplatin	Platinol	80-100 mg/m^2 I.V., day 1
	etoposide (VP-16)	VePesid	80-120 mg/m^2 I.V., days 1-3 *Repeat cycle q 21-28 days.*
VC	vinorelbine	Navelbine	30 mg/m^2 I.V., days 1, 8, 15, and 22
	cisplatin	Platinol	120 mg/m^2 I.V., days 1 and 29; then give one dose q 6 wk *Repeat cycle q 28 days.*
Ovarian cancer			
Carbo–Tax	paclitaxel	Taxol	175 mg/m^2 I.V. over 3 hr, day 1
	carboplatin	Paraplatin	Area under the curve 7.5 targeted by Calvert equation, day 1 (after paclitaxel) *Repeat cycle q 21 days.*
CC	carboplatin	Paraplatin	300-350 mg/m^2 I.V., day 1
	cyclophosphamide	Cytoxan	600 mg/m^2 I.V., day 1 *Repeat cycle q 28 days.*
CP	cyclophosphamide	Cytoxan	600-1,000 mg/m^2 I.V., day 1
	cisplatin	Platinol	60-80 mg/m^2 I.V., day 1 *Repeat cycle q 21-28 days.*

CHEMOTHERAPY ACRONYMS AND PROTOCOLS *(continued)*

INDICATION AND ACRONYM	GENERIC DRUG NAME	TRADE DRUG NAME	DOSAGE
Prostatic cancer			
FL	flutamide	Eulexin	250 mg P.O. t.i.d.
	with		
	leuprolide acetate	Lupron	1 mg S.C. daily
	or		
	leuprolide acetate	Lupron Depot	7.5 mg I.M. q 28 days
	or		
	leuprolide acetate	Lupron Depot	22.5 mg I.M. q 3 mo
FZ	flutamide	Eulexin	250 P.O. q 8 hr
	goserelin acetate	Zoladex	3.6-mg implant S.C. q 28 days or 10.8-mg implant S.C. q 12 wk
MP	mitoxantrone	Novantrone	12 mg/m^2 by short I.V. infusion q 3 wk
	prednisone	Deltasone	5 mg P.O. b.i.d.
Small–cell lung cancer			
ACE (CAE)	doxorubicin	Adriamycin	45 mg/m^2 I.V., day 1
	cyclophos- phamide	Cytoxan	1 g/m^2 I.V., day 1
	etoposide (VP-16)	VePesid	50 mg/m^2 I.V., days 1-5 *Repeat cycle q 21 days.*
CAV	cyclophos- phamide	Cytoxan	1 g/m^2 I.V., day 1
	doxorubicin	Adriamycin	40-50 mg/m^2 I.V., day 1
	vincristine	Oncovin	1-1.4 mg/m^2 (2 mg maximum) I.V., day 1 *Repeat cycle q 21 days.*

(continued)

CHEMOTHERAPY ACRONYMS AND PROTOCOLS *(continued)*

INDICATION AND ACRONYM	GENERIC DRUG NAME	TRADE DRUG NAME	DOSAGE
Small–cell lung cancer *(continued)*			
EP	cisplatin	Platinol	75–100 mg/m² I.V., day 1
	etoposide (VP-16)	VePesid	75–100 mg/m² I.V., days 1–3 *Repeat cycle q 21-28 days.*
Soft-tissue sarcoma			
AD	doxorubicin	Adriamycin	45–60 mg/m² I.V., day 1
	dacarbazine	DTIC-Dome	200–250 mg/m² I.V., days 1–5 *Repeat cycle q 21 days.*
CYVADIC	cyclophos– phamide	Cytoxan	500 mg/m² I.V., day 1
	vincristine	Oncovin	1 mg/m² (2 mg max- imum) I.V., days 1 and 5
	doxorubicin	Adriamycin	50 mg/m² I.V., day 1
	dacarbazine	DTIC-Dome	250 mg/m² I.V., days 1–5 *Repeat cycle q 21 days.*
MAID	mesna	Mesnex	2.5 g/m² by continu- ous I.V. infusion, days 1–4
	doxorubicin	Adriamycin	15 mg/m² by contin- uous I.V. infusion, days 1–4
	ifosfamide	Ifex	2 g/m² by continu- ous I.V. infusion, days 1 to 3
	dacarbazine	DTIC-Dome	250 mg/m² by con- tinuous I.V. infu- sion, days 1–4 *Repeat cycle q 21 days.*

CHEMOTHERAPY ACRONYMS AND PROTOCOLS (continued)

INDICATION AND ACRONYM	GENERIC DRUG NAME	TRADE DRUG NAME	DOSAGE
Testicular cancer			
BEP	bleomycin	Blenoxane	30 units I.V., days 2, 9, and 16
	etoposide (VP-16)	VePesid	100 mg/m² , days 1–5
	cisplatin	Platinol	20 mg/m² I.V., days 1–5 *Repeat cycle q 21 days.*
VelP	vinblastine	Velban	0.11 mg/kg I.V., days 1 and 2
	ifosfamide	Ifex	1.2 g/m²/day by continuous I.V. infusion, days 1–5
	cisplatin	Platinol	20 mg/m² I.V. over 1 hr, days 1–5
	mesna	Mesnex	400 mg I.V. 15 min before ifosfamide, day 1; then 1.2 g daily by continuous I.V. infusion, days 1 to 5 *Repeat cycle q 21 days.*
VIP	etoposide (VP-16)	VePesid	75 mg/m² I.V., days 1–5
	ifosfamide	Ifex	1.2 g/m² by continuous I.V. infusion, days 1–5
	cisplatin	Platinol	20 mg/m² I.V., days 1–5
	mesna	Mesnex	400 mg I.V. 15 min before ifosfamide, day 1; then 1.2 g daily by continuous I.V. infusion, days 1–5 *Repeat cycle q 21 days.*

GUIDELINES FOR HANDLING CHEMOTHERAPY DRUGS

If you prepare or handle chemotherapy drugs without taking the proper precautions, you face a significant risk of reproductive abnormalities, hematologic problems, and possible damage to your liver and skin. You may foster certain environmental dangers as well. That's why it's important for you to follow the guidelines established by the Occupational Safety and Health Administration (OSHA). They help ensure the safety of both handler and environment.

The OSHA guidelines include two basic requirements:
■ All health care workers who handle chemotherapy drugs should be specifically trained, with an emphasis on reducing exposure during handling.
■ The drugs must be prepared in a class II or III biological safety cabinet.

Safety equipment
To protect yourself and the environment, wear a face shield or goggles, a long-sleeved gown, surgical gloves made from latex (or nitrile, if you're allergic to latex), with cuffs long enough to pull over the cuffs of your gown. Wear a disposable gown made of lint-free, low-permeability fabric with a closed front, long sleeves, and elastic or knotted cuffs if you're preparing or giving

drugs. Make sure you have eyewash, a plastic absorbent pad, alcohol wipes, sterile gauze pads, shoe covers, and an impervious container with the label CAUTION: BIOHAZARD for disposing of any unused drug or equipment.

Also, keep a chemotherapy spill kit handy. It should contain a water-resistant, nonpermeable, long-sleeved gown with cuffs and back closure; shoe covers; two pairs of high-grade, extra-thick latex gloves (for double-gloving); goggles; a mask; a disposable dustpan and plastic scraper (for collecting broken glass); plastic-lined or absorbent towels; a container of desiccant powder or granules (to absorb wet contents); two disposable sponges; a puncture- and leak-proof container labeled BIOHAZARD WASTE; and detergent for cleaning the spill area.

Precautions for drug preparation
Prepare the prescribed chemotherapy drugs according to product instructions, with special attention to compatibility, stability, and reconstitution technique.
■ Wash your hands before and after drug preparation and administration. Prepare the drug in a class II or III biological safety cabinet. Wear protective garments, including gloves, as re-

GUIDELINES FOR HANDLING CHEMOTHERAPY DRUGS
(continued)

quired by your facility's policy. Don't wear these garments outside the preparation area. Never eat, drink, smoke, or apply cosmetics in the drug preparation area.

■ Before and after preparing the drug, clean the inside of the cabinet according to the drug manufacturer's instructions. When finished, discard cleaning products in a leakproof chemical or biohazard waste container, according to facility policy. Then cover the work surface with a clean, plastic absorbent pad to minimize contamination by droplets or spills. Change the pad at the end of each shift and after any spill.

■ All drug preparation equipment and any unused drug are hazardous waste. Dispose of them according to facility policy. Place all chemotherapy waste products in leakproof, sealable, plastic bags or another suitable container, and make sure the container is appropriately labeled.

Special considerations
Reduce exposure to chemotherapy drugs by following these guidelines:

■ Remember that systemic absorption can occur if contaminated materials are ingested or inhaled or if they come in contact with the skin. You can accidentally inhale a drug while opening a vial, clipping a needle, expelling air from a syringe, or discarding excess drug that splashes. Drug absorption also can result from handling contaminated feces or body fluids.

■ Prime I.V. bags containing chemotherapy drugs in an approved class II or III biological safety cabinet. Leave the blower on 24 hours a day, 7 days a week.

■ If the safety cabinet doesn't have a hood, prepare drugs in a quiet, well-ventilated work space, away from heating or cooling vents and other staff. Wear a respirator that has a high-efficiency filter.

■ If you must prime the drug at the administration site, either prime the I.V. line with a fluid that doesn't contain the drug or use a backflow-closed system. Discard used supplies with other chemotherapy waste.

■ Vent vials with a hydrophobic filter, or use negative-pressure techniques. Use a needle with a hydrophobic filter to remove the solution from vials. Break an ampule by wrapping a sterile gauze pad or alcohol wipe around its neck to decrease the risk of droplet contamination.

■ Use only syringes and I.V. sets with luer-lock fittings.

(continued)

GUIDELINES FOR HANDLING CHEMOTHERAPY DRUGS
(continued)

- Mark all chemotherapy drugs with CHEMOTHERAPY HAZARD labels.
- Don't clip needles, break syringes, or remove needles from syringes used in drug preparation. Use a gauze pad when removing syringes and needles from I.V. bags of chemotherapy drugs.
- Place used syringes, needles, and other sharp or breakable items in a puncture-proof container.
- Change gloves every 30 minutes and whenever you spill a drug solution or puncture or tear a glove. Wash your hands before putting on and after removing gloves.
- If the drug touches your skin, wash the area thoroughly with soap (not a germicidal agent) and water. If the drug gets in your eye, hold your eyelid open and flood the eye with water or isotonic eyewash for at least 5 minutes. Obtain a medical evaluation as soon as possible after accidental exposure.
- Use a chemotherapy spill kit to clean up a major spill.
- Discard disposable gowns and gloves in an appropriately marked, waterproof receptacle whenever they become contaminated or whenever you leave the work area.

- Never place food or drinks in a refrigerator that contains chemotherapy drugs.
- Understand individual drug excretion patterns because they vary significantly. Take appropriate precautions when handling a chemotherapy patient's body fluids, especially if he's receiving a drug that's excreted in an active state.
- Wear disposable latex or nitrile gloves when handling body fluids or soiled linens of patients who have received chemotherapy drugs in the past 48 hours. Give men a urinal with a tight-fitting lid. Before flushing the toilet, place a waterproof pad over the toilet bowl to prevent splashing. Place soiled linens in designated isolation linen bags.
- Remember that women who are pregnant, trying to conceive, or breast-feeding should be extremely careful when handling chemotherapy drugs.
- Document each exposure incident according to facility policy.
- Have the biological safety cabinet examined every 6 months and whenever it's moved by a company that specializes in certifying such equipment.

Home care considerations

Remember these guidelines when giving chemotherapy to a patient at home:

GUIDELINES FOR HANDLING CHEMOTHERAPY DRUGS
(continued)

- If chemotherapy drugs aren't provided by the home care agency pharmacy, contact the patient to confirm that he obtained them from a hospital pharmacy or a specialized retail pharmacy. The drug should be packaged in a sealed plastic bag.

- Determine that the home care agency has received precertification or authorization from the patient's insurance company for home administration of these drugs. If the patient's chemotherapy treatment requires a 24-hour continuous infusion, it's typically given through a portable infusion pump. Make sure all infusion equipment is available and ready for use, or bring it with you.

- Teach the patient or caregiver to wear two pairs of latex or nitrile gloves when handling chemotherapy equipment, contaminated linens or bedclothes, or body fluids.

- Instruct the patient or caregiver to place soiled linens in a separate washable pillowcase and to launder the pillowcase twice, with the soiled linen inside, separate from other household items.

- Teach the patient or caregiver how to manage a chemotherapy spill. Provide a spill kit or help assemble one. Give the patient a phone number with 24-hour availability, and tell him to contact the prescriber about questions, concerns, or a spill.

- Advise the patient or caregiver to arrange for pickup and proper disposal of contaminated waste, and help make these arrangements.

- Urge the patient or caregiver to place all treatment equipment in a leakproof container before disposal.

- Tell the patient or caregiver to dispose of waste products in the toilet, emptying the container close to the water to minimize splashing, and then to close the lid and flush two or three times.

RISKS OF TISSUE DAMAGE

Some chemotherapy drugs cause severe damage if they come in contact with body tissues. When administering chemotherapy, make sure you know whether the drug you're giving is a vesicant, an irritant, or a nonvesicant.

Vesicants

Vesicants cause a reaction so severe that blisters form and tissue is damaged or destroyed. Examples of vesicants include the following:
- dactinomycin
- daunorubicin
- doxorubicin
- idarubicin
- mechlorethamine
- mitomycin
- mitoxantrone
- nitrogen mustard
- vinblastine
- vincristine
- vinorelbine.

Irritants

Irritants can cause a local venous response, with or without a skin reaction. Examples of irritants include the following:
- dacarbazine
- streptozocin.

Nonvesicants

Nonvesicants don't cause tissue irritation or damage, although exposure poses other risks. Examples of nonvesicants include the following:
- asparaginase
- bleomycin
- carboplatin
- cyclophosphamide
- cytarabine
- floxuridine
- fluorouracil
- ifosfamide.

PREVENTING ERRORS

Follow these precautions to prevent errors in chemotherapy administration:

- Only qualified personnel should write orders or administer chemotherapy. With rare exceptions, the administration of chemotherapy isn't an emergency procedure.
- All orders should be double-checked by the person preparing and giving the drugs.
- Repeatedly check the "five rights" of drug administration (right drug, right patient, right time, right dosage, right route).
- Question any aspect of the order that's contrary to customary practice or to what the patient has received in the past, especially when unusually high doses or unusual schedules are involved.
- Don't allow any distractions while checking an order or giving treatment.
- Orders for chemotherapy should be written only by the attending physician or oncology fellow who is responsible for the patient's care and most familiar with the drug regimen and dosing schedule.

PREVENTING INFILTRATION

Follow these guidelines when giving vesicants:

- Use a distal vein that allows successive proximal venipunctures.
- Avoid using the hand, antecubital space, damaged areas, or areas with compromised circulation.
- Don't probe or "fish" for veins.
- Place a transparent dressing over the site.
- Start the push delivery or the infusion with normal saline solution.
- Inspect the site for swelling and erythema.
- Tell the patient to report burning, stinging, pain, pruritus, or temperature changes near the site.
- After drug administration, flush the line with 20 ml of normal saline solution.

MANAGING COMPLICATIONS OF CHEMOTHERAPY

This table identifies some common adverse effects of chemotherapy and offers ways to minimize them.

ADVERSE EFFECT	SIGNS AND SYMPTOMS	INTERVENTIONS
Anemia	Dizziness, fatigue, pallor, and shortness of breath after minimal exertion; low hemoglobin and hematocrit; may develop slowly over several courses of treatment	■ Monitor hemoglobin, hematocrit, and red blood cell count; report dropping values; remember that dehydration from nausea, vomiting, and anorexia will cause hemoconcentration, yielding falsely high hematocrit readings. ■ Be prepared to administer a blood transfusion or erythropoietin. ■ Instruct the patient to take frequent rests, increase intake of iron-rich foods, and take a multivitamin with iron as prescribed.
Leukopenia	Susceptibility to infections; neutropenia (an absolute neutrophil count less than 1,500 cells/mm³)	■ Watch for the nadir, the point of lowest blood cell count (usually 7 to 14 days after last treatment). ■ Be prepared to administer colony-stimulating factors. ■ Institute neutropenic precautions in the hospitalized patient. ■ Include the following information in patient and family teaching: good hygiene practices, signs and symptoms of infection, the importance of checking the patient's temperature regularly, how to prepare a low-microbe diet, and how to care for vascular access devices. ■ Instruct the patient to avoid crowds, people with colds or respiratory infections, and fresh fruit, fresh flowers, and plants.

MANAGING COMPLICATIONS OF CHEMOTHERAPY

(continued)

ADVERSE EFFECT	SIGNS AND SYMPTOMS	INTERVENTIONS
Thrombocy-topenia	Bleeding gums, increased bruising, petechiae, hypermenorrhea, tarry stools, hematuria, coffee-ground emesis	■ Monitor platelet count: fewer than 50,000 cells/mm³ means a moderate risk of excessive bleeding; less than 20,000 cells/mm³ means a major risk and the patient may need a platelet transfusion. ■ Avoid unnecessary I.M. injections or venipunctures; if either is needed, apply pressure for at least 5 minutes; then apply a pressure dressing to the site. ■ Instruct patient to shave with an electric razor, avoid blowing his nose, stay away from irritants that would trigger sneezing, not use rectal thermometers, and avoid situations in which he could receive cuts or bruises. ■ Instruct patient to report sudden headaches (which could indicate potentially fatal intracranial bleeding).
Alopecia	Hair loss that may include eyebrows, lashes, and body hair	■ Minimize shock and distress by warning patient of the possibility of hair loss, discussing why hair loss occurs, and describing how much hair loss to expect. ■ Emphasize the need for appropriate head protection against sunburn and heat loss in the winter. ■ For patients with long hair, suggest cutting the hair shorter before treatment because washing and brushing cause more hair loss.

24 / PAIN MANAGEMENT

Assessing and managing your patients' pain is as much an art as it is a science. In this chapter, you'll find the following selection of assessment tools and handy reviews of common analgesic drugs:

- PQRST: The alphabet of pain assessment
- Differentiating acute and chronic pain
- Pain behavior checklist
- Using a numeric rating scale
- Using a visual analog scale
- Using the Wong-Baker faces scale
- Selected nonopioid analgesic combination products
- Selected opioid analgesic combination products

PQRST: The alphabet of pain assessment

Using the PQRST mnemonic device helps you better characterize your patient's pain. Simply ask these questions.

Provocative or palliative
Ask the patient:
- What provokes or worsens your pain?
- What relieves or causes the pain to subside?

Quality or quantity
Ask the patient:
- What does the pain feel like? Is it aching, intense, knifelike, burning, cramping?
- Are you having pain right now? If so, is it more or less severe than usual?
- To what degree does the pain affect your normal activities?
- Do you have other symptoms along with the pain, such as nausea or vomiting?

Region and radiation
Ask the patient:
- Where is your pain?
- Does the pain radiate to other parts of your body?

Severity
Ask the patient:
- How severe is your pain? How would you rate it on a scale of 0 to 10, with 0 being no pain and 10 being the worst pain imaginable?
- How would you describe the intensity of your pain at its least? At its worst? Right now?

Timing
Ask the patient:
- When did your pain begin?
- At what time of day is your pain least? What time is it worst?
- Is the onset sudden or gradual?
- Is the pain constant or intermittent?

DIFFERENTIATING ACUTE AND CHRONIC PAIN

Acute pain may cause certain physiologic and behavioral changes that you won't observe in a patient with chronic pain.

TYPE OF PAIN	PHYSIOLOGIC EVIDENCE	BEHAVIORAL EVIDENCE
Acute	■ Increased respirations ■ Increased pulse ■ Increased blood pressure ■ Dilated pupils ■ Diaphoresis	■ Restlessness ■ Distraction ■ Worry ■ Distress
Chronic	■ Normal respirations, pulse, blood pressure, and pupil size ■ No diaphoresis	■ Reduced or absent physical activity ■ Despair, depression ■ Hopelessness

PAIN BEHAVIOR CHECKLIST

A pain behavior is something a patient uses to communicate pain, distress, or suffering. Place a check in the box next to each behavior you observe or infer while talking with your patient.

❏ Grimacing
❏ Moaning
❏ Sighing
❏ Clenching teeth
❏ Holding or supporting the painful body area
❏ Sitting rigidly
❏ Shifting posture or position frequently
❏ Moving in a guarded or protective manner
❏ Moving very slowly
❏ Limping
❏ Taking medication

❏ Using a cane, cervical collar, or other prosthetic device
❏ Walking with an abnormal gait
❏ Requesting help with walking
❏ Stopping frequently while walking
❏ Lying down during the day
❏ Avoiding physical activity
❏ Being irritable
❏ Asking such questions as "Why did this happen to me?"
❏ Asking to be relieved from tasks or activities

USING A NUMERIC RATING SCALE

This 10-point numeric rating scale can help you quantify your patient's pain. Explain that 0 means no pain and 10 means the worst pain imaginable. Then ask the patient to choose a number on the scale that represents his current level of pain. You may want to give the patient a copy of the scale and have him circle the number that best represents his pain level.

No pain   0   1   2   3   4   5   6   7   8   9   10   **Worst pain imaginable**

USING A VISUAL ANALOG SCALE

To use the visual analog scale, ask the patient to place an X on the scale to indicate his current level of pain, as shown below.

No pain   **Pain as bad as it can be**

USING THE WONG-BAKER FACES SCALE

A pediatric or an adult patient with language difficulties may not be able to describe the pain he's feeling. In such instances, use the pain intensity scale below. Ask your patient to choose the face that best represents the severity of his pain on a scale from 0 to 10.

0	2	4	6	8	10
No hurt	Hurts a little bit	Hurts a little more	Hurts even more	Hurts a whole lot	Hurts worst

From Wong, D.L., Hockenberry-Eaton, M., Wilson, D., Winkelstein, M.L., Schwartz, P.: *Wong's Essentials of Pediatric Nursing*, 6th ed. St. Louis: Mosby, Inc., 2001. Reprinted by permission.

SELECTED NONOPIOID ANALGESIC COMBINATION PRODUCTS

Many common analgesics are combinations of two or more generic drugs. This table reviews common nonopioid analgesics.

TRADE NAMES	GENERIC DRUGS	INDICATIONS AND ADULT DOSAGES
Alka-Seltzer Plus Cold & Sinus Caplets, Allerest No-Drowsiness Tablets, Coldrine, Ornex No Drowsiness Tablets, Sinus-Relief Tablets, Sinutab Without Drowsiness	■ acetaminophen 325 mg ■ pseudoephedrine hydrochloride 30 mg	For common cold, nasal congestion, sinus congestion, sinus pain. Give 2 tablets q 6 hours. Maximum, 8 tablets in 24 hours.
Esgic, Femcet, Fioricet, Fiorpap, Isocet, Repan, Triad	■ acetaminophen 325 mg ■ butalbital 50 mg ■ caffeine 40 mg	For headache, mild to moderate pain, migraine. Give 1-2 tablets or capsules q 4 hours. Maximum, 6 tablets or capsules in 24 hours.
Anacin, Gensan, P-A-C Analgesic Tablets	■ aspirin 400 mg ■ caffeine 32 mg	For headache, mild pain, myalgia. Give 2 tablets q 6 hours. Maximum, 8 tablets in 24 hours.
Ascriptin, Magnaprin	■ aluminum hydroxide 50 mg ■ aspirin 325 mg ■ calcium carbonate 50 mg ■ magnesium hydroxide 50 mg	For fever, mild to moderate pain. Give 1-2 tablets q 4 hours.
Ascriptin A/D, Magnaprin Arthritis Strength Caplets	■ aluminum hydroxide 75 mg ■ aspirin 325 mg ■ calcium carbonate 75 mg ■ magnesium hydroxide 75 mg	For mild to moderate pain. Give 1-2 tablets q 4 hours.

* Available in Canada only

SELECTED NONOPIOID ANALGESIC COMBINATION PRODUCTS *(continued)*

TRADE NAMES	GENERIC DRUGS	INDICATIONS AND ADULT DOSAGES
Aspirin-free Anacin PM, Excedrin P.M., Extra Strength Tylenol P.M., Sominex Pain Relief	■ acetaminophen 500 mg ■ diphenhydramine 25 mg	For allergic rhinitis, headache, insomnia from pain or pruritus. Give 1 tablet at bedtime.
Axocet, Bucet, Butex Forte, Phrenilin Forte, Tencon	■ acetaminophen 650 mg ■ butalbital 50 mg	For headache, mild to moderate pain. Give 1 tablet or capsule q 4 hours. Maximum, 4 tablets or capsules in 24 hours.
Bayer Select Head Cold Caplets, Dristan Cold Caplets, Sinus Excedrin Extra Strength, Sudafed Severe Cold Formula	■ acetaminophen 500 mg ■ pseudoephedrine hydrochloride 30 mg	For common cold, nasal and sinus congestion, sinus pain. Give 2 tablets q 6 hours. Maximum, 8 tablets in 24 hours.
Bufferin AF NiteTime, Excedrin P.M. Caplets, Excedrin P.M. Geltabs, Excedrin P.M. Tablets	■ acetaminophen 500 mg ■ diphenhydramine citrate 38 mg	For insomnia from pain or pruritus. Give 1 tablet at bedtime.
Cama Arthritis Pain Reliever	■ aluminum hydroxide 150 mg ■ aspirin 500 mg ■ magnesium oxide 150 mg	For mild to moderate pain. Give 1-2 tablets q 4 hours. Maximum, 8 tablets in 24 hours.
Comtrex Allergy-Sinus, Sine-Off Allergy/Sinus Maximum Strength, Sine-Off Medicine Caplets, Sine-Off Tablets, Sinutab Maximum Strength	■ acetaminophen 500 mg ■ chlorpheniramine maleate 2 mg ■ pseudoephedrine hydrochloride 30 mg	For allergic rhinitis, common cold, flu symptoms. Give 2 tablets q 4 hours. Maximum, 8 tablets in 24 hours.

* Available in Canada only

(continued)

SELECTED NONOPIOID ANALGESIC COMBINATION PRODUCTS (continued)

TRADE NAMES	GENERIC DRUGS	INDICATIONS AND ADULT DOSAGES
Esgic–Plus	■ acetaminophen 500 mg ■ butalbital 50 mg ■ caffeine 40 mg	For headache, migraine, mild to moderate pain. Give 1–2 tablets or capsules q 4 hours. Maximum, 6 tablets or capsules in 24 hours.
Excedrin Extra Strength, Excedrin Migraine	■ acetaminophen 250 mg ■ aspirin 250 mg ■ caffeine 65 mg	For headache, migraine. Give 2 tablets q 4 hours. Maximum, 8 tablets in 24 hours.
Fiorinal, Fiortal, Lanorinal	■ aspirin 325 mg ■ butalbital 50 mg ■ caffeine 40 mg	For headache, mild to moderate pain. Give 1–2 tablets or capsules q 4 hours. Maximum, 6 tablets or capsules in 24 hours.
Phrenilin	■ acetaminophen 325 mg ■ butalbital 50 mg	For headache, mild to moderate pain. Give 1–2 tablets q 4 hours. Maximum, 6 tablets in 24 hours.
Midrin	■ acetaminophen 325 mg ■ dichloralphenazone 100 mg ■ isometheptene mucate 65 mg	For migraine, tension headache. For migraine, give 2 capsules initially; then 1 capsule q 1 hour to a maximum of 5 capsules in 12 hours. For tension headache, give 1–2 capsules q 4 hours to a maximum of 8 capsules in 24 hours.
Sinutab	■ acetaminophen 325 mg ■ chlorpheniramine 2 mg ■ pseudoephedrine hydrochloride 30 mg	For allergic rhinitis, common cold, flu symptoms. Give 2 tablets q 6 hours. Maximum, 8 tablets in 24 hours.
Tecnal*	■ aspirin 330 mg ■ butalbital 50 mg ■ caffeine 40 mg	For headache, mild to moderate pain. Give 1–2 tablets or capsules q 4 hours. Maximum, 6 tablets or capsules in 24 hours.

* Available in Canada only

SELECTED NONOPIOID ANALGESIC COMBINATION PRODUCTS (continued)

TRADE NAMES	GENERIC DRUGS	INDICATIONS AND ADULT DOSAGES
Vanquish	■ acetaminophen 194 mg ■ aluminum hydroxide 25 mg ■ aspirin 227 mg ■ caffeine 33 mg ■ magnesium hydroxide 50 mg	For minor aches and pains. Give 2 caplets q 4 hours. Maximum, 12 caplets in 24 hours.

* Available in Canada only

SELECTED OPIOID ANALGESIC COMBINATION PRODUCTS

Many common analgesics are combinations of two or more generic drugs. This table reviews common opioid analgesics.

TRADE NAMES AND CONTROLLED SUBSTANCE SCHEDULE	GENERIC DRUGS	INDICATIONS AND ADULT DOSAGES
Aceta with Codeine, Tylenol with Codeine No. 3 CSS III	■ acetaminophen 300 mg ■ codeine phosphate 30 mg	For fever, mild to moderate pain. Give 1-2 tablets q 4 hours. Maximum, 12 tablets in 24 hours.
Alor 5/500 Tablets, Azdone, Damason-P, Lortab ASA, Panasal 5/500 CSS III	■ aspirin 500 mg ■ hydrocodone bitartrate 5 mg	For moderate to moderately severe pain. Give 1-2 tablets q 4 hours. Maximum, 8 tablets in 24 hours.
Anexsia 7.5/650, Lorcet Plus CSS III	■ acetaminophen 650 mg ■ hydrocodone bitartrate 7.5 mg	For arthralgia, bone pain, dental pain, headache, migraine, moderate pain. Give 1-2 tablets q 4 hours. Maximum, 6 tablets in 24 hours.
Capital with Codeine Suspension, Tylenol with Codeine Elixir CSS V	■ acetaminophen 120 mg ■ codeine phosphate 12 mg/5 ml	For mild to moderate pain. Give 15 ml q 4 hours.
Darvocet-N 50 CSS IV	■ acetaminophen 325 mg ■ propoxyphene napsylate 50 mg	For mild to moderate pain. Give 1-2 tablets q 4 hours. Maximum, 12 tablets in 24 hours.
Darvocet-N 100, Propacet 100 CSS IV	■ acetaminophen 650 mg ■ propoxyphene napsylate 100 mg	For mild to moderate pain. Give 1 tablet q 4 hours. Maximum, 6 tablets in 24 hours.

SELECTED OPIOID ANALGESIC COMBINATION PRODUCTS *(continued)*

TRADE NAMES AND CONTROLLED SUBSTANCE SCHEDULE	GENERIC DRUGS	INDICATIONS AND ADULT DOSAGES
Empirin with Codeine No. 3 *CSS III*	■ aspirin 325 mg ■ codeine phosphate 30 mg	For fever, mild to moderate pain. Give 1-2 tablets q 4 hours. Maximum, 12 tablets in 24 hours.
Empirin with Codeine No. 4 *CSS III*	■ aspirin 325 mg ■ codeine phosphate 60 mg	For fever, mild to moderate pain. Give 1 tablet q 4 hours. Maximum, 6 tablets in 24 hours.
Fioricet with Codeine *CSS III*	■ acetaminophen 325 mg ■ butalbital 50 mg ■ caffeine 40 mg ■ codeine phosphate 30 mg	For headache, mild to moderate pain. Give 1-2 capsules q 4 hours. Maximum, 6 capsules in 24 hours.
Fiorinal with Codeine *CSS III*	■ aspirin 325 mg ■ butalbital 50 mg ■ caffeine 40 mg ■ codeine phosphate 30 mg	For headache, mild to moderate pain. Give 1-2 tablets or capsules q 4 hours. Maximum, 6 tablets or capsules in 24 hours.
Lorcet 10/650 *CSS III*	■ acetaminophen 650 mg ■ hydrocodone bitartrate 10 mg	For moderate to moderately severe pain. Give 1 tablet q 4 hours. Maximum, 6 tablets in 24 hours.
Lortab 2.5/500 *CSS III*	■ acetaminophen 500 mg ■ hydrocodone bitartrate 2.5 mg	For moderate to moderately severe pain. Give 1-2 tablets q 4 hours. Maximum, 8 tablets in 24 hours.
Lortab 5/500 *CSS III*	■ acetaminophen 500 mg ■ hydrocodone bitartrate 5 mg	For moderate to moderately severe pain. Give 1-2 tablets q 4 hours. Maximum, 8 tablets in 24 hours.

(continued)

SELECTED OPIOID ANALGESIC COMBINATION PRODUCTS (continued)

TRADE NAMES AND CONTROLLED SUBSTANCE SCHEDULE	GENERIC DRUGS	INDICATIONS AND ADULT DOSAGES
Lortab 7.5/500 CSS III	■ acetaminophen 500 mg ■ hydrocodone bitartrate 7.5 mg	For moderate to moderately severe pain. Give 1 tablet q 4 hours. Maximum, 8 tablets in 24 hours.
Lortab 10/500 CSS III	■ acetaminophen 500 mg ■ hydrocodone bitartrate 10 mg	For moderate to moderately severe pain. Give 1 tablet q 4-6 hours. Maximum, 6 tablets in 24 hours.
Percocet CSS II	■ acetaminophen 325 mg ■ oxycodone hydrochloride 5 mg	For moderate to moderately severe pain. Give 1-2 tablets q 4 hours. Maximum, 12 tablets in 24 hours.
Percocet 2.5/325 CSS II	■ acetaminophen 325 mg ■ oxycodone hydrochloride 2.5 mg	For moderate to moderately severe pain. Give 1-2 tablets q 4-6 hours. Maximum, 12 tablets in 24 hours.
Percocet 7.5/500 CSS II	■ acetaminophen 500 mg ■ oxycodone hydrochloride 7.5 mg	For moderate to moderately severe pain. Give 1-2 tablets q 4-6 hours. Maximum, 8 tablets in 24 hours.
Percocet 10/650 CSS II	■ acetaminophen 650 mg ■ oxycodone hydrochloride 10 mg	For moderate to moderately severe pain. Give 1-2 tablets q 4-6 hours. Maximum, 6 tablets in 24 hours.
Percodan–Demi CSS II	■ aspirin 325 mg ■ oxycodone hydrochloride 2.25 mg ■ oxycodone terephthalate 0.19 mg	For moderate to moderately severe pain. Give 1-2 tablets q 6 hours. Maximum, 8 tablets in 24 hours.
Percodan, Roxiprin CSS II	■ aspirin 325 mg ■ oxycodone hydrochloride 4.5 mg ■ oxycodone terephthalate 0.38 mg	For moderate to moderately severe pain. Give 1 tablet q 6 hours. Maximum, 4 tablets in 24 hours.

SELECTED OPIOID ANALGESIC COMBINATION PRODUCTS *(continued)*

TRADE NAMES AND CONTROLLED SUBSTANCE SCHEDULE	GENERIC DRUGS	INDICATIONS AND ADULT DOSAGES
Phenaphen/ Codeine No. 3 *CSS III*	■ acetaminophen 325 mg ■ codeine phosphate 30 mg	For fever, mild to moderate pain. Give 1-2 tablets q 4 hours. Maximum, 12 tablets in 24 hours.
Phenaphen/ Codeine No. 4 *CSS III*	■ acetaminophen 325 mg ■ codeine phosphate 60 mg	For fever, mild to moderate pain. Give 1 tablet q 4 hours. Maximum, 6 tablets in 24 hours.
Propoxyphene Napsylate/ Acetaminophen *CSS IV*	■ acetaminophen 650 mg ■ propoxyphene napsylate 100 mg	For mild to moderate pain. Give 1 tablet q 4 hours. Maximum, 6 tablets in 24 hours.
Roxicet *CSS II*	■ acetaminophen 325 mg ■ oxycodone hydrochloride 5 mg	For moderate to moderately severe pain. Give 1-2 tablets q 4 hours. Maximum, 12 tablets in 24 hours.
Roxicet 5/500, Roxilox *CSS II*	■ acetaminophen 500 mg ■ oxycodone hydrochloride 5 mg	For moderate to moderately severe pain. Give 1-2 tablets q 4-6 hours. Maximum, 8 tablets in 24 hours.
Roxicet Oral Solution *CSS II*	■ acetaminophen 325 ■ oxycodone hydrochloride 5 mg/5 ml	For moderate to moderately severe pain. Give 5-10 ml q 4-6 hours. Maximum, 60 ml in 24 hours.
Talacen *CSS IV*	■ acetaminophen 650 mg ■ pentazocine hydrochloride 25 mg	For mild to moderate pain. Give 1 tablet q 4 hours. Maximum, 6 tablets in 24 hours.
Talwin Compound *CSS IV*	■ aspirin 325 mg ■ pentazocine hydrochloride 12.5 mg	For moderate pain. Give 2 tablets q 6 hours. Maximum, 8 tablets in 24 hours.

(continued)

SELECTED OPIOID ANALGESIC COMBINATION PRODUCTS (continued)

TRADE NAMES AND CONTROLLED SUBSTANCE SCHEDULE	GENERIC DRUGS	INDICATIONS AND ADULT DOSAGES
Tylenol with Codeine No. 2 CSS III	■ acetaminophen 300 mg ■ codeine phosphate 15 mg	For fever, mild to moderate pain. Give 1-2 tablets q 4 hours. Maximum, 12 tablets in 24 hours.
Tylenol with Codeine No. 3 CSS III	■ acetaminophen 300 mg ■ codeine phosphate 30 mg	For fever, mild to moderate pain. Give 1-2 tablets q 4 hours. Maximum, 12 tablets in 24 hours.
Tylenol with Codeine No. 4 CSS III	■ acetaminophen 300 mg ■ codeine phosphate 60 mg	For fever, mild to moderate pain. Give 1 tablet q 4 hours. Maximum, 6 tablets in 24 hours.
Tylox CSS II	■ acetaminophen 500 mg ■ oxycodone hydro-chloride 5 mg	For moderate to moderately severe pain. Give 1 tablet q 6 hours. Maximum, 4 tablets in 24 hours.
Vicodin CSS III	■ acetaminophen 500 mg ■ hydrocodone bitar-trate 5 mg	For moderate to moderately severe pain. Give 1-2 tablets q 4 hours. Maximum, 8 tablets in 24 hours.
Vicodin ES CSS III	■ acetaminophen 750 mg ■ hydrocodone bitar-trate 7.5 mg	For moderate to moderately severe pain. Give 1 tablet q 4-6 hours. Maximum, 5 tablets in 24 hours.
Vicodin HP CSS III	■ acetaminophen 660 mg ■ hydrocodone bitar-trate 10 mg	For mild to moderate pain. Give 1 tablet q 4 hours. Maximum, 6 tablets in 24 hours.
Wygesic CSS IV	■ acetaminophen 650 mg ■ propoxyphene nap-sylate 65 mg	For moderate to moderately severe pain. Give 1 tablet q 4-6 hours. Maximum, 6 tablets in 24 hours.

SELECTED OPIOID ANALGESIC COMBINATION PRODUCTS (continued)

TRADE NAMES AND CONTROLLED SUBSTANCE SCHEDULE	GENERIC DRUGS	INDICATIONS AND ADULT DOSAGES
Zydone *CSS III*	■ acetaminophen 400 mg ■ hydrocodone bitartrate 5 mg	For moderate to moderately severe pain. Give 1 tablet q 4–6 hours. Maximum, 6 tablets in 24 hours.
Zydone 7.5 *CSS III*	■ acetaminophen 400 mg ■ hydrocodone bitartrate 7.5 mg	For moderate to moderately severe pain. Give 1 tablet q 4–6 hours. Maximum, 6 tablets in 24 hours.
Zydone 10 CSS III	■ acetaminophen 400 mg ■ hydrocodone bitartrate 10 mg	For moderate to moderately severe pain. Give 1 tablet q 4–6 hours. Maximum, 6 tablets in 24 hours.

PART VI

HERBAL THERAPY

COMMON
HERBAL SUPPLEMENTS

ALOE

Aloe Gel, Aloe Latex, Aloe Vera, Cape Aloe

Available forms

Available as dried latex for internal use, extract capsules, juice (99.7% of whole leaf aloe vera juice), tincture (1:10, 50% alcohol), and topical gel.

- *Extract capsules:* 75 mg, 100 mg, 200 mg
- *Topical gel:* 98%, 99.5%, 99.6%, and 100% purity strengths

Actions and components

A solid residue is obtained by evaporating aloe latex. It contains aloinosides, which irritate the large intestine, increasing peristalsis, thereby producing a laxative effect. Water and electrolyte reabsorption is inhibited. Aloe can cause potassium loss.

Aloe gel is a clear, thin, viscous material obtained by crushing the mucilaginous cells found in the leaf. The gel contains a polysaccharide similar to guar gum.

The gel's wound-healing ability comes from its moisturizing effect, which prevents air from drying the wound. Mucopolysaccharides and sulfur and nitrogen compounds also stimulate healing.

Aloe gel may work as an antibacterial against *Staphylococcus aureus*, *Escherichia coli*, and *Mycobacterium tuberculosis*, but information is conflicting.

Aloe also contains bradykinase, which is a protease inhibitor that relieves pain and decreases swelling and redness. The anti-itching effect of aloe may be related to the antihistamine properties of magnesium lactate.

Uses

Used orally, aloe latex is a potent cathartic. It's used to treat constipation; to provide evacuation relief for patients with anal fissures, hemorrhoids, or recent anorectal surgery; and to prepare a patient for diagnostic testing of the GI tract.

Aloe gel is used to treat minor burns and skin irritation and to aid in wound healing. It may also be effective as an antibacterial.

Dosage and administration

■ *Laxative:* 100 to 200 mg of aloe capsules, 50 mg of aloe extract, or 1 to 8 ounces of juice h.s. Or, 30 ml of aloe gel or 15 to 60 gtt of aloe tincture (1:10, 50% alcohol), p.r.n.

■ *Topical use:* Apply gel liberally three to five times daily, p.r.n.

Adverse reactions

CV: arrhythmias, edema.
GI: cramps, diarrhea.
GU: albuminuria, hematuria, nephropathy.
Metabolic: electrolyte abnormalities, weight loss.
Musculoskeletal: muscle weakness, accelerated bone deterioration.
Skin: nummular eczematous, papular dermatitis.

Interactions
HERB-DRUG

■ *Antiarrhythmics, cardiac glycosides such as digoxin:* May lead to toxic reaction. Monitor patient closely.

■ *Beta blockers, corticosteroids, diuretics:* May enhance potassium loss. Check potassium level.

■ *Disulfiram:* Any herbal preparation that contains alcohol can precipitate a disulfiram-like reaction. Discourage use together.

HERB-HERB

■ *Licorice:* Increases risk of potassium deficiency. Discourage use together.

Effects on lab test results
■ May decrease potassium level.

Cautions
Patients with intestinal obstruction, Crohn's disease, ulcerative colitis, appendicitis, or abdominal pain of unknown origin; pregnant women; and children younger than age 12 should avoid taking aloe orally.

Products derived from the latex of aloe's outer skin should be used cautiously.

Nursing considerations
■ Explore patient's knowledge of this herb.

■ Aloe's laxative effects are apparent within 10 hours of taking it.

■ Monitor patient for signs of dehydration. Elderly patients are particularly at risk.

■ Monitor electrolyte levels, especially potassium, after long-term use.

■ If patient is using aloe topically, monitor wound for healing.

Patient teaching

■ Advise patient to consult a health care provider before using an herbal preparation because another treatment may be available.

■ Tell patient that when filling a new prescription he should inform pharmacist of any herbal or dietary supplement he's taking.

■ Caution patient that his condition could worsen if he delays seeking medical diagnosis and treatment.

Alert If patient is taking a diuretic, a corticosteroid, digoxin, or another drug to control his heart rate, he shouldn't take aloe without consulting a health care provider.

■ Advise patient to reduce dose if cramping occurs after a single dose, and not to take aloe for longer than 1 or 2 weeks at a time without consulting a health care provider.

■ Advise patient to notify a health care provider immediately if he experiences symptoms of dehydration, including weak-ness, thirst, decreased urination, dry mouth, or confusion.

ANGELICA

Nature's Answer Angelica Root Liquid

Available forms

Available as liquid extract, tincture, and essential oil.

Actions and components

The root and fruit seeds of angelica are used to extract the medicinally active part of the plant. Angelica contains alpha-angelica lactone, which augments calcium binding and calcium turnover. Its action may involve increasing the contraction-dependent calcium pool to be released on systolic depolarization. The coumarins and furanocoumarins may induce photosensitivity and may be photocarcinogenic and mutagenic.

Uses

Angelica seed is used as a diuretic and diaphoretic. It's also used to treat conditions of the kidneys and the urinary, GI, and respiratory tracts as well as rheumatic and neuralgic symptoms.

Angelica root is used orally for loss of appetite, GI spasm, and flatulence. It has been used topically to treat neuralgia. Other uses include treatment for coughs and bronchitis, anorexia, dyspepsia with intestinal cramping, and menstrual, liver, and gallbladder complaints.

Angelica seed has also been used as a flavoring in gin, some regional wines, candied leaves, and cake and pastry decorations.

Dosage and administration
- *Crude root:* 4.5 g P.O. daily.
- *Essential oil:* 10 to 20 gtt P.O. daily.
- *Liquid extract (1:1):* 0.5 to 3 g P.O. daily.
- *Tincture (1:5):* 1.5 g P.O. daily.

Adverse reactions
Skin: photosensitivity reactions.

Interactions
HERB-DRUG
- *Antacids, H₂ blockers, proton pump inhibitors, sucralfate:* Angelica may increase acid production in the stomach and so may interfere with absorption of these drugs. Advise patient to separate administration times.
- *Anticoagulants:* Potentiated effects of anticoagulants with excessive doses of angelica. Monitor patient for bleeding.

HERB-LIFESTYLE
Sun exposure: Increases risk of photosensitivity reactions. Advise patient to wear protective clothing and sunscreen and to limit direct exposure to sunlight.

Effects on lab test results
- None reported.

Cautions
Pregnant and breast-feeding patients should avoid angelica because it may stimulate menstruation and the uterus.

Nursing considerations
- Explore patient's knowledge of this herb.
- Monitor patient for persistent diarrhea, which may be a sign of something more serious.
- Assess patient for dermatologic reactions.
- Photodermatosis is possible after contact with the plant juice or plant extract.

Patient teaching
- Advise patient to consult a health care provider before using an herbal preparation because another treatment may be available.

■ Tell patient that when filling a new prescription he should inform pharmacist of any herbal or dietary supplement he's taking.

■ Caution patient not to delay seeking medical treatment for symptoms that may be related to a serious medical condition.

■ Advise patient not to take angelica if pregnant or if taking a gastric acid blocker or anticoagulant.

■ Advise patient to notify his health care provider if he develops a skin rash.

BILBERRY

Bilberry, Bilberry Fruit, Bilberry Power, Bilberry Tincture, Dried Bilberry

Available forms

Available as dried fruit, 10% decoction for topical use, dry extract (25% anthocyanosides) in an 80-mg capsule, and fluid extract 1:1.

Actions and components

The fruit of the bilberry contains 5% to 10% tannins, which act as an astringent; these tannins may help treat diarrhea.

The anthocyanidins in bilberry help prevent angina episodes, reduce capillary fragility, and stabilize tissues that have collagen-like tendons and ligaments. They also inhibit platelet aggregation and thrombus formation by interacting with vascular prostaglandins.

The anthocyanidins also help regenerate rhodopsin, a light-sensitive pigment found on the rods of the retina, so bilberry may help treat degenerative retinal conditions, macular degeneration, poor night vision, glaucoma, and cataracts.

Bilberry may have vasoprotective, antiedemic, and hepatoprotective properties because of its antioxidant effects from anthocyanidins. The anthocyanidin pigment in the herb may increase the gastric mucosal release of prostaglandin E_2, accounting for the antiulcerative and gastroprotective effects.

Uses

Used to treat acute diarrhea and mild inflammation of the mucous membranes of the mouth and throat. Used to provide symptomatic relief from vascular disorders (including capillary weakness, venous insufficiency, and hemorrhoids) and to prevent macular degeneration. Also used for its potential ability to protect the liver.

Dosage and administration

■ *Dried fruit:* 4 to 8 g P.O. with water several times daily.

■ *Fluid extract:* 2 to 4 ml P.O. t.i.d.

■ *For eye disorders:* 80 to 160 mg dry extract (25% anthocyanosides) P.O. t.i.d.

■ *For inflammation:* 10% decoction. Prepared by boiling 5 to 10 g of crushed dried fruit in 5 ounces of cold water for 10 minutes and then straining while hot. Applied topically as an astringent.

■ *For treatment of acute diarrhea:* 20 to 60 g of dried fruit P.O. daily.

Adverse reactions

None known.

Interactions

HERB-DRUG

■ *Warfarin:* May cause additive effects. Monitor patient for bleeding or loss of therapeutic anticoagulation.

Effects on lab test results

■ May decrease glucose level.

Cautions

The herb is unsuitable in patients with a bleeding disorder because it may inhibit platelet aggregation.

Nursing considerations

■ Explore patient's knowledge of this herb.

■ Because bilberry may reduce a diabetic patient's glucose level, dosage of conventional antidiabetics may need to be adjusted if patient is also using this herb.

■ Consistent dosing of bilberry is needed when using the herb to treat vascular or ocular conditions.

■ Bilberry should be safe for pregnant and breast-feeding patients to use.

■ Bilberry may be taken without regard to food.

Patient teaching

■ Advise patient to consult a health care provider before using an herbal preparation because another treatment may be available.

■ Tell patient that when filling a new prescription he should inform pharmacist of any herbal or dietary supplement that he's taking.

■ Tell patient that bilberry may be taken without regard to food.

■ Advise any patient using the dried fruit to take each dose with a full glass of water.

■ If patient is using bilberry to treat diarrhea, advise him to consult a health care provider if the condition doesn't improve in 3 to 4 days.

CAPSICUM

Topical products
Capsin (0.025% or 0.075% lotion), Capzasin-P (0.025% cream), Dolorac (0.025% cream in emollient base), No Pain-HP (0.075% roll-on), Pain Doctor (0.025% cream with methyl-salicylate and menthol), Pain-X (0.05% gel), R-Gel (0.025% gel), Zostrix (0.025% cream in emollient base), Zostrix-HP (0.075% cream in emollient base)

Oral products
Cajun Seasoning, Capsicool, Cayenne, Cayenne Extra Hot, Cayenne Pepper Capsules, Kidney Blend, Tincture of Capsicum

Available forms
Available as cayenne pepper capsules, extract, and topical preparation.

Actions and components
The active component of capsicum (capsaicin) is isolated from the membrane and seeds of the pepper.

Topically applied capsaicin depletes substance P from peripheral sensory neurons and blocks its synthesis and transport. Substance P is a neurotransmitter involved in transmitting pain and itch sensations from the periphery to the CNS, and may have vasodilating effects. The effects may be similar to cutting or ligating a nerve.

Oral capsicum may interfere with gastric basal acid output and may inhibit platelet aggregation, but it doesn't alter PT or PTT. High-dose capsicum therapy may decrease coagulation (because of higher antithrombin III levels), lower plasma fibrinogen levels, and increase fibrinolytic activity.

Capsaicin also is highly irritating to mucous membranes and eyes.

Uses
The FDA has approved topical capsicum for temporary relief from pain caused by rheumatoid arthritis, osteoarthritis, postherpetic neuralgia (shingles), and diabetic neuropathy. The herb is being tested for treatment of psoriasis, intractable pruritus, vitiligo, phantom limb pain, mastectomy pain, Guillain-Barré syndrome, neurogenic bladder, vulvar vestibulitis,

apocrine chromhidrosis, and reflex sympathetic dystrophy. It's also used in personal defense sprays.

Oral capsicum is used for various GI complaints, including dyspepsia, flatulence, ulcers, and stomach cramps. It's used to treat hypertension and improve circulation. It's also used in some weight-loss and metabolic-enhancement products.

Dosage and administration
■ *Oral:* In adults, up to 3 g P.O. daily, as a spice on food.
■ *Topical:* For adults and children age 2 and older, capsicum is applied topically to affected area, not more than t.i.d. or q.i.d. Hands should be washed immediately after applying capsicum.

Adverse reactions
EENT: eye irritation, corneal abrasion.
GI: oral burning, diarrhea, gingival irritation, bleeding gums.
Respiratory: cough, *bronchospasm*, respiratory irritation.
Skin: burning sensation, stinging sensation, erythema, contact dermatitis.

Interactions
HERB-DRUG
■ *ACE inhibitors:* Increases risk of cough when applied topically. Monitor patient closely.
■ *Anticoagulants:* May alter anticoagulant effects. Monitor PT and INR closely; advise patient to avoid using herb and drug together.
■ *Antiplatelet drugs, heparin and low–molecular-weight heparin, warfarin:* May cause additive effects. Discourage use together. If herb and drug must be used together, monitor patient for bleeding.
■ *Aspirin, salicylic acid compounds:* Reduces bioavailability of these drugs. Discourage use together.
■ *Disulfiram:* Herbal products prepared with alcohol may cause a disulfiram-like reaction. Discourage use together.
■ *Theophylline:* Increases absorption when taken with capsicum. Discourage use together.

HERB-HERB
■ *Feverfew, garlic, ginger, ginkgo, ginseng:* These anticoagulant or antiplatelet herbs may increase the anticoagulant effects of cayenne, thus increasing bleeding tendencies. Discourage use together.

Effects on lab test results
None reported.

Cautions
Pregnant patients should avoid use because herb's effects on the fetus aren't known. Patients with irritable bowel syndrome shouldn't use herb because of its irritant and peristaltic effects. Breast-feeding patients and those hypersensitive to herb should avoid use.

Patients with asthma who use capsicum may experience bronchospasm.

Nursing considerations
■ Explore patient's knowledge of this herb.

■ Alcoholic extracts may be unsuitable for children, alcoholic patients, patients with liver disease, and those taking disulfiram or metronidazole.

■ Topical product shouldn't be used on broken or irritated skin or covered with a tight bandage.

■ Treat adverse skin reactions to topically applied capsaicin by washing the area thoroughly with soap and water. Soaking the area in vegetable oil after washing provides a slower onset but longer duration of relief than cold water. Vinegar water irrigation is moderately success-ful. Rubbing alcohol may also help.

■ EMLA (a topical emulsion of lidocaine and prilocaine) provides pain relief in about 1 hour to skin that has been severely irritated by capsaicin.

🌀 ALERT Capsicum shouldn't be taken orally for more than 2 days and then shouldn't be consumed again for 2 weeks.

Patient teaching
■ Advise patient to consult a health care provider before using an herbal preparation because another treatment may be available.

■ Tell patient that when filling a new prescription he should inform pharmacist of any herbal or dietary supplement he's taking.

■ Advise patient not to take this herb if she is pregnant, breast-feeding, or planning a pregnancy.

■ If patient is applying capsicum topically, explain that it may take 1 to 2 weeks to achieve maximum pain control.

■ If patient is using capsicum topically, instruct him to wash his hands before and immediately after applying it and to avoid contact with eyes. Advise contact lens wearer to wash his hands and to use gloves or an applicator if handling lenses after applying capsicum.

■ If patient is using capsicum topically, advise him not to apply it to broken or irritated skin and instruct him not to tightly bandage any area to which he has applied it.

■ Inform patient not to delay treatment for an illness that doesn't improve after taking capsicum. If he is applying it topically, advise him to promptly contact his health care provider if the condition worsens or if symptoms persist for 2 to 4 weeks.

■ Tell patient to store capsicum in a tightly sealed container, away from light.

CHAMOMILE

Azulon, Chamomile Flowers, Chamomile Tea, Kid Chamomile, Standardized Chamomile Extract, Wild Chamomile

Available forms

Available as capsules, fresh or dried flowerheads of *Matricaria recutita* and *Chamaemelum nobile*, liquid extract, raw herb, tea, and topical cream.

■ *Capsules:* 350 to 400 mg/ capsule (standardized to contain 1% apigenin and 0.5% essential oil).

■ *Liquid extracts:* The strength of the liquid extracts available is usually 1:1 or 1:1.5. Some liquid extracts contain between 10% and 63% grain alcohol. Nature's Answer makes a liquid extract for children that contains glycerin, not alcohol.

■ *Raw herb:* Frontier offers whole German chamomile flowers for making teas or massage oils.

■ *Teas:* Made from dried chamomile flowers. Most chamomile teas are organic and caffeine free.

Actions and components

Contains a volatile oil that consists of up to 50% alpha-bisabolol. Bisabolol reduces inflammation and is an antipyretic. It also shortens the healing times of superficial burns and ulcers and inhibits development of ulcers. The essential oil also has antibacterial and slight antiviral effects.

Chamazulene, a minor component of the oil, has anti-inflammatory and antioxidant effects. The flavonoids apigenin and luteolin also contribute to the anti-inflammatory effect. Unlike the benzodiazepines, apigenin is primarily responsible for the anxiolytic and slight sedative effect through action on the CNS benzodiazepine receptors. Apigenin doesn't produce anticonvulsant effects.

Bisabolol, bisabolol oxides A and B, and the essential oil of chamomile are probably best known for their antispasmodic effects. Other compounds in chamomile that exert antispasmodic effects include apigenin, quercetin, luteolin, and the coumarins umbelliferone and herniarine.

Uses

Used orally to treat diarrhea, anxiety, restlessness, stomatitis, hemorrhagic cystitis, flatulence, and motion sickness.

Used topically to stimulate skin metabolism, reduce inflammation, encourage the healing of wounds, and treat cutaneous burns. Also used for its antibacterial and antiviral effects.

Teas are mainly used for sedation or relaxation.

Dosage and administration

Adults: 1:1 or 1:1.5 liquid extract in 10% to 70% alcohol, 1 to 4 ml t.i.d.

Children age 2 and older: 1:4 strength alcohol-free extract, 1 to 4 ml t.i.d.

Children ages 2 to 4: ⅛ to ¼ teaspoon directly or in water or juice b.i.d. to t.i.d.

Children weighing 41 to 54 kg (90 to 119 lb): 1 to 2 teaspoons directly or in water or juice b.i.d. to t.i.d.

Children weighing 27 to 41 kg (60 to 90 lb): ½ to 1 teaspoon directly or in water or juice b.i.d. to t.i.d.

Children weighing 14 to 27 kg (31 to 60 lb): ¼ to ½ teaspoon directly or in water or juice b.i.d. to t.i.d.

■ *Raw herb:* Used in massage oils, p.r.n.

■ *Teas:* For GI upset, tea is taken t.i.d. to q.i.d. between meals. **Adults and children older than age 6:** Prepared by pouring boiling water over 1 tablespoon of chamomile or one chamomile tea bag, covering it for 5 to 10 minutes, and then (if using bulk herbs) straining it. For inflammation of the mucous membranes in the mouth and throat, tea is used as a wash or gargle. For young children, tea should be diluted.

Children ages 5 to 6: 100 to 120 ml daily to q.i.d.

Children ages 3 to 4: 50 to 80 ml daily to q.i.d.

Children ages 1 to 2: 20 to 40 ml daily to q.i.d.

Adverse reactions

EENT: conjunctivitis, eyelid angioedema.
GI: nausea, vomiting.
Skin: eczema, contact dermatitis.
Other: *anaphylaxis.*

Interactions

HERB-DRUG

■ *CNS depressants:* May have additive effects. Discourage use together.

■ *Drugs metabolized by cytochrome P-450 3A4 such as alprazolam, atorvastatin, diazepam, ketoconazole, verapamil:* May increase levels of drugs metabolized by cytochrome P-450 3A4 because chamomile is a weak inhibitor of this enzyme. Monitor drug concentrations and effects of using this herb with these drugs.

■ *Warfarin:* The coumarin content of chamomile may antagonize or potentiate the effect of an anticoagulant. Discourage use together.

Effects on lab test results

None reported.

Cautions

Patients with known or suspected allergy to chamomile or related members of the Compositae family should avoid use because of the potential for anaphylaxis. Pregnant patients should avoid use because chamomile may trigger menstruation or a miscarriage.

Herb shouldn't be used in teething babies and in children younger than age 2.

Safety in breast-feeding patients and those with liver or kidney disorders hasn't been established; therefore, these patients should avoid use.

Nursing considerations

■ Explore patient's knowledge of this herb.

🌀 ALERT *People sensitive to ragweed and chrysanthemums or other Compositae family members (arnica, yarrow, feverfew, tansy, artemisia) may be more susceptible to contact allergies and anaphylaxis. Patients with hay fever or bronchial asthma caused by pollens are more susceptible to anaphylactoid reactions.*

■ Signs and symptoms of anaphylaxis include shortness of breath, swelling of the tongue, rash, tachycardia, and hypotension.

Patient teaching

■ Advise patient to consult a health care provider before using an herbal preparation because another treatment may be available.

■ Tell patient that when filling a new prescription he should inform pharmacist of any herbal or dietary supplement he's taking.

■ Advise patients who are pregnant or planning pregnancy not to use chamomile.

■ If patient is taking a blood thinner, advise him not to use chamomile because it may thin the blood too much.

■ Advise patient that chamomile may enhance an allergic reaction or make existing symptoms worse in susceptible patients.

■ Instruct parent not to give chamomile to any child before checking with a knowledgeable practitioner.

■ Advise patient to avoid herb if taking CNS depressants.

ECHINACEA

Coneflower Extract, EchinaCare Liquid, Echinacea, Echinacea Angustifolia Herb, Echinacea Extract, Echinacea Fresh Freeze Dried, Echinacea Glycerite, Echinacea Herbal Comfort, Echinacea Red Root Supreme, Echinacea Root Complex, Echinacea Root Extract, Echinacea Xtra, Echina Fresh, EchinaGuard Liquid, EchinaGuard Pro, Echinex, Enhanced Echinacea, Standardized Echinacea Extract

Available forms

Available as capsules, glycerite, expressed juice, hydroalcoholic extract, lozenges, tablets, tea, tinctures (1:5, 15% to 90% alcohol), and whole dried root.

■ *Capsules:* 125 mg, 250 mg, 355 mg, 500 mg

■ *Hydroalcoholic extracts:* 50%

■ *Tablets:* 335 mg

Actions and components

Obtained from the dried rhizomes and roots of *Echinacea angustifolia* and *E. pallida* and the roots or above-ground parts of *E. purpurea*. Extracts of echinacea contain numerous components, including alkylamides, caffeic acid derivatives, polysaccharides, essential oils, chicoric acids, flavonoids, and glycoproteins.

Echinacea—most notably the lipophilic fraction in the roots and leaves—may enhance immune system function. When taken internally, echinacea may increase the number of circulating leukocytes, enhance phagocytosis, stimulate cytokine production, and trigger the alternate complement pathway. In vitro, some components are directly bacteriostatic and exhibit antiviral activity. Applied topically, echinacea can exert local anesthetic, antimicrobial, and anti-inflammatory activity, and it can stimulate fibroblasts.

Echinacea's effects on cytokines may result in antitumorigenic activity.

Uses

Used to stimulate the immune system and to treat acute and chronic upper respiratory tract infections and urinary tract infections. Used also to heal wounds, including abscesses, burns, eczema, and skin ulcers. May be used as an adjunct to a conventional antineoplastic and may provide prophylaxis against upper respiratory tract infections and the common cold.

Dosage and administration

■ *Capsules containing powdered* E. pallida *root extract:* Equivalent to 300 mg P.O. t.i.d.
■ *Expressed juice of* E. purpurea *(2.5:1, 22% alcohol):* 6 to 9 ml P.O. daily. When used external-

ly, juice should be used for no longer than 8 weeks.
■ *Hydroalcoholic tincture (15% to 90% alcohol):* 3 to 4 ml P.O. t.i.d.
■ *Tea:* Prepared by simmering ¼ teaspoon of coarsely powdered herb in 1 cup of boiling water for 10 minutes. For colds, the dosage is 1 cup of freshly made tea taken several times daily.
■ *Whole dried root:* 1 to 2 g P.O. t.i.d.

Adverse reactions

CNS: fever.
EENT: taste disturbance.
GI: nausea, vomiting, minor GI complaints.
Skin: diuresis.
Other: allergic reaction, ***tachyphylaxis.***

Interactions
HERB-DRUG

■ *Amprenavir, other protease inhibitors:* May advance HIV or AIDS (because the herb depresses CD4+ cells and increases HIV replication). Advise patient to avoid use together.
■ *Disulfiram, metronidazole:* May cause a disulfiram-like reaction if herbal preparation contains alcohol. Advise patient to avoid use together.
■ *Immunosuppressants such as cyclosporine, corticosteroids, and*

methotrexate: Decreases drug effectiveness. Advise patient to avoid use together.

■ *Prednisone:* May interfere with drug's immunosuppressive effect. Monitor patient for therapeutic effect. Advise patient to avoid use together.

HERB-LIFESTYLE

■ *Alcohol use:* May enhance CNS depression if herbal preparation contains alcohol. Advise patient to avoid use together.

Effects on lab test results
None reported.

Cautions
Patients with HIV infection, AIDS, tuberculosis, collagen disease, multiple sclerosis, or another autoimmune disease shouldn't use this herb; nor should patients who are pregnant or breast-feeding.

Nursing considerations
■ Explore patient's knowledge of this herb.

■ Daily dose depends on the preparation and potency, but patient shouldn't take the herb for more than 8 weeks. Consult specific manufacturer's instructions for parenteral administration, if applicable.

■ Echinacea is considered supportive treatment for infection; it shouldn't be used in place of antibiotic therapy.

■ Tinctures and extracts contain 15% to 60% alcohol and may be unsuitable for children, patients with a history of alcoholism or liver disease, or patients taking certain drugs.

■ Some active components may be water-insoluble.

■ Echinacea is usually taken at the first sign of illness and continued for up to 14 days. Prolonged use isn't recommended.

■ Herbalists recommend using liquid preparations because they believe echinacea functions in the mouth and should come in direct contact with the lymph tissues at the back of the throat.

Patient teaching
■ Advise patient to consult a health care provider before using an herbal preparation because another treatment may be available.

■ Tell patient that when filling a new prescription he should inform pharmacist of any herbal or dietary supplement he's taking.

■ If patient has a chronic illness, advise him not to put off seeking appropriate medical evaluation, because doing so may delay diagnosis of a potentially serious medical condition.

■ If patient has a history of alcoholism or liver disease, inform him that some herbal products contain alcohol.

■ Advise patient that prolonged use can result in either overstimulation or suppression of the immune system. Echinacea shouldn't be used for more than 14 days as supportive treatment of infection.

■ Inform patient that the herb should be stored away from direct light.

■ Warn patients to keep all herbal products away from children and pets.

EUCALYPTUS

Eucalyptamint, Eucalyptus Oil, Eucalyptus Rub

Available forms

Available as dried herb, eucalyptus leaf, essential oil, tincture, and tea bags.

Actions and components

The primary component of eucalyptus oil is the volatile substance 1,8-cineol (cineole). Oil preparations are standardized to contain 80% to 90% cineole.

The effectiveness of the herb as an expectorant is attributed to the local irritant action of the volatile oil.

Uses

Used internally and externally as an expectorant. Used to treat nasal congestion. Also used topically to treat sore muscles and rheumatism.

The essential oil (external use only) can be used in massage blends for sore, aching muscles and in foot baths or saunas, steam inhalations, chest rubs, room sprays, bath blends, and air diffusions.

Dosage and administration

■ *Leaf:* Average dosage is 4 to 6 g P.O. daily, divided q 3 to 4 hours.

■ *Oil:* For internal use, average dosage is 0.3 to 0.6 g P.O. daily. For external use, oil with 5% to 20% concentration or a semi-solid preparation with 5% to 10% concentration.

■ *Tea:* Prepared using one of two methods: For the infusion method, 6 ounces of dried herb is steeped in boiling water for 2 to 3 minutes and then strained; for the decoction method, 6 to 8 ounces of dried herb is placed in boiling water, boiled for 3 to 5 minutes, and then strained.

■ *Tincture:* 3 to 4 g P.O. daily.

Adverse reactions

CNS: dizziness.
GI: nausea, vomiting, diarrhea.
Respiratory: *bronchospasm.*

Interactions

HERB-DRUG

■ *Antidiabetics:* Causes enhanced effects. Advise patient to avoid use together unless under the direct supervision of a health care provider.
■ *Disulfiram, metronidazole:* May cause a disulfiram-like reaction if herbal preparation contains alcohol. Advise patient to avoid use together.
■ *Drugs metabolized by the liver:* May alter drug effects. (Eucalyptus oil induces detoxification of the liver's enzyme systems.) Monitor patient for drug effectiveness and toxic reaction.

HERB-HERB

■ *Herbs that cause hypoglycemia (basil, glucomannan, Queen Anne's lace):* Decreased glucose level. Monitor patient for this effect.

Effects on lab test results

■ May decrease glucose level.

Cautions

Patients who are allergic to eucalyptus or its vapors, who are pregnant or breast-feeding, or who have liver disease or intestinal tract inflammation shouldn't use this herb.

Essential oil preparations shouldn't be applied to an infant's or a child's face because of the risk of severe bronchospasm.

Nursing considerations

■ Explore patient's knowledge of this herb.
■ Eucalyptus oil, also known as eucalyptol, is steam-distilled from the twigs and long leathery leaves of the eucalyptus tree. Eucalyptus folium contains the dried leaves of older *E. globulus* trees. The leaves are collected after the tree has been cut down and allowed to dry in the shade.
■ Monitor patient for allergic reaction.
■ Tinctures and extracts contain 15% to 60% alcohol and may be unsuitable for children, patients with a history of alcoholism or liver disease, or patients taking certain drugs.
■ In susceptible patients, particularly infants and children, applying eucalyptus preparations to the face or inhaling vapors can cause asthmalike attacks.
■ If patient is diabetic, monitor glucose level.

■ Oral administration may cause nausea, vomiting, and diarrhea.

🌀 *ALERT* *Taken internally, a few drops of oil for children and 4 to 5 ml of oil for adults can cause poisoning. Signs of poisoning include hypotension, circulatory dysfunction, and cardiac and respiratory failure.*

■ If poisoning or overdose occurs, don't induce vomiting because of risk of aspiration. Administer activated charcoal, and treat symptomatically.

■ If patient is taking any drug that's metabolized in the liver, monitor its effectiveness.

Patient teaching

■ Advise patient to consult a health care provider before using an herbal preparation because another treatment may be available.

■ Tell patient that when filling a new prescription he should inform pharmacist of any herbal or dietary supplement he's taking.

■ If patient has trouble breathing or develops hives or a rash, advise him to immediately stop taking the herb and to check with his health care provider.

■ Inform patient of the herb's adverse effects.

■ If patient has a history of alcoholism or liver disease, inform him that some herbal products contain alcohol.

■ Advise patient with diabetes that glucose level may be altered.

■ Advise patient to use caution when performing activities that require mental alertness until he knows how the herb affects his CNS.

■ Instruct caregiver not to apply eucalyptus preparations to the face of a child or infant, especially around the nose.

■ Warn patient to keep all herbal products away from children and pets.

EVENING PRIMROSE OIL

Evening Primrose Oil Capsules, Mega Primrose Oil, Royal Brittany Evening Primrose Oil

Available forms

Available as capsules, liquid, oil, and tablets (evening primrose complex).

■ *Capsules:* 50 mg, 500 mg, 1,300 mg
■ *Gelcaps:* 500 mg, 1,300 mg
■ *Liquid, oil:* 2 ounces, 4 ounces

Actions and components

Contains the amino acid tryptophan and a high concentration of essential fatty acids, in particular *cis*-linoleic acid (CLA) and gamma-linoleic acid (GLA). The variety of evening primrose grown for commercial purposes produces oil with 72% CLA and 9% GLA. These fatty acids are prostaglandin precursors.

Conversion of the prostaglandin precursors into prostaglandins is the basis for using this oil to stimulate cervical ripening, prevent heart disease, and reduce signs and symptoms of rheumatoid arthritis. Its efficacy in other clinical conditions may result from its supply of fatty acids.

Uses

Primarily used to treat mastalgia and premenstrual syndrome. Used by midwives to stimulate cervical ripening during pregnancy at or near term and to ease childbirth. Also used to manage cyclic mastitis and neurodermatitis. Used as a dietary stimulant.

In Europe, used to treat eczema and diabetic neuropathy, although recent evidence doesn't support its use for these conditions. Also used to treat hypercholesterolemia, rheumatoid arthritis, inflammatory bowel disease, Raynaud's disease, Sjögren's syndrome, chronic fatigue syndrome, endometriosis, obesity, prostate disease, hyperactivity in children, and asthma.

Dosage and administration

■ *Cyclic mastitis:* 3 g P.O. daily in two or three divided doses.
■ *Diabetic neuropathy:* 4 to 6 g P.O. daily.
■ *Eczema in children:* 2 to 4 g P.O. daily.
■ *Oral use:* The usual dose is based on GLA content. Typical dose is 1 to 2 capsules (0.5 to 1 g) t.i.d.
■ *Rheumatoid arthritis:* 5 to 10 g daily.

Adverse reactions

CNS: headache.
GI: nausea, diarrhea, bloating, vomiting, flatulence.
Other: allergic reaction (including breathing problems, hives, itchy or swollen skin, and rash).

Interactions

HERB-DRUG
■ *Drugs that lower the seizure threshold, such as phenothiazines and tricyclic antidepressants:* May cause additive or synergistic effect, thus lowering the seizure threshold and increasing the

risk of seizures. Advise patient to avoid use together.

Effects on lab test results
None reported.

Cautions
Patients who are allergic to evening primrose oil or who are pregnant or breast-feeding shouldn't use this herb, nor should those who have a history of epilepsy or are taking a tricyclic antidepressant, a phenothiazine, or another drug that lowers the seizure threshold.

Nursing considerations
■ Explore patient's knowledge of this herb.

■ The fatty oil, extracted from the seeds of the evening primrose plant by a cold-extraction process, is available with a standardized fatty acid content.

ALERT *Evening primrose oil may unmask previously undiagnosed seizures, especially when taken with a drug that treats depression or schizophrenia.*

■ Drug effects may be delayed 4 to 6 weeks (with maximum benefit in 4 to 8 months) for cyclic mastitis and premenstrual syndrome, 3 to 4 months for eczema and decreased pruritus, and 3 to 6 months for diabetic neuropathy.

■ Vitamin E may be given with evening primrose oil to prevent toxic metabolites from forming.

■ Drug should be taken with food to decrease adverse GI reactions.

Patient teaching
■ Advise patient to consult a health care provider before using an herbal preparation because another treatment may be available.

■ Tell patient that when filling a new prescription he should inform pharmacist of any herbal or dietary supplement he's taking.

■ Tell patient to discontinue the herb if he has signs or symptoms of an allergic reaction, such as breathing problems, hives, itchy or swollen skin, or rash.

■ If patient is pregnant or breast-feeding, advise her to consult her health care provider before using the herb.

■ Advise patient to take herb with food to minimize adverse GI reactions.

■ Warn patient to keep all herbal products away from children and pets.

FENNEL

Fennel, Fennel Herb Tea, Fennel Seed

Available forms
Available as essential oil, honey syrup, and seeds.

Actions and components
Fennel oil is obtained from the ripe or dried seeds of either sweet or bitter fennel. The composition of the oil varies slightly, depending on the source.

Fennel oil extracted from bitter fennel is made up of 50% to 75% trans-anetholes, 12% to 33% fenchone, and 2% to 5% estragole; fennel oil extracted from sweet fennel, 80% to 90% trans-anetholes, 1% to 10% fenchone, and 3% to 10% estragole. Additional components are present in smaller quantities. Fennel oil stimulates GI motility, and at high levels it has antispasmodic activity. The anethole and fenchone components have a secretolytic effect on the respiratory tract, probably because of fennel's local irritant effects on the respiratory tract.

Uses
Used as an expectorant to manage cough and bronchitis. Also used to treat mild, spastic disorders of the GI tract, feelings of fullness, and flatulence. Fennel syrup has been used to treat upper respiratory tract signs and symptoms in children.

Dosage and administration
■ *Essential oil:* 0.1 to 0.6 ml P.O. daily (equivalent to 0.1 to 0.6 g of fennel).
■ *Honey syrup with 0.5 g fennel oil/kg:* 10 to 20 g P.O. daily.
■ *Seeds:* Crushed or ground; used for teas, tealike products, and internal use. Daily dose is 5 to 7 g.

Adverse reactions
CNS: *seizures,* hallucinations.
GI: nausea, vomiting.
Respiratory: *pulmonary edema.*
Skin: photosensitivity reactions, contact dermatitis.
Other: allergic reaction.

Interactions
HERB–DRUG
■ *Anticonvulsants, drugs that lower the seizure threshold:* Increases risk of seizures. Monitor patient closely.

HERB-LIFESTYLE

■ *Sun exposure:* Increases risk of photosensitivity. Advise patient to wear protective clothing and sunscreen and to limit exposure to direct sunlight.

Effects on lab test results

None reported.

Cautions

Patients with sensitivity to fennel, celery, or similar foods and herbs should avoid use, as should pregnant patients and those with a history of seizures. The herb shouldn't be used for small children.

Diabetic patients should be cautious when using honey syrup because of the sugar content.

Nursing considerations

■ Explore patient's knowledge of this herb.

■ Verify that patient isn't allergic to celery, fennel, or similar spices and herbs.

ALERT Don't confuse fennel with poison hemlock. Hemlock can cause vomiting, paralysis, and death.

■ If patient decides to take the herb while undergoing anticonvulsant therapy, monitor him closely.

■ Most adverse reactions are caused by fennel oil.

Patient teaching

■ Advise patient to consult a health care provider before using an herbal preparation because another treatment may be available.

■ Tell patient that when filling a new prescription he should inform pharmacist of any herbal or dietary supplement he's taking.

■ If patient is taking an anticonvulsant, advise him to avoid using this herb.

■ If patient has diabetes, make sure he's aware of the sugar content of the product.

ALERT Caution patient not to take this herb for longer than 2 weeks.

■ Tell patient to stop taking this herb and to contact health care provider immediately if he experiences difficulty breathing, hives, or a rash.

■ Warn patient to keep all herbal products away from children and pets.

FEVERFEW

Feverfew, Feverfew Extract, Feverfew Extract Complex, Feverfew Leaf, Feverfew Leaf and Flower, Feverfew LF and FL-GBE, Feverfew Power, Fresh Freeze-Dried Feverfew, Migracare

Feverfew Extract, Migracin, MigraSpray, MygraFew, Partenelle, Tanacet

Available forms

Available as capsules, dried leaves, liquid, powder, seeds, and tablets.

■ *Capsules containing leaf extract:* 250 mg
■ *Capsules containing pure leaf:* 380 mg

Actions and components

Feverfew has more than 35 chemical components. Of these, sesquiterpene lactones are the most well known and studied, and parthenolide, a germacranolide, is the most abundant of them. Monoterpenes, such as camphor; flavonoids, such as luteolin and apigenin; and volatile oils, including angelate, costic acid, and pinene are also found in feverfew. Traces of melatonin appear in pure leaves and commercial preparations of the herb.

Parthenolide is thought to be the major component responsible for the pharmacologic effects of feverfew. It inhibits prostaglandin synthesis, platelet aggregation, serotonin release from platelets, release of granules from polymorphonuclear leukocytes, histamine release from mast cells, and phagocytosis. Parthenolide may have thrombolytic, cytotoxic, and antibacterial activity and may cause contraction and relaxation of vascular smooth muscle.

Monoterpenes, and possibly melatonin, may be responsible for feverfew's sedative and mild tranquilizing effects.

Uses

Used most commonly to prevent or treat migraine headaches and to treat rheumatoid arthritis. Used to treat asthma, psoriasis, menstrual cramps, digestion problems, and intestinal parasites; to debride wounds; and to promote menstrual flow. Also used as a mouthwash after tooth extraction, a tranquilizer, an abortifacient, and an external antiseptic and insecticide.

Dosage and administration

■ *Infusion:* Prepared by steeping 2 teaspoons of feverfew in a cup of water for 15 minutes. For a stronger infusion, double the amount of feverfew, and allow it to steep for 25 minutes. Infusion dose is 1 cup t.i.d.; stronger infusions are used for washes.
■ *Migraines:* 125 mg of dried leaf preparation daily; *Tanacetum parthenium* content should be standardized to contain at

least 0.2% parthenolide, equivalent to 250 mcg of feverfew.

■ *Powder:* Recommended daily dose is 50 mg to 1.2 g.

Adverse reactions
CNS: dizziness.
CV: tachycardia.
EENT: mouth ulcerations (from chewing fresh leaf).
GI: GI upset.
Skin: contact dermatitis, rash, abnormal change in the skin.

Interactions
HERB-DRUG
■ *Anticoagulants, antiplatelet drugs including aspirin, and thrombolytics:* Inhibits prostaglandin synthesis and platelet aggregation, thus increasing risk of bleeding. Monitor patient for abnormal bleeding.

■ *Iron:* May decrease iron absorption. Instruct patient to separate administration times by at least 2 hours.

Effects on lab test results
■ May increase PT, INR, and PTT.

Cautions
Pregnant women shouldn't use this herb because of its potential abortifacient properties, nor should patients who are breast-feeding. Patients allergic to members of the daisy, or Aster-

aceae, family—including yarrow, southernwood, wormwood, chamomile, marigold, goldenrod, coltsfoot, and dandelion—and patients who have had previous reactions to feverfew shouldn't take it internally. The herb shouldn't be given to children younger than age 2.

Patients taking an anticoagulant, such as warfarin or heparin, should be cautious when using the herb.

Nursing considerations
■ Explore patient's knowledge of this herb.

■ If patient is taking an anticoagulant, monitor appropriate coagulation values—such as INR, PTT, and PT. Observe patient for abnormal bleeding.

■ Rash or contact dermatitis may indicate sensitivity to feverfew. Patient should discontinue use immediately.

■ Abruptly stopping the herb may cause postfeverfew syndrome, which is characterized by tension headaches, insomnia, joint stiffness and pain, and lethargy.

Patient teaching
■ Advise patient to consult a health care provider before using an herbal preparation because another treatment may be available.

■ Tell patient that when filling a new prescription he should inform pharmacist of any herbal or dietary supplement he's taking.

■ If patient is pregnant or breast-feeding, or planning to become pregnant, advise her not to use this herb.

■ Inform patient that combining the herb with an anticoagulant, such as warfarin or heparin, or an antiplatelet, such as aspirin or another NSAID, can increase the risk of abnormal bleeding.

■ Caution patient that a rash or an abnormal change in the skin may indicate an allergy to feverfew. Instruct patient to stop taking the herb if a rash appears.

■ Advise patient not to stop taking herb abruptly.

■ Warn patient to keep all herbal products away from children and pets.

FLAX

Dakota Flax Gold, Flax Seed Oil, Flax Seed Whole

Available forms

Available as capsules, flour, fresh flowering plant, oil, and whole seeds. Also, many cereals, pancake and muffin mixes, and eggs contain flax.

■ *Capsules:* 1,000 mg; 1,300 mg

Actions and components

Contains mucilages, cyanogenic glycosides, 10% to 25% linoleic acid, oleic acid proteins (albumin), xylose, galactose, rhamnose, and galacturonic acid. Cyanogenic acids, with the activity of a certain enzyme, have the potential to release cyanide. Linolenic, linoleic, and oleic acids are classified as omega fatty acids.

The mucilaginous fiber absorbs and expands. The omega fatty acid component may decrease total cholesterol and low-density lipoprotein levels and may decrease platelet aggregation.

Uses

Taken internally to treat diarrhea, constipation, diverticulitis, irritable bowel, colons damaged by laxative abuse, gastritis, enteritis, and bladder inflammation. It may help to remove heavy metals from the body.

Used externally to remove foreign objects from the eye. Also used as a poultice for skin inflammation.

Dosage and administration

■ *For gastritis, enteritis:* 1 tablespoon of whole or bruised seed, not ground, mixed with 5 ounces of liquid and taken b.i.d. or t.i.d. Or, 5 to 10 g of whole seed soaked in cold water for 30 minutes; liquid is then discarded, the seeds are ground, and 2 to 4 tablespoons are used as linseed gruel.

■ *Ophthalmic:* A single moistened flaxseed is placed under the eyelid until the foreign object sticks to the mucous secretion from the seed.

■ *Topical:* 30 to 50 g of the flour is used for a hot poultice or compress.

Adverse reactions

GI: *intestinal obstruction,* diarrhea, flatulence, nausea.

Interactions

HERB-DRUG

■ *Oral drugs:* Alters or blocks drug absorption, resulting from the herb's fibrous content and binding potential. Instruct patient to separate administration times by at least 2 hours.

Effects on lab test results

None reported.

Cautions

Patients with an ileus, an esophageal stricture, or an acute inflammatory illness of the GI tract shouldn't use this herb, nor should patients who are pregnant, breast-feeding, or planning to become pregnant.

Nursing considerations

■ Explore patient's knowledge of this herb.

■ When flax is used internally, it should be taken with more than 5 ounces of liquid per tablespoon of flaxseed.

■ Cyanogenic glycosides may release cyanide; however, the body only metabolizes these to a certain extent. At therapeutic doses, flax doesn't elevate cyanide ion level.

■ Even though flax may decrease a patient's cholesterol level or increase bleeding time, it's unnecessary to monitor cholesterol level or platelet aggregation.

Patient teaching

■ Advise patient to consult a health care provider before using an herbal preparation because another treatment may be available.

■ Tell patient that when filling a new prescription he should inform pharmacist of any herbal or dietary supplement he's taking.

■ Warn patient not to treat chronic constipation or other GI disturbances or eye injury with flax before seeking medical evaluation, because doing so can delay diagnosis of a potentially serious medical condition.

■ If patient is pregnant or breast-feeding or planning to become pregnant, advise her not to use flax.

■ Instruct patient to drink plenty of water when taking flaxseed.

■ Instruct patient not to take any drug for at least 2 hours after taking flax.

■ Tell patient to refrigerate flax oil and protect flaxseeds from light.

■ Warn patient to keep all herbal products away from children and pets.

GARLIC

Garlicin, Garlic Powermax, Garlinase 4000, GarliPure, Garlique, Garlitrin 4000, Kwai, Kyolic Liquid, Sapec, Wellness GarliCell

Available forms

Available as aqueous extract (1:1), capsules, fermented garlic, fresh cloves, garlic oil macera-tion (1:1), powdered cloves, softgel capsules, solid garlic extract, and tablets.

Actions and components

Medicinal ingredients of garlic are obtained from the bulb of the *Allium sativum* plant. The aroma, flavor, and medicinal properties are mainly from sulfur compounds, including alliin, ajoens, and allicin. Also found in garlic are vitamins, minerals, and the trace elements germanium and selenium.

Garlic inhibits lipid synthesis, thus decreasing cholesterol and triglyceride levels. It works as an anticoagulant by inhibiting platelet aggregation, which is probably the work of allicin and ajoens. It lowers blood pressure, and it lowers the glucose level by increasing circulating insulin and glycogen storage in the liver. As an antibacterial, garlic acts against both gram-positive and gram-negative organisms, including *Helicobacter pylori* (the causative organism in many peptic ulcers and certain gastric cancers). It may also have antifungal and antitumorigenic effects.

Uses

Used most commonly to decrease total cholesterol and triglyceride levels and to increase the high-density lipoprotein level. Also used to help prevent atherosclerosis because of its effect on blood pressure and platelet aggregation. Used to decrease the risk of cancer, especially of the GI tract; to decrease the risk of stroke and heart attack; and to treat cough, colds, fevers, and sore throats.

Used orally and topically to fight infection through antibacterial and antifungal effects.

Dosage and administration

Cholesterol reduction: 900 mg of dried power, 2 to 5 mg of allicin, or 2 to 5 g of fresh clove. Average dose is 4 g of fresh garlic or 8 mg of essential oil daily.

Adverse reactions

CNS: headache, insomnia, fatigue, vertigo.
CV: tachycardia, orthostatic hypotension
GI: heartburn, flatulence, nausea, vomiting, bloating, diarrhea.
Metabolic: hypothyroidism.
Respiratory: asthma, shortness of breath.
Skin: contact dermatitis, burns.
Other: hypersensitivity reactions, facial flushing, body odor, bad breath.

Interactions
HERB-DRUG
■ *Acetaminophen, other drugs metabolized by the enzyme CYP2E1 (a member of the CYP450 system):* Causes decreased drug metabolism. Monitor patient for drug effectiveness and toxic reaction.
■ *Anticoagulants, NSAIDs, prostacyclin:* May increase bleeding time. Advise patient to avoid use together.
■ *Antidiabetics:* Causes decreased glucose level. Advise patient to be cautious if using the herb and drug together. Monitor patient's glucose level.
■ *Disulfiram, metronidazole:* May cause a disulfiram-like reaction if herbal preparation contains alcohol. Advise patient to avoid use together.
■ *Ritonavir:* May cause severe GI toxicity. Advise patient to avoid use together.

HERB-HERB
■ *Herbs with anticoagulant effects, such as feverfew and ginkgo:* Increases bleeding time. Advise patient to avoid use together.
■ *Herbs that exert antihyperglycemic effects, such as glucomannan:* Decreases glucose level. Advise patient to be cautious if using these herbs together. Monitor patient's glucose level.

Effects on lab test results

- May decrease glucose, cholesterol, and triglyceride levels.
- May increase PT, INR, and PTT.

Cautions

People who are allergic to garlic shouldn't use this herb. Pregnant or breast-feeding women should avoid amounts greater than those used in cooking.

Patients with severe hepatic or renal disease should use caution with garlic, as should those using garlic for young children.

Nursing considerations

- Explore patient's knowledge of this herb.
- Garlic isn't recommended for postsurgical patients or those with diabetes, insomnia, pemphigus, organ transplants, or rheumatoid arthritis.
- Tinctures and extracts contain 15% to 60% alcohol and may be unsuitable for children, patients with a history of alcoholism or liver disease, or patients taking certain drugs.
- Consuming excessive amounts of raw garlic increases the risk of adverse reactions.
- Monitor patient for signs and symptoms of bleeding.
- Garlic may lower glucose level. If patient is taking an antidiabetic, watch for signs and symptoms of hypoglycemia, and monitor glucose level.

🌀 *ALERT Garlic oil shouldn't be used to treat inner ear infections in children.*

Patient teaching

- Advise patient to consult a health care provider before using an herbal preparation.
- Tell patient that when filling a prescription he should inform pharmacist of any herbal or dietary supplement he's taking.
- If patient has a chronic illness, urge him not to put off medical evaluation, because doing so may delay diagnosis of a serious medical condition.
- If patient has a history of alcoholism or liver disease, inform him that some herbal products contain alcohol.
- Urge patient to consume garlic in moderation to minimize the risk of adverse reactions, especially if he's scheduled for upcoming surgery.
- If patient is using garlic to lower his cholesterol levels, advise him to notify his health care provider and to have his cholesterol levels monitored.
- If patient is diabetic, advise him to carefully monitor his glucose level.
- If patient is taking an anticoagulant, explain that garlic may increase the risk of bleeding.

■ If patient is using garlic as a topical anesthetic, advise him to avoid prolonged use because it could burn the skin surface.

■ Warn patient to keep all herbal products away from children and pets.

GINGER

Alcohol-Free Ginger Root, Caffeine-Free Ginger Root, Ginger Aid Tea, Ginger Kid, GingerMax, Ginger Powder, Ginger Root, Quanterra Stomach Comfort, Zintona

Available forms

Available as candied ginger root, fresh root, oil, powdered spice, syrup, tablet, tea, and tincture.

■ *Capsules:* 250 mg, 410 mg, 550 mg

Actions and components

Ginger's medicinal components are derived from the rhizome or root of the plant *Zingiber officinale*. Its pungent properties also contribute to its pharmacologic activities. Ginger contains cardiotonic compounds known as gingerols, volatile oils, and other compounds, such as (6)-, (8)-, and (10)-shogaol, (6)- and (10)-dehydrogingerdione, (6)- and (10)-gingerdione, zingerone, and zingibain.

The root has antiemetic effects from its carminative and absorbent properties and from its ability to enhance GI motility. In large doses, the root has positive inotropic effects on the CV system. Ginger's ability to inhibit prostaglandin, thromboxane, and leukotriene biosynthesis may have an anti-inflammatory effect; its ability to inhibit prostaglandins and thromboxane, an antimigraine effect; its ability to inhibit platelet aggregation, antithrombotic effects. The volatile oil may have antimicrobial effects.

Uses

Used most commonly as an antiemetic in those with motion sickness, morning sickness, or generalized nausea. Used to treat colic, flatulence, and indigestion. Used to treat hypercholesterolemia, burns, ulcers, depression, impotence, and liver toxicity. Used as an anti-inflammatory for those with arthritis and as an antispasmodic. Also used for its antitumorigenic activity in patients with cancer.

Dosage and administration

■ *As an antiemetic:* 2 g of fresh powder P.O. taken with some liquid. Total daily recommended dose is 2 to 4 g of dried rhizome powder.

- *For arthritis:* 1 to 2 g daily.
- *For migraine headache or arthritis:* Up to 2 g daily.
- *For motion sickness:* 1 g P.O. 30 minutes before travel, then 0.5 to 1 g q 4 hours; may also begin treatment 1 to 2 days before trip.
- *For nausea caused by chemotherapy:* 1 g before chemotherapy.
- *Infusion:* Prepared by steeping 0.5 to 1 g of herb in boiling water and then straining after 5 minutes (1 teaspoon is equivalent to 3 g of drug).

Adverse reactions
CNS: CNS depression.
CV: *arrhythmias*.
GI: heartburn.

Interactions
HERB-DRUG
- *Anticoagulants, other drugs that can increase bleeding time:* May further increase bleeding time. Advise patient to avoid use together.
- *Disulfiram, metronidazole:* May cause a disulfiram-like reaction if herbal preparation contains alcohol. Advise patient to avoid use together.

HERB-HERB
- *Herbs that may increase bleeding time:* May further increase bleeding time. Advise patient to avoid use together.

Effects on lab test results
- May increase bleeding time with large doses.

Cautions
Patients with gallstones or an allergy to ginger shouldn't use ginger. Patients who are pregnant or who have a bleeding disorder shouldn't use large amounts of the herb.

Patients taking a CNS depressant or an antiarrhythmic should use caution when taking the herb and drug together.

Nursing considerations
- Explore patient's knowledge of this herb.
- Adverse reactions are uncommon.
- Tinctures and extracts contain 15% to 60% alcohol and may be unsuitable for children, patients with a history of alcoholism or liver disease, or patients taking certain drugs.
- Monitor patient for signs and symptoms of bleeding. If patient is taking an anticoagulant, monitor PTT, PT, and INR closely.

■ Use in pregnant patients is questionable, although small amounts used in cooking are safe. It's unknown if ginger appears in breast milk.

■ Ginger may interfere with the intended therapeutic effect of conventional drugs.

■ If overdose occurs, monitor patient for arrhythmias and CNS depression.

Patient teaching

■ Advise patient to consult a health care provider before using an herbal preparation because another treatment may be available.

■ Tell patient that when filling a new prescription he should inform pharmacist of herbal or dietary supplements he's taking.

■ If patient has a history of alcoholism or liver disease, warn that some herbal products contain alcohol.

■ If patient is pregnant, advise her to consult with a knowledgeable practitioner before using ginger medicinally.

■ Instruct patient to look for signs and symptoms of bleeding, such as nosebleeds or excessive bruising.

■ Warn patient to keep all herbal products away from children and pets.

GINKGO

Bioginkgo, Gincosan, Ginkgo Go!, Ginkgo Liquid Extract, Ginkgo Power, Ginko Capsules, Ginkyo, Quanterra Mental Sharpness

Available forms

Available as tablets, capsules, and liquid preparations.

Actions and components

Medicinal parts include dried or fresh leaves and the seeds separated from the fleshy outer layer. Flavonoids and terpenoids of ginkgo extracts are antioxidants that serve as free radical scavengers. Other actions may include arterial vasodilation, increased tissue perfusion and cerebral blood flow, and decreased arterial spasm, blood viscosity, and platelet aggregation. Ginkgo may help manage cerebral insufficiency, dementia, and circulatory disorders.

Uses

Primarily used to manage cerebral insufficiency, dementia, and circulatory disorders such as intermittent claudication. Also used to treat headaches, asthma, colitis, impotence, depression, altitude sickness, tinnitus, cochlear deafness, vertigo, premenstrual syndrome, macular degeneration, diabetic retinopathy, and allergies.

Used as an adjunctive treatment for pancreatic cancer and schizophrenia. Also used with physical therapy to decrease pain during ambulation in Fontaine stage IIb peripheral arterial disease (with at least 6 weeks of treatment).

In Germany, standardized ginkgo extracts must contain 22% to 27% ginkgo flavonoids and 5% to 7% terpenoids.

Dosage and administration
■ *Tablets and capsules:* 40 to 80 mg P.O. t.i.d.
■ *Tincture (1:5 tincture of crude ginkgo leaf):* 0.5 ml P.O. t.i.d.

Adverse reactions
CNS: headaches, dizziness, *subarachnoid hemorrhage.*
CV: palpitations.
GI: nausea, vomiting, flatulence, diarrhea.
Hematologic: *bleeding.*
Other: allergic reaction.

Interactions
HERB-DRUG
■ *Anticoagulants, antiplatelet drugs, high doses of vitamin E:* May increase risk of bleeding. Advise patient to avoid use together.
■ *Carbamazepine, phenobarbital, phenytoin:* May decrease drug effectiveness. Advise patient to avoid use together.
■ *Disulfiram, metronidazole:* May cause a disulfiram-like reaction if herbal preparation contains alcohol. Advise patient to avoid use together.
■ *Drugs that lower seizure threshold, such as bupropion; tricyclic antidepressants:* May further decrease the seizure threshold. Advise patient to avoid use together.
■ *MAO inhibitors:* May potentiate drug activity. Advise patient to be cautious if using the herb and drug together.
■ *SSRIs:* May reverse the sexual dysfunction linked to these drugs. Advise patient to consult health care provider before taking herb for sexual dysfunction resulting from SSRI use.
■ *Trazodone:* May cause coma (can occur after only four doses of ginkgo). Advise patient to avoid use together.

HERB-HERB
Garlic, other herbs that increase bleeding time: May potentiate anticoagulant effects. Advise patient to be cautious if using the herb and drug together.

Effects on lab test results
None reported.

Cautions
Patients with a history of an allergic reaction to ginkgo or its components or with risk factors for intracranial hemorrhage (such as hypertension or diabetes) shouldn't use ginkgo, nor should patients receiving an antiplatelet drug or an anticoagulant, because of the increased risk of bleeding.

The neurotoxin ginkgo toxin is present in leaf and seeds; patients prone to seizures also should avoid using the herb.

Ginkgo shouldn't be used in the perioperative period or before childbirth.

Nursing considerations
■ Explore patient's knowledge of this herb.
■ Ginkgo extracts are considered standardized if they contain 24% ginkgo flavonoids and 6% terpenoids.
■ Tinctures and extracts contain 15% to 60% alcohol and may be unsuitable for children, patients with a history of alcoholism or liver disease, or patients taking certain drugs.
■ Treatment should continue for at least 6 weeks, but for no more than 3 months.

⟳ ALERT Seizures have been reported in children who ate more than 50 seeds.
■ Patients must be monitored for possible adverse reactions, such as GI problems, headaches, dizziness, allergic reactions, and serious bleeding.
■ Toxicity may cause atonia and adynamia.

Patient teaching
■ Advise patient to consult a health care provider before using an herbal preparation because another treatment may be available.
■ Tell patient that when filling a new prescription he should inform pharmacist of any herbal or dietary supplement he's taking.
■ If patient has a history of alcoholism or liver disease, inform him that some herbal products contain alcohol.
■ Inform patient that the therapeutic and toxic components of ginkgo can vary significantly from product to product. Advise him to obtain ginkgo from a reliable source.
■ If patient is scheduled for upcoming surgery, advise him to stop using ginkgo at least 2 weeks beforehand.
■ Warn patient to keep all herbal products away from children and pets.

GINSENG

American Ginseng, American Ginseng Root, Centrum Ginseng, Chinese Red Panax Ginseng, Concentrated Ginseng Extract, Gin-Action, Ginsai, Ginsana, Ginseng Concentrate, Ginseng Natural, Ginseng Power Max 4X, Ginseng Solution, Ginseng Up, Korean Ginseng Power-Herb, Korean Ginseng Root, Korean White Ginseng, Lynae Ginse-Cool

Available forms

Available as powdered root, tablets, capsules, and tea.

Actions and components

The dried root is medicinal. It contains triterpenoid saponins called ginsenosides that appear to be the active ingredients responsible for the plant's immunomodulatory effects. Ginsenosides seem to increase natural-killer cell activity, stimulate interferon production, accelerate nuclear RNA synthesis, and increase motor activity.

Ginsenosides also have been found to protect against stress ulcers, to decrease the glucose level, to increase high-density lipoprotein level, and to affect CNS activity by acting as a depressant, anticonvulsant, analgesic, and antipsychotic.

Uses

Used for fatigue and lack of concentration and to treat atherosclerosis, bleeding disorders, colitis, diabetes, depression, and cancer. Also used to help recover health and strength after sickness or weakness.

Dosage and administration

■ *Powdered root:* For a healthy patient, 0.5 to 1 g of the root P.O. daily in two divided doses for 15 to 20 days. The morning dose is usually taken 1 to 2 hours before breakfast; the evening dose, 2 hours after dinner. If a second course of therapy is desired, patient must wait at least 2 weeks before starting ginseng again.

For a geriatric or sick patient, 0.4 to 0.8 g of the root P.O. daily taken continuously.

■ *Solid extracts in tablets and capsules:* 100 to 300 mg P.O. t.i.d.

■ *Tea:* 1 cup daily to t.i.d. for 3 to 4 weeks. Prepared by steeping 3 g of herb in a cup of boiling water for 5 to 10 minutes.

Adverse reactions

CNS: headache, insomnia, dizziness, restlessness, nervousness.

CV: hypertension, hypotension.
GI: diarrhea, vomiting.
GU: estrogen-like effects, such as vaginal bleeding and mastalgia.
Other: ginseng abuse syndrome (increased motor and cognitive activity, significant diarrhea, nervousness, insomnia, hypertension, edema, skin eruptions).

Interactions
HERB–DRUG
■ *Anticoagulants, antiplatelet drugs:* May decrease drug effects. Monitor PT and INR.

■ *Antidiabetics, insulin:* Increases hypoglycemic effects. Monitor glucose level.

■ *CNS stimulants, corticosteroids:* May cause excessive CNS stimulation. Monitor patient, and advise him not to take these drugs near bedtime.

■ *Drugs metabolized by CYP3A4:* May result in inhibition of this enzyme system. Monitor patient for effects and toxicity.

■ *Estrogen:* May cause additive estrogenic effect. Monitor patient.

■ *Furosemide:* May decrease diuretic effect. Advise patient to avoid use together; otherwise, furosemide dosage may need to be reduced.

■ *Ibuprofen:* May increase risk of bleeding from decreased platelet aggregation. Advise patient to avoid using herb and drug together. If patient uses them together, monitor him for signs of unusual bleeding or bruising.

■ *Phenelzine and other MAO inhibitors:* May cause headache, irritability, and visual hallucinations. Advise patient to avoid using herb and drug together.

Effects on lab test results
■ May decrease glucose level.
■ May decrease PT and INR.

Cautions
Patients with a history of an allergic reaction to ginseng or its components shouldn't use it, nor should patients taking an MAO inhibitor.

Patients receiving an anticoagulant or an antiplatelet drug and those with a manic-depressive disorder, psychosis, diabetes, or a cardiovascular disorder should be cautious if using the herb.

Nursing considerations
■ Explore patient's knowledge of this herb.
■ The German Commission E doesn't recommend using ginseng for more than 3 months.
■ Ginseng is believed to strengthen the body and increase resistance to disease.

ALERT *Patients who take large doses (more than 3 g daily for up to 2 years) may develop ginseng abuse syndrome: increased motor and cognitive activity, significant diarrhea, nervousness, insomnia, hypertension, edema, and skin eruptions.*

Patient teaching

■ Advise patient to consult a health care provider before using an herbal preparation because another treatment may be available.

■ Tell patient that when filling a new prescription he should inform pharmacist of herbal and dietary supplements he takes.

■ Inform patient that therapeutic and toxic elements of ginseng can vary significantly from product to product. Advise him to obtain ginseng from a reliable source.

■ Warn patient to keep all herbal products away from children and pets.

GOLDENSEAL

Golden Seal Extract, Golden Seal Extract 4:1, Golden Seal Power, Golden Seal Root, Nu Veg Golden Seal Herb, Nu Veg Golden Seal Root

Available forms

Available as capsules, dried ground root powder, cream, tablets, tea, tincture, and water ethanol extracts.

■ *Capsules, tablets:* 250 mg, 350 mg, 400 mg, 404 mg, 470 mg, 500 mg, 535 mg, 540 mg

Actions and components

Consists of rhizome and roots of *Hydrastis canadensis*. Major chemical elements are the alkaloids hydrastine and berberine. Also contains other alkaloids, volatile oils, chlorogenic acid, phytosterols, and resins.

May have anti-inflammatory, antihemorrhagic, immunomodulatory, and muscle relaxant properties. Decreases hyperphagia and polydipsia linked to streptozocin diabetes in mice. Exhibits inconsistent uterine hemostatic properties. Hydrastine causes peripheral vasoconstriction. Berberine can decrease the anticoagulant effect of heparin; it stimulates bile secretion and has some antineoplastic and antibacterial activity. Berberine also can stimulate cardiac function in lower doses or inhibit it at higher doses.

Uses

Used to treat postpartum hemorrhage and improve bile secretion. Also used to treat urinary tract infections, dysmenorrhea, hemorrhoids, constipation, and flatulence. Also used as a digestive aid and expectorant. Used topically on wounds and genital herpes lesions.

Dosage and administration

- *Alcohol and water extract:* 250 mg P.O. t.i.d.
- *Dried rhizome:* 0.5 to 1 g in 1 cup of water t.i.d.
- *Expectorant:* 250 to 500 mg P.O. t.i.d.
- *To relieve symptoms of mouth sores and sore throat:* 2 to 4 ml of tincture (1:10 in 60% ethanol) swished or gargled t.i.d.
- *Topical use:* Small amount of cream, ointment, or powder applied to wound once daily. Wound should be cleaned at least once daily.

Adverse reactions

CNS: sedation, reduced mental alertness, hallucinations, delirium, paresthesia, paralysis.
CV: hypotension, hypertension, *asystole, heart block.*
EENT: mouth ulceration.
GI: nausea, vomiting, diarrhea, abdominal cramps.
Hematologic: megaloblastic anemia from decreased vitamin B absorption, *leukopenia.*

Respiratory: *respiratory depression.*
Skin: contact dermatitis.

Interactions
HERB-DRUG
Acid-reducing drugs, such as H₂ antagonists, antacids, and proton pump inhibitors: May increase stomach acid and thus interfere with drug action. Advise patient to avoid use together.

- *Anticoagulants:* May decrease anticoagulant effect. Advise patient to avoid use together.
- *Antidiabetics, insulin:* May increase hypoglycemic effect. Advise patient to be cautious if using the herb and drug together.
- *Antihypertensives:* May increase or decrease hypotensive effect. Advise patient to avoid use together.
- *Beta blockers, calcium channel blockers, digoxin:* May increase or decrease cardiac effect. Advise patient to avoid use together.
- *Cephalosporins, disulfiram, metronidazole:* May cause a disulfiram-like reaction if herbal preparation contains alcohol. Advise patient to avoid use together.
- *CNS depressants such as benzodiazepines:* May increase sedative effects. Advise patient to avoid use together.

Herb-lifestyle

■ *Alcohol use:* May increase sedative effects. Advise patient to avoid use together.

Effects on lab test results

■ May decrease bilirubin level.
■ May decrease PTT.

Cautions

Patients with hypertension, heart failure, or an arrhythmia shouldn't use this herb, nor should patients who are pregnant or breast-feeding or who have severe renal or hepatic disease. The herb shouldn't be given to infants because it increases their bilirubin levels.

Nursing considerations

■ Explore patient's knowledge of this herb.
■ Tinctures and extracts contain 15% to 60% alcohol and may be unsuitable for children, patients with a history of alcoholism or liver disease, or patients taking certain drugs.
■ The German Commission E hasn't endorsed the use of goldenseal for any condition because of potential toxicity and lack of well-documented efficacy.
■ Goldenseal is less effective than ergot alkaloids in treating postpartum hemorrhage.
■ Berberine can decrease the duration of diarrhea caused by various pathogens such as *Vibrio cholerae, Shigella, Salmonella, Giardia,* and some Enterobacteriaceae.
■ Monitor patient for signs and symptoms of vitamin B deficiency, such as megaloblastic anemia, paresthesia, seizures, cheilosis, glossitis, and seborrheic dermatitis.
■ Monitor patient for adverse cardiovascular, respiratory, and neurologic effects. If patient has a toxic reaction, induce vomiting and perform gastric lavage. After lavage, administer activated charcoal and treat symptoms.

Patient teaching

■ Advise patient to consult a health care provider before using an herbal preparation because another treatment may be available.
■ Tell patient that when filling a new prescription he should inform pharmacist of herbal and dietary supplements he takes.
■ If patient has a history of alcoholism or liver disease, caution that some herbal products contain alcohol.
■ Advise patient not to use goldenseal because of its toxicity and lack of documented efficacy, especially if he has cardiovascular disease.

　　 Alert *High doses may lead to vomiting, slowed heart rate,* *high blood pressure, respiratory depression, exaggerated reflexes, seizures, and death.*

■ Advise patient to avoid activities that require mental alertness until he knows how the product affects his CNS.

■ Warn patient to keep herbal products away from children and pets.

GRAPESEED

Antistax, Grape Seed Extract, Mega Juice, NutraPack

Available forms
Available as tablets, capsules, drops, cream, and grape liquid concentrate.

Actions and components
Obtained by grinding the seeds of red grapes. Extract contains procyanidins, also called proanthocyanidins, or flavonoids, which are free radical scavengers. Procyanidins inhibit proteolytic enzymes, including hyaluronidase, collagenase, elastase, and beta-glucuronidase. By this mechanism, they help stabilize collagen.

Grapeseed oil contains essential fatty acids and vitamin E. Its antioxidant properties may exceed those of vitamin C or E.

Grapeseed extract also has anticarcinogenic effects. It prevents oxidative damage to cholesterol and may lower the cholesterol level. It protects collagen lining the walls of the arteries and stabilizes the vasculature. It also protects the eyes against oxidative damage and prevents diabetic retinopathy and macular degeneration.

Grapeseed may also prevent dental caries by inhibiting *Streptococcus mutans* and glucan formation from sugar.

Uses
Used to prevent cardiovascular disease and cancer and to treat venous insufficiency, bruising, edema, and allergic rhinitis.

Dosage and administration
Capsules or tablets: Initially, 75 to 300 mg P.O. daily for 3 weeks; then 40 to 80 mg daily.
Liquid concentrate: 1 tablespoon mixed in 1 cup of water P.O.

Adverse reactions
Hepatic: *hepatotoxicity.*

Interactions
HERB-DRUG
■ *Warfarin:* May increase bleeding potential. Advise patient to avoid use together.

Effects on lab test results

■ May increase liver enzyme levels. May decrease cholesterol levels.

Cautions

Patients with liver dysfunction should be cautious when using the herb.

Nursing considerations

■ Explore patient's knowledge of this herb.

■ If patient has liver dysfunction, monitor liver enzyme test results.

■ Grapeseed may interfere with the intended therapeutic effect of conventional drugs.

■ Grapeseed extract may have antiplatelet effects. If a patient is scheduled for surgery, he should stop the supplement 2 to 3 days beforehand. Monitor PT and INR.

Patient teaching

■ Advise patient to consult a health care provider before using an herbal preparation because another treatment may be available.

■ Tell patient that when filling a new prescription he should inform pharmacist of herbal and dietary supplements he takes.

■ Warn patient not to use grapeseed to treat venous insufficiency or a circulatory disorder before seeking medical evaluation, because doing so may delay diagnosis of a potentially serious medical condition.

■ Warn patient to keep herbal products away from children and pets.

KAVA

Combination products
Alcohol-Free Kava-Kava, Kavacin, Kava Plus, Kava Kava Root, Kava Tone, St. John's Wort Plus, Standardized Kava Extract, Veggie Capsules

Available forms

Available as capsules, soft gel caps, liquid spray, and tea bags.

Actions and components

Obtained from dried rhizome and root of *Piper methysticum*, a member of the black pepper family (Piperaceae). Kava contains seven major and several minor kava lactones, both aqueous and lipid soluble. Pharmacologic effects result from lipid-soluble lactones. Their mechanism of action differs from that of benzodiazepines and opiate agonists. Kava affects the limbic system, modulating emotional processes to produce anxiolytic effects. Kava lactones inhibit

MAO type B, producing psychotropic effects. They also inhibit voltage-gated calcium and sodium channels, producing anticonvulsant and skeletal muscle relaxant effects. The kava lactone kawain inhibits cyclooxygenase and thromboxane synthase, producing antithrombotic effects on human platelets.

Uses

Used for anxiety, stress, and restlessness. Used orally to produce sedation, to promote wound healing, and to treat headaches, seizure disorders, the common cold, respiratory tract infection, tuberculosis, and rheumatism. Also used for urogenital infections, including chronic cystitis, venereal disease, uterine inflammation, menstrual problems, and vaginal prolapse. Some herbal practitioners consider kava an aphrodisiac. Kava juice is used to treat skin diseases, including leprosy, and as a poultice for intestinal problems, otitis, and abscesses.

Dosage and administration

■ *Anxiety:* 50 to 70 mg purified kava lactones t.i.d., equivalent to 100 to 250 mg of dried kava root extract per dose. (By comparison, the traditional bowl of raw kava beverage contains about 250 mg of kava lactones.) Other sources cite 60 to 120 mg of kava lactones daily as a conservative dose.

■ *Restlessness:* 180 to 210 mg of kava lactones taken as a tea 1 hour before bedtime. The typical dose in this form is 1 cup t.i.d. Prepared by simmering 2 to 4 g of the root in 5 ounces boiling water for 5 to 10 minutes and then straining.

Adverse reactions

CNS: mild euphoric changes characterized by feelings of happiness, fluent and lively speech, and increased sensitivity to sounds; morning fatigue; headache.

EENT: visual accommodation disorders, pupil dilation, disorders of oculomotor equilibrium, initial numbing or astringent effect (with use of beverage).

GI: mild GI disturbances, mouth numbness.

GU: hematuria.

Hepatic: *hepatitis, cirrhosis, fatal liver failure.*

Respiratory: pulmonary hypertension.

Skin: scaly rash.

Interactions
HERB-DRUG

■ *Antiplatelet drugs, MAO type B inhibitors:* May cause additive effects. Monitor patient closely.

■ *Barbiturates, benzodiazepines:* May potentiate CNS depressant effects, leading to toxicity. Advise patient to avoid use together.

■ *Levodopa:* May reduce drug effectiveness in patients with Parkinson's disease because of dopamine antagonism. Advise patient to be cautious if using the herb and drug together.

■ *Hepatotoxic drugs:* Causes additive effects. Advise patient to avoid use together.

HERB-HERB

■ *Calamus, calendula, California poppy, capsicum, catnip, celery, couchgrass, elecampane, German chamomile, goldenseal, gotu kola, hops, Jamaican dogwood, lemon balm, sage, sassafras, shepherd's purse, Siberian ginseng, skullcap, stinging nettle, St. John's wort, valerian, wild lettuce, yerba maté:* Causes additive sedative effects. Monitor patient closely.

HERB-LIFESTYLE

■ *Alcohol use:* Increases risk of CNS depression and liver damage. Warn patient to avoid use together.

Effects on lab test results

■ May increase liver enzyme and high-density lipoprotein levels. May decrease albumin, total protein, bilirubin, and urea levels.

■ May increase RBCs in urine. May decrease platelet and lymphocyte counts.

Cautions

ALERT *Several patients have developed cirrhosis, hepatitis, and liver failure after taking kava; some needed transplantation. People with liver disease shouldn't take this herb; others should use caution and be alert for signs of liver damage.*

Patients sensitive to kava or its components shouldn't use the herb, nor should those who have Parkinson's disease or who are breast-feeding. Depressed or bipolar patients shouldn't use it because of possible sedative activity; those with endogenous depression, because of possibly increased risk of suicide; and pregnant women, because of possible loss of uterine tone. The herb shouldn't be given to children younger than age 12.

Nursing considerations

■ Explore patient's knowledge of this herb.

■ Patient shouldn't take kava with sedative-hypnotics, anxiolytics, MAO inhibitors, other psychotropic drugs, levodopa, or antiplatelet drugs without first consulting a health care provider.

■ Adverse effects of kava are mild at suggested dosages. They may occur at start of therapy but are transient.

■ Oral use is probably safe for up to 3 months, but taking the herb for longer than that may be habit forming.

■ Kava can cause drowsiness and may impair motor reflexes.

■ Patients should avoid taking herb with alcohol because of increased risk of CNS depression and liver damage.

■ Periodic monitoring of liver enzyme levels and CBC may be needed.

■ Patients who regularly use high doses of kava are more likely to complain of poor health: 20% are underweight with decreased levels of albumin, total protein, bilirubin, and urea; decreased platelet and lymphocyte counts; increased HDL levels and RBC counts; hematuria; puffy faces; scaly rashes; and some evidence of pulmonary hypertension. However, these signs and symptoms resolve several weeks after the herb is stopped. Toxic doses can cause progressive ataxia, muscle weakness, and ascending paralysis, all of which usually resolve when herb is stopped. Extreme use (more than 300 g per week) may increase GGT levels.

Patient teaching

■ Advise patient to consult a health care provider before using an herbal preparation because another treatment may be available.

■ Tell patient that when filling a new prescription he should inform pharmacist of herbal and dietary supplements he takes.

■ Urge patient to seek medical diagnosis before taking kava.

🌀 ALERT Tell patient to immediately stop taking herb and to contact a health care provider if evidence of liver damage occurs, such as jaundice, nausea, vomiting, or abdominal pain.

■ Because usual doses can affect motor function, advise patient to use caution when performing activities that require mental alertness until he knows how the herb affects his CNS.

■ Tell patient that oral use is probably safe for up to 3 months but that using the herb for longer than that may be habit forming.

🌀 ALERT Caution patient never to use kava above the recommended dosage and to use it only under the supervision of a qualified health care provider.

■ Warn patient to avoid taking this herb with alcohol because of increased risk of CNS depression and liver damage.

■ Warn patient to keep all herbal products away from children and pets.

MILK THISTLE

Liver Formula with Milk Thistle, Milk Thistle Extract, Milk Thistle Phytosome, Milk Thistle Plus, Milk Thistle Power, Milk Thistle Super Complex, Silybin Phytosome, Silymarin Milk Thistle, Simply Milk Thistle, Thisilyn

Available forms

Obtained from seeds of *Silybum marianum*. Available as capsules, soft gels, liquid, extract, tincture, and I.V. silymarin (I.V. form unavailable in the United States).

■ *Capsules:* 70 mg, 120 mg, 175 mg, 280 mg, 350 mg, 525 mg, 1,050 mg
■ *Liquid caps:* 75 mg, 150 mg
■ *Liquid extract:* 1:1, 1:2 (70% silymarin extract)
■ *Softgels:* 100 mg, 150 mg
■ *Tablets:* 50 mg, 500 mg
■ *Tincture:* 80 mg, 140 mg

Actions and components

Contains silymarin, which consists of hepatoprotective flavonolignans, including silibinin (silybin), isosilibinin, silidyanin, and silychristin. Silymarin stabilizes liver cell membranes and acts as an antioxidant by scavenging free radicals. It also stimulates protein synthesis in the liver, promoting liver cell generation. Silymarin's anti-inflammatory and immunomodulatory activity may add to its protective actions. Silibinin blocks toxin binding on liver cell membranes, reducing severe liver damage. It also reduces intracellular forms of prostate-specific antigen and inhibits cell growth via G_1 arrest in the cell cycle in hormone-refractory prostate cancer.

Milk thistle components reduce histamine release from basophils through membrane stabilization, inhibit T-lymphocyte activation, increase neutrophil motility, and alter polymorphonuclear leukocyte function. Silibinin administration decreases biliary cholesterol levels. Milk thistle reduces insulin resistance in patients with alcoholic cirrhosis.

Uses

Used for dyspepsia, liver damage from chemicals, *Amanita* mushroom poisoning, supportive therapy for inflammatory liver disease and cirrhosis, loss of appetite, prostate disorders, and gallbladder and spleen disorders. It's also used as a liver protectant.

Dosage and administration

■ *Dried fruit or seed:* 12 to 15 g P.O. daily.

■ *Injection (not available in the United States) for* Amanita phalloides *mushroom poisoning:* 20 to 50 mg/kg I.V. over 24 hours, divided into four doses infused over 2 hours each.

■ *Oral:* Doses of extract vary from 70 to 1,050 mg of silibinin (70% silymarin extract) P.O. daily in divided doses.

Adverse reactions

GI: nausea, vomiting, diarrhea.

Interactions

HERB–DRUG

■ *Aspirin:* May improve aspirin metabolism in patients with liver cirrhosis. Advise patient to consult his health care provider before using the herb.

■ *Cisplatin:* May prevent kidney damage by cisplatin. Tell patient to consult a health care provider before using the herb.

■ *Disulfiram, metronidazole:* May cause a disulfiram-like reaction if herbal preparation contains alcohol. Advise patient to avoid using herb and drug together.

■ *Hepatotoxic drugs:* May prevent liver damage from butyrophenones, phenothiazines, phenytoin, acetaminophen, or halothane. Advise patient to consult his health care provider before using the herb.

■ *Tacrine:* Reduces adverse cholinergic effects from the herb. Advise patient to consult his health care provider before using the herb.

Effects on lab test results

■ May decrease liver enzyme and glucose levels.

■ May increase clotting times.

Cautions

Patients who are pregnant or breast-feeding and those sensitive to the herb shouldn't use it. Those with decompensated liver disease also should avoid use.

Nursing considerations

■ Explore patient's knowledge of this herb.

■ Mild allergic reactions may occur, especially in those allergic to members of the Asteraceae family, including ragweed, chrysanthemums, marigolds, and daisies.

🌀 *ALERT Don't confuse milk thistle seeds or fruit with other parts of the plant or with blessed thistle (Cnicus benedictus).*

■ Silymarin has poor water solubility; efficacy when prepared as a tea is questionable.

Patient teaching

■ Advise patient to consult a health care provider before using an herbal preparation because another treatment may be available.

■ Tell patient that when filling a new prescription he should inform pharmacist of herbal and dietary supplements he takes.

■ Although no chemical interactions have been reported in clinical studies, advise patient that herb may interfere with therapeutic effects of conventional drugs.

■ If patient is pregnant or breast-feeding, advise her to avoid using this herb.

■ Tell patient to stay alert for allergic reactions, especially if he's allergic to ragweed, chrysanthemums, marigolds, or daisies.

■ Tell patient to report evidence of low glucose levels.

■ Warn patient to stop taking the herb and notify his health care provider if he notices easy bruising or bleeding from gums, which may be signs of overdose.

■ Warn patient not to take herb for liver inflammation or cirrhosis before seeking medical evaluation, because doing so

may delay diagnosis of a potentially serious medical condition.

■ Tell patient to keep the herb at room temperature, away from heat and moisture.

■ Warn patient to keep all herbal products away from children and pets.

NETTLE

Freeze-Dried Nettle Capsules, Fresh Nettle Leaf, Nettle Blend, Nettle Leaf, Nettle Leaf Tea, Nettle Organic Tea, Nettle Root, Nettle Seed

Available forms

Available as tea, tablets, capsules, tincture, and liquid extract.

■ *Capsules:* 50 mg, 100 mg

Actions and components

Obtained from fresh or dried roots and aboveground parts of *Urtica dioica, U. urens,* and their hybrids. Contains acids, amines, histamine, flavonoids, choline acetyltransferase, and lectins. Aqueous extract yields five immunologically active polysaccharides and some lectins, which may also have anti-inflammatory and immunostimulant properties. The lectin agglutinin has antifungal activity.

Two of the five polysaccharides have antihemolytic effects. Nettle leaves have diuretic, analgesic, and immunomodulating pharmacologic actions in vivo.

Uses
Used to treat allergic rhinitis, osteoarthritis, rheumatoid arthritis, kidney stones, asthma, BPH, eczema, hives, bursitis, tendinitis, laryngitis, sciatica, and premenstrual syndrome. Also used as a diuretic, an expectorant, a general health tonic, a blood builder and purifier, a pain reliever and anti-inflammatory, and a lung tonic for ex-smokers. Nettle is being investigated for treatment of hay fever and irrigation of the urinary tract.

Dosage and administration
■ *Allergic rhinitis:* 600 mg freeze-dried leaf P.O. at onset of signs and symptoms.
■ *Benign prostatic hyperplasia:* 4 g root extract P.O. daily, or 600 to 1,200 mg P.O. encapsulated extract daily.
■ *Fresh juice:* 5 to 10 ml P.O. t.i.d.
■ *Infusion:* 1.5 g powdered nettle in cold water; heated to boiling for 1 minute, and then steeped covered for 10 minutes and strained (1 teaspoon = 1.3 g herb). Dose is 1 to 4 g.
■ *Liquid extract (1:1 in 25% alcohol):* 2 to 8 ml P.O. t.i.d.
■ *Osteoarthritis:* 1 leaf applied to affected area daily.
■ *Rheumatoid arthritis:* 8 to 12 g leaf extract P.O. daily.
■ *Tea:* 1 tablespoon fresh young plant steeped in 1 cup boiled water for 15 minutes. 3 or more cups taken daily.
■ *Tincture (1:5 in 45% alcohol):* 2 to 6 ml P.O. t.i.d.

Adverse reactions
CV: edema.
GI: gastric irritation, gingivostomatitis.
GU: decreased urine formation; oliguria; increased diuresis in patients with arthritic conditions and those with myocardial or chronic venous insufficiency.
Skin: topical irritation, burning sensation, urticaria.

Interactions
HERB-DRUG
■ *Diclofenac:* Increases anti-inflammatory effect of diclofenac. Monitor patient for effect.
■ *Disulfiram, metronidazole:* May cause a disulfiram-like reaction if herbal preparation contains alcohol. Advise patient to avoid using the herb and drug together.

HERB-LIFESTYLE

■ *Alcohol use:* May cause additive effect from liquid extract and tincture. Advise patient not to use the herb and alcohol together.

Effects on lab test results

■ May decrease BUN and creatinine levels. May alter electrolyte levels.

Cautions

Patients with fluid retention caused by reduced cardiac or renal activity, patients sensitive to herb, and patients who are pregnant or breast-feeding shouldn't use the herb.

Nursing considerations

■ Explore patient's knowledge of this herb.

■ Tinctures and extracts typically contain between 15% and 60% alcohol and may be unsuitable for children, patients with a history of alcoholism or liver disease, or patients taking certain drugs.

■ Nettle is reported to be an abortifacient and may affect the menstrual cycle.

■ Allergic reactions from internal use are rare.

Patient teaching

■ Advise patient to consult a health care provider before us-ing an herbal preparation because another treatment may be available.

■ Tell patient that when filling a new prescription he should inform pharmacist of herbal or dietary supplements he's taking.

■ If patient has a history of alcoholism or liver disease, warn that some herbal products contain alcohol.

■ Warn patient that skin contact may cause external adverse reactions, such as burning and stinging, which could last for 12 hours or more.

■ Advise patient to monitor fluid balance by checking his weight regularly.

■ Advise patient to notify her health care provider before continuing to use the herb if she suspects or knows that she's pregnant or if she plans to become pregnant. Also advise her not to take the herb if she breast-feeds.

■ Inform patient that capsules and extracts should be stored at room temperature, away from heat and direct light.

■ Warn patient to keep all herbal products away from children and pets.

PASSION FLOWER

Passion Flower, Alcohol Free Passion Flower Liquid

Available forms
Available as fruits, flowers, extracts, capsules, tincture, and tea.
- *Capsules:* 400 mg
- *Liquid:* 1:1 (in 25% alcohol)

Actions and components
Obtained from leaves, fruits, and flowers of *Passiflora incarnata*. Contains indole alkaloids, including harman and harmine, flavonoids, and maltol. Indole alkaloids are the basis of many biologically active substances, such as serotonin and tryptophan. Exact effect of these alkaloids is unknown; however, they can cause CNS stimulation via MAO inhibition, thereby decreasing intracellular metabolism of norepinephrine, serotonin, and other biogenic amines. Flavonoids can reduce capillary permeability and fragility. Maltol can cause sedative effects and potentiate hexobarbital and anticonvulsive activity.

Uses
Used as a sedative, a hypnotic, an analgesic, and an antispasmodic for treating muscle spasms caused by indigestion, menstrual cramping, pain, or migraines. Also used for neuralgia, generalized seizures, hysteria, nervous agitation, and insomnia. Crushed leaves and flowers are used topically for cuts and bruises.

Dosage and administration
- *Dried herb:* 250 mg to 1 g P.O., two to three 100-mg capsules P.O. b.i.d., or one 400-mg capsule P.O. daily.
- *For cuts and bruises:* Crushed leaves and flowers are applied topically, p.r.n.
- *For anxiety:* 100 mg P.O. b.i.d. to t.i.d.
- *For hemorrhoids:* Prepared by soaking 20 g dried herb in 200 ml of simmering water, straining, and then cooling before use. Applied topically, as indicated.
- *For insomnia:* 200 mg P.O. h.s.
- *Infusion:* 5 ounces (150 ml) of hot water poured over 0.25 to 2 g of herb. Strained after standing for 10 minutes. Taken b.i.d. or t.i.d., with a final dose about 30 minutes before h.s.
- *Liquid extract (1:1 in 25% alcohol):* 0.5 to 1 ml P.O. t.i.d.
- *Solid extract:* Taken in doses of 150 to 300 mg/day P.O.

■ *Tincture (1:8 in 45% alcohol):* 0.5 to 2 ml P.O. t.i.d. or ¼ to 1 teaspoon P.O. t.i.d.

Adverse reactions

CNS: drowsiness, headache, flushing, agitation, confusion, psychosis.
CV: tachycardia, hypotension, *ventricular arrhythmias.*
GI: nausea, vomiting.
Respiratory: asthma.
Other: allergic reaction, *shock.*

Interactions

HERB-DRUG
■ *Anticoagulants, antiplatelet drugs:* May increase risk of bleeding. Advise patient to avoid using the herb and drug together.
■ *CNS depressants:* May cause additive effect. Advise patient to avoid using the herb and drug together.
■ *Disulfiram, metronidazole:* May cause a disulfiram-like reaction if herbal preparation contains alcohol. Advise patient to avoid using the herb and drug together.
■ *Hexobarbital, phenobarbital:* May increase sleeping time or potentiation of other barbiturate effects. Monitor patient's level of consciousness carefully.
■ *Isocarboxazid, moclobemide, phenelzine, selegiline, tranylcypromine:* May potentiate drug action. Advise patient to avoid using herb and drug together.

Effects on lab test results
■ May alter PT and INR.

Cautions

Excessive doses may cause sedation and may potentiate MAO inhibitor therapy. Pregnant patients shouldn't take this herb.

Nursing considerations
■ Explore patient's knowledge of this herb.
■ No adverse reactions have been observed with recommended doses.
■ Monitor patient for adverse CNS reactions.
■ Tinctures and extracts typically contain between 15% and 60% alcohol and may be unsuitable for children, patients with a history of alcoholism or liver disease, and patients taking certain drugs.

⟳ *ALERT A disulfiram-like reaction may produce nausea, vomiting, flushing, headache, hypotension, tachycardia, ventricular arrhythmias, and shock leading to death.*

Patient teaching
■ Advise patient to consult a health care provider before using an herbal preparation be-

cause another treatment may be available.

■ Tell patient that when filling a new prescription he should inform pharmacist of herbal or dietary supplements he's taking.

■ Advise patient to use caution when performing activities that require mental alertness until he knows how the herb affects his CNS. Also advise him to avoid taking the herb with alcohol or other CNS depressants.

■ If patient has a chronic illness, advise against delaying medical evaluation because it may delay diagnosis of a potentially serious medical condition.

■ Advise patient to notify her health care provider before continuing to use the herb if she suspects or knows that she's pregnant or if she plans to become pregnant.

■ Warn patient to keep all herbal products away from children and pets.

St. John's wort

Alterra, Hypercalm, Kira, Quanterra Emotional Balance, St. John's Wort Extracts, Tension Tamer

Available forms

Available as tablets, pellets, capsules of standardized extract, powdered or dried herb, liquid extract, tincture, and transdermal forms. Also available in various combination products.

■ *Capsules (extended-release, standardized at 0.3% hypericin):* 450 mg, 900 mg, 1,000 mg

■ *Capsules (standardized at 0.3% hypericin):* 125 mg, 150 mg, 250 mg, 300 mg, 350 mg, 370 mg, 375 mg, 400 mg, 424 mg, 434 mg, 450 mg, 500 mg, 510 mg

■ *Extract:* 1:1

■ *Injection:* 1%

■ *Liquid:* 250 mg/ml, 300 mg/5 ml

■ *Liquid dilutions:* 3x, 6x, 30x, 12c, 30c

■ *Pellets:* 3x, 6x, 12x, 12c, 30c

Tablets (standardized at 0.3% hypericin): 100 mg, 150 mg, 300 mg, 450 mg

■ *Tincture:* 1:10

■ *Transdermal:* 900 mg/24 hr

Actions and components

Obtained from *Hypericum perforatum*. Contains naphthodianthrones, including hypericin and pseudohypericin; hyperoside; quercitrin; rutin; isoquercitrin; bioflavonoids, including amentoflavone; 1,3,6,7-tetrahydroxy-xanthone;

hyperforin; adhyperforin; aliphatic hydrocarbons, including 2-methyloctane and undecane; dodecanol; mono- and sesquiterpenes, including alphapinene and caryophyllene; 2-methyl-3-but-3-en-2-ol, oligomeric procyanidines; catechin tannins; and caffeic acid derivatives, including chlorogenic acid. St. John's wort may have a slight inhibitory effect on MAO with more inhibition of the reuptake of serotonin, dopamine, and norepinephrine. Hypericin inhibits catecholmethyltransferase and receptors for adenosine, benzodiazepines, GABA-A, GABA-B, and inositol triphosphate. Hypericin has antiviral activity and other constituents have shown antibacterial activity; can also stimulate or inhibit the cytochrome P-450 enzyme system.

Uses

Used orally for mild to moderate depression, anxiety, restlessness, sciatica, and viral infections, including herpes simplex virus types 1 and 2, hepatitis C, influenza virus, murine cytomegalovirus, poliovirus, and Epstein-Barr. Has also been used to treat bronchitis, asthma, gallbladder disease, nocturnal enuresis, gout, and rheumatism, although it hasn't proven effective in these cases. Used topically for contusions, inflammation, myalgia, burns, hemorrhoids, vitiligo, herpetic lesions, and shingles. In traditional Chinese medicine, used as a gargle for tonsillitis and as a lotion for dermatoses.

Dosage and administration

■ *Capsules or tablets for mild to moderate depression:* Initially, 300 mg P.O. t.i.d.; maintenance, 300 to 600 mg P.O. daily.

■ *For depression:* 2 to 4 g dried herb P.O. daily, or 0.2 to 1 mg hypericin.

■ *For wounds, bruising, and swelling:* Applied topically to affected area.

■ *Liquid extract:* 2 to 4 ml P.O. daily.

■ *Tea:* 2 or 3 g of dried herb in boiling water.

■ *Tincture:* 2 to 4 ml P.O. daily.

Adverse reactions

CNS: fatigue, neuropathy, restlessness, headache.

GI: digestive complaints, fullness sensation, constipation, diarrhea, nausea, abdominal pain, dry mouth.

Skin: photosensitivity reaction, pruritus.

Other: delayed hypersensitivity.

Interactions
HERB–DRUG

■ *Amitriptyline; chemotherapy drugs; cyclosporine; digoxin; drugs metabolized by the cytochrome P-450 enzyme system; hormonal contraceptives; protease inhibitors, including amprenavir, indinavir, nelfinavir, ritonavir, saquinavir; theophylline; warfarin:* Decreases effectiveness, requiring possible dosage adjustment. Drug therapy may fail when these drugs are used with St. John's wort. Advise patient to avoid using together. If patient stops taking the herb during drug therapy, check blood drug levels because they may rise.

■ *Anesthetics:* May have synergistic or unpredictable effects. Discourage use together.

■ *MAO inhibitors, including phenelzine and tranylcypromine:* May increase effects and cause possible toxicity and hypertensive crisis. Advise patient to avoid using together.

■ *Nonnucleoside reverse transcriptase inhibitors, such as delavirdine, efavirenz, nevirapine:* May enhance metabolism of these drugs, causing treatment failure. Advise patient to avoid using together.

■ *Reserpine:* Antagonizes effects of reserpine. Advise patient to avoid using together.

■ *Selective serotonin reuptake inhibitors, such as citalopram, fluoxetine, paroxetine, sertraline:* Increases risk of serotonin syndrome: confusion, agitation, tachycardia, hypertension, nausea, hyperreflexia, muscle rigidity, restlessness, diaphoresis and, rarely, death. Advise patient to avoid using together.

HERB–HERB

■ *Herbs with sedative effects, such as calamus, calendula, California poppy, capsicum, catnip, celery, couch grass, elecampane, German chamomile, goldenseal, gotu kola, Jamaican dogwood, kava, lemon balm, sage, sassafras, skullcap, shepherd's purse, Siberian ginseng, stinging nettle, valerian, wild carrot, wild lettuce:* May enhance effects of either herb. Monitor patient closely, and advise him to avoid using together.

HERB–FOOD

■ *Tyramine-containing foods such as beer, cheese, dried meats, fava beans, liver, yeast, and wine:* May cause hypertensive crisis when used together. Advise patient to separate administration times.

HERB–LIFESTYLE

■ *Alcohol use:* May increase sedative effects. Advise patient to avoid using together.

■ *Sun exposure:* May increase risk of photosensitivity reactions. Urge patient to avoid unprotected sun exposure.

Effects on lab test results
None reported.

Cautions
Pregnant patients and men and women planning pregnancy shouldn't take St. John's wort because of the mutagenic risk to developing cells and fetus. Transplant patients maintained on cyclosporine therapy should avoid this herb because of the risk of organ rejection.

Nursing considerations
■ Find out why patient is using this herb.

■ Herb should be used with caution, if at all, in patients at high risk for, or who have had, skin cancer related to photosensitivity.

■ St. John's wort is effective in treating mild to moderate depression. Recommended duration of trial for depression is 4 to 6 weeks. Monitor patient for response to herbal therapy, as evidenced by improved mood and lessened depression. If no improvement occurs, a different therapy should be considered.

■ By using standardized extracts, patient can better control dosage. Formulations of standardized 0.3% hypericin and hyperforin-stabilized version of the extract have been used.

■ St. John's wort interacts with many prescription or OTC products. Patient must consider possible interactions before taking herb with other products.

■ Because St. John's wort decreases the effect of certain prescription drugs, watch for signs of drug toxicity if patient stops using the herb. Drug dosage may need to be reduced.

■ Serotonin syndrome may cause dizziness, nausea, vomiting, headache, epigastric pain, anxiety, confusion, restlessness, and irritability.

■ Because St. John's wort has mutagenic effects on sperm cells and oocytes and adversely affects reproductive cells, it shouldn't be used by pregnant patients or those planning pregnancy (including men).

■ Topically, the volatile plant oil is an irritant. Monitor affected site for adverse effects and improvement.

■ Monitor patient for sedative effects and GI complaints.

Patient teaching

■ Advise patient to consult a health care provider before using an herbal preparation because a standard treatment that has been proven effective may be available.

■ Tell patient that when filling a new prescription he should remind pharmacist of any herbal and dietary supplements he's taking.

■ Advise patient to discontinue herb several weeks before elective surgery.

■ Encourage patient to discuss depression and to seek professional psychiatric help, as indicated.

■ If patient takes St. John's wort for mild to moderate depression, explain that several weeks may pass before beneficial effects occur. Tell patient that a new therapy may be needed if no improvement occurs after 4 to 6 weeks.

■ Inform patient that St. John's wort interacts with many prescription and OTC products and may reduce their effectiveness.

■ Tell patient that St. John's wort may cause increased sensitivity to direct sunlight. Recommend protective clothing, sunscreen, and limited sun exposure.

■ Urge patient to wait a certain amount of time (to be determined by a health care provider) between stopping an antidepressant and starting St. John's wort.

■ Tell patient to report adverse effects to a health care provider.

■ Warn patient to keep all herbal products away from children and pets.

SAW PALMETTO

Centrum Saw Palmetto, Herbal Sure Saw Palmetto, Permixon, PlusStrogen, Premium Blend Saw Palmetto, Proactive Saw Palmetto, Propalmex, Quanterra Prostate, Saw Palmetto Power, Standardized Saw Palmetto ExtractCap, Super Saw Palmetto

Available forms

Available as tablets, capsules, fresh and dried berries, and as extracts.
Extracts: 60% to 70% grain alcohol

Actions and components

Obtained from berries of *Serenoa repens*. Contains fatty acids, fatty acid esters, sitosterols, and phytosterols. Exact mechanism of action isn't known, but sitosterols may inhibit conversion of testosterone to dihydrotestosterone (DHT), reducing prostate enlargement. May also inhibit androgenic activity by competing with DHT for androgen receptors, affecting testosterone metabolism and may have antiestrogenic effect, which may also contribute to its use with benign prostatic hyperplasia (BPH). The antispasmodic activity is related to the inhibition of calcium influx and activation of the sodium/calcium exchanger. Herb also has anti-inflammatory and astringent properties and inhibits prolactin and growth factor–induced cell proliferation. Said to improve urine flow rate and postvoid residual urine and relieve nocturia by up to 73% in BPH.

Uses

Used to treat symptoms of BPH (stages I and II) and coughs and congestion from colds, bronchitis, or asthma. Also used as a mild diuretic, urinary antiseptic (for urinary tract infections and interstitial cystitis), and astringent.

Dosage and administration

■ *Average daily dose:* 160 mg P.O. b.i.d. or 320 mg P.O. daily (1 or 2 g fresh berries or 320 mg of lipophilic extract).
■ *Decoction of berries:* 1 or 2 g of fresh berries in 1 cup of water, boiled, then simmered for 5 minutes. Taken t.i.d., possibly for longer than 3 months but less than 6 months.

Adverse reactions

CNS: headache.
CV: hypertension.
GI: nausea, abdominal pain, diarrhea.
GU: urine retention.
Musculoskeletal: back pain.

Interactions

HERB–DRUG

■ *Adrenergics, hormones, hormone-like drugs:* May block alpha receptors, estrogen, and androgen. Drug dosages may need adjustment if patient takes this herb. Monitor patient closely.

Effects on lab test results

None reported.

Cautions

Pregnant or breast-feeding women and women of childbearing age shouldn't use this herb. Adults and children with hormone-dependent illnesses other than BPH or breast cancer should avoid this herb.

Nursing considerations

■ Find out why patient is using the herb.

■ Herb should be used cautiously for conditions other than BPH because data about its effectiveness in other conditions are lacking.

■ Obtain a baseline prostate-specific antigen (PSA) test before patient starts taking herb because it may cause a false-negative PSA result. PSA laboratory values didn't change significantly in clinical trials using dosages of 160 to 320 mg daily.

■ Saw palmetto may not alter prostate size. Some sources report that herb does reduce prostate swelling and further progression.

Patient teaching

■ Advise patient to consult a health care provider before using an herbal preparation because a standard treatment that has been proven effective may be available.

■ Tell patient that when filling a new prescription he should remind pharmacist of any herbal and dietary supplements he's taking.

■ Warn patient not to take herb for bladder or prostate problems before seeking medical attention because this could delay diagnosis of a potentially serious medical condition.

■ Tell patient to take herb with food to minimize GI effects.

■ Caution patient to promptly notify health care provider about new or worsened adverse effects.

■ Warn women to avoid herb if pregnant or planning pregnancy or if breast-feeding.

VALERIAN

Herbal Sure Valerian Root, NuVeg Valerian Root, Quanterra Sleep, Valerian Root

Available forms

Available as dried root, essential oil, tea, tincture, extract, capsules, tablets, and combination products.

■ *Capsules:* 100 mg, 250 mg, 380 mg, 400 mg, 445 mg, 475 mg, 493 mg, 495 mg, 500 mg, 530 mg, 550 mg, 1,000 mg

■ *Tablets:* 160 mg, 550 mg

Actions and components

Obtained from *Valeriana officinalis.* Multiple constituents, including essential oils, seem to contribute to sedating properties of valerian. Valeric acid, the main component of the root, inhibits the enzyme system responsible for breaking down the neurotransmitter GABA, thus increasing its level in the brain. Valerian may also have mild pain relief properties and some hypotensive effects.

Uses

Used to treat menstrual cramps, restlessness and sleep disorders from nervous conditions, and other symptoms of psychological stress, such as anxiety, nervous headaches, and gastric spasms. Used topically as a bath additive for restlessness and sleep disorders.

Dosage and administration

■ *Bath additive:* 100 g of root mixed with 2 L of hot water and added to one full bath.

■ *For hastening sleep and improving sleep quality:* 400 to 800 mg root P.O. up to 2 hours before bedtime. Some patients need 2 to 4 weeks of use for significant improvement. Maximum dosage is 15 g daily.

■ *For restlessness:* 220 mg of extract P.O. t.i.d.

■ *Tea:* 1 cup P.O. b.i.d. to t.i.d., and h.s.

■ *Tincture (1:5 in 45% to 50% alcohol):* 15 to 20 gtt in water several times daily.

Adverse reactions

CNS: headache, morning drowsiness, uneasiness, restlessness.
CV: cardiac disturbances.
GI: GI complaints.
Skin: contact allergies.
Other: withdrawal symptoms, including increased agitation and decreased sleep.

Interactions

HERB-DRUG

Barbiturates, benzodiazepines: May have additive CNS effects. Monitor patient closely.

HERB-HERB

■ *Herbs with sedative effects, such as catnip, hops, kava, passion flower, skullcap:* May potentiate sedative effects. Monitor patient closely.

HERB-LIFESTYLE

■ *Alcohol use:* May potentiate sedative effects. Advise patient to avoid using together.

Effects on lab test results

None reported.

Cautions

Pregnant or breast-feeding women should avoid this herb.

Patients with acute or major skin injuries, fever, infectious diseases, cardiac insufficiency, or hypertonia shouldn't bathe with valerian products.

Nursing considerations

■ Find out why patient is using the herb.

■ Valerian seems to have a more pronounced effect on those with disturbed sleep or sleep disorders.

🌀 **ALERT** *Evidence of valerian toxicity includes difficulty walking, hypothermia, and increased muscle relaxation.*

■ Withdrawal symptoms, such as increased agitation and decreased sleep, can occur if valerian is abruptly stopped after prolonged use.

■ Monitor CNS status and patient response to herb.

■ Monitor patient for cardiac disturbances and GI complaints.

Patient teaching

■ Advise patient to consult a health care provider before using an herbal preparation because a standard treatment that has been proven effective may be available.

■ Tell patient that when filling a new prescription he should remind pharmacist of any herbal and dietary supplements he's taking.

■ If patient takes valerian, tell him to do so 1 or 2 hours before his desired bedtime. Explain that patient may not feel herb's effect for 2 to 4 weeks.

■ Inform patient that most adverse effects occur only after long-term use.

■ Instruct patient to promptly notify a health care provider about adverse effects.

■ Warn patient not to take herb for insomnia before seeking medical attention because doing so may delay diagnosis of a potentially serious medical condition.

■ If patient takes valerian for a long time, caution that amount should be tapered to avoid withdrawal symptoms, which may include increased agitation and decreased sleep.

■ Instruct patient to avoid hazardous activities until he knows how herb affects his CNS.

■ Tell patient to protect herb from light and to keep tincture in a tightly closed plastic container at room temperature.

■ Warn patient to keep all herbal products away from children and pets.

26 / SAFER HERBAL THERAPY

If your patient chooses to take herbal supplements, you can help to reduce the risk of toxic or unwanted effects by reviewing the resources provided in this chapter:

- Toxic herbs
- Herb-drug interactions
- Monitoring patients using herbs

TOXIC HERBS

The Food and Drug Administration considers these herbs unsafe because the plants contain poisonous components.

COMMON NAME	BOTANICAL NAME
arnica	*Arnica montana*
belladonna	*Atropa belladonna*
bittersweet	*Solanum dulcamara*
bloodroot	*Sanguinaris canadensis*
broom-tops	*Cytisus scoparius*
buckeye	*Aesculus hippocastanum*
ephedra	*Ephedra sinica*
heliotrope	*Heliotropium eropaeum*
hemlock	*Conium maculatum*
henbane	*Hyoscyamus niger*
jimsonweed	*Datura stramonium*
lily of the valley	*Convallaria majalis*
lobelia	*Lobelia inflata*
mandrake	*Mandragora officinarum*
mayapple	*Podophyllum peltatum*
mistletoe	*Phoradendron flavescens*
periwinkle	*Vinca major, Vinca minor*
snakeroot	*Eupatorium rugosum*
tonka bean	*Dipteryx odorata, Coumarouna odorata*
wahoo bark	*Euonymus atropurpureus*
wormwood	*Artemisia absinthium*
yohimbe	*Corynanthe yohimbe*

HERB-DRUG INTERACTIONS

HERB	DRUG	POSSIBLE EFFECTS
aloe (dried juice from leaf [latex])	antiarrhythmics, cardiac glycosides	Ingestion of aloe juice may lead to hypokalemia, which may potentiate cardiac glycosides and antiarrhythmics.
	licorice, thiazide diuretics, other potassium-wasting drugs such as corticosteroids	May cause additive effect of potassium wasting with thiazide diuretics and other potassium-wasting drugs.
	orally administered drugs	May decrease absorption of drugs because of more rapid GI transit time.
	stimulant laxatives	May increase risk of potassium loss.
bilberry	anticoagulants, antiplatelets	Decreases platelet aggregation.
	hypoglycemics, insulin	May increase serum insulin levels, causing hypoglycemia; additive effect with diabetes drugs.
capsicum	ACE inhibitors	May cause cough.
	anticoagulants, antiplatelets	Decreases platelet aggregation and increases fibrinolytic activity, prolonging bleeding time.
	antihypertensives	May interfere with antihypertensives by increasing catecholamine secretion.
	aspirin, NSAIDs	Stimulates GI secretions to help protect against NSAID-induced GI irritation.
	CNS depressants such as barbiturates, benzodiazepines, opioids	Increases sedative effect.
	cocaine	Concomitant use (including exposure to capsicum in pepper spray) may increase effects of cocaine and risk of adverse reactions, including death.

(continued)

HERB–DRUG INTERACTIONS (continued)

HERB	DRUG	POSSIBLE EFFECTS
capsicum (continued)	H$_2$ blockers, proton-pump inhibitors	Decreases effects resulting from the increased catecholamine secretion by capsicum.
	hepatically metabolized drugs	May increase hepatic metabolism of drugs by increasing G6PD and adipose lipase activity.
	MAO inhibitors	May decrease effectiveness because of increased acid secretion by capsicum.
	theophylline	Increases absorption of theophylline, possibly leading to higher serum levels or toxicity.
chamomile	anticoagulants	Warfarin constituents may enhance anticoagulant therapy and prolong bleeding time.
	drugs requiring GI absorption	May delay drug absorption.
	drugs with sedative properties, such as benzodiazepines	May cause additive effects and adverse reactions.
	iron	Tannic acid content may reduce iron absorption.
echinacea	hepatotoxics	Hepatotoxicity may increase with drugs known to elevate liver enzyme levels.
	immunosuppressants	Echinacea may counteract immunosuppressant drugs.
	warfarin	Increases bleeding time without increased INR.
ephedra (ma huang)	amitriptyline	May decrease hypertensive effects of ephedrine.
	caffeine	Increases risk of stimulatory adverse effects of ephedra and caffeine and risk of hypertension, myocardial infarction, stroke, and death.

HERB-DRUG INTERACTIONS *(continued)*

HERB	DRUG	POSSIBLE EFFECTS
ephedra (ma huang) *(continued)*	CNS stimulants, caffeine, theophylline	Causes additive CNS stimulation.
	dexamethasone	Increases clearance and decreases effectiveness of dexamethasone.
	digoxin	Increases risk of arrhythmias.
	hypoglycemics	Decreases hypoglycemic effect because of hyperglycemia caused by ma huang.
	MAO inhibitors	Potentiates MAO inhibitors.
	oxytocin	May cause hypertension.
	theophylline	May increase risk of stimulatory adverse effects.
evening primrose oil	anticonvulsants	Lowers seizure threshold.
	antiplatelets, anticoagulants	Increases risk of bleeding and bruising.
feverfew	anticoagulants, antiplatelets	May decrease platelet aggregation and increase fibrinolytic activity.
	methysergide	May potentiate methysergide.
garlic	anticoagulants, antiplatelets	Enhances platelet inhibition, leading to increased anticoagulation.
	antihyperlipidemics	May have additive lipid-lowering properties.
	antihypertensives	May cause additive hypotension.
	cyclosporine	May decrease effectiveness of cyclosporine. May induce metabolism and decrease drug to subtherapeutic levels; may cause rejection.
	hormonal contraceptives	May decrease efficacy of contraceptives.

(continued)

HERB-DRUG INTERACTIONS *(continued)*

HERB	DRUG	POSSIBLE EFFECTS
garlic *(continued)*	insulin, other drugs causing hypoglycemia	May increase serum insulin levels, causing hypoglycemia, an additive effect with antidiabetics.
	nonnucleotide reverse transcriptase inhibitors	May affect metabolism of these drugs.
	saquinavir	Decreases saquinavir levels, causing therapeutic failure and increased viral resistance.
ginger	anticoagulants, antiplatelets	Inhibits platelet aggregation by antagonizing thromboxane synthetase and enhancing prostacyclin, leading to prolonged bleeding time.
	antidiabetics	May interfere with diabetes therapy because of hypoglycemic effects.
	antihypertensives	May antagonize antihypertensive effect.
	barbiturates	May enhance barbiturate effects.
	calcium channel blockers	May increase calcium uptake by myocardium, leading to altered drug effects.
	chemotherapy	May reduce nausea from chemotherapy.
	H_2 blockers, proton-pump inhibitors	May decrease effectiveness because of increased acid secretion by ginger.
ginkgo	anticoagulants, antiplatelets	May enhance platelet inhibition, leading to increased anticoagulation.
	anticonvulsants	May decrease effectiveness of anticonvulsants.
	drugs that lower seizure threshold	May further reduce seizure threshold.
	insulin	Ginkgo leaf extract can alter insulin secretion and metabolism, affecting blood glucose levels.

HERB–DRUG INTERACTIONS *(continued)*

HERB	DRUG	POSSIBLE EFFECTS
ginkgo *(continued)*	thiazide diuretics	Ginkgo leaf may increase blood pressure.
ginseng	alcohol	Increases alcohol clearance, possibly by increasing activity of alcohol dehydrogenase.
	anabolic steroids, hormones	May potentiate effects of hormone and anabolic steroid therapies. Estrogenic effects of ginseng may cause vaginal bleeding and breast nodules.
	antibiotics	Siberian ginseng may enhance effects of some antibiotics.
	anticoagulants, antiplatelets	Decreases platelet adhesiveness.
	antidiabetics	May enhance blood glucose–lowering effects.
	antipsychotics	Because of CNS stimulant activity, avoid use with antipsychotics.
	digoxin	May falsely elevate digoxin levels.
	furosemide	May decrease diuretic effect.
	immunosuppressants	May interfere with immunosuppressive therapy.
	MAO inhibitors	Potentiates action of MAO inhibitors. May cause insomnia, headache, tremors, and hypomania.
	stimulants	May potentiate stimulant effects.
	warfarin	Causes antagonism of warfarin, resulting in a decreased INR.
goldenseal	antihypertensives	Large amounts of goldenseal may interfere with blood pressure control.
	CNS depressants, such as barbiturates, benzodiazepines, opioids	Increases sedative effect.

(continued)

HERB-DRUG INTERACTIONS (continued)

HERB	DRUG	POSSIBLE EFFECTS
goldenseal (continued)	diuretics	Causes additive diuretic effect.
	general anesthetics	May potentiate hypotensive action of general anesthetics.
	heparin	May counteract anticoagulant effect of heparin.
	H$_2$ blockers, proton-pump inhibitors	May decrease effectiveness because of increased acid secretion by goldenseal.
grapeseed	warfarin	Increases effects and INR because of tocopherol content of grapeseed.
green tea	acetaminophen, aspirin	May increase effectiveness of these drugs by as much as 40%.
	adenosine	May inhibit hemodynamic effects of adenosine.
	beta-adrenergic agonists (albuterol, isoproterenol, metaproterenol, terbutaline)	May increase the cardiac inotropic effect of these drugs.
	clozapine	May cause acute exacerbation of psychotic symptoms.
	disulfiram	Increases risk of adverse effects of caffeine; decreases clearance and increases half-life of caffeine.
	ephedrine	Increases risk of agitation, tremors, and insomnia.
	hormonal contraceptives	Decreases clearance by 40% to 65%. Increases effects and adverse effects.
	lithium	Abrupt caffeine withdrawal increases lithium levels; may cause lithium tremor.
	MAO inhibitors	Large amounts of green tea may precipitate hypertensive crisis.

HERB–DRUG INTERACTIONS (continued)

HERB	DRUG	POSSIBLE EFFECTS
green tea (continued)	mexiletine	Decreases caffeine elimination by 50%. Increases effects and adverse effects.
	verapamil	Increases plasma caffeine levels by 25%; increases effects and adverse effects.
	warfarin	Causes antagonism resulting from vitamin content of green tea.
hawthorn berry	cardiovascular drugs	May potentiate or interfere with conventional therapies for congestive heart failure, hypertension, angina, and arrhythmias.
	CNS depressants	Causes additive effects.
	coronary vasodilators	Causes additive vasodilator effects when used with such agents as theophylline, caffeine, papaverine, sodium nitrate, adenosine, and epinephrine.
	digoxin	Causes additive positive inotropic effect, with risk of digitalis toxicity.
kava	alcohol	Potentiates depressant effect of alcohol and other CNS depressants.
	benzodiazepines	Use with benzodiazepines has resulted in comalike states.
	CNS stimulants or depressants	May hinder therapy with CNS stimulants.
	hepatotoxic drugs	May increase risk of liver damage.
	levodopa	Decreases effectiveness because of dopamine antagonism by kava.
licorice	antihypertensives	Decreases effect of antihypertensive therapy. Large amounts of licorice cause sodium and water retention and hypertension.

(continued)

HERB–DRUG INTERACTIONS (continued)

HERB	DRUG	POSSIBLE EFFECTS
licorice (continued)	aspirin	May protect against aspirin-induced damage to GI mucosa.
	corticosteroids	Causes additive and enhanced effects of corticosteroids.
	digoxin	Licorice causes hypokalemia, which predisposes to digitalis toxicity.
	hormonal contraceptives	Increases fluid retention and potential for increased blood pressure resulting from fluid overload.
	hormones	Interferes with estrogen or antiestrogen therapy.
	insulin	Causes hypokalemia and sodium retention when used together.
	spironolactone	Decreases effects of spironolactone.
melatonin	CNS depressants, such as barbiturates, benzodiazepines, opioids	Increases sedative effect.
	fluoxetine	Improves sleep in some patients with major depressive disorder.
	fluvoxamine	May significantly increase melatonin levels; may decrease melatonin metabolism.
	immunosuppressants	May stimulate immune function and interfere with immunosuppressive therapy.
	isoniazid	May enhance effects of isoniazid against some *Mycobacterium* species.
	nifedipine	May decrease effectiveness of nifedipine; increases heart rate.
	verapamil	Increases melatonin excretion.

HERB-DRUG INTERACTIONS (continued)

HERB	DRUG	POSSIBLE EFFECTS
milk thistle	drugs causing diarrhea	Increases bile secretion and often causes loose stools. May increase effect of other drugs commonly causing diarrhea. May have liver membrane-stabilization and antioxidant effects, leading to protection from liver damage from various hepatotoxic drugs, such as acetaminophen, phenytoin, ethanol, phenothiazines, butyrophenones.
nettle	anticonvulsants	May increase sedative adverse effects; may increase risk of seizure.
	anxiolytics, hypnotics, opioids	May increase sedative adverse effects.
	warfarin	Antagonism resulting from vitamin K content of aerial parts of nettle.
	iron	Tannic acid content may reduce iron absorption.
passion flower	CNS depressants, such as barbiturates, benzodiazepines, opioids	Increases sedative effect.
St. John's wort	5-HT$_1$ agonists (triptans)	Increases risk of serotonin syndrome.
	alcohol, opioids	Enhances the sedative effect of opioids and alcohol.
	anesthetics	May prolong effect of anesthesia drugs.
	barbiturates	Decreases barbiturate-induced sleep time.
	cyclosporine	Decreases cyclosporine levels below therapeutic levels, threatening transplanted organ rejection.

(continued)

HERB–DRUG INTERACTIONS (continued)

HERB	DRUG	POSSIBLE EFFECTS
St. John's wort (continued)	digoxin	May reduce serum digoxin concentrations, decreasing therapeutic effects.
	HIV protease inhibitors, indinavir, non-nucleoside reverse transcriptase inhibitors (NNRTIs)	Induces cytochrome P-450 metabolic pathway, which may decrease therapeutic effects of drugs that use this pathway for metabolism. Use of St. John's wort and protease inhibitors or NNRTIs should be avoided because of the potential for subtherapeutic antiretroviral levels and insufficient virologic response that could lead to resistance or class cross-resistance.
	hormonal contraceptives	Increases breakthrough bleeding when taken with hormonal contraceptives; decreases serum levels and effectiveness of contraceptives.
	irinotecan	Decreases serum irinotecan levels by 50%.
	iron	Tannic acid content may reduce iron absorption.
	MAO inhibitors, nefazodone, SSRIs, trazodone	Causes additive effects with SSRIs, MAO inhibitors, and other antidepressants, potentially leading to serotonin syndrome, especially when combined with SSRIs.
	photosensitizing drugs	Increases photosensitivity.
	reserpine	Antagonizes effects of reserpine.
	sympathomimetic amines, such as pseudoephedrine	Causes additive effects.
	theophylline	May decrease serum theophylline levels, making the drug less effective.
	warfarin	May alter INR. Reduces effectiveness of anticoagulant, requiring increased dosage of drug.

HERB-DRUG INTERACTIONS *(continued)*

HERB	DRUG	POSSIBLE EFFECTS
valerian	alcohol	Claims no risk for increased sedation with alcohol, although debated.
	CNS depressants, sedative hypnotics	Enhances effects of sedative hypnotic drugs.
	iron	Tannic acid content may reduce iron absorption.

MONITORING PATIENTS USING HERBS

Altered laboratory values and changes in a patient's condition can signal unwanted effects of an herb. This table helps you focus your assessments so that you can better meet the needs of a patient who is using an alternative medicine

HERB	WHAT TO MONITOR	EXPLANATION
aloe	■ Serum electrolyte levels ■ Weight patterns ■ BUN and creatinine levels ■ Heart rate ■ Blood pressure ■ Urinalysis	Aloe possesses cathartic properties that inhibit water and electrolyte reabsorption, which may lead to potassium depletion, weight loss, and diarrhea. Long-term use may lead to nephritis, albuminuria, hematuria, and cardiac disturbances.
bilberry	■ Weight patterns ■ CBC ■ Blood glucose level ■ Triglyceride level ■ Liver function tests ■ INR, PT, PTT	Bilberry contains flavonoids and chromium, which are thought to have blood glucose- and triglyceride-lowering effects. Continued intoxication may lead to wasting, anemia, and jaundice.
capsicum	■ Liver function tests ■ BUN and creatinine levels ■ PT, PTT	Oral administration of capsicum can lead to gastroenteritis and hepatic or renal damage.
cat's claw	■ Blood pressure ■ Lipid panel ■ Serum electrolyte levels	Cat's claw can potentially cause hypotension through inhibition of the sympathetic nervous system and its diuretic properties. May also lower cholesterol level.
chamomile (German, Roman)	■ Menstrual changes ■ Pregnancy	Chamomile has been reported to cause changes in menstrual cycle and is a known teratogen in animals.
echinacea	■ Temperature	When echinacea is used parenterally, dose-dependent, short-term fever, nausea, and vomiting can occur.

HERB	WHAT TO MONITOR	EXPLANATION
ephedra	■ Blood pressure ■ Heart rate ■ BUN and creatinine levels ■ Weight patterns	Ephedra's active ingredient, ephedrine, stimulates the CNS in a similar manner to that of amphetamine. Adverse effects include hypertension, tachycardia, and kidney damage.
evening primrose oil	■ Pregnancy ■ CBC ■ Lipid profile	Evening primrose elevates plasma lipid levels and reduces platelet aggregation. It may increase the risk of pregnancy complications, including rupture of membranes, oxytocin augmentation, arrest of descent, and vacuum extraction.
fennel	■ Liver function tests ■ Blood pressure ■ Serum calcium level ■ Blood glucose level	Fennel contains trans-anethole and estrogole. Trans-anethole has estrogenic activity, whereas estrogole is a procarcinogen with the potential to cause liver damage. Adverse effects include photodermatitis and allergic reactions, particularly in those sensitive to carrots, celery, and mugwort.
feverfew	■ CBC ■ Pregnancy ■ Sleep patterns ■ INR, PT, PTT	Feverfew may inhibit blood platelet aggregation and decrease neutrophil and platelet secretory activity. It can cause uterine contractions in full-term, pregnant women. Adverse effects include mouth ulceration, tongue irritation and inflammation, abdominal pain, indigestion, diarrhea, flatulence, nausea, and vomiting. Post-feverfew syndrome includes nervousness, headache, insomnia, joint pain, stiffness, and fatigue.

(continued)

MONITORING PATIENTS USING HERBS *(continued)*

HERB	WHAT TO MONITOR	EXPLANATION
flaxseed	■ Lipid panel ■ Blood pressure ■ Serum calcium level ■ Blood glucose level ■ Liver function tests	Flaxseed possesses weak estrogenic and antiestrogenic activity. May reduce platelet aggregation and serum cholesterol level. Oral administration with inadequate fluid intake can cause intestinal blockage.
garlic	■ Blood pressure ■ Lipid panel ■ Blood glucose level ■ CBC ■ PT and PTT	Garlic is linked to hypotension, leukocytosis, inhibition of platelet aggregation, and decreased blood glucose and cholesterol levels. Postoperative bleeding and prolonged bleeding time can occur.
ginger	■ Blood glucose level ■ Blood pressure ■ Heart rate ■ Respiratory rate ■ Lipid panel ■ ECG ■ INR, PT, PTT	Ginger contains gingerols, which have positive inotropic properties. Adverse effects include platelet inhibition, hypoglycemia, hypotension, hypertension, and stimulation of respiratory centers. Overdoses cause CNS depression and arrhythmias.
ginkgo	■ Respiratory rate ■ Heart rate ■ PT and PTT	Consumption of ginkgo seed may cause difficulty breathing, weak pulse, seizures, loss of consciousness, and shock. Ginkgo leaf is linked to infertility, as well as GI upset, headache, dizziness, palpitations, restlessness, lack of muscle tone, weakness, bleeding, subdural hematoma, subarachnoid hemorrhage, and a bleeding iris.

MONITORING PATIENTS USING HERBS (continued)

HERB	WHAT TO MONITOR	EXPLANATION
ginseng (American, Panax, Siberian)	■ BUN and creatinine levels ■ Blood pressure ■ Serum electrolyte levels ■ Liver function tests ■ Serum calcium level ■ Blood glucose level ■ Heart rate ■ Sleep patterns ■ Menstrual changes ■ Weight patterns ■ PT, PTT, and INR ■ Blood pressure	Ginseng contains ginsenosides and eleutherosides that can affect blood pressure, CNS activity, platelet aggregation, and coagulation. A reduction in glucose and hemoglobin A1C levels has also been reported. Adverse effects include drowsiness, mastalgia, vaginal bleeding, tachycardia, mania, cerebral arteritis, Stevens-Johnson syndrome, cholestatic hepatitis, amenorrhea, decreased appetite, diarrhea, edema, hyperpyrexia, pruritus, hypotension, palpitations, headache, vertigo, euphoria, and neonatal death.
goldenseal	■ Respiratory rate ■ Heart rate ■ Blood pressure ■ Liver function tests ■ Mood patterns	Goldenseal contains berberine and hydrastine. Berberine improves bile secretion and bilirubin level, increases coronary blood flow, and stimulates or inhibits cardiac activity. Hydrastine causes hypotension, hypertension, increased cardiac output, exaggerated reflexes, seizures, paralysis, and death from respiratory failure. Other adverse effects include digestive disorders, constipation, excitatory states, hallucinations, delirium, GI upset, nervousness, depression, dyspnea, and bradycardia.
kava	■ Weight patterns ■ Lipid panel ■ CBC ■ Blood pressure ■ Liver function tests ■ Urinalysis ■ Mood changes ■ Sleep patterns	Kava contains arylethylene pyrone constituents that have CNS activity. It also has antianxiety effects. Long-term use may lead to weight loss, increased HDL cholesterol levels, hematuria, increased RBCs, decreased platelet count, decreased lymphocyte levels, reduced protein levels, and pulmonary hypertension.

(continued)

MONITORING PATIENTS USING HERBS *(continued)*

HERB	WHAT TO MONITOR	EXPLANATION
milk thistle	■ Liver function tests	Milk thistle contains flavono-lignans, which have liver-protective and antioxidant effects.
nettle	■ Blood glucose level ■ Blood pressure ■ Weight patterns ■ BUN and creatinine levels ■ Serum electrolyte levels ■ Heart rate ■ PT and INR	Nettle contains significant amounts of vitamin C, vitamin K, potassium, and calcium. Nettle may cause hyperglycemia, decreased blood pressure, decreased heart rate, weight loss, and diuretic effects.
passion flower	■ Liver function tests ■ Amylase level ■ Lipase level	Passion flower may contain cyanogenic glycosides, which can cause liver and pancreas toxicity.
St. John's wort	■ Vision ■ Menstrual changes ■ INR, PT, PTT ■ Sleep patterns	Changes in menstrual bleeding and a reduction in fertility may be caused by St. John's wort. Other adverse effects include GI upset, fatigue, dry mouth, dizziness, headache, delayed hypersensitivity, phototoxicity, and neuropathy. St. John's wort may also increase the risk of cataracts.
SAM-e	■ Blood pressure ■ Heart rate ■ BUN and creatinine levels	SAM-e contains homocysteine, which requires folate, cyanocobalamin, and pyridoxine for metabolism. Increased levels of homocysteine are linked to CV and renal disease.
saw palmetto	■ Liver function tests	Saw palmetto inhibits conversion of testosterone to dihydrotestosterone and may inhibit growth factors. Adverse effects include cholestatic hepatitis, erectile or ejaculatory dysfunction, and altered libido.

MONITORING PATIENTS USING HERBS (continued)

HERB	WHAT TO MONITOR	EXPLANATION
valerian	■ Blood pressure ■ Heart rate ■ Sleep patterns ■ Liver function tests	Valerian contains valerenic acid, which increases gamma–butyric acid and decreases CNS activity. Adverse effects include cardiac disturbances, insomnia, chest tightness, and hepatotoxicity.

INDEX

A

abacavir, 42-44
  for human immunodeficiency
    virus infection, 425
Abbreviations, xi-xii
  drug names and, 268
ABO blood groups, 238-239t
Absorption, altered, as drug-drug
    interaction, 330
acarbose, 77-79
  for diabetes, 385-386
ACE inhibitors. *See* Angiotensin-
    converting enzyme in-
    hibitors.
acebutolol, 17-18, 33-35, 46-47,
    48-49t, 49
Acetaminophen overdose, 309
  antidote for, 314t
acetazolamide, 25-27
acetylcysteine as acetaminophen
    toxicity antidote, 314t
activated charcoal as antidote, 314t
acyclovir, 42-44
  for herpes simplex, 452
Addisonian crisis. *See* Adrenal crisis.
Addison's disease, 381. *See also*
    Adrenal hypofunction.
Additive effects, 327
Adenocarcinoma, chemotherapy
    protocol for, 623t
Adenovirus, 494-495t. *See also*
    Pneumonia.
Administration route, incorrect,
    medication errors and, 276-
    277

Adrenal crisis, 381-382. *See also*
    Adrenal hypofunction.
Adrenal hypofunction, 381-382
  drug therapy for, 382-384
Adrenergics, geriatric patients and,
    118t
Adrenocorticoids, geriatric patients
    and, 118t
Adverse reactions, 297-298, 299-
    304t, 304
  dose-related, 297-298
  English-Spanish phrase translator
    for, 137
  geriatric patients and, 118-127t
  misinterpretation of, as age-
    related changes, 128-129t
Age-related changes, misinterpreta-
    tion of adverse reactions as,
    128-129t
Agranulocytosis as drug reaction,
    299-300t
Air bubbles in pump tubing, med-
    ication errors and, 276
Air embolism
  as central venous therapy compli-
    cation, 236t
  as I.V. therapy complication, 232t
albumin, transfusing, 242-243t
albuterol, 486
Alcohol toxicity, interventions for,
    320t
alemtuzumab, 590
alendronate
  for osteoporosis, 478-479
  for Paget's disease, 481

t refers to a table; i refers to an illustration.

t refers to a table; i refers to an illustration.

t refers to a table; i refers to an illustration.

t refers to a table; i refers to an illustration.